T0269204

Cooperative Breeding in Vertebrates

Cooperative breeders are species in which individuals beyond a pair assist in the production of young in a single brood or litter. Although relatively rare, cooperative breeding is widespread taxonomically and continues to pose challenges to our understanding of the evolution of cooperation and altruistic behavior.

Bringing together long-term studies of cooperatively breeding birds, mammals, and fishes, this book provides a synthesis of current studies in the field. The chapters are organized by individual studies of particular species or (in the case of mole-rats) two closely related cooperatively breeding species. Each focuses not only on describing behavior and ecology but also on testing evolutionary hypotheses for the form and function of the diverse and extraordinary cooperative breeding lifestyles that have been discovered. This unique and comprehensive text will be of interest to graduate students and researchers of behavioral ecology and the evolution of cooperation.

Walter D. Koenig is Senior Scientist at the Cornell Lab of Ornithology and the Department of Neurobiology and Behavior at Cornell University. He has studied cooperative breeding in acorn woodpeckers for more than 40 years. He is co-editor of *Cooperative Breeding in Birds: Long-Term Studies of Ecology and Behavior* (Cambridge, 1990) and *Ecology and Evolution of Cooperative Breeding in Birds* (Cambridge, 2004), and has published widely, primarily in the fields of population and behavioral ecology.

Janis L. Dickinson is Arthur A. Allen Director of Citizen Science at the Cornell Lab of Ornithology and Professor in the Department of Natural Resources at Cornell University. Her work has primarily been in the fields of sexual selection and social behavior in insects and birds; she has studied the behavioral ecology of western bluebirds for more than 25 years and is also co-editor of *Ecology and Evolution of Cooperative Breeding in Birds* (Cambridge, 2004). Her current interests include understanding how socially networked Web environments can be designed to support collaborative conservation actions.

Cooperative Breeding in Vertebrates

Studies of Ecology, Evolution, and Behavior

Edited by

Walter D. Koenig

Janis L. Dickinson
The Cornell Lab of Ornithology,
Cornell University

with illustrations by

Stef den Ridder

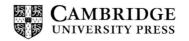
CAMBRIDGE
UNIVERSITY PRESS

CAMBRIDGE
UNIVERSITY PRESS

University Printing House, Cambridge CB2 8BS, United Kingdom

One Liberty Plaza, 20th Floor, New York, NY 10006, USA

477 Williamstown Road, Port Melbourne, VIC 3207, Australia

314-321, 3rd Floor, Plot 3, Splendor Forum, Jasola District Centre, New Delhi - 110025, India

79 Anson Road, #06-04/06, Singapore 079906

Cambridge University Press is part of the University of Cambridge.

It furthers the University's mission by disseminating knowledge in the pursuit of education, learning and research at the highest international levels of excellence.

www.cambridge.org
Information on this title: www.cambridge.org/9781107642126

© Cambridge University Press 2016

First published 2016
First paperback edition 2018

A catalogue record for this publication is available from the British Library

Library of Congress Cataloging in Publication data
Cooperative breeding in vertebrates : studies of ecology, evolution, and behavior / edited by Walter D. Koenig, Janis L. Dickinson, The Cornell Lab of Ornithology, Cornell University; with illustrations by Stef den Ridder.
    pages   cm
Includes index.
ISBN 978-1-107-04343-5 (hardback)
1. Parental behavior in animals.   2. Animal societies.   I. Koenig, Walter D., 1950– editor.   II. Dickinson, Janis L., 1955– editor.
QL762.C66   2016
591.56′3–dc23   2015028165

ISBN 978-1-107-04343-5 Hardback
ISBN 978-1-107-64212-6 Paperback

Contents

The color plate section is situated between
pages 158 and 159.

Contributors

Çağlar Akçay
Department of Biological Sciences
Virginia Tech University
Blacksburg, Virginia, U.S.A.

Vittorio Baglione
Department of Agroforestry and Sustainable Forest
Management Research Institute
University of Valladolid
Palencia, Spain

Nigel C. Bennett
Department of Zoology and Entomology
University of Pretoria
Pretoria, South Africa

Reed Bowman
Archbold Biological Station
Venus, Florida, U.S.A.

Lyanne Brouwer
Division of Evolution, Ecology & Genetics
Research School of Biology
Australian National University
Canberra, Australia

Terry Burke
Department of Animal and Plant Sciences
University of Sheffield
Sheffield, U.K.

Daniela Canestrari
Department of Biology of Organisms and Systems
University of Oviedo
Oviedo, Spain
and
Research Unit of Biodiversity (CSIC, UO, PA)
University of Oviedo
Campus de Mieres, Edificio de Investigación
Mieres, Spain

Michael A. Cant
Centre for Ecology and Conservation
University of Exeter, Penryn Campus
Cornwall, U.K.

Tim Clutton-Brock
Department of Zoology
Downing Street
University of Cambridge
Cambridge, U.K.

Andrew Cockburn
Division of Evolution, Ecology & Genetics
Research School of Biology
Australian National University
Canberra, Australia

Janis L. Dickinson
Cornell Lab of Ornithology
Cornell University
Ithaca, New York, U.S.A.

Hannah Dugdale
Department of Animal and Plant Sciences
University of Sheffield
Sheffield, U.K.
and
Behavioural and physiological ecology
Groningen Institute for evolutionary Life Sciences
University of Groningen
Groningen, The Netherlands

Jan Ekman
Department of Ecology and Genetics
Uppsala University
Uppsala, Sweden

Stephen T. Emlen
Department of Neurobiology and Behavior
Cornell University
Ithaca, New York, U.S.A.

Chris G. Faulkes
School of Biological and Chemical Sciences
Queen Mary, University of London
London, U.K.

Elise D. Ferree
Keck Science Department
Claremont Colleges
Claremont, California, U.S.A.

John W. Fitzpatrick
Cornell Lab of Ornithology
Cornell University
Ithaca, New York, U.S.A.

Victoria Garcia
Department of Biological Sciences
Virginia Tech
Blacksburg, U.S.A.

Michael Griesser
Anthropological Institute and Museum
University of Zurich
Zurich, Switzerland

Ben J. Hatchwell
Department of Animal and Plant Sciences
University of Sheffield
Sheffield, U.K.

Joseph Haydock
Department of Biology
Gonzaga University
Spokane, Washington, U.S.A.

Walter D. Koenig
Cornell Lab of Ornithology
Cornell University
Ithaca, New York, U.S.A.

Jan Komdeur
Behavioural and Physiological Ecology
Groningen Institute for Evolutionary Life Sciences
University of Groningen
Groningen, The Netherlands

Mark Liu
Biodiversity Research Center
Academia Sinica
Taipei, Taiwan

Regina H. Macedo
Departamento de Zoologia – IB
Universidade de Brasilia
Brasilia, Brazil

Marta Manser
Institute of Evolutionary Biology and Environmental
Studies
University of Zürich
Zürich, Switzerland

Nicolas Margraf
Division of Evolution, Ecology & Genetics
Research School of Biology
Australian National University
Canberra, Australia

Paul G. McDonald
Behavioural and Physiological Ecology Research Centre
School of Environmental and Rural Science
University of New England
Armidale, New South Wales, Australia

Hazel J. Nichols
School of Natural Sciences and Psychology
Liverpool John Moores University
James Parsons Building, Byrom Street
Liverpool, U.K.

Helen L. Osmond
Division of Evolution, Ecology & Genetics
Research School of Biology
Australian National University
Canberra, Australia

David S. Richardson
School of Biological Sciences and Nature Seychelles
University of East Anglia
Norwich Research Park
Norwich, U.K.

Amanda R. Ridley
Centre for Evolutionary Biology
University of Western Australia
Crawley, Western Australia

Dustin R. Rubenstein
Department of Ecology, Evolution and Environmental
Biology
Columbia University
New York, U.S.A.

Andrew F. Russell
Centre for Ecology and Conservation
University of Exeter, Penryn Campus
Cornwall, U.K.
and
Fowlers Gap Arid Zone Station
School of Biological Earth and Environmental Sciences
University of New South Wales
Sydney, Australia

Sheng-Feng Shen
Biodiversity Research Center
Academia Sinica
Taipei, Taiwan

Caitlin A. Stern
Santa Fe Institute
Santa Fe, New Mexico, U.S.A.

Michael Taborsky
Department of Behavioural Ecology
University of Bern
Hinterkappelen, Switzerland

Faye J. Thompson
Centre for Ecology and Conservation
University of Exeter, Penryn Campus
Cornwall, U.K.

Martijn van de Pol
Division of Evolution, Ecology & Genetics
Research School of Biology
Australian National University
Canberra, Australia
and
Department of Animal Ecology
Netherlands Institute of Ecology
NIOO-KNAW, Wageningen, The Netherlands

Emma Vitikainen
Centre for Ecology and Conservation
University of Exeter, Penryn Campus
Cornwall, U.K.

Eric L. Walters
Department of Biological Sciences
Old Dominion University
Norfolk, Virginia, U.S.A.

Jeffrey R. Walters
Department of Biological Sciences
Virginia Tech
Blacksburg, Virginia, U.S.A.

Jonathan Wright
Centre for Biodiversity Dynamics
Department of Biology
Norwegian University of Science and Technology
Trondheim, Norway

Hsiao-Wei Yuan
School of Forestry and Resource Conservation
National Taiwan University
Taipei, Taiwan

Introduction

Janis L. Dickinson and Walter D. Koenig

(a)

(b)

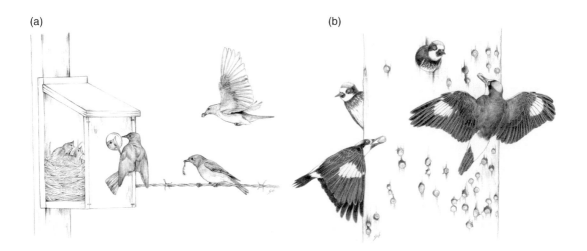

Cooperative breeding was described by naturalists as early as the nineteenth century (Boland and Cockburn 2002) and refers to breeding associations with three or more individuals collectively raising young in a single brood or litter. Breeding in groups was little more than a biological curiosity, however, until nearly 30 years after Skutch (1935) first introduced "helpers at the nest" to refer to individuals that forgo breeding to help raise young that are not their own. In the 1960s, evolutionary studies of animal social behavior were quickly transformed by the realization that selection acts mainly on individuals and only rarely on groups (Williams 1966). This insight spawned the field of behavioral ecology,

and, in particular, kin selection and inclusive fitness theory (Hamilton 1963, 1964), which provided a firm theoretical basis for understanding the paradox of helping and other forms of cooperative breeding that appeared to involve a sacrifice in personal reproduction. This book provides examples of studies that test specific predictions based on individual selection and inclusive fitness theory, using a combination of experimental and observational studies designed to measure the socioecological drivers and fitness consequences of giving up at least a share of personal reproduction to help others breed.

Relatively quickly after Hamilton's seminal papers, cooperative breeders became subjects of several

Cooperative Breeding in Vertebrates: Studies of Ecology, Evolution, and Behavior, eds W. D. Koenig and J. L. Dickinson.
Published by Cambridge University Press. © Cambridge University Press 2016.

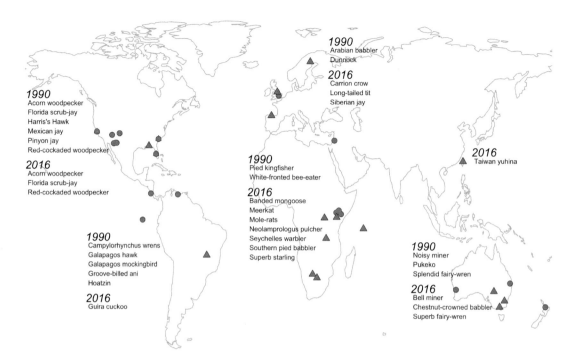

Figure I.1. The geographic distribution of studies represented in Stacey and Koenig (1990; circles) and this book (2016; triangles).

long-term studies, many of which were summarized species by species in Stacey and Koenig (1990) and topic by topic in Koenig and Dickinson (2004). This latter volume reviewed theory and evidence by summarizing the literature across a range of relevant topics. The book we introduce here returns to the earlier model, examining advances based on population studies of vertebrate species across the globe (Figure I.1) with the goal of exploring the ways in which new theory and empirical evidence have altered our perspective on cooperation over the last 25 years. We believe that new insights usually come from exploring the diversity and complexity of animal societies within the context of theory; our hope is that having summaries of these studies all in one place will generate new thinking, while helping to foster generalities and illuminate holes in current thinking.

The chapters in this book include contributions from both new and more senior researchers; three chapters are updates of studies summarized earlier in Stacey

and Koenig (1990), demonstrating the added value that comes with increased longevity of studies in this field. The remaining studies highlight the many advances that have been made with the addition of new, and often exceptional, study systems and experimental approaches.

Results from such studies indicate that what we know today about cooperative breeding may not be representative of the different kinds of systems that are out there, making it difficult to draw general conclusions. Within the complexity that has been uncovered, however, are both consistent patterns and new gems of ideas that help push the field forward. It is only in bringing together and synthesizing the evidence that already exists that a story begins to emerge for each species, allowing us to get a sense of what matters in a system, what the important design features are, and how natural selection has shaped them variously among species. We have particularly enjoyed seeing the insights that emerge when researchers have the opportunity to tell the whole story in one place, rather than piecemeal in technical publications.

What has happened since the last collection of long-term studies was published in 1990? While reproductive skew theory had already been around for a while (Vehrencamp 1983), it really took hold, generating an array of models and ideas that improved understanding of the extent of reproductive sharing in animal societies and the complexities surrounding measuring and modeling reproductive division of labor (Magrath et al. 2004). Although the original insights provided by reproductive skew theory have proven problematic for most cooperatively breeding vertebrates (Haydock and Koenig 2002; Magrath et al. 2004), the interplay between empirical studies and theory continues to produce new generalizations and understanding of how and why reproductive sharing varies across taxa.

Study systems chosen as exceptions appear early in the book, beginning with a species that exhibits delayed dispersal in the absence of cooperative breeding (Chapter 1), as well as two cases of cooperative breeders that have fluid systems of helping that become possible when localized dispersal of offspring leads to breeding in kin neighborhoods (Chapters 2 and 3). Chapters 2 through 13 focus on cooperatively breeding birds in which relatedness and kin selection are generally critical to the evolution of cooperative behaviors, although beyond that they encompass a wide range of social organizations ranging from socially and genetically monogamous pairs with helpers (Chapters 4, 5, and 7) to species with helpers in which extra-pair matings are common (Chapters 2, 8, and 12), species organized into complex and in some cases multileveled groups (Chapters 9, 10, and 11), and cooperatively polygamous groups with helpers (Chapters 6, 12, and 13). In addition to these are chapters covering species of vertebrates in which individuals cooperating with one another are apparently *not* related, with the idea that these can provide strong, complementary tests of alternative hypotheses for the evolution of cooperation (Chapters 14 and 15).

Great strides have been made in understanding cooperation in non-avian vertebrates, including fishes (Chapter 16) and mammals (Chapters 17, 18, and 19), with several of these studies combining field research with field and laboratory experiments to test important hypotheses concerning the evolution of helping behavior that are difficult to address in the field alone. In bringing these newer studies together with the three landmark, older studies, which were largely focused on such classic ecological constraints as habitat and cavities (Chapters 4, 5, and 13), it becomes possible to assess current understanding of cooperative breeding in vertebrates and to develop the broad perspective needed to foster new thinking. Significantly, the 19 studies summarized here include some of the most extensive and detailed population studies of wild living vertebrates ever undertaken.

Perhaps the most important technical advance since the 1990 volume is the widespread availability of molecular tools to assess parentage, especially the advent of hypervariable microsatellites, which allow study-wide parentage assignment. While Nick Davies' (1990) dunnock (*Prunella modularis*) chapter was the only study to integrate molecular parentage assignment in the previous book, molecular tools are commonly used today, allowing for assessment of such critical measures as relatedness, incest, inbreeding, reproductive skew, and, of course, inclusive fitness.

Since Hamilton (1963, 1964), the primary body of theory informing studies of social behavior has been inclusive fitness theory, which compares the direct fitness benefits of producing offspring with the indirect fitness benefits of helping relatives produce additional offspring over what they might otherwise produce, weighted by relatedness (Brown 1980). The minimal predictions of inclusive fitness theory are that helpers should prefer, or at least be more likely to aid, relatives over nonrelatives, that the inclusive fitness advantages of helping should be greater than what helpers (as individuals) might otherwise achieve (i.e., Hamilton's rule, which infers that helping must be better than actual outside options), and that if breeding is the better option, helpers should breed independently when they have the opportunity to do so.

The studies presented here provide a breadth of evidence supporting the importance of indirect fitness benefits, which often, but not always, act in concert with limitations on independent breeding to drive decisions to help or cobreed with relatives. In general, studies of cooperative breeders indicate that even when indirect fitness benefits are small, they can still be an important driver of helping behavior – because the outside options are even worse. Most of the chapters in this book present strong evidence for the importance of kinship and kin recognition in the behavioral choices that individuals make, especially choices of whether to help and whom to help (Chapters 2, 3, 7, and 11). Explicit tests of Hamilton's rule (Chapters 2 and 3) provide insights that further demonstrate the value of kin selection and inclusive fitness thinking. This large body of evidence supporting the importance of kin selection to helping stands in direct opposition to challenges based on modeling efforts and spotty interpretation of empirical evidence (Nowak et al. 2010).

Unsurprisingly, relatedness and indirect fitness benefits are much less prevalent among same-sex cobreeders in species that exhibit cooperative polygamy, over half of which are thought to involve cobreeding by nonrelatives (Riehl 2013). Such partnerships among nonrelatives are, of course, driven by direct fitness benefits, rather than indirect fitness benefits arising through collateral kinship (Hartley and Davies 1994). Here we feature two cooperative breeders, both joint-nesting, that exhibit cobreeding by nonkin (Chapters 14 and 15). Despite these examples, studies of species whose cooperative behavior is not based on kinship remain relatively rare, and even ruminating about why unrelated males might help raise offspring of nonkin is intriguing: reciprocity; potential to inherit a mate; experience; high costs of floating or maintaining a territory as an individual?

At a time when funding is challenging to obtain and granting agencies are shying away from the complexity of demographic studies in favor of the "ooh, shiny" payoffs that can arise from short-term, mechanistic questions (Zuk and Balenger 2014), we hope this book inspires renewed interest in long-term studies of social behavior for their value in addressing lifetime fitness consequences of behaviors, their corrective potential (most authors in this book would, we think, agree that their ideas and evidence have changed significantly since they first began their study), their importance to conservation (Chapters 4, 5, and 12), and their capacity to uncover the complexities underlying the evolution of social behavior. Ideally, long-term studies of social behavior knit together multiple approaches by integrating ecology, life-history theory, behavioral genetics, physiology, and behavior, while forging new connections by measuring the traits, trajectories, and demography of individual agents. Such efforts provide important fodder for new theory and ideas.

Most importantly, in an age when there is a large focus on analyzing existing data, we believe this book illustrates the vital interplay between natural history observations and the development of new ideas, which when situated within a rich domain of accumulated knowledge can be tested rigorously and in ways that advance our understanding of the evolution of social complexity. All of the authors in this book are dedicated naturalists whose propensity to take on the unforgiving commitment of embarking on the long-term study of marked populations of animals is integral to the insights they have had and the discoveries they continue to make.

Acknowledgments

We thank all of our authors for their insights and willingness to cooperate on this joint venture. We particularly wish to thank the Cornell Lab of Ornithology's Bartels Science Illustration Intern, Stef den Ridder, for the artwork that graces the beginning of each chapter and Diane Tessaglia-Hymes for her help in arranging Stef's visit and allowing us to enjoy Stef's talents. We also wish to thank the National Science Foundation, which has supported much of our work over the years.

REFERENCES

Boland, C. R. J. and Cockburn, A. (2002). Short sketches from the long history of cooperative breeding in Australian birds. *Emu*, 102, 9–17.

Brown, J. L. (1980). Fitness in complex avian social systems. In: *Evolution of Social Behavior: Hypotheses and Empirical Tests*, ed. H. Markl. Weinheim: Dahlem Konferenzen Verlag, pp. 115–128.

Davies, N. B. (1990). Dunnocks: cooperation and conflict among males and females in a variable mating system.

In: *Cooperative Breeding in Birds: Long-term Studies of Ecology and Behavior*, ed. P. B. Stacy and W. D. Koenig. Cambridge: Cambridge University Press, pp. 457–485.

Hamilton, W. D. (1963). The evolution of altruistic behavior. *Am. Nat.*, 97, 354–356.

Hamilton, W. D. (1964). The genetical evolution of social behaviour. I and II. *J. Theor. Biol.* 7, 1–52.

Hartley I. and Davies, N. B. (1994). Limits to cooperative polyandry in birds. *Proc. R. Soc. London B*, 257, 67–73.

Haydock, J. and Koenig, W. D. (2002). Reproductive skew in the polygynandrous acorn woodpecker. *Proc. Natl. Acad. Sci. (USA)*, 99, 7178–7183.

Koenig, W. D. and Dickinson, J. L., eds. (2004). *Ecology and Evolution of Cooperative Breeding in Birds*. Cambridge: Cambridge University Press.

Magrath, R. D., Johnstone, R. A., and Heinsohn, R. G. (2004). Reproductive skew. In: *Ecology and Evolution of Cooperative Breeding in Birds*, ed. W. D. Koenig and J. L. Dickinson. Cambridge: Cambridge University Press, pp. 157–176.

Nowak, M. A., Tarnita, C. E., and Wilson, E. O. (2010). The evolution of eusociality. *Nature*, 466, 1057–1062.

Riehl, C. (2013). Evolutionary routes to non-kin cooperative breeding in birds. *Proc. R. Soc. London B*, 208, 20132245.

Skutch, A. F. (1935). Helpers at the nest. *Auk*, 52, 257–273.

Stacey, P. B. and Koenig, W. D., eds. (1990). *Cooperative Breeding in Birds: Long-term Studies of Ecology and Behavior*. Cambridge: Cambridge University Press.

Vehrencamp S. L. (1983). Optimal degree of skew in cooperative societies. *Am. Zool.*, 23, 327–335.

Williams, G. C. (1966). *Adaptation and Natural Selection: A Critique of Some Current Evolutionary Thought*. Princeton, NJ: Princeton University Press.

Zuk, M. and Balenger, S. L. (2014). Behavioral ecology and genomics: new directions, or just a more detailed map? *Behav. Ecol.*, 25, 1277–1282.

1

Siberian jays: Delayed dispersal in the absence of cooperative breeding

Jan Ekman and Michael Griesser

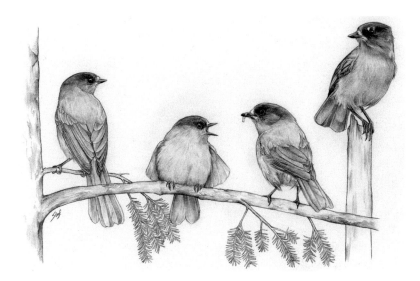

Introduction

In most cases, helping-at-the-nest is associated with delayed dispersal, leading to widespread interest in the selective factors causing offspring to stay and delay breeding on their natal territory. Today, with the identification of a number of species where offspring delay dispersal without ever helping, we have the opportunity to examine a more comprehensive set of fitness benefits of delayed dispersal in cases where it appears to be beneficial even in the absence of helping (Ekman 2006). Here we discuss one such species, the Siberian

jay (*Perisoreus infaustus*), which has been studied extensively as an exceptional case of delayed dispersal in the absence of cooperative breeding.

Our work with the Siberian jay contributes to the field of cooperative breeding by demonstrating how benefits of cooperation other than helping-at-the-nest can select for family-group living. Many studies of the mechanisms facilitating cooperative breeding emphasize the role of offspring as donors of help and breeding parents as recipients of benefits. Given that offspring are an evolutionary asset of the parents, however, parents clearly have an incentive to provide

Cooperative Breeding in Vertebrates: Studies of Ecology, Evolution, and Behavior, eds W. D. Koenig and J. L. Dickinson.
Published by Cambridge University Press. © Cambridge University Press 2016.

care for them in cases where offspring extend their association with parents. Such care could be instrumental in prolonging the time offspring remain in the family, thus facilitating family cohesion. Family-group living evolves as a transactional process, balancing the inclusive fitness costs and benefits among family members. As such, family life involves concession of resources, competition, and cooperation, especially rivalry among siblings (Mock and Parker 1997). Understanding the evolution of delayed dispersal thus requires examination of both cooperative and competitive interactions.

Models explaining why sexually mature offspring remain with their parents on their natal territory have emphasized the role of constraints on access to breeding opportunities and variation in habitat quality (Brown 1969, 1978; Koenig and Pitelka 1981; Emlen 1982). While ecological constraints may explain dispersal decisions within populations, and may account for the delayed onset of independent reproduction, they do not make predictions regarding where offspring will wait prior to gaining breeder status. Thus, we know little about what, in the absence of immediately available breeding opportunities, drives offspring to remain philopatric on their natal territory rather than "floating" – which is generally assumed to involve roaming between territories or groups – or settling in a group of unrelated birds.

We also know relatively little about within-species variation in dispersal timing, as this subject has received much less attention in cooperatively breeding species than the behavior of offspring delaying dispersal. Indeed, variation in dispersal timing, where some offspring disperse while others remain and help, occurs in many, perhaps most, cooperatively breeding species (Riehl 2013), and it has been well documented in a number of thoroughly studied species including southern pied babblers *Turdoides bicolor* (Ridley et al. 2008; Chapter 7) and the Arabian babbler *Turdoides squamiceps* (Zahavi 1990). Models accounting for delayed dispersal based on ecological constraints generally consider independent breeding to be the alternative and do not consider variation in pathways to breeder status among siblings. Given that in the Siberian jay some offspring wait as nonbreeders on the

natal territory while others wait as nonbreeders outside it (Ekman et al. 1994), it is possible to examine the factors that determine how offspring decide between these alternatives and to explore the ultimate fitness consequences of decisions favoring family living and ultimately cooperative breeding.

Study site

Our study site is located outside the village of Arvidsjaur, northern Sweden, about 100 km south of Arctic Circle (Figure 1.1). It is part of the vast continuous taiga biome of northern Scandinavia. Accordingly, the climate is boreal with warm summers and temperatures up to +30°C, cold winters with temperatures down to –40°C (exceptionally to –50°C), and annual precipitation of about 600 mm. The study site is usually snowbound from October until the beginning of May. Scots pine (*Pinus sylvestris*) and Norway spruce (*Picea abies*) are the dominant tree species while deciduous trees (birch *Betula pubescens*, aspen *Populus tremula*, willow *Salix* spp.) are less abundant. In wetter locations marshes occur, forming a natural mosaic of forests with marshes.

Our study started in 1989 and the study site was chosen because Siberian jays in this area had been ringed for several decades, nests had been located, and population trends monitored by a local amateur (Lindgren 1975; Griesser and Lagerberg 2012). Our study site consists of two separate areas in continuous habitat (Figure 1.1). The southern area (53 km²; 37 km² when excluding clear-felled areas, plantations, and lakes) is located in intensively managed forests. In this area the primeval forest is interspersed with clear-felled areas and plantations. The northern area is located in a nature reserve (Reivo, 30 km²) with continuous primeval forests unaffected by forestry for over the last 200 years. Managed forests are dominated by the commercially valuable pines, making forests more open as Scots pine has branches in the crown of the tree while spruce often has branches almost down to ground level. This difference in habitat openness strongly influences the breeding success and survival of Siberian jays (see the "Role of vegetation structure").

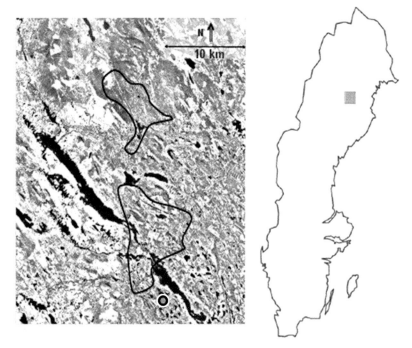

Figure 1.1. Aerial image of the study area (encircled by dark lines). The location of the study site in Sweden is indicated on the map with a black circle; the village of Arvidsjaur is indicated with a gray circle.

Group structure

Siberian jay groups form around a strictly monoga-mous breeding pair (Gienapp and Merila 2010). Group sizes vary from 2 to 5 individuals (mean: 2.7, range of mean = 2.05–3.43, $N = 20$ years) at the start of the breed-ing season (March) and between 2 to 6 individuals (mean: 3.25, range of mean = 2.46–3.67) in September, after the breeding season (Figure 1.2). Extra birds con-sist of a mixture of philopatric offspring and unrelated immigrants (Ekman et al. 1994; Lillandt et al. 2003), with the majority being the latter (66% of nonbreeders in breeding groups, 62% in winter groups; Figure 1.3). Extra birds accompany around 80% of breeders and the most common group composition is a pair of adult breed-ers accompanied only by immigrants. Most extra birds are first-winter birds or yearlings, with an equal sex ratio among both philopatric and immigrants (Table 1.1).

Groups inhabit territories with ill-defined borders that are partly determined by unsuitable habitats such

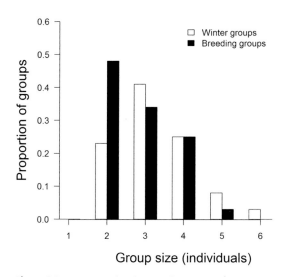

Figure 1.2. Frequency distribution of group sizes ($N = 376$ groups; open symbols: groups during the non-breeding season ("winter"); filled symbols: breeding groups).

Table 1.1. Age and sex-ratio of extra birds in winter (September) groups (N = 270 groups)

	Age		
Extra bird category	Number of individuals		Proportion first winter birds
	Juveniles	Older individuals	
Philopatric	143	75	0.65
Immigrant	117	28	0.80

	Sex-ratio		
Extra bird category	Number individuals		Sex ratio (males/females)
	Males	Females	
Philopatric	57	59	0.97
Immigrant	70	67	1.04

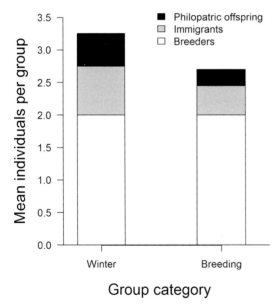

Figure 1.3. The average number of members of each category in winter (assessed in September) and breeding groups (N = 376).

as open bogs, clear-felled areas, and lakes. Territories are stable and many have remained the same over the entire study period. The managed, southern area harbors 35 groups, and the unmanaged, northern area 28 groups, which corresponds to an average territory size

of 1.1 km² in both areas. Once they have settled down to breed, jays rarely shift territories, with shifts having been observed in only 3 of 346 (< 1%) breeding attempts (Griesser et al. 2007). The direction of territory shifts is always from low quality to high quality neighboring territories, which will typically yield higher breeding success (Ekman et al. 2001).

Natal dispersal

Dispersal timing and distance

Siberian jay offspring almost always become breeders by dispersing away from their natal territory, although the timing and distance of dispersal varies considerably (Ekman et al. 2002; Griesser et al. 2014). Offspring only inherit their natal territory if both parents disappear within a short period of time, a rare event that we have witnessed only twice in 20 years. Bimodality in both age and distance is the defining feature of dispersal strategies in the Siberian jay (Ekman et al. 2001, 2002).

One category of offspring (early dispersers) leaves the parental territory between four and eight weeks after fledging (Figure 1.4a). These early dispersers settle as immigrants in groups of unrelated birds without immediately acquiring breeder status or, more rarely, find a vacancy allowing them to become breeders at

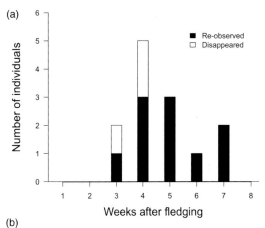

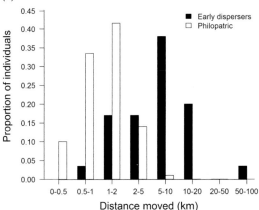

Table 1.2. The increase with age in the fraction of individuals having started to breed

Age (years)	Proportion of population breeding	
	Dispersers	Philopatric
1	0.32	0.21
2	0.78	0.70
3	1	0.87
4	1	0.96
5	1	1

Figure 1.4. (a) The timing of dispersal for early dispersers observed from newly fledged birds with radio transmitters. Filled bars: birds re-observed after dispersal outside the natal territory ($N = 10$). Open bars: birds disappearing without being re-observed ($N = 3$). From Ekman et al. (2002) (b) The frequency distribution of dispersal distances of philopatric offspring ($N = 90$; open symbols) and early dispersers (immigrants; $N = 27$; filled symbols). From Griesser et al. (2014).

the age of one (Table 1.2) (Ekman et al. 1994; Griesser et al. 2008). Out of 31 color-banded fledglings observed daily during the months after fledging (22 of these also carried a radio transmitter) we confirmed 10 early dispersers (seven with radio transmitter and three through re-observation: Figure 1.4a). Three birds disappeared during the same period for which we could not confirm whether they dispersed or died (Ekman

et al. 2002). Out of the seven early-dispersing birds with radio transmitters, six settled permanently in a new territory within two days. The seventh made a temporary stop in a new group before moving to settle permanently with another group a week after dispersing. The mean (± standard error [S.E.]) dispersal distance of early dispersers was 9.0 ± 2.6 km, corresponding to having traversed 7.0 ± 2.2 territories ($N = 27$ birds all ringed as nestlings; 12 followed with radio transmitters) (Figure 1.4b). The longest dispersal distance of an untagged disperser was 72 km (Griesser et al. 2014). The majority of early dispersers became breeders either by inheriting breeding position in the group where they initially settled or by filling a vacancy in a neighboring group (Figure 1.5a).

Those offspring that have not dispersed by the age of eight weeks remain on their natal territories at least through the first winter (philopatric offspring). In 75% of successful broods, at most one, and rarely more, offspring delayed dispersal (Figure 1.5b). Philopatric offspring disperse only when they acquire a breeding position except for cases of parent–offspring reproductive conflict, thus making the age of dispersal equal to the age at first reproduction. In contrast to delayed dispersers, philopatric offspring dispersed on average only 1.25 km before settling ($N = 97$; visual re-observations only) (Figure 1.4b) traversing on average 1.2 ± 0.1 territories (Figure 1.6). Philopatric offspring delay dispersal longer and initiate first breeding for later than early dispersers (Table 1.2). Molecular estimates based on 23 microsatellite markers support distance estimates from the direct methods we have described above (Griesser et al. 2014).

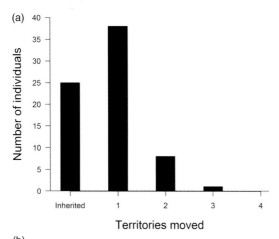

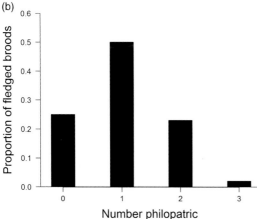

Figure 1.5. (a) The number of territories moved by early-dispersing immigrants that became breeders (*N* = 72). (b) The frequency distribution of philopatric offspring from broods that produced fledged offspring (*N* = 117 broods).

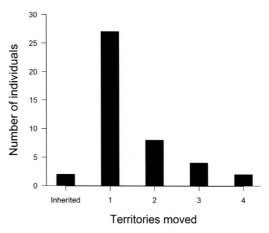

Figure 1.6. The number of territories moved by philopatric offspring on becoming breeders (*N* = 43).

Sibling rivalry and dispersal pathway

The bimodal timing of dispersal among Siberian jay brood mates implies that delayed dispersal is not an obligate response to a specific set of conditions that promote philopatry. A main proximate factor determining variation in the timing of dispersal is sibling rivalry as expressed in within-brood dominance (Ekman et al. 2002). Aggressive behavior within dyads of siblings, consisting of bill clicking and displacements, was consistently directed toward the sibling becoming an early disperser. Aggression eventually leads to the subordinate dispersing six to eight weeks after aggression escalates (Griesser et al. 2008).

Constraints on breeding

Delayed breeding is a response to constraints on access to breeding openings with larger proportions of birds becoming nonbreeding extra birds at high population densities (Figure 1.7). There is a strong preference to breed in less open forest where nests can be well hidden from nest predators; breeders in territories with poor protection readily abandon if given access to a better territory (Ekman et al. 2001). Yet this constraint on breeding at high population densities does not carry over into larger proportions of fledglings becoming philopatric. Most broods have only one philopatric offspring (Figure 1.5b) and it is rare to see two philopatric offspring of the same sex (1.3% for sons and 3.7% for daughters compared to 24% of broods with two opposite sex philopatric offspring). Apparently, reproductive conflict and a tendency to avoid sharing the natal territory with a same-sex sibling leads to departure of subordinate siblings, as described in the prior section, and helps to maintain a relatively even sex bias in dispersal (Table 1.1).

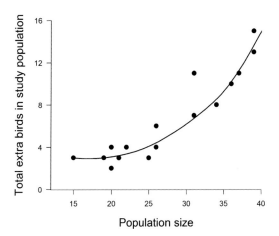

Figure 1.7. The total number of extra birds (philopatric offspring and nonbreeder immigrants) in the study site each year plotted against total population size.

Survival and reproductive value

First winter survival

Enhanced survivorship by philopatric offspring has been reported in two studies of first-winter survival (October to February; Ekman et al. 2000; Griesser et al. 2006). Visual mark-recapture data showed that first-winter survival was higher for philopatric offspring than among immigrants in groups where both parents were present compared to those where one or both parents had disappeared. Only a minority of disappearances could be accounted for by retrievals of dead birds (Ekman et al. 2000). Then, in a second study using radio-tagged birds, data over two winters revealed that philopatric juveniles had higher survival than immigrant (early disperser) juveniles (Figure 1.8), and confirmed that predators killed all juveniles that disappeared during winter (Griesser et al. 2006). Thus philopatric offspring survive better, with winter survivorship of 0.73–0.79 compared to 0.36–0.67 for immigrants.

Reproductive value of adults

Despite the finding that philopatric offspring postpone the onset of reproduction longer than immigrants

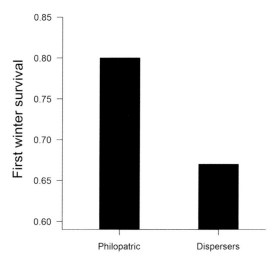

Figure 1.8. First-winter survival (October to February; 2001–2002 and 2002–2003) of philopatric offspring ($N = 34$) and immigrants ($N = 39$) with radio transmitters; all individuals (dead or surviving) were accounted for. From Griesser et al. (2006).

(Table 1.2), the reproductive value of philopatric offspring is still higher at all ages (Figure 1.9a). Philopatric offspring are compensated for the loss of breeding opportunities early in life by higher breeding success and better adult survival (Ekman et al. 1999). The breeding success of philopatric offspring is higher at all ages (non-overlapping Bayesian credible intervals of estimates except for yearlings). Brood size varies from 1 to 5 eggs (mean ± S.E. = 3.1 ± 0.31, $N = 96$). Nest success is poor and the number of fledged offspring per breeding attempt levels off with age at about 1.5 fledglings for philopatric offspring compared to 0.92 fledglings for early dispersers (Figure 1.9b). This difference is mainly a result of the probability of nests escaping predation and thus fledging offspring as discussed in relation to the quality of breeding site quality below. Furthermore, philopatric offspring survive better than early dispersers not only when in the company of their parents during their first winter (Griesser et al. 2006), but throughout their lifetime (Figure 1.9c). The average expected lifespan of birds recruited to the adult population was 4.35 years for philopatric offspring, corresponding to an annual survival rate of 0.77, and a

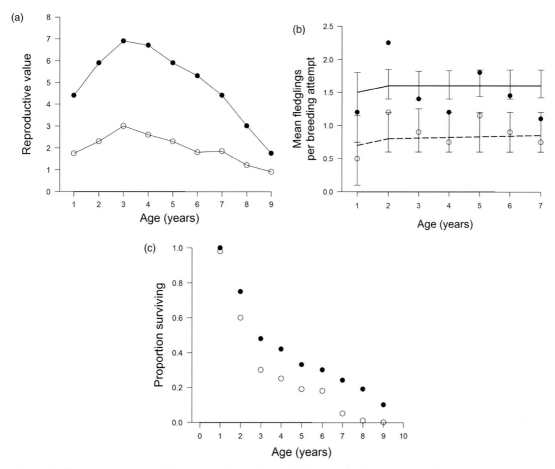

Figure 1.9. (a) Reproductive value of philopatric offspring (*N* = 47; filled symbols) and early dispersers (immigrants, *N* = 62; open symbols). (b) Mean number of fledglings per breeding attempt (includes failed nests) by age for philopatric (*N* = 153; filled symbols) and early dispersers (immigrants; *N* = 112; open symbols). Regression fitted by Bayesian technique with 95% credible intervals indicated for the estimate at each age. (c) Survivorship of birds recruited to the adult population at age 1 for philopatric offspring (*N* = 47; filled symbols) and early dispersers (immigrants; *N* = 62; open symbols).

lifespan of 3.11 years for early dispersers, corresponding to an annual survival rate of 0.68. The fit of a negative exponential decay curve to data with an exception for the first year (r^2 = 0.98 for philopatric and 0.84 for early dispersers) points to constancy of mortality risk (in particular for philopatric offspring), which indicates that the average rates are meaningful representations of adult survival.

Breeding

Role of vegetation structure

Nest predation is the main threat to reproductive success, being more important than brood reduction as a source of loss (Eggers et al. 2005). The risk of nest failure varies dramatically between years. The

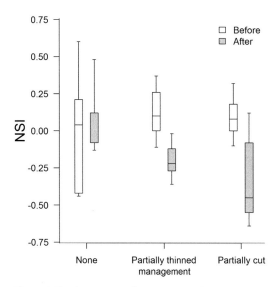

Figure 1.10. The response of nest success to thinning and partial cutting of the forest on Siberian jay territories. Nest success is expressed as NSI (Nest Success Index), which is a weighted index expressing the success rate in a territory in proportion to the population average success rate. Note the value for the first and second quartile is identical for "None, After." From Griesser et al. (2007).

annual variation in proportion of successful breeding attempts ranged from 0.08 to 0.94 (Griesser et al. 2014), and was the main cause of annual variation in population numbers (total number of adults breeders + extra birds on study site). Video surveillance of nests indicates that other corvid species, including the European jay *Garrulus glandarius*, hooded crow *Corvus corone*, raven *C. corax*, and magpie *Pica pica*, are the main nest predators. As Siberian jays are smaller than their main nest predators (adult body weight of Siberian jay is 75–90 g compared to 150–1300 g for its main nest predators), they are unable to defend nests effectively. Instead, Siberian jays rely on cryptic behavior and cover provided by the vegetation to obstruct the visibility of predators hunting using visual cues (Eggers et al. 2005, 2008).

Given the threat to eggs and nestlings from visually oriented predators, it is not surprising that foliage structure has a strong effect on breeding success (Ekman et al. 2001; Griesser et al. 2007). Pines provide little protection for jay nests, while breeding success is high in dense stands of spruce with live branches low (< 2 m) to the ground. The poor visibility in such habitats facilitates concealment of the nest and allows parents to provision nestlings without giving away the nest location (Eggers et al. 2006). This effect is demonstrated by the dramatic increase in nest loss observed in thinned areas where all understory is removed (Figure 1.10). This functional linkage between forest openness and predation risk is supported by evidence of an interaction in which there is a stronger influence of habitat structure on nest loss in areas with high than low abundances of nest predators (Eggers et al. 2005). Habitat preferences of breeders match this association between habitat structure and higher perceived predation risk. When exposed to an increased perceived risk by playbacks of corvid calls, Siberian jay parents shifted to nesting in more dense forest even if this move resulted in nestlings being exposed to the thermoregulatory cost of a colder microclimate (Eggers et al. 2006).

Dispersal pathways and access to habitat

Unsurprisingly, territories with a high proportion of unthinned spruce forests are more likely to be occupied (Griesser and Lagerberg 2012) and Siberian jay parents search out such habitat for nesting sites (Ekman et al. 2001). There is an order of magnitude difference in the variation of spruce density across different territories, however, and the success of breeders can be linked to whether they obtain territories with high densities of spruce, which confers a lower risk of losing eggs and nestlings to predators. In particular, given that early dispersing subordinate offspring fail to secure high-quality territories (Table 1.3), it appears that access to higher quality breeding habitat through delayed and then localized dispersal results in high probability of successful reproduction for delayed dispersers, and this in turn selects for competition among brood mates over which individual gets to remain on the natal territory.

Table 1.3. Nest success and tree density at nest site of breeders with different dispersal history

Extra bird category	Nesting success; Proportion nest with fledged offspring (credible interval)	Spruce density at nest site (Trees with branches below 2 m per100 m² ± credible interval)
Philopatric	0.52 (0.44–0.59)	8.30 ± 0.45
Immigrant	0.32 (0.25–0.41)	6.15 ± 0.20

Prolonged parental care

Parental nepotism and foraging

Siberian jays are opportunistic scavengers and scatter-hoarders, traits likely to have evolved under conditions of cold, harsh winters where birds capitalized on carcasses of large animals killed by wolves and wolverines, but today include feeding on road kills and food left by humans. Within-group conflicts are an important component of competition for such concentrated food resources. The level of conflict ranges from peacefully feeding together to displacement and aggressive chasing, including long-distance pursuits (Ekman et al. 1994). Levels of aggression are affected by kinship: breeders are nepotistic and share food resources nonaggressively with their philopatric offspring, while breeders frequently displace and chase away immigrant group members (Figure 1.11).

The difference in the level of aggression that breeders display toward their retained offspring compared to immigrants profoundly affects the behavior of nonbreeders while foraging (Griesser 2003). Parental tolerance allows philopatric offspring to feed until they are sated or cannot carry more food to store (mean bout length = 21 s). In contrast, immigrants are often displaced and their feeding bouts are regularly interrupted by aggression from breeders or philopatric offspring. Thus, feeding bouts of immigrants follow a negative exponential distribution with a constant failure rate, suggesting an equally high risk of being interrupted at any time. Such interruptions also affect risk-taking behavior: a typical feeding bout of philopatric offspring starts with them scanning the environment for predators or other

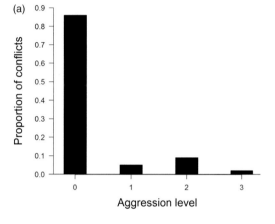

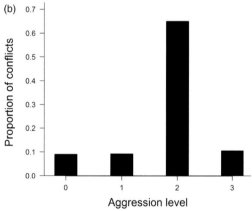

Figure 1.11. The level of aggression directed by parents toward (a) philopatric offspring (N = 1,219 interactions), and (b) immigrants (early dispersers); N = 857 interactions). Scores of aggression level are 0: no aggression, amicably feeding together; 1: tolerated on food, but not allowed to feed; 2: displaced from food; 3: displaced from food and chased. After Ekman et al. (1994).

dangers before they start to feed, whereas immigrants are more risk prone and, in order to maximize their foraging time, do not scan for danger prior to feeding.

Parental nepotism and predator protection

Philopatric offspring benefit not only from more predictable access to food, but also from the antipredator behavior of their parents, which differs depending on the nature of the threat. The first line of defense is increased vigilance by parents when foraging with retained offspring (Griesser 2003). When a predator appears, warning calls alert group members to its presence, the identity of the predator, and the level of threat it poses (Griesser and Ekman 2004, 2005; Griesser 2008, 2009). The role of parental nepotism becomes especially crucial should a predator launch a surprise attack, because warning calls in such circumstances provide unaware individuals the chance to escape (Griesser 2013). Female breeders are particularly nepotistic in this situation and give warning calls primarily while feeding together with offspring (Griesser and Ekman 2004).

Parental presence

The important role that parental presence plays in the decision of offspring to remain philopatric is demonstrated by their response to the loss of a parent, which is to disperse. After the experimental removal of a breeder male ($N = 6$ groups) in late August or early September and his subsequent replacement by a new unrelated male, philopatric offspring of both sexes ($N = 10$) lost their preferential treatment and seven philopatric offspring dispersed within a month (Ekman and Griesser 2002). The dispersal of such first year birds is outside the ordinary dispersal period (early dispersers: mid-June to mid-July; philopatric offspring: beginning in March after winter). This confirms the role that parents and their nepotistic behavior play in influencing the decision made by offspring to delay dispersal and stay in the natal territory.

Conclusions

Siberian jays offer the unusual conditions needed to examine not only the fitness consequences of delayed dispersal, but also the processes through which those benefits come about. Both extended philopatry and immediate dispersal (early dispersers) are pathways to becoming a breeder, but these two different strategies are associated with significant differences in several key life history traits, including dominance within the brood, age of dispersal, dispersal mode and distance, social environment, age of first reproduction, and lifetime reproductive success (Ekman et al. 1999, 2001, 2002). Siberian jays not only delay dispersal, they also delay breeding. In Siberian jays, postponing the onset of independent reproduction is a superior strategy despite the fact that philopatric offspring are older when they start to breed. The lack of a lifetime penalty for delayed breeding emphasizes the role of life-history trade-offs in demonstrating that philopatric individuals are compensated for the loss of reproductive success they suffer early in life.

Breeding is constrained by availability of high quality nesting sites in Siberian jays with larger proportions of individuals becoming nonbreeders at high densities (Figure 1.7). While postponement of breeding is fundamental to behavior of delaying dispersal, alternative dispersal pathways show that remaining in the natal territory is not an obligate response to constraints on breeding. A shortage of high quality breeding opportunities cannot account for the differences in behavior between siblings, or for why some remain philopatric in the first place. The dispersal pathway represents life-history decisions in the quest to become breeder where the adaptive value of philopatry depends on how it compares to alternatives. Life-history decisions are circumscribed by a variety of constraints, and limited breeding resources is but one of these. Within-brood dominance is another constraint affecting siblings unequally and accounting for their differences in dispersal pathway and ultimately reproductive value. Further, replacement of a breeder usually leads to dispersal of retained offspring. This means that subordinate individuals and those that are orphaned by one parent are simultaneously exposed to both ecological constraints on breeding and social constraints on delayed dispersal.

Delayed dispersal in the Siberian jay cannot be understood without considering both the behavior of parents and offspring. The presence of parents and their behavior toward offspring are essential factors in understanding the benefits of philopatry (Ekman and Griesser 2002). The role of prolonged brood care, which appears to be so important for delayed dispersal in Siberian jays, remains a largely unexplored question in cooperatively breeding species. Yet parents are found only in the natal territory, and thus prolonged brood care is a unique benefit available only to philopatric offspring, which can render the family group a safe haven until the offspring is ready to become a breeder (Kokko and Ekman 2002). In reverse, the role of kinship appears crucial to explaining the prolonged brood care in the Siberian jay, particularly in terms of parents gaining making direct fitness gain from favoring more closely related individuals by directing behaviors of food sharing and predator protection selectively toward those group members returning a higher inclusive fitness payoff of such acts (Ekman et al. 1994; Griesser et al. 2006).

While delayed dispersal certainly requires parental tolerance of young on the natal territory when breeding is constrained, it is within-brood conflict that accounts for individual differences in dispersal pathways in Siberian jays (Ekman et al. 2002). The within-brood dominance of an offspring has a legacy lasting throughout its lifetime as reflected in the age of first breeding, habitat choice, and eventually breeding success. Delayed dispersal occurs based upon an inherent asymmetry in phenotypic quality among siblings and this asymmetry is thus the proximate mechanism accounting for unequal access to resources later in life. In particular, the decision by early dispersers to start breeding at an earlier age than philopatric siblings and in more open habitat despite these options being less likely to result in successful breeding can be seen as a best-of-a-bad-job life-history strategy where poor competitive ability limits access to high-quality resources (Ekman et al. 2001). Given the profound and lasting fitness effects of within-brood dominance, seeking to understand its developmental basis is likely to provide new insights into how this early trajectory toward fitness remains stable throughout a bird's lifetime.

Philopatric offspring may suffer a cost of lost reproduction from having to postpone the start of reproduction, but the adaptive value of delaying dispersal can only be assessed relative to realistic alternatives. In the Siberian jay, the alternative is not independent breeding, but being an early disperser. Siberian jays may be far from unique in that offspring follow alternative dispersal pathways. Immigrants to family groups containing philopatric offspring have been recorded in a large proportion of social species, many of which breed cooperatively (Riehl 2013). Little is known about their history and fate compared to the wealth of information available for philopatric offspring. Yet early dispersers are pivotal to an understanding of the adaptive value of delayed dispersal by representing the alternative.

Acknowledgments

This study owes its origin to the inspiration from Malte Andersson. It would not have been possible without the generosity of Folke Lindgren inviting us to use his study area around Arvidsjaur, sharing his rich experiences with the jays, and introducing us to the logistics of working in a boreal environment. The late Gunnar Pavval and his wife Ingrid generously provided the perfect base camp and a host of entertaining acquaintances over the years. A number of field assistants have helped collect data, and the late Anders Bylin, a master at making campfires and trapping birds, shared many enjoyable days in the field. The prompt and accurate service of Kerstin Santesson provided invaluable help taking over molecular analyses after earlier work by Håkan Tegelström. Jonathan Barnaby and Hanna Kokko share our passion for the jays and provided many ideas. Thesis work by Sönke Eggers, Magdalena Nystrand, Tobias Sahlman, Peter Halvarsson, Alexandros Panagoulis, and Radoslav Koszma each contributed to the story. The owner of the Reivo Nature Reservation and the governmental forest company Sveaskog AB kindly allowed us to work on their land. The study was supported by the Swedish Natural Science Research, the Swedish Nature Conservancy, and Uppsala University. To all these we are most grateful.

REFERENCES

Brown J. L. (1969). Territorial behavior and population regulation in birds. *Wilson Bull.*, 81, 293–329.

Brown J. L. (1978). Avian communal breeding systems. *Annu. Rev. Ecol. Syst.*, 9, 123–155.

Eggers S., Griesser M., Andersson T., and Ekman J. (2005). Nest predation and habitat change interact to influence Siberian jay numbers. *Oikos*, 111, 150–158.

Eggers S., Griesser M., Nystrand M., and Ekman J. (2006). Predation risk induces changes in nest-site selection and clutch size in the Siberian jay. *Proc. R. Soc. London B*, 273, 701–706.

Eggers S., Griesser M., and Ekman J. (2008). Predator-induced reductions in nest visitation rates are modified by forest cover and food availability. *Behav. Ecol.*, 19, 1056–1062.

Ekman J. (2006). Family living among birds. *J. Avian Biol.*, 37, 289–298.

Ekman J. and Griesser M. (2002). Why offspring delay dispersal: experimental evidence for a role of parental tolerance. *Proc. R. Soc. London B*, 269, 1709–1713.

Ekman J., Sklepkovych B., and Tegelström H. (1994). Offspring retention in the Siberian jay (*Perisoreus infaustus*): the prolonged brood care hypothesis. *Behav. Ecol.*, 5, 245–253.

Ekman J., Bylin A., and Tegelström H. (1999). Increased lifetime reproductive success for Siberian jay (*Perisoreus infaustus*) males with delayed dispersal. *Proc. R. Soc. London B*, 266, 911–915.

Ekman J., Bylin A., and Tegelström H. (2000). Parental nepotism enhances survival of retained offspring in the Siberian jay. *Behav. Ecol.*, 11, 416–420.

Ekman J., Eggers S., Griesser M., and Tegelström H. (2001). Queuing for preferred territories: delayed dispersal of Siberian jays. *J. Anim. Ecol.*, 70, 317–324.

Ekman J., Eggers S., and Griesser M. (2002). Fighting to stay: the role of sibling rivalry for delayed dispersal. *Anim. Behav.*, 64, 453–459.

Emlen S. T. (1982). The evolution of helping. 1. An ecological constraints model. *Am. Nat.*, 119, 29–39.

Gienapp P. and Merila J. (2010). High fidelity: no evidence for extra-pair paternity in Siberian jays (*Perisoreus infaustus*). *PLoS One*, 5(8), e12006.

Griesser M. (2003). Nepotistic vigilance behavior in Siberian jay parents. *Behav. Ecol.*, 14, 246–250.

Griesser M. (2008). Referential calls signal predator behavior in a group-living bird species. *Curr. Biol.*, 18, 69–73.

Griesser M. (2009). Mobbing calls signal predator category in a kin group-living bird species. *Proc. R. Soc. London B*, 276, 2887–2892.

Griesser M. (2013). Do warning calls boost survival of signal recipients? Evidence from a field experiment in a group-living bird species. *Front. Zool.*, 10, 49.

Griesser M. and Ekman A. (2004). Nepotistic alarm calling in the Siberian jay, *Perisoreus infaustus*. *Anim. Behav.*, 67, 933–939.

Griesser M. and Ekman J. (2005). Nepotistic mobbing behaviour in the Siberian jay, *Perisoreus infaustus*. *Anim. Behav.*, 69, 345–352.

Griesser M. and Lagerberg S. (2012). Long-term effects of forest management on territory occupancy and breeding success of an open-nesting boreal bird species, the Siberian jay. *For. Ecol. Manage.*, 271, 58–64.

Griesser M., Nystrand M., and Ekman J. (2006). Reduced mortality selects for family cohesion in a social species. *Proc. R. Soc. London B*, 273, 1881–1886.

Griesser M., Nystrand M., Eggers S., and Ekman J. (2007). Impact of forestry practices on fitness correlates and population productivity in an open-nesting bird species. *Conserv. Biol.*, 21, 767–774.

Griesser M., Nystrand M., Eggers S., and Ekman J. (2008). Social constraints limit dispersal and settlement decisions in a group-living bird species. *Behav. Ecol.*, 19, 317–324.

Griesser M., Halvarsson P., Sahlman T., and Ekman J. (2014). What are the strengths and limitations of direct and indirect assessment of dispersal? Insights from a long-term field study in a group-living bird species. *Behav. Ecol. Sociobiol.*, 68, 485–497.

Koenig W. D. and Pitelka F. A. (1981). Ecological factors and kin selection in the evolution of cooperative breeding in birds. In: *Natural Selection and Social Behavior: Recent Research and New Theory*, ed. R. D. Alexander and D. W. Tinkle. New York: Chiron Press, pp. 261–280.

Kokko H. and Ekman J. (2002). Delayed dispersal as a route to breeding: territorial inheritance, safe havens, and ecological constraints. *Am. Nat.*, 160, 468–484.

Lillandt B. G., Bensch S., and von Schantz T. (2003). Family structure in the Siberian jay as revealed by microsatellite analyses. *Condor*, 105, 505–514.

Lindgren F. (1975). Iakttagelser rörande lavskrikan (*Perisoreus infaustus*) – huvudsakligen dess häckningsbiologi. *Fauna och Flora*, 70, 193–232.

Mock D. W. and Parker G. A. (1997). *Sibling Rivalry*. Oxford: Oxford University Press.

Ridley A. R., Raihani N. J., and Nelson-Flower M. J. (2008). The cost of being alone: the fate of floaters in a population of cooperatively breeding pied babblers *Turdoides bicolor*. *J. Avian Biol.*, 39, 389–392.

Riehl C. (2013). Evolutionary routes to non-kin cooperative breeding in birds. *Proc. R. Soc. London B*, 280, 20132245.

Zahavi A. (1990). Arabian babbler: the quest for social status in a cooperative breeder. In: *Cooperative Breeding in Birds: Long-term Studies of Ecology and Behavior*, ed. P. B. Stacey and W. D. Koenig. Cambridge: Cambridge University Press, pp. 105–130.

2

Western bluebirds: Lessons from a marginal cooperative breeder

Janis L. Dickinson, Çağlar Akçay, Elise D. Ferree, and Caitlin A. Stern

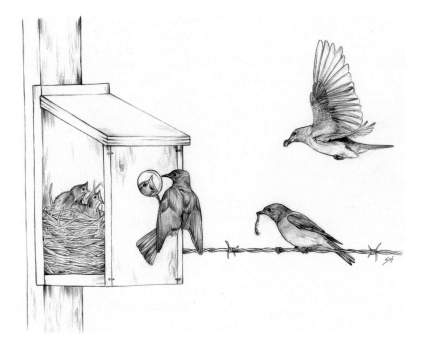

Introduction

As in many species of cooperative breeders, western bluebirds, *Sialia mexicana*, have adult male offspring that help at nests of close relatives. They are unusual in maintaining helping at a low level; only 11% of sons help and, when they do, they feed at nests of one or both parents, nestmate brothers, or rarely, grandfathers. On average, only 7% of pairs have helpers, although the range is 3–16% depending upon the year (Dickinson et al. 1996). Helping is facultative, with males able to switch from helping to breeding and back again within a season (Dickinson and Akre 1998). While their most common behavior is to breed in pairs,

Cooperative Breeding in Vertebrates: Studies of Ecology, Evolution, and Behavior, eds W. D. Koenig and J. L. Dickinson.
Published by Cambridge University Press. © Cambridge University Press 2016.

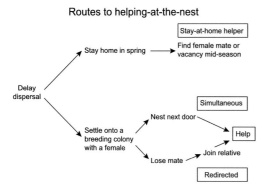

Figure 2.1. Routes to helping behavior in western bluebirds.

three characteristics render western bluebirds useful for understanding the evolution and maintenance of helping behavior as a facultative trait.

First, the mode of helping is unusually fluid: in addition to the typical "stay-at-home" helpers, which delay dispersal, remain on their natal territory, and then help as yearlings, western bluebirds have "redirected helpers," which help mid-season after their mate is killed or their nest fails (Figure 2.1). This makes the territorial system of western bluebirds more similar to that of colonial white-fronted bee-eaters (*Merops bullockoides*) in Kenya (Emlen and Wrege 1989) or Galápagos mockingbirds (*Mimus parvulus;* Curry and Grant 1990) than to the acorn woodpeckers (*Melanerpes formicivorus*) with which they often share cavity trees and space (Chapter 13). Western bluebirds also have a third type of helper, "simultaneous breeder-helpers," which breed adjacent to their parents and feed at both their parents' nest and their own nest within a single day. This cross-territorial helping was our first hint that western bluebirds favor kin even while living on different territories. A strength of the study system is that we have been able to follow birds as they adopt these different options to gain important insights into each option's relative fitness benefits.

Second, although western bluebirds are marginal cooperative breeders in spring, they exhibit high levels of kin-based sociality in winter, living in stable family groups on their territories (Kraaijeveld and Dickinson 2001). This has afforded us the opportunity to examine

the drivers and fitness consequences of delayed and localized dispersal, which we hypothesize provide the permissive conditions for kin-based helping. Benefits can include nepotism as well as access to abundant or familiar resources and space (Ekman et al. 2001). While relatively few western bluebird males ever help, many stay home on their natal territories during their first winter, and among these, a large proportion also settle near their parents and brothers, where they have the opportunity to interact in complex neighborhoods comprised of a mix of kin and nonkin.

Third, western bluebirds are an example of a cooperative breeder in which fitness measures for males are significantly influenced by extra-pair paternity (Dickinson and Akre 1998). This has made assessing the benefits of helping tricky, but it also means that males potentially exercise outside options, seeking copulations with females outside the group in which they reside. This can feed back on the fitness benefits of philopatry and of living near kin in interesting and complex ways, influencing the structure of the fitness payoffs of helping, having sons help, or breeding close to kin (Dickinson et al. 1996; Stern 2012). Together, these attributes of western bluebirds, discovered over many years, make for an informative case study in the field of cooperative breeding.

Natural history and methods

Taxonomic affiliation and distribution

Western bluebirds are one of three species in the genus, *Sialia*, which is restricted to North America. Their distribution runs from British Columbia and southwestern Alberta to Northern Baja and Mexico's volcanic belt with a large gap in the great basin of the western United States (Guinan et al. 2008). Western bluebirds are partially separated from mountain bluebirds (*S. currucoides*) by elevation, and from eastern bluebirds (*S. sialis*) by geography, although there are contact zones, such as in eastern Texas, where all three species co-occur. Western bluebirds are short-distance, partial migrants, and populations vary from being exclusively migratory to being altitudinal migrants or year-round residents.

Adults eat a variety of berries in fall and winter, and they rely heavily on juniper berries in some parts of the southwestern United States (Balda 1987). Western bluebirds also consume mistletoe *(Phoradendron* spp*.)* throughout most of their range and, in general, mistletoe appears to be an important winter food resource (Guinan et al. 2008). The population we studied is resident year-round in the mistletoe-rich oak savanna of central coastal California.

Study site and methods

At Hastings Reservation, a University of California, Berkeley field station in the Santa Lucia Mountains of central California's outer coast range, western bluebirds inhabit blue oak (*Quercus douglasii*) savanna – one of the largest old-growth forests remaining in North America (Stahle 2002) – and are rarely found in the intermingled patches of chaparral and mixed hardwood forest. They nest in secondary cavities and, in our study system, nest boxes, which they occupy almost as greedily as do other bluebird species. Boxes with a 3.8 cm-diameter entrance-hole were first put up on our study site in 1983–1985 by Walt Koenig, who until 1989 oversaw color-banding and monitoring of 363 nest boxes scattered over 700 hectares of oak woodland.

Starting in 1990, we initiated a rigorous sampling scheme, which included observing nests for provisioning rates and assessing group composition at three evenly-spaced intervals over the course of the nesting cycle. We also measured nestlings at 6 and 14 days of age, and banded new adults once nestlings were 9 days old, creating a powerfully consistent set of measurements. From 1985 to 2001 densities on Hastings and the adjacent Oak Ridge Ranch ranged from 36 pairs in an el niño year to 130 pairs 3 years later, placing the upper limit of nest box occupancy by western bluebirds at 36%. During this period, the Hastings study area stood at 7 km² and was little changed until 2002, when we lost access to the section that was located on Oak Ridge Ranch and added a section of another, more distant ranch (Rana Creek). Most of our experimental work was conducted after 2001, making the 1985–2001 data the most valuable for long-term demography.

Western bluebirds are the primary nest box occupants on our study area, comprising 67% of occupants with the other 33% comprising deer mice, five other cavity-nesting bird species, bumblebees, and vespid wasps. About half of nest boxes were empty most years and western bluebirds had up to seven nest boxes within their territories. Radio-tracking studies indicated that territories comprise a disproportionately large amount of grassland and, within territories, birds spend proportionally more time in edges than expected by chance (C. Marx and J. Dickinson, unpubl. MS). These results, based on GIS analysis and randomization tests, indicate that western bluebirds are an open habitat and edge-loving species.

When we started our study, it was generally thought that western bluebirds travel in mobile flocks in winter, tracking resources and thermal regimes, with some altitudinal migrants moving uphill to visit their territories on warm, winter days (Guinan et al. 2008). Our discovery that they live on their territories year-round was incidental and developed over time as we began to accumulate observations of color-banded birds coming to water troughs in family groups and appearing in winter precisely where they had been the prior spring. Once we began observing family groups systematically, their cohesiveness and their connection to mistletoe became apparent (Kraaijeveld and Dickinson 2001).

Upon further investigation, it turned out that Grinnell and Storer (1924), prominent early California ornithologists closely associated with Hastings Reservation, had pointed out that mistletoe berries are commonly eaten by western bluebirds in winter and that "the presence of this plant may govern local occurrence." Even though they presented no quantitative data supporting their claims, they took extensive field notes, making a fine example of the unparalleled wealth of knowledge these and other early naturalists accumulated during long trips on foot and horseback observing birds and other organisms throughout California.

Oak mistletoe (*Phoradendron villosum*) provided a new context for understanding the socioecological factors influencing delayed and localized dispersal and, ultimately, helping at the nest (Figure 2.2). Of the

(a)   (b)

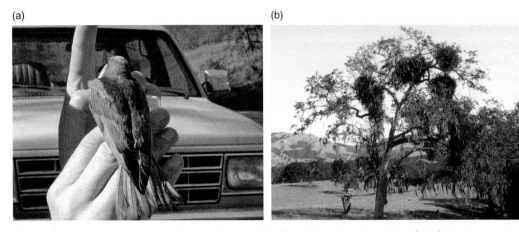

Figure 2.2. Western bluebird male with rufous back patch (left) and blue oak with mistletoe (right). See plate section for color figure.

handful of berry types consumed by western blue-birds at Hastings, mistletoe and toyon (*Heteromeles arbutifolia*) are the only two that provide a constant berry supply all winter long. As toyon is neither common nor clumped at our study site, mistletoe was the only candidate with the constancy and abundance to support winter territoriality. Early analysis revealed that nestbox occupancy rates declined exponentially with distance from the nearest mistletoe, dropping off to near zero at a distance of 50 m (r_s = -0.35, N = 50 boxes, P = 0.03). This led us to map, photograph, and quantify mistletoe within 200 m of all nest boxes on our study areas, which amounted to quantifying mistletoe volume on 3377 trees (Dickinson and McGowan 2005).

Mean winter territory size is between 1.27 and 3.85 ha, depending on the year (Kraaijeveld and Dickinson 2001; Dickinson et al. 2014). We also found that mistletoe volume is spatially autocorrelated to a distance of 250 m. This means, when sons disperse next door to their parents, as often occurs, they will acquire a territory similar in quality to that of their parents (Wilson et al. 2014). Having a quantifiable resource that is apparently so important – all individuals caught have mistletoe seeds in their feces in winter – provided us with the opportunity to study the social and ecological drivers of delayed dispersal.

Breeding behavior and sexual selection

Both sexual competition and kin-biased helping are important components of the breeding system of western bluebirds at Hastings, allowing for an integrated understanding of sexual selection and cooperative breeding. About 45% of nests have extra-pair young (Dickinson and Akre 1998), and paired males guard their mates assiduously by following females during the peak receptive period (10 days before and during laying), when they begin to accept over 80% of within-pair copulation attempts (Dickinson and Leonard 1996). When their mate was detained for an hour during the laying period, most females (86%) were joined by intruder males, often from neighboring territories, whereas females whose mate was caught and released immediately were joined only 5% of the time; these results demonstrate a 17-fold effectiveness of mate guarding (Dickinson 1997).

Female receptivity to such attempts favors males that are older, but not necessarily larger, than the female's social mate (Dickinson 2001) and this preference is consistent with the finding that older males are most successful at gaining extra-pair paternity (Ferree and Dickinson 2011). How, though, do females tell which males are older? Based on spectrometry of five body regions, we discovered a strong positive relationship between head plumage brightness, male age, and nestling mass (Budden and Dickinson 2009, Figure 2.2). Older males not only had brighter heads, they were in better condition. The ruddy patch on a male's back provides additional information on age, becoming increasingly mottled over successive molts; in the oldest males, it is often entirely replaced with blue feathers. Although we have not tested for preferences and paternity advantages based on male plumage color, plumage not only carries information on age, it also provides information directly relevant to fitness.

How do older males that gain extra-pair paternity fare, given that extra-pair copulations mean leaving the territory and, in many cases, leaving the male's own mate unguarded (Dickinson and Leonard 1996)? Males successful at siring extra-pair offspring do not tend to lose paternity in their own nests and have roughly double the annual reproductive success of those without extra-pair paternity, resulting in a Bateman gradient that is positive for males and level for females (Ferree and Dickinson 2014). They also fare well in terms of offspring quality. Extra-pair chicks grow faster than their within-pair nestmates. This kind of result was originally interpreted as evidence for good genes, albeit with caveats (Kempanaers et al. 1992). In western bluebirds this difference is a result of extra-pair chicks appearing earlier in the laying and hatch sequence, and thus represents a phenotypic, rather than a genetic effect (Ferree et al. 2010). Whether the phenotypic effect arises from maternal effects or from the timing of extra-pair males' copulation attempts is yet to be determined and separating paternal from maternal effects is likely to prove quite difficult.

Although adult males are slightly larger than females, early eggs are as likely to be female as male. Unlike female fledglings, male fledglings often remain in the area where they were born and their fitness can be tracked over the course of their adult lives. Those that are relatively heavy on day 14, and are present on the study area as adults, tend to live longer than lighter nestlings (Dickinson 2004a), creating a positive feedback loop in which older males have extra-pair sons that grow faster and are more likely to reap extra-pair paternity advantages as they become old males.

Despite a sex ratio of unity at fledging (Koenig and Dickinson 1996), female removal studies indicate a shortage of adult females in the population (Dickinson 2004a). The first hint of such a shortage was the observation that replacement males frequently come in to take over a vacancy when a paired male is removed or killed. Replacement males, when they come in during laying, tend to contribute half the feeding trips to the nest, just as the parental male would, but those coming in later follow the female around, behaving as if paired, and even feed the female on occasion, but usually do not feed nestlings (Dickinson and Weathers 1999).

A high proportion of females (78%) acquired a replacement mate, usually a yearling male, following experimental removal of their mate. In contrast, only 17% of males acquired a new mate following female removal; instead, they helped, became a replacement mate, or held their territory alone (Dickinson 2004a). This is in contrast with matched controls where we removed the nest and eggs, but not the female mate, in which 83% of males renested. Failure to renest was thus due to a female shortage, not seasonal timing. The shortage of females suggests that local competition represents a cost of philopatry for males, which is augmented by the fact that they will compete with their fathers and brothers for mates (Dickinson 2004a).

Dispersal and family group formation

Delayed dispersal of males emerges against a backdrop of male philopatry and female-biased dispersal, which is typical for passerine birds (Greenwood 1980). While it is not currently feasible to track long-distance dispersal of small birds with sufficient numbers and resolution to gather fitness data, it is possible to compare immigrants with birds born on the study area and assess their survival and reproductive success after they settle to breed as yearlings. Focusing on immigrants and philopatric individuals does not allow us to address the costs of movement and settlement, the costs of competing locally with relatives for limited breeding vacancies, nor the benefits of cooperating with local kin (Dobson 2013). What it can do is help address why sons tend to be philopatric and breed near their natal sites when

Table 2.1. Post-settlement fitness comparisons for immigrant and local males and females of western bluebirds over their lifetimes based on data from birds that were yearlings in 1985–1998

Sex and type	Number of years bred	Total number of nests	Number of nests that fledged	Total number of young that fledged
Local male N = 158	1.84 ± 0.10	2.27 ± 0.11	1.90 ± 0.09	5.84 ± 2.07
Immigrant male N = 267	1.65 ± 0.10	2.00 ± 0.20	1.36 ± 0.11	5.36 ± 1.56
Mann-Whitney *U*-test	**W = 19913** **P = 0.23**	**W = 19523** **P = 0.13**	**W = 20951** **P = 0.76**	**W = 21393** **P = 0.94**
Local female, n = 74	1.57 ± 0.15	1.86 ± 0.25	1.20 ± 0.22	4.62 ± 3.26
Immigrant female, n = 309	1.89 ± 0.09	2.32 ± 0.18	1.58 ± 0.11	6.28 ± 2.00
Mann-Whitney *U*-test	**W = 13138** **P = 0.03***	**W = 13117** **P = 0.04***	**W = 13570** **P = 0.01***	**W = 13544** **P = 0.01***

A Mann-Whitney U-test was used in place of a GLMM due to issues of false Convergence.

most daughters disperse. Conveniently, western bluebird adults can be classified as yearlings or older by plumage, allowing us to distinguish and follow immigrants that bred as yearlings from their first breeding attempt through the next four years, truncating the data set to remove any birds not observed long enough to get four years of breeding data.

In western bluebirds, sons compete locally for mates, and this leads to occasional adoption of the lesser fitness option of helping. Even so, these costs could be offset by survival and breeding advantages of staying home. Assuming that incest is equally costly for both sexes, if these advantages are greater for males than for females, then females should be the more dispersive sex. Instead, we found that immigrant females had higher breeding success than did local females, and these advantages were evident in the number of years they bred, their total number of nests, the number of their nests that fledged at least one offspring, and the total number of young they fledged over four breeding seasons (Table 2.1). Although locally dispersing sons had higher success than immigrants in each of these fitness categories, we found no statistical difference for any of these four metrics of lifetime reproductive success for males. While some studies have revealed

advantages of philopatry for males (Bensch et al. 1998), our study effectively shows disadvantages of philopatry for females, at least after settlement. This finding is surprising and provides a novel reason why females tend to be the more dispersive sex. It also shows that male philopatry is not costly after settlement in our population, even including helpers in the analysis, but neither is it beneficial for male western bluebirds. Male philopatry is not so much selected for as not selected against, whereas female philopatry appears to be disadvantageous, favoring females becoming the more dispersive sex.

Western bluebirds delay dispersal beyond the period of parental dependence typical for altricial birds. Such delayed dispersal begins with offspring, usually sons, remaining on their natal territories for winter, while most daughters leave the study area permanently in late summer. The departing daughters are replaced by young immigrant females achieving a mean group sex ratio of unity (Figure 2.3; Table 2.2). In spring, we found that 57% of local sons and 61% of immigrant females dispersed locally to breed, usually pairing up in their winter group (Kraaijeveld and Dickinson 2001). Daughters that had not dispersed in late summer usually left the study area the following spring, and the

Table 2.2. The number and proportion of first winter males and females that remained in their natal group, moved groups, or immigrated from outside the study area

Sex	Natal group	Moved groups	Immigrant
First-winter males	35 (70%)	12 (24%)	3 (6%)
First-winter females	14 (25%)	13 (24%)	28 (51%)

Source: From Kraaijeveld and Dickinson (2001).

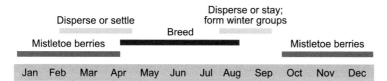

Figure 2.3. The annual cycle of dispersal and breeding of western bluebirds relative to mistletoe berry availability.

15% that remained for winter usually bred quite far from their natal territory (mean ± standard error distance = 2.5 ± 0.4 km). After these two steps of dispersal, about 25% of fledgling sons and 5% of fledgling daughters remain on the study area as yearlings, with remaining daughters being farther from home than sons.

This pattern of dispersal means that sons live in kin neighborhoods, where they have opportunities for prolonged interactions with close relatives even after dispersing onto independent breeding territories (Kraaijeveld and Dickinson 2001; Stern 2012). A major focus of our work has been to examine what causes sons to remain in their natal groups for winter and what governs the steps they take after that, including dispersing locally to breed, helping, and other kin-based interactions occurring across territories.

Composition and stability of winter groups

In winter, western bluebirds live in bisexual territorial groups of up to 18 individuals. Groups form in late summer and are usually stable until young birds settle onto independent breeding territories in spring. Although group stability is the norm, a reproductive vacancy will occasionally open up on a nearby territory in winter, such as when a breeder female is widowed. In such cases, we have observed males from adjacent territories switch into the new group, presumably because there is a nonincestuous breeding opportunity with an older female on an established territory.

Winter group compositions are variable, ranging from a pair of breeders that failed to fledge young the previous spring to complex family groups, usually with sons, living parents, and immigrant females (Kraaijeveld and Dickinson 2001). Figure 2.4 shows group sizes based on year-round field work in 2000–2006, during which the modal group size was six birds, in contrast with 1996–1997, for which we reported a modal group size of four birds (Kraaijeveld and Dickinson 2001). We also see blended families consisting of fledged young, a widowed male, and his new mate, or groups of orphans and widows. Coalescence sometimes occurs, where families come back together for winter to form groups comprised of a father, son, both their mates, and their surviving offspring from the prior spring. Group members travel together, often to watering sites, and they signal with a steady *pew* call as they fly above the trees or when they fly as a group from tree to tree prior to roosting. Groups roost communally in mistletoe or, on cold nights, in nest boxes, but only rarely roost together with a nearby group.

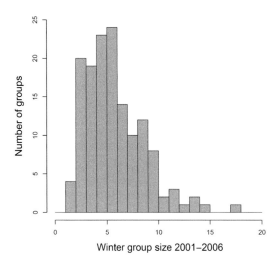

Figure 2.4. Winter group sizes from 2001 to 2006.

The helping system

Adult helpers are always male, whereas females comprise 14% of juvenile helpers assisting at their parents' second nests (Dickinson et al. 1996). Adult male helpers both increase food delivery to nestlings and lighten the feeding loads for both their parents. In contrast, juvenile helpers do not have a significant effect on feeding rates at nests, whether we consider total feeds per hour (work done) or total feeds per nestling per hour (amount of food received per nestling). Juvenile helpers only contributed 21% of the feeding trips to the nest, and while this could have led to nestlings receiving more food, the effect of their effort was canceled because the parental male fed less frequently. As second nests with juvenile helpers had fewer fledglings than second nests without helpers, juvenile helpers either elect to help under dire circumstances or they are "hinderers" rather than helpers. Given that juvenile helpers are qualitatively different from adult helpers and do not give up breeding in order to help, we do not include juvenile helpers in any of our analyses of fitness consequences of helping, and always keep the two separate when analyzing their effects on feeding. All further discussion of helping here focuses on adult helpers.

Most groups with helpers have just one, but we have seen up to three adult helpers at a nest, including sons born in different years. While there are more younger than older adult helpers, this is due to demography. The probability of helping does not appear to decline with age for males whose parents are both still alive, rather, the opportunity to help parents declines with age due to the ~50% annual mortality of adults (Dickinson et al. 1996). Adult females, which never help, are statistically less likely to help than are adult males, even when both their parents are alive.

Helpers assist at nests of their parents, a parent and stepparent, and occasionally brothers or a grandfather. In one case, we observed a son lose his mate and begin helping at his father's nest; then, when the father's nest failed, both father and son traveled 0.46 km to the grandfather's nest to help, and remained there to help in the subsequent year. This example points to one of the most intriguing aspects of the western bluebird system: the persistence of familial relationships across territories and years, a feature that allows for cross-territorial aid-giving and recognition of relatives long after those relatives have left home.

We have never found helpers to have paternity at helped nests, even when they are with their father or brother and an unrelated female and thus would not be committing incest. As such, western bluebirds represent a case of absolute reproductive skew, in which auxiliaries are always nonbreeding helpers. Usually helper status is enforced through incest avoidance, but in the much rarer cases where the mother has been replaced and incest is possible, it is likely enforced by reproductive competition. Based on this information, we refer to all auxiliaries as helpers.

Drivers of delayed and localized dispersal

While delayed dispersal is commonly associated with helping (Emlen 1978; Brown 1987), we distinguish delayed dispersal from the maintenance of family connections, which is the minimal requirement for facultative kin-based helping. In a migratory population of western bluebirds with helpers in Montana, simply placing an extra box on the breeding territory increases

Formation of kin neighborhoods

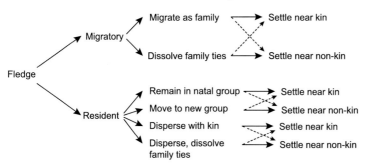

Figure 2.5. How western bluebird kin neighborhoods form.

the likelihood that fathers and sons or brothers nest next door to each other in spring (Duckworth and Badyaev 2007). Such families must migrate together, or at least return to the same locale after migration. This and other examples of offspring breeding near parents, despite not remaining on the natal territory year-round, falsify the idea that delayed dispersal is necessary for kin-based helping, and demonstrate that there are multiple routes to remaining with family (Figure 2.5). While migrants may have greater exposure to outside options, it is settling near kin, rather than delayed dispersal per se, that provides the fundamental conditions for facultative, kin-based helping. Our resident population at Hastings offers the opportunity to examine the drivers and fitness consequences of the steps leading to such localized dispersal. We start by examining which factors influence whether sons remain in the natal group during the winter, and their tendencies to settle onto local breeding territories in spring.

We focus on two potentially important drivers of delayed dispersal, following Ekman and Rosander (1992), who considered delayed dispersal as a transaction between parents and their offspring in which parents have complete control. They assumed that parents, as dominants, will gauge the benefit:cost ratio of conceding resources to offspring in determining whether young birds should remain on the natal territory. A corollary of this assumption is that the frequency of delayed dispersal should scale with the amount of depletable resources that parents have available to

share, since having sons stay home incurs a cost for parents when resources are limited, and is thus a form of parental effort. These ideas informed the "prolonged brood care hypothesis" leading to evidence that parental tolerance on the natal territory (Ekman and Griesser 2002) and active protection of offspring (Griesser 2003; Griesser and Ekman 2004, 2005) provide fitness advantages for retained offspring that they cannot get anywhere else (Ligon 1981; Fitzpatrick and Woolfenden 1986). The prolonged brood care hypothesis provides a nonexclusive alternative to the hypotheses that birds delay dispersal, stay on the natal territory, and help due to habitat saturation, a shortage of marginal habitat, spatio-temporal variation in environmental factors influencing reproduction, and other kinds of ecological constraints (Emlen 1982a, 1982b).

We teased apart the effects of resources and parents using behavioral observations combined with demographic data. First, we asked whether parents are nepotistic in winter groups and whether mistletoe is a causal factor in delayed dispersal. Then we analyzed the importance of resources and parents within the same analysis, following sons through the fall and spring steps of dispersal and through their first spring as a breeder.

Group defense, nepotism, and intersexual aggression in winter groups

Although winter-group-living entails both cooperation and competition, it also allows western bluebirds to reduce the costs of territoriality by sharing the effort required for territorial defense. Individuals in winter groups invested less time defending against a caged "intruder" as group size increased, while the constancy of defense (the total time at least one bird was on the intruder's cage) was similar across group sizes (Kleiber et al. 2007). This indicates that one benefit of being in a group is that it allows individuals to reduce their effort without lowering the constancy of defense. While members of both sexes and all ages exhibited aggression when presented with a caged male or female, breeder males and females were more aggressive toward same-sex than opposite-sex intruders. Variance in male aggression was apparent in the frequency with which they hopped while on or next to the cage, whereas variance in female aggression was apparent in the total duration of time they spent standing on or next to the cage.

Observations of winter groups at mealworm feeders, for which access to food was restricted to just one corner of the feeder, provided evidence of nepotism. Mothers, but not fathers, were less aggressive to their own offspring than to immigrant young of the year that had joined their winter group (Dickinson et al. 2009). In addition, experienced breeders of both sexes were more aggressive to same-sex than to opposite-sex group members. Experienced breeder males were more than 12 times as aggressive to their sons, with which they compete for mates, than females were toward their daughters, which are likely to leave the study area after winter. Males were as aggressive toward their own sons as toward immigrant males, perhaps because both sons and immigrant males are potential competitors for nonincestuous matings and extra-pair fertilizations.

In general, group defense and intragroup aggression were variously influenced by sexual competition, nepotism (kinship), individual benefits, and group benefits. While we observed nepotism by female parents, we cannot rule out the possibility that male parents are also nepotistic outside the feeding context, for example through vigilance or alarm calling.

The importance of mistletoe

Western bluebirds not only feed on mistletoe berries, they disperse the seeds, making it ambiguous as to whether the birds are there because of the mistletoe or the mistletoe is aggregated on territories because of the birds, whose settlement patterns might be due to something else entirely. In order to separate cause and effect, we designed an experiment to test the importance of mistletoe abundance to delayed dispersal. The experiment involved removing half the mistletoe from 13 territories and comparing retention of offspring over the winter with that of control territories where we spent time on the territories, but did not remove any mistletoe. We mapped territories and selected dyads of territories that were closely matched by mistletoe volume, allocating one of each pair at random to the experimental removal and control treatments. As mistletoe is not producing berries during the time when fall dispersal occurs, differential access to food was not a factor in the experiment.

By watching through the summer, we observed that offspring did not suffer aggression from their parents, and only rarely experienced aggression from siblings, indicating that sons on mistletoe-reduced territories were probably not evicted by their parents (Dickinson and McGowan 2005). Nonetheless, by autumn only 10% of experimental territories had retained sons compared to 80% of control territories (Figure 2.6). We saw no such difference for daughters, which were retained on about one-third of territories in both treatment and control groups. Mistletoe removal did not affect whether parents stayed on their territories for winter, indicating that sons will leave their parents behind if mistletoe volume on the natal territory is low enough. Because resources and nepotism are expected to covary, we could not rule out presence of parents as also playing an important role in delayed dispersal.

Resources and parents as drivers of delayed dispersal

We examined the combined effects of resources (mistletoe) and parental presence on delayed dispersal of sons based on six years of data with 3–4 censuses of each group per month throughout the winter. We used mistletoe volume within 100 m of the central nest box on the winter territory, or the breeding nest box in spring, as measures of territory quality, since this

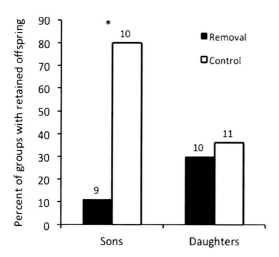

Figure 2.6. Western bluebird sons, but not daughters, were less likely to stay home through the winter on territories where half their parents' mistletoe was removed (removal) than when mistletoe was left intact (control).

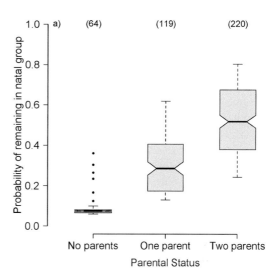

Figure 2.7. The relationship between retention of sons in family groups and the number of parents still present.

measure is highly correlated with mistletoe volume on mapped territories (Dickinson et al. 2014). Parental presence was a strong predictor of delayed dispersal of sons and sons were more likely to stay home when both parents were present than when just one parent was present (Figure 2.7). In contrast with the mistletoe removal experiment, delayed dispersal did not increase with mistletoe volume on the natal territory the prior spring except in cases where only the mother was alive (GLMM, binomial, $\beta = 0.66$, $N = 76$, $z = 2.4$, $P = 0.02$).

This surprising result prompted us to reconsider the mistletoe removal experiment. After removal, the mean volume of mistletoe on territories in the experiment was 40.0 ± 8.1 m^3 (range 5.8–89.6 m^3), much lower than the mean of 70.7 ± 11.1 m^3 (range 0–291 m^3) on territories examined in the observational study. This raises the possibility that our experimental removal pushed a large share of territories below some critical threshold volume of mistletoe. This idea is supported by our prior assessment that the threshold volume of mistletoe for parents to stay is 28 m^3, 1.96 standard errors above the mean volume measured for territories that parents vacated for winter (15.9 ± 6.5 m^3). If sons in a relatively small group of four birds stayed, they would do so

along with parents and so their threshold would have to be 50% higher, or at least 42 m^3, in order to achieve the same per capita mistletoe volume. In the mistletoe removal experiment, the per capita mistletoe volume did not differ between controls and experimental territories after late summer dispersal. Together these disparate results are consistent with threshold-based decision rules that could potentially lead to an ideal free distribution (Fretwell and Lucas 1970) of western bluebird sons on their group's territories during the winter. Such an ideal-free distribution would suggest that within-group competition is driving sons to leave home, rather than the between-lineage competition that appears to be so important for Florida scrub-jays (*Aphelocoma coerulescens*, Chapter 5).

Also consistent with an ideal free distribution is the high level of overwinter survival for immigrants, local dispersers, and delayed dispersers alike, which we estimated at 95% for first winter birds using an R-Mark analysis of survival in groups monitored from September to the beginning of March. Our winter survival estimates are among the highest reported for any bird species (Karr et al. 1990), suggesting that the oak savanna habitat in upper Carmel Valley is relatively unbeatable, at least in winter. Survival was high (95%) and the variance in survival was so low that it was not possible to detect an effect of resources and parents on overwinter survival. Our findings are consistent with Koenig and Pitelka's (1981) hypothesis that delayed dispersal is beneficial for birds living in high quality habitats where there is a steep drop off in territory quality and little in the way of marginal habitat. Delayed dispersal is likely influenced by variance in landscape composition at much larger geographic scales, which favors delayed and localized dispersal on our study site.

During the second step of dispersal, when birds settle onto breeding territories, both social and resource drivers of localized dispersal are apparent. The tendency to disperse locally to breed after surviving through the winter increased with winter mistletoe volume when males remained in their natal group for winter, but not when they wintered in new groups (Dickinson et al. 2014, Figure 2.8). Males overwintering with nonrelatives were more likely to leave the study area from high than low mistletoe volume territories after winter as if there is a tendency for nonnatal males to lose the competition for breeding space when they winter on territories of high quality. We also observed an effect of parents, with sons being more likely to remain on the study area in spring if they overwintered in their natal group with than without parents (Figure 2.8), an effect that is compounded by sons without parents largely disappearing from the study area prior to forming winter groups in fall (Figure 2.7). This large effect of resources and parents on whether or not sons stay on the study area to breed paints a different picture of drivers of dispersal than do findings from a study of migratory western bluebirds in Montana, for which the pattern is that males with kin disperse farther to their first breeding site, although less so when nearby kin are less aggressive and nest boxes more abundant (Aguillon and Duckworth 2015). Given that the population is migratory, the Montana study dealt with birds that ended up on the study area in spring, following migration, rather than addressing effects of winter resources and parents on localized dispersal.

As in the Florida scrub-jay (Woolfenden and Fitzpatrick 1984, chapter 4), western bluebird sons exhibit "territorial budding" in which they acquire

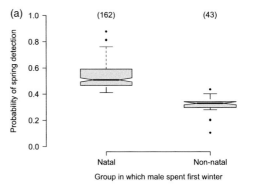

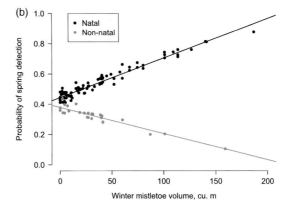

Figure 2.8. The influence of (a) parents and (b) mistletoe volume on the presence of yearlings on the study area after wintering in a local group. Gray dots or bars indicate nonnatal males and black dots or bars indicate males that stayed home for winter.

some mistletoe from their parents when they settle next door in spring. The mistletoe volume on spring breeding territories of sons increased as a function of the volume on their family's winter territory, revealing a benefit of settling locally from a high volume territory (Dickinson et al. 2014). When they nested next door to their parents, sons acquired 81% of their spring mistletoe volume by budding off a portion of their parents' winter territory, although parents conceded proportionally less mistletoe per unit area than they kept for themselves. It could be beneficial for sons to have mistletoe of their own, because they will not inherit their parents' territory unless both parents die simultaneously, which is rare. By conceding some of the winter territory to their sons, parents ensure that those sons will "own" at least some mistletoe as they enter their second winter, which could become important if one or both parents are replaced.

Natal dispersal decisions do not appear to affect reproductive success of sons in their first spring. We observed no effect of parents or mistletoe volume on reproductive success or opportunities for extra-pair fertilizations after winter, indicating that fitness effects of mistletoe and social benefits of remaining with parents, if they exist, will only be detected with analysis of lifetime fitness and a data set spanning more than five years (Dickinson et al. 2014). An additional benefit of delayed dispersal is that sons do not have to face the aggression costs of entering a new group or breeding arena. In contrast, the effect of parental presence on delayed and localized dispersal suggests that nepotism by parents is far more important to why sons remain at home than we previously thought. It is possible, too, that sons delay and disperse near parents, in part, because this affords them the insurance of being able to help when they are unable to breed.

Fitness benefits of helping

We first examined the fitness consequences of helping based on 11 years of data, separating direct and indirect fitness benefits (Brown 1980). Direct fitness benefits accrue through the helper's survival and personal reproduction, whereas indirect fitness benefits arise by increasing the survival and personal reproduction of relatives. In our study, we sought to test Hamilton's rule (Hamilton 1963) by comparing the combined direct and indirect fitness benefits for helpers with the direct fitness of nonhelpers in the same age class (Dickinson et al. 1996).

Direct fitness benefits

Helpers are truly nonbreeding helpers and do not gain paternity in the nests at which they help (Dickinson and Akre 1998). Even though helpers carried a lighter load by feeding less frequently than they would have as breeders, we detected no direct fitness benefits one

year later that could be attributed to this decreased workload (Dickinson et al. 1996). Age-specific survival was not statistically different for helpers compared to same-aged breeders. Neither were helpers more likely than nonhelping offspring (breeders) to breed next door or nearer to their parents, for this is something afforded offspring by delayed dispersal, regardless of whether they help. The nestlings fed by helpers did not help them later on and, despite being older when they first bred, helpers fledged fewer young in their first nests and had lower proportional nesting success over their (truncated) lifetimes than did nonhelpers. Helpers did not outperform breeders in the number of years they bred, the number of nesting attempts they had, the number or proportion of successful nests they produced, or the number of young they fledged over their lifetime. By all measures of direct fitness, helping was either equivalent to or worse than breeding independently; however, lifetime fledging success was equivalent for helpers and nonhelpers, because survival of helpers was slightly, but not statistically, higher. Delayed fitness benefits of helping are still possible and may be revealed with additional years of data, especially if age-dependent extra-pair paternity is included (see "Extra-pair paternity").

Indirect fitness benefits

We examined two types of indirect fitness benefits: those accruing through increased survival of parents, allowing them to produce more young over their lifetimes, and those arising through increased survival of nestlings in helped versus unhelped nests. The minimum age for birds to have adult offspring helping is two years old (third year birds). Considering only parents in their third year or older, the probability that either was present the next year was ~50% regardless of whether or not they had help (Dickinson et al. 1996). In spite of load-lightening that occurs with help, we have detected no short-term effects of help on parental survival.

In the absence of survival benefits for parents receiving aid, does helping produce indirect fitness benefits in the current nest? Helpers gained indirect fitness benefits, increasing both the growth rate and the fledging

Table 2.3. Annual inclusive fitness (offspring equivalents) of sons, their mother, and father as a function of the type of helper

Son's status	Son's annual inclusive fitness	Mother's annual inclusive fitness	Father's annual inclusive fitness
Redirected helper	0.08	2.94	2.10
Nonbreeding helper	0.41	3.38	2.41
Breeder	3.02	4.03	2.95
Simultaneous breeder-helper	3.75	5.32	3.86

Source: From Dickinson (2004).
Note that both sons and their parents do best when the son is a breeder.

success at their parents' nests by an average of 1.12 offspring (Dickinson et al. 1996). This increase was not due to differences in clutch size, but was comprised of a statistical increase in the probability of having a successful nest and, among successful nests, an increase in the number of offspring fledged. The incidence of second nests was not affected by helping; second nests are rare and do not significantly alter overall success, but young at helped nests were heavier at 14 days of age than those at unhelped nests, and mass at 14 days leads to longer lifespans for nestlings that initiate breeding on the study area (Dickinson 2004a).

Extra-pair paternity

Given that about 45% of females have extra-pair young in their nests, how does extra-pair paternity alter direct and indirect fitness estimates? Using multilocus fingerprinting and genealogies based upon paternity exclusion to estimate relatedness, we detected no biases in paternity that would favor helping; helpers were as likely to be extra-pair offspring as were their nonhelping counterparts, and nests with helpers were as likely to have extra-pair young as were their counterparts without helpers (Dickinson and Akre 1998).

Incorporating measures of relatedness derived from paternity exclusion reduces the indirect fitness benefit of helping, measured as offspring equivalents, but it also reduces the direct fitness benefit of breeding independently. Using these adjusted inclusive fitness estimates to compare the fitness of the different types of helpers, we demonstrated that males breeding on their

own or those that were simultaneous breeder-helpers had higher annual inclusive fitness than did males staying home and helping or those that became redirected helpers after nest failure (Table 2.3). Redirected helpers had the lowest inclusive fitness because they had no direct fitness in the current year and also had only a small impact on their parents' nest.

Together, these data indicate that both sons and their parents have higher annual inclusive fitness when the son is a breeder than when he is a nonbreeding helper, which counters arguments that parents should adjust their sex ratios to increase the likelihood of having a nonbreeding helper (Dickinson 2004a). This fitness disadvantage for parents of having a helper rather than a breeder son suggests that everyone is making the best of a bad job when sons help, except possibly stepparents, and they are far less likely to have assistance from helpers than are social parents (Table 2.4).

The weak link in this argument is that relatedness of a helper to helped nestlings versus young in their own nest is only part of the picture. Given that extra-pair paternity increases with male age, it is still possible that population-wide paternity assignment will reveal delayed benefits of helping, both through increased opportunities for extra-pair paternity of helpers later in life (future direct fitness benefits) and increased opportunities for extra-pair paternity of their parents (future indirect fitness benefits). These benefits can arise through increased survival or increased stamina, both of which may come about through load-lightening that occurs when helpers assume one-third of the feeding obligations at a nest. Such benefits are consistent with

Table 2.4. Targets of help showing that helpers are much more likely to help when both parents are alive than when one or no parents are alive

Present on study area	Helped	Did not help	% helping	Relatedness to nestlings
Both parents	24	56	30%	0.50
Only father	3	48	6%	0.25
Only mother	1	75	1%	0.25
No parents	4	110	3%	0.25

Source: From Dickinson et al. (1996).
Helpers with no parents assist brothers.

the age-dependent extra-pair paternity observed in western bluebirds, and form the basis of a new hypothesis, the "delayed extra-pair benefits" hypothesis, which can only be tested with population-wide parentage assignment over a large number of contiguous years (we calculate this to be 16 years for western bluebirds, which occasionally live to be 8 years old). This hypothesis stands in opposition to the monogamy hypothesis (Boomsma 2009) in recognizing that extra-pair paternity affects a would-be helper's relatedness to both his own and helped nestlings (Dickinson et al. 1996, Figure 2.6). It provides a novel, functional explanation for the occurrence of kin-based helping in species with moderate-to-high levels of extra -pair paternity.

Hamilton's rule and helping by western bluebirds

Hamilton's rule states that helping should evolve when the benefit (B) of helping times the relatedness (r) between the helper and recipient is greater than the cost of helping (C), that is, $rB > C$ (Hamilton 1963). Empirically, we can test Hamilton's rule using our measure of the frequency with which males were able to acquire a new mate when their female was removed. This measure allows us to calculate C based on what a male without a mate could expect if he did not help and instead tried to breed. As only one of six males remated when females were removed, this probability is 0.167 (Dickinson 2004a).

Given that the annual inclusive fitness of breeder males in the same age classes as helpers is 2.41 offspring equivalents, the cost of staying home to help is

0.167×2.41, or 0.40 offspring equivalents early in the season. Combining direct and indirect fitness benefits for all types of helpers, including those that had nests of their own while they helped, helpers gained 0.92 offspring equivalents. This is more than twice the expected annual inclusive fitness for males without a mate and its magnitude is largely attributable to simultaneous breeder-helpers. When we consider stay-at-home helpers, which gain only indirect fitness benefits, their annual inclusive fitness is just slightly higher than the costs of helping (0.42 versus 0.40). Redirected helpers do even worse at 0.19 offspring equivalents, but it is fair to assume that their likelihood of breeding is near zero as they elect to help mid- or late-season. Given that western bluebirds retain the ability to breed opportunistically, their decision to help does not keep them from increasing their annual fitness should a reasonable breeding opportunity arise. This ability to keep options open may reduce the costs of helping. On the other hand, none of these measures takes into consideration the potential for delayed fitness benefits, including delayed extra-pair benefits (discussed above), which are likely to be important in this system.

Kin recognition and kin discrimination

Our first hint that western bluebirds discriminate familiar kin was based on seeing that males of all ages help and always help relatives. Second, males help regardless of whether they have bred next door to their parents or not and they sometimes help brothers and grandfathers, suggesting that they can discriminate kin independent of the natal location. Third, simultaneous breeder-helpers help only on territories with at least one first-order relative. Fourth, males are six times more likely to help when both parents are alive than when just one parent is alive, indicating that they prefer helping to raise full-sibs over half-sibs (Table 2.4). Recently, we have discovered that males provide cross-territorial assistance to relatives in response to caged intruders and playbacks of distress screams (Stern 2012). Based on readings of radio frequency identification (RFID) tags, they frequently visit each other's nest boxes during the breeding season; thus far, we have recorded 28 visits by 19 males and 15 visits by 15 females to nest boxes that were not their own (C. Stern, C. Akçay, and J. Dickinson unpubl. data). In our sample, all adult males that had kin available visited at least one relative's box; in contrast, no adult females with kin available visited a relative's box. Together, these behaviors indicate that living in kin neighborhoods elicits different behaviors for males than females, and requires sophisticated kin recognition and not simply association of kinship with the natal territory.

On the other hand, the effects of extra-pair parentage on helping, described above, indicate that helpers determine who they are and who their parents are based on social experience at the nest or in the winter group, rather than actual genetic relationship (Dickinson and Akre 1998). Western bluebird males are not able to tell extra-pair young in the nest and do not reduce their parental feeding rates, even after being experimentally exposed to their mate accepting extra-pair copulations from an intruding male (Dickinson 2003). Similarly, helpers show no reduction in feeding effort when their relatedness is cut in half due to feeding offspring of a parent and step-parent or because they themselves were extra-pair young in the nest (Dickinson 2004b). Neither do nestlings behave as if they can tell their kin, including their parents; we observed juveniles help after fledging from a nonrelative's nest to which they had been fostered shortly beforehand (Dickinson et al. 1996). While it is rare for helpers to assist birds not associated with their natal nest, when they help older brothers or other relatives they may still be using prior experience. Three males that we know of helped grandfathers or brothers that were not in their natal group. In each of these cases a bridging relative, one that had

been at the nest with both of them, was alive, suggesting that bridging relatives may "introduce" unfamiliar relatives to each other or that they treat as relatives individuals present in their family group in winter.

Given that western bluebirds can discriminate kin based on prior experience, we used song playback to determine whether males use song to differentiate kin from nonkin. Western bluebirds have a simple song consisting of two basic types of notes, the *pew* and the *chuck*, which are given in variable sequence at a ratio of about nine *pews* for every two *chucks*. Most of the male's singing is done in the dark, during the predawn chorus, when they sing with a constancy that makes them relatively easy to record. Using a balanced design, we played male song from equidistant kin and nonkin near each focal male's nest box on alternate days, and found that males responded significantly more aggressively toward songs of nonkin compared to kin (Akçay et al. 2013). Surprisingly, and in contrast to long-tailed tits, *Aegithalos caudatus* (Chapter 3), males do not appear to use family-specific signatures to recognize kin (Akçay et al. 2014). Levels of note-sharing are high among neighbors, whether kin or nonkin, and drop off significantly with distance such that non-neighbors rarely show note sharing even if they are related. Even in the absence of note sharing, as between non-neighboring kin, western bluebirds seem to be able to discriminate kin vocalizations.

How can birds identify kin from vocalizations if there is no kin signature? It is likely that western bluebirds learn their relatives' signatures during their interactions with them while tied to the natal territory, either at the nestling and fledgling stages or in winter groups. In any case, the lack of kin signature in the songs suggests that kin recognition is but one function of a much broader recognition system associated with social cognition and discrimination of individuals, whether relatives or nonrelatives. We hypothesize that song variation may even allow birds to store a spatial vocal map of their neighborhood, labeling each individual as kin or nonkin, distinguishing neighbors from strangers, and perhaps tagging individuals with status information, such as age.

While helping has been reported as heritable in western bluebirds in a study controlling for parental age and food supplementation in spring (Charmantier et al. 2007), this finding included both juvenile and adult helpers in the analysis, and may have conflated territory quality and demography with heritability. Because helpers are as likely as nonhelpers to be extrapair young (Dickinson and Akre 1998), heritability studies based on population-wide assignment of parentage could get around these issues.

Conclusions, future directions, and a new hypothesis

After 30 years of studying western bluebirds, we were most surprised by the overriding importance of parental presence to delayed and localized dispersal. Because parental influence on delayed and localized dispersal is both paternal and maternal, and extends into the breeding season, the benefits almost certainly go beyond the maternal nepotism we see in winter groups. For example, tug-of-war models of kin-nonkin interactions suggest that spatial proximity of male kin during the breeding season, when combined with potential for extra-pair fertilizations, can increase the likelihood that extra-pair paternity in nests of young males, if it occurs, will involve relatives (Stern 2012). In such cases, breeding by a young male is effectively an extension of the helping system in that sons would be raising their father's offspring in their own nest.

How might extended social interactions with parents be beneficial for breeding sons, given that territorial inheritance is rare? First, parents concede a share of their winter territory, which allows sons to start off with mistletoe of their own. Then, if sons fail to attract a mate or lose their nest and mate, they can get a small indirect benefit from helping at their parents' nest. Finally, if during rare events fathers come to the aid of sons (Stern 2012), this can increase survival or allow them to hold onto a territory, which would augment future breeding success. Although helping is consistent with Hamilton's rule, it is clear from the fitness data that most helpers do not delay dispersal in order to help; rather they use it to augment inclusive fitness when they cannot breed independently. Delayed

benefits, especially delayed extra-pair benefits, have yet to be analyzed and may play a critical role in the evolution of helping in western bluebird and other species with extra-pair paternity.

Currently, the most fruitful direction to move in with this study population is to further integrate the two bodies of work we have carried out over the years. First, we have demonstrated dramatic increases in male reproductive success with age, based on females' extra-pair mate choice favoring older males, and the doubling of reproductive success we see in males successful at extra-pair fertilization (Dickinson 2001; Ferree et al. 2014). We have yet to measure delayed fitness benefits, which requires about 16 years' of demographic data with population-wide assignment of paternity. Our hypothesis is that delayed benefits arising through extra-pair paternity counter-balance the early costs of helping; this hypothesis predicts that helping on the natal territory increases survival of the helper. If the delayed extra-pair benefits hypothesis is supported, it will provide a novel explanation for why kin-based cooperation occurs in species with moderate-to-high levels of extra-pair paternity, like western bluebirds and even such paragons of promiscuity as the fairy-wrens (*Malurus cyaneus*; Chapter 8).

It remains to be seen whether parental effects on delayed and localized dispersal, such as we see in western bluebirds, are restricted to species in which helping is relatively rare, or also can also be important in species with much higher levels of helping. If, as our data suggest, helpers are making the best of a bad job, then what do their other options look like? What are the true costs of dispersal and at what scale does spatial variation in resource abundance matter to survival and lifetime reproductive success? These questions will only be answerable by tracking dispersal over long distances and expanding this study to include analysis of partial and complete migration once such tracking tools are widely available.

Acknowledgments

We thank Walt Koenig, bequeathor of bluebirds, Hastings enthusiast, and all around funny guy, for his encouragement of this study. We also thank the owners of Oak Ridge and Rana Creek Ranches and the staff and directors of the Museum of Vertebrate Zoology and Hastings Reserve for tremendous logistical support. Walt Koenig and Maria Smith provided helpful comments on the manuscript. A huge number of fun and excellent field interns and research students brought enthusiasm, dedication, and a willingness to volunteer for room and board. Some great (now senior) colleagues have also collaborated on this study, including Marty Leonard and Andy Horn, with whom we shared toddler care, Andy McGowan, collaborator on the mistletoe experiment, Amber Budden, uber-organized "colouration guru," and Joey Haydock, co-creator of the Hastings DNA Lab. We also thank the Fuller Evolutionary Genetics Lab at Cornell for hosting and providing intellectual support for the microsatellite work. Finally, we were fortunate to have NSF funding (and a bit of NIH funding) for over half the years of this 30-year effort. A long-term study is like a Cape Breton fiddle set. It begins with an aire, moves on to a march, builds to a strathspey where the only reasonable bodily response is to hop up and down vigorously, and finishes with a reel, plenty of swing tempered with anticipation of the ending. It is our great hope that our interns, students, and postdocs will have opportunities as sweet as those we have had.

REFERENCES

Aguillon, S. A. and Duckworth, R. A. (2015). Kin aggression and resource availability influence phenotype-dependent dispersal in a passerine bird. *Behav. Ecol. Sociobiol.*, 69, 625–633.

Akçay, C., Swift, R. J., Reed, V. A., and Dickinson, J. L. (2013). Vocal kin recognition in kin neighborhoods of western bluebirds. *Behav. Ecol.*, 24, 898–905.

Akçay, C., Hambury, K. L., Arnold, A. J., Nevins, A. M., and Dickinson, J. L. (2014). Song-sharing with neighbors and relatives in a cooperatively breeding songbird. *Anim. Behav.*, 92, 55–62.

Balda, R. P. (1987). Avian impacts on pinyon-juniper woodland. In: *Proceedings Pinyon-Juniper Conference*, ed. R. L. Everett. Ogden, Utah: USDA Forest Service Intermountain Res. Station Gen. Tech. Rep. INT-125, pp. 525–533.

Bensch, S., Hasselquist, D., Nielsen, B., and Hansson, B. (1998). Higher fitness for philopatric than for immigrant males in a semi-isolated population of great reed warblers. *Evolution*, 52, 877–883.

Boomsma, J. J. (2009). Lifetime monogamy and the evolution of eusociality. *Phil. Trans. R. Soc. London B*, 364, 3191–3207.

Brown, J. L. (1980). Fitness in complex avian social systems. In: *Evolution of Social Behavior: Hypotheses and Empirical Tests*, ed. H. Markl. Weinheim: Verlag Chemie, pp. 115–128.

Brown, J. L. (1987). *Helping and Communal Breeding in Birds: Ecology and Evolution*. Princeton, NJ: Princeton University Press.

Budden, A. E. and Dickinson, J. L. (2009). Signals of quality and age: the information content of multiple plumage ornaments in male western bluebirds, *Sialia mexicana*. *J. Avian Biol.*, 40, 18–27.

Charmantier, A., Keyser, A. J., and Promislow, D. E. L. (2007). First evidence for heritable variation in cooperative breeding behaviour. *Proc. R. Soc. London B*, 274, 1757–1761.

Curry, R. L. and Grant, P. R. (1990). Galapagos mockingbirds: territorial cooperative breeding in a climatically variable environment. In: *Cooperative Breeding in Birds: Long-term Studies of Ecology and Behavior*, ed. P. B. Stacey and W. D. Koenig. Cambridge: Cambridge University Press, pp. 291–331.

Dickinson, J. L. (1997). Male detention affects extra-pair copulation frequency and pair behavior in western bluebirds. *Anim. Behav.*, 53, 561–571.

Dickinson, J. L. (2001). Extrapair copulations in western bluebirds: female receptivity depends on male age. *Behav. Ecol. Sociobiol.*, 50, 423–429.

Dickinson, J. L. (2003). Male share of provisioning is not influenced by actual or apparent loss of paternity in western bluebirds. *Behav. Ecol.*, 14, 360–366.

Dickinson, J. L. (2004a). Facultative sex ratio adjustment by western bluebird mothers with stay-at-home helpers-at-the-nest. *Anim. Behav.*, 68, 373–380.

Dickinson, J. L. (2004b). A test of the importance of direct and indirect fitness benefits for helping decisions in western bluebirds, *Behav. Ecol.*, 15, 233–238.

Dickinson, J. L. and Akre, J. J. (1998). Extrapair paternity, inclusive fitness, and within-group benefits of helping in western bluebirds. *Mol. Ecol.*, 7, 95–105.

Dickinson, J. L. and Leonard, M. L. (1996). Mate attendance and copulatory behavior in western bluebirds. *Anim. Behav.*, 52, 981–992.

Dickinson, J. L. and McGowan, A. (2005). Resource wealth drives family group living in western bluebirds. *Proc. R. Soc. London B*, 272, 2423–2428.

Dickinson, J. L. and Weathers, W. W. (1999). Replacement males in the western bluebird: opportunity for paternity, chick-feeding rules, and fitness consequences of male parental care. *Behav. Ecol. Sociobiol.*, 45, 201–209.

Dickinson, J. L., Koenig, W. D. and Pitelka, F. A. (1996). Fitness consequences of helping behavior in the western bluebird. *Behav. Ecol.*, 7, 168–177.

Dickinson, J. L., Euaparadorn, M., Greenwald, K., Mitra, C., and Shizuka, D. (2009). Cooperation and competition: nepotistic tolerance and intra-sexual aggression in western bluebird winter groups. *Anim. Behav*, 77, 867–872.

Dickinson, J. L., Ferree, E. D., Stern, C. A., Swift, R. J., and Zuckerberg, B. (2014). Delayed dispersal in western bluebirds: teasing apart the importance of resources and parents. *Behav. Ecol.*, 25, 843–851.

Dobson, F. S. (2013). The enduring question of sex-biased dispersal: Paul J. Greenwood's (1980) seminal contribution. *Anim. Behav.*, 85, 299–304.

Duckworth, R. A. and Badyaev, A. V. (2007). Coupling of dispersal and aggression facilitates the rapid range expansion of a passerine bird. *Proc. Natl. Acad. Sci. (USA)*, 104, 15017–15022.

Ekman, J. and Griesser, M. (2002). Why offspring delay dispersal: experimental evidence for a role of parental tolerance. *Proc. R. Soc. London B*, 269, 1709–1714.

Ekman, J. and Rosander, B. (1992). Survival enhancement through food sharing: a means for parental control of natal dispersal. *Theor. Pop. Biol.*, 42, 117–129.

Ekman, J., Baglione, V., Egger, S., and Griesser, M. (2001). Delayed dispersal: living under the reign of nepotistic parents. *Auk*, 118, 1–10.

Emlen, S. T. (1978). The evolution of cooperative breeding in birds. In: *Behavioral Ecology: An Evolutionary Approach*, ed. J. R. Krebs and N. B. Davies. Sunderland, MA: Sinauer, pp. 245–281.

Emlen, S. T. (1982a). The evolution of helping. I. An ecological constraints model. *Am. Nat.*, 119, 29–39.

Emlen, S. T. (1982b). The evolution of helping. II. The role of behavioral conflict. *Am. Nat.*, 119, 40–53.

Emlen, S. T. and Wrege, P. H. (1989). A test of alternate hypotheses for helping behavior in white-fronted bee-eaters of Kenya. *Behav. Ecol. Sociobiol.*, 25, 303–319.

Ferree, E. D. and Dickinson, J. L. (2011). Natural extrapair paternity matches receptivity patterns in unguarded females: evidence for importance of female choice. *Anim. Behav.*, 82, 11670–1173.

Ferree, E. D. and Dickinson, J. L. (2014). Male western bluebirds that sire extra-pair young are successful within-pair sires as well. *Anim. Behav.*, 90, 11–19.

Ferree, E. D., Dickinson, J. L., Rendell, W., Stern, C., and Porter, S. (2010). Hatch order drives an extrapair chick advantage in western bluebirds. *Behav. Ecol.*, 21, 802–807.

Fitzpatrick, J. W. and Woolfenden, G. E. (1986). Demographic routes to cooperative breeding in some New World Jays. In: *Evolution of Animal Behavior*, ed. M. H. Nitecki and J. A. Kitchell. Oxford: Oxford University Press, pp. 137–160.

Fretwell, S. D. and Lucas, H. L., Jr. (1970). On territorial behavior and other factors influencing habitat distribution in birds. I. Theoretical Development. *Acta Biotheor.*, 19, 16–36.

Greenwood, P. J. (1980). Mating systems, philopatry and dispersal in birds and mammals. *Anim. Behav.*, 28, 1140–1162.

Griesser, M. (2003). Nepotistic vigilance behaviour in Siberian jay parents. *Behav. Ecol.*, 14, 246–250.

Griesser, M. and Ekman, J. (2004). Nepotistic alarm calling in the Siberian jay, *Perisoreus infaustus. Anim. Behav.*, 67, 933–939.

Griesser, M. and Ekman, J. (2005). Nepotistic mobbing behaviour in the Siberian jay, *Perisoreus infaustus. Anim. Behav.*, 69, 345–352.

Grinnell, J. and Storer, T. I. (1924). *Animal Life in the Yosemite*. Berkeley: University of California Press.

Guinan, J. A., Gowaty, P. A., and Eltzroth, E. K. (2008). Western bluebird (*Sialia mexicana*). In: *The Birds of North America Online*, ed. A. Poole. Ithaca, NY: Cornell Lab of Ornithology. http://bna.birds.cornell.edu/bna/species/510

Hamilton, W. D. (1963). The evolution of altruistic behavior. *Am. Nat.*, 97, 354–356.

Karr, J. R., Nichols, J. D., Klimkiewicz, M. K., and Brawn, J. D. (1990). Survival rates of birds of tropical and temperate forests: will the dogma survive? *Am. Nat.*, 136, 277–291.

Kempanaers, B., Verheyen, G. R., Van den Broeck, M., Burke, T., Van Broeckhoven, C., et al. (1992). Extra-pair paternity results from female preference for high-quality males in the blue tit. *Nature*, 357, 494–496.

Kleiber, D., Kyle, K., Rockwell, S., and Dickinson, J. (2007). Sexual competition explains patterns of individual investment in territorial aggression in western bluebird winter groups. *Anim. Behav.*, 73, 763–770.

Koenig, W. D. and Dickinson, J. L. (1996). Nestling sex-ratio variation in western bluebirds. *Auk*, 113, 902–910.

Koenig, W. D. and Pitelka, F. A. (1981). Ecological factors and kin selection in the evolution of cooperative breeding in birds. In: *Natural Selection and Social Behavior: Recent Research and New Theory*, ed. R. D. Alexander and D. W. Tinkle. New York: Chiron Press, pp. 261–280.

Kraaijeveld, K. and Dickinson, J. L. (2001). Family-based winter territoriality in western bluebirds: the structure and dynamics of winter groups. *Anim. Behav.*, 61, 109–117.

Ligon, J. D. (1981). Demographic patterns and communal breeding in the green woodhoopoe, *Phoeniculus purpureus*. In: *Natural Selection and Social Behavior: Recent Research and New Theory*, ed. R. D. Alexander and D. Tinkle. New York: Chiron Press, pp. 231–243.

Stahle, D. W. (2002). The unsung ancients. *Nat. Hist.*, 111(1), 48–53.

Stern, C. A. (2012). Cooperation and competition in kin associations. Ph.D. thesis, Cornell University, Ithaca, New York.

Wilson, E. A., Sullivan, P. J., and Dickinson, J. L. (2014). Spatial distribution of oak mistletoe as it relates to habits of oak woodland frugivores. *PlosOne*, 9, e111947.

Woolfenden, G. E. and Fitzpatrick, J. W. (1984). *The Florida Scrub Jay: Demography of a Cooperative-Breeding Bird*. Princeton, NJ: Princeton University Press.

3

Long-tailed tits: Ecological causes and fitness consequences of redirected helping

Ben J. Hatchwell

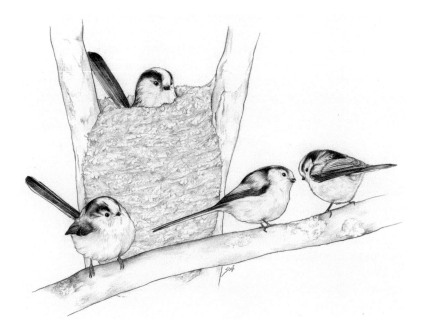

Introduction

The avifauna of the United Kingdom is severely impoverished for anyone enthused by the idea of studying avian cooperative breeding. An exception is the long-tailed tit (*Aegithalos caudatus*), one of very few regular cooperative breeders in northern Europe. Lack and Lack (1958), Riehm (1970), Gaston (1973), and Glen and Perrins (1988) described the essentials of this bird's

cooperative breeding system, but when casting around for a tractable study system it was not just a question of them being the only possible candidate, I became convinced that long-tailed tits had received far less attention than they deserved. Long-tailed tits were already known to have an unusual cooperative breeding system in which helping is redirected; that is, failed breeders move to the nest of another pair to help them care for their offspring. Such behavior has often been

Cooperative Breeding in Vertebrates: Studies of Ecology, Evolution, and Behavior, eds W. D. Koenig and J. L. Dickinson.
Published by Cambridge University Press. © Cambridge University Press 2016.

suggested as a potential route to the evolution of more sophisticated cooperative breeding systems (Brown 1987; Ligon and Burt 2004), suggesting that they sit somewhere along the continuum between cooperative and noncooperative species. Consequently, I thought it likely that long-tailed tits would have something interesting to say about the evolutionary trajectory toward sociality, especially the ecological and life history traits that promote helping.

Second, the apparent simplicity of their life history and breeding system appealed to me. Complex social systems may take many generations to unravel and few researchers can set out safe in the knowledge that they will have the luxury of long-term funding. Two decades later, I still regard this as a key virtue of long-tailed tits, allowing us to investigate not only the fitness consequences of their cooperative behavior, but also to investigate experimentally some of the mechanisms underlying their decision-making.

Phylogeny and natural history

Long-tailed tits are members of the Aegithalidae, a family comprising 13 species (del Hoyo et al. 2008). The bushtit (*Psaltriparus minimus*) of North America and the pygmy tit (*Psaltria exilis*) of Java are geographic outliers and, along with the two species of *Leptopoecile* tit-warblers, have uncertain affinity to the family. The remaining nine species are all members of the genus *Aegithalos* whose core distribution is in the montane regions and forests of central and eastern Asia. The long-tailed tit is an exception, however, having a broad distribution stretching from Europe to Japan and from the Middle East to Siberia. Bushtits and three species of *Aegithalos* are known to be cooperative breeders, but other members of the family are poorly known and may also be cooperative.

Long-tailed tits are small (7–8 g), sexually monomorphic birds of woodland and scrub habitats. They are primarily insectivorous throughout the year, finding most of their food by gleaning from leaves, twigs, and branches. In Britain they are common birds that are increasingly found in towns and cities. During the nonbreeding season, from June to March in the United

Kingdom, long-tailed tits live in flocks of about 10–20 birds that forage together over large overlapping home ranges. Flock composition is fluid with some dispersal between flocks and occasional amalgamation of neighboring flocks, but they typically comprise males and females, juveniles and adults, relatives and nonrelatives, and philopatric and immigrant birds (Hatchwell et al. 2001a; McGowan et al. 2007). Flock members roost together in linear huddles, often using the same perch on successive nights.

Pair formation usually takes place within flocks and from February onward, flocks start to break up during warm, sunny days. At the start of the breeding season all members of the population attempt to breed in monogamous pairs. Long-tailed tits are not territorial and each pair occupies a breeding home range that was usually part of their winter range and that overlaps substantially the ranges of neighboring pairs. Nest-building starts in February or March, nests usually being placed within 2–3 m of the ground in thorny bushes such as gorse (*Ulex europaeus*), holly (*Ilex aquifolium*), hawthorn (*Crataegus monogyna*) or bramble (*Rubus fruticosus*). A minority of nests are placed high in the forks of trees, especially birch (*Betula* spp.), or in the upper braches of conifers. The nest is built by both sexes and is an elaborate structure of moss and fibers bound together with spider silk collected from egg cocoons, with the exterior covered by flakes of lichen; the resulting structure is a ball (about 15 cm high × 10 cm wide) with a small entrance hole near the top. The nest is lined by up to 2,500 feathers collected from an extensive area around the nest. First nests take about 38 days to build, but replacement nests, which are of poorer quality, are built in just 11 days (McGowan et al. 2004).

Typical clutch size is 9–11 with eggs being laid daily. Males follow females closely during her fertile period, although copulation is rarely observed. Females start incubation on the day that the last egg is laid and she incubates alone in bouts lasting an average of 24 min., interspersed with bouts of foraging (accompanied by the male) lasting about 12 min.; males also feed females on the nest (Hatchwell et al. 1999a). After about 15 days of incubation, eggs hatch more or less synchronously. Females brood nestlings for the first 5–6 days of the nestling period, during which time males do the majority of provisioning, but thereafter males and females feed the brood at similar rates. Nestlings fledge when 16–17 days old and are fed by the adults for a further 2–3 weeks. Long-tailed tits are single-brooded, never raising more than one brood a year.

This life history is typical of many temperate passerines. The twist in the tale of the long-tailed tit is what happens when a pair fails to breed successfully. Most long-tailed tit nests – 72% – fail due to corvid or mustelid predation at some stage between nest completion and fledging. When this occurs early in the breeding season, failed breeders attempt to breed again, but otherwise pairs abandon breeding for that year and some choose to become helpers at a nearby nest belonging to another pair. As a result of the high nest predation rate, a mean (± S.D.) of 15.2% ± 5.2 (range 5.4–27.0%, $N = 17$ years) of all adults become helpers and about half of all successful nests have helpers, each helped nest having a mean of 1.8 ± 0.36 helpers (range 1.2–2.5, $N = 17$ years; Hatchwell et al. 2013). Thus, long-tailed tits have a "redirected" cooperative breeding system in which helpers care for broods belonging to other pairs following the failure of their own nests.

History of the study and general methods

I started studying long-tailed tits in the Rivelin Valley, Sheffield, U.K., in 1994. The area of the study site was increased from 1.5 km² to 2.5 km² in 1995, but thereafter the study site, which comprises farmland, scrub, and deciduous woodland, was unchanged. We followed standard field protocols each year from 1994 to 2014, with the exception of 2001 when an episode of national hysteria during an epidemic of foot-and-mouth disease restricted access to the study site. The population comprised 25–72 pairs, and each season we color-banded over 95% of all adults, catching any immigrants during nest-building or when they moved into the study area as helpers. We located nests by following nest-building pairs and monitored all nests until failure or fledging. All nests that reached the nestling phase were observed, usually for 1 hr, every other day from day 2 (hatch day = day 0) until fledging to record the identity and provisioning rate of adults attending a nest.

Nestlings were banded when they were 11 days old. Blood samples were taken from all birds when first captured and standard measurements recorded.

A second population (Melton Wood, Doncaster), established and monitored using similar protocols from 1996 to 2003, was used for experimental manipulations that were likely to have individual life history or population genetic consequences, but we generally avoided such experiments in the Rivelin population, focusing instead on short-term behavioral experiments. The genetic parentage and relatedness data described in this chapter are based either on analyses conducted up to 2006 using nine microsatellite primers (Simeoni et al. 2007), or more recent analyses using 19 microsatellite loci.

Helping behavior

Who helps?

The Rivelin Valley population is not closed, so some birds turn up as helpers for which we have no prior information that season. Therefore, we cannot be certain that all helpers are failed breeders, but evidence suggests that this is the case. First, helpers are not observed at early nests, and their appearance at nests follows the time in the breeding season when renesting by failed breeders is abandoned (MacColl and Hatchwell 2002).

Second, 96% ($N = 126$ birds) of ringed birds that appeared as helpers were failed breeders, the remaining 4% being birds with unknown history that year. A small proportion of these failed breeders had lost their breeding partner due to divorce (4%) or death (3%), but in most cases their nests had been depredated. In the Rivelin Valley, helpers moved an average distance of 340 m from their last breeding attempt to the nest where they helped. This compares to a mean inter-nest distance of 170 m in a year of typical density, suggesting that helpers do not simply pick the nearest available nest at which to redirect their care (see "Kin-directed helping"). Interestingly, the decision of whether to renest or to abandon breeding and help is not simply a function of stage of the breeding season, but also the stage at which nest failure occurs. If a nest fails after a brood has hatched and parents have started provisioning, sometimes for as little as a day, then they rarely renest, even though other pairs that failed at an earlier stage may be doing so at the same time. Thus, an apparently irreversible physiological switch must occur when pairs start to provision nestlings that prevents further breeding attempts (Hatchwell et al. 2004).

Helping is male-biased. An average of 38% of failed male breeders became helpers, while only 9% of failed female breeders do, giving an overall helper sex ratio of 84% males (Sharp et al. 2011). This is not a consequence of a biased population sex ratio among adults, and while the brood sex ratio is marginally male-biased (53% male, N = 195 broods), this is not significantly different from parity either. In addition, we found no evidence for facultative adjustment of sex ratio by individual females according to the presence of potential or actual helpers (Nam et al. 2011).

These results are not consistent with the repayment hypothesis (Emlen et al. 1986), which predicts that either breeders or helpers may prefer to invest in the helping sex, but given that all adults first become breeders, and, on average, only 15% of adults subsequently become helpers, an equilibrium sex ratio of parity may be optimal. Moreover, in a redirected helping system the presence of helpers during the nestling phase is unpredictable at the time of egg-laying, so adaptive adjustment of brood sex ratio by females in relation to the presence of helpers may not be possible, even if the physiological capacity to do so exists.

How do helpers help?

Helpers rarely help another pair until the nestling phase and when they do their principal contribution is to provision nestlings. The absence of territoriality means that helpers cannot contribute to territory defense, and although they may alarm call and mob when predators approach, their behavior is apparently ineffective in deterring those predators because the probability of nests being depredated is unrelated to the presence of helpers (Hatchwell et al. 2004).

From the start of the study, we have systematically observed provisioning behavior at almost all hatched

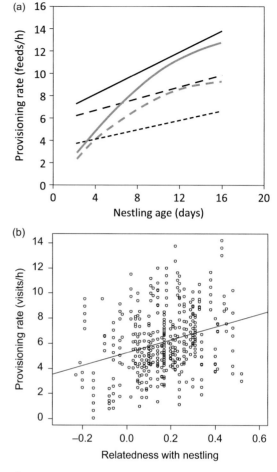

Figure 3.1. Provisioning behavior of parent and helper long-tailed tits: (a) provisioning rates of males (black lines) and females (grey lines), when unassisted by helpers (continuous lines), helped (dashed lines) and as helpers (dotted line) in relation to nestling age (adapted from MacColl and Hatchwell 2003a); (b) provisioning rates of helpers in relation to mean helper-brood relatedness. From Nam et al. (2010).

broods. The general pattern of care described in MacColl and Hatchwell (2003a; Figure 3.1a) has been consistent over the years of the study. All carers increase their provisioning rate for older nestlings and for larger brood sizes, and fathers provision nestlings at a higher rate than mothers, although this effect is largely a consequence of females brooding young nestlings. Helpers provision nestlings less frequently than parents, on average feeding 75% as much as parents at the same nest. Parents reduce their provisioning rate as the number of carers at a nest increases (see "Load-lightening"), but this compensatory reduction in effort is only partial, so the total provisioning rate increases linearly as the number of helpers increases (see "Indirect fitness benefits"). Therefore, although the provisioning effort of helpers is lower than that of parents, all carers follow similar provisioning rules in terms of their response to nestling demand and workforce.

Nevertheless, there is considerable variation among individuals in their provisioning behavior and we have used a quantitative genetic approach to partition this variation into its direct genetic and environmental components, and the indirect social effects of individuals with whom they interact, which in turn will have genetic and environmental components. These analyses showed that an individual's effort is repeatable within and across nests (MacColl and Hatchwell 2003b), but this variation is not solely attributable to heritable genetic effects, but also to direct environment effects (condition) and indirect social effects of other carers at the same nest (Adams et al. 2015). This social effect on individual investment is consistent with the finding that parents responded to experimentally manipulated provisioning rates of their partners (Hatchwell and Russell 1996).

Kin-directed helping

Glen and Perrins (1988) found that help in long-tailed tits is usually directed toward relatives, and this has been substantiated in our study. Estimates of helper–breeder pedigree relatedness show that 77% of helpers assisted at a nest belonging to at least one first- or second-order relative (Nam et al. 2010). An annual adult mortality rate of about 45% (Meade et al. 2010), coupled with a divorce rate of 49–65% for surviving pairs (Hatchwell et al. 2000; Simeoni 2011), means that failed breeders only rarely (6% of helpers) get the opportunity to feed full siblings. Rather, the most frequent helper–offspring relatedness is 0.25, the helper assisting at a nest belonging to one of their siblings (42%), a parent (14%), or a son or daughter (11%). The other related helpers in this sample were second-order relatives of a breeder

(5%), with helper–offspring relatedness $r = 0.125$. The absence of pedigree relatedness ($r = 0$) for the remaining 23% of helpers was confirmed using genotype data. Thus, assuming that breeders have complete parentage of their broods, the average relatedness of helpers to nestlings estimated from pedigrees is 0.17, close to the estimated helper–brood relatedness of $r = 0.16$ ($N = 186$ helpers) using microsatellite genotypes (Hatchwell et al. 2014). Therefore, helpers generally assist at a nest belonging to kin, although relatedness is lower than that found in many cooperatively breeding species.

This kin association could arise if populations are highly kin-structured and failed breeders simply feed at a nearby nest. Many failed breeders do not become helpers despite having active nests nearby, however, and a minority of helpers care at the nearest available nest (Russell and Hatchwell 2001). To test whether kin-directed help is a result of active discrimination, we conducted an experiment in which failed breeders were presented with a choice between nests belonging to potential recipient pairs that either included a closely related breeder ($r = 0.5$), or an unrelated or distantly related breeder ($r < 0.125$). The distance between the focal failed breeder's nest and the nests of potential related and unrelated recipients did not differ significantly. There were two key findings of this study. First, failed breeders only became helpers for pairs from their current social group; that is, if they had dispersed away from their natal area they did not return there to help. Second, when choosing between nests belonging to kin and nonkin within the same social group, 16 of 17 (94%) failed breeders chose to help kin. Thus, long-tailed tits exhibit strong kin preference in their helping behavior.

We have since shown that long-tailed tits are capable of more sophisticated investment decisions with respect to kinship. Helpers also provision broods at a higher rate when they are more closely related to the brood, as determined from either genotypes of pedigrees (Nam et al. 2010; Figure 3.1b). It is perhaps significant that some of the strongest evidence for kin discrimination, and thus for the importance of kin selection, in cooperatively breeding birds comes from species with redirected helping (Emlen and Wrege 1988; Lessells 1990; Dickinson et al. 1996) where

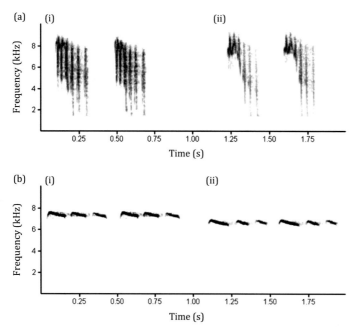

Figure 3.2. Sonograms of long-tailed tit calls: (a) *churr* calls; (b) *triple* calls. Sonograms show two calls of each type from each of two birds (i) and (ii). From Sharp and Hatchwell (2005).

helpers choose between multiple potential recipients when deciding who to help.

Kin recognition

How do long-tailed tits achieve these feats of kin discrimination, which eclipse the known discriminatory ability of helpers in any other cooperatively breeding bird species (Cornwallis et al. 2009)? This is an important question for two reasons. First, as described later, there are substantial fitness payoffs in being able to direct care toward kin. Second, the short dispersal distances of males and some females, coupled with the high rate of re-pairing each year, generates a substantial risk of inbreeding even in an open population (Simeoni 2011). Both are likely to exert selection for an effective kin recognition mechanism.

Our work has focused on vocal cues as the most likely mode of kin recognition. Long-tailed tits have a small vocal repertoire that includes five main call types and a rarely heard song (Cramp and Perrins 1993); we studied the long-range contact call (*triple*), and a more

complex call (*churr*) that is used when birds interact closely either within a pair or with members of other pairs or flocks, and which also functions as a low intensity alarm call (Figure 3.2).

Sharp and Hatchwell (2005) showed using spectrographic cross-correlation that the triple and churr calls are individually distinctive with greater inter-bird variation than within-bird variation; in both cases, frequency parameters provided the most effective basis for discrimination. Moreover, for both call types there was a degree of family specificity, with variation in the calls of siblings being less than that of nonsiblings (Sharp and Hatchwell 2006).

To test the ability of long-tailed tits to discriminate between the calls of kin and nonkin we played *churr* calls recorded from kin and nonkin to focal pairs close to their nest during the nestling period, when potential helpers were likely to be available. Calls were played back either unmanipulated or following manipulation by raising or lowering the frequency domain of the call. Vocal and behavioral responses to playback of unmanipulated kin calls differed significantly from the responses elicited by the other three treatments (Sharp et al. 2005). This experiment does not demonstrate that *churr* call frequency is the only cue used to discriminate kin from nonkin, but it does show that these calls encode information allowing such discrimination to occur.

A question arising from this experiment is how vocalizations encode information on relatedness. Are calls genetically determined signals of kinship, or are they learned during development? To distinguish between these alternatives, half-broods were cross-fostered between synchronous nests belonging to nonkin when 4–5 days old (Sharp et al. 2005). The calls of nestlings and adults are very similar by the time of fledging (Sharp and Hatchwell 2006), and analysis of the *churr* calls of philopatric recruits from these broods in the following year revealed that the calls of foster siblings were as similar as those of true siblings reared together and that both were more similar than the calls of true siblings reared apart. Furthermore, the calls of fostered chicks (as adults) were more similar to the calls of their foster parents than they were to their true genetic parents. These results indicate a substantial learned component to these vocalizations.

A learned mechanism of kin recognition is an effective means of discriminating kin providing that social and genetic relationships are closely correlated. This is the case in long-tailed tits because extra-pair paternity is low (< 7% of nestlings) and intraspecific brood parasitism is negligible (Hatchwell et al. 2002). Moreover, broods are associated exclusively with their parents and any helpers during the nestling period, and this close association usually continues during the period of postfledging dependence.

Two other findings support the notion that the rearing period is a critical phase in the development of kin recognition cues that are subsequently used in helping decisions. First, in the years following our cross-fostering experiments, a small sample of failed breeders helped unrelated foster siblings reared in the same nest (Hatchwell et al. 2001b). Second, in 89% (*N* = 64) of cases with complete information on associations during the putative learning period, helpers assisted a breeder with whom they had been associated in some capacity during the nestling phase, usually as a sibling, offspring, parent, helper, or recipient of help, and in a further 5% of cases helpers assisted a sibling of one of the carers that fed it as a nestling (Sharp et al. 2005). The latter result suggests that birds may not only recognize kin with which they were directly associated, but perhaps also indirectly through assessment of shared call characteristics. Indeed, such assessment could also be involved in the fine-scale adjustment of investment according to the relatedness of helpers to the brood (Nam et al. 2010; Figure 3.1b).

Fitness benefits of helping

Two consistent themes have emerged from our work assessing the fitness consequences of helping behavior: substantial indirect fitness gains from helping, and an absence of direct fitness benefits.

Indirect fitness

Care for kin creates the opportunity for long-tailed tit helpers to gain indirect fitness benefits in two ways: their care increases the number of recruits that a helped pair produces, and the presence of helpers allows breeders to reduce their reproductive costs ("load-lightening"; Crick 1992).

Productivity

Helpers have no effect on either the probability of a nest failing due to predation or the survival of nestlings in nondepredated broods. The latter is counterintuitive given the positive effect of helpers on the total provisioning rate of broods, but there is little scope for helpers to influence brood size because the starvation rate of long-tailed tit nestlings is low (< 3%, *N* = 133 broods) even when fed by parents alone (Hatchwell et al. 2004). However, although the extra food provided by helpers does not affect the quantity of fledglings, it does influence their quality because the recruitment of fledged offspring into the adult population is positively correlated with the number of helpers that provisioned them (Figure 3.3). The scale of this helper effect on productivity is dramatic: a male fledgling raised by its parents

Table 3.1. Productivity of long-tailed tit breeders and helpers in relation to numbers of helpers

	Number of helpers at the nest			
	0	1	2	3+[a]
Recruitment probability (%)[b]	12	19	27	41
Number of recruits per brood[c]	1.07	1.69	2.40	3.65
Productivity (genetic equivalents)[d]				
Breeders	0.51	0.81	1.15	1.75
Helpers	0.18	0.29	0.41	0.62
Marginal effect of helpers (genetic equivalents)				
Breeders[e]	-	+0.30	+0.64	+1.24
Per helper[f]	-	+0.11	+0.12	+0.11

[a] mean number of helpers at nests with 3+ helpers = 3.86.
[b] recruitment rates taken from Hatchwell et al. (2004).
[c] brood size at fledging = 8.9.
[d] coefficients of relatedness: parent-offspring = 0.48, helper-offspring = 0.17.
[e] productivity with helpers – productivity without helpers.
[f] (productivity with n helpers – productivity without helpers)/n.
Source: Adapted from Hatchwell et al. (2004).

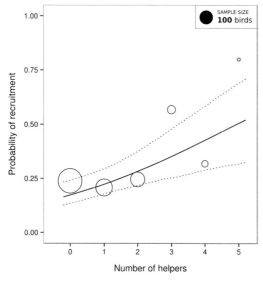

Figure 3.3. The effect of the number of helpers on the probability of fledgling recruitment. Observed values are shown as circles scaled by sample size, and the fitted line (±95% confidence interval) shows recruitment probability for males ($N = 672$) from a multilevel logistic regression. From Hatchwell et al. (2014).

alone has about a 15% chance of recruiting as a breeder, but this probability rises to > 40% for male fledglings raised by their parents plus four or more helpers, an astonishingly high recruitment rate for a small temperate passerine.

The marginal effect of helpers on fledgling recruitment can be used to compare the relative merits of breeding and helping (Table 3.1). Assuming average relatedness of 0.17 between helpers and the brood, each helper adds 0.11 genetic equivalents to the next generation, compared to 0.51 genetic equivalents from breeding without helpers. Why, then, don't failed breeders persist in trying to breed independently rather than becoming a helper?

An answer to this question is suggested by the marked seasonal decline in brood size and probability of fledgling recruitment. MacColl and Hatchwell (2002) modeled the expected fitness payoffs for a failed breeder adopting the alternative strategies of breeding or helping at different stages through the breeding season. This model predicted that although breeding was on average a better option than helping, there was a strong seasonal decline in expected fitness from breeding. In contrast, while the expected fitness from helping was generally lower and still declined seasonally, the fitness return was realized more quickly because following nest failure a helper can immediately start helping at an active nest without the need to make a new nest, lay eggs, incubate a clutch, and feed nestlings. Therefore, although the payoff from breeding was initially higher than that of helping, later in the season the expected payoff from helping exceeded that of breeding and failed breeders are predicted to switch from breeding independently to helping kin (Figure 3.4). The time of the predicted switch in strategy closely fits the behavior observed in our population. It is significant that this model assumes the only benefit from helping is that gained indirectly through the increased productivity of relatives.

We now know more about the relatedness of helpers to offspring (mean $r = 0.17$ rather than 0.25 in the model) and about the effect of ecological conditions on the phenology of breeding (Gullet et al. 2013a), so the details of this model could be modified, but such minor changes would not alter the main conclusion that temporal constraints have driven the evolution of redirected helping of kin in long-tailed tits.

Load-lightening

Breeders with helpers provision their brood at a lower rate than those without helpers (Meade et al. 2010). This could arise if helpers target parents with low provisioning rates, thereby maximizing their impact on the marginal fitness of broods. However, contrary to this hypothesis, when a helper is temporarily removed, breeders increase their provisioning effort and then reduce their effort again when the helper is returned and starts helping again, thereby demonstrating a causal link between helpers and reduced parental provisioning (Hatchwell and Russell 1996).

Given the positive effect of additional food on offspring recruitment, this parental strategy makes sense only if the reduction in their provisioning rate reduces their reproductive costs and enhances their fitness. This prediction was tested by Meade et al. (2010) using adult survival data collected over 14 years. We first confirmed previous findings that both sexes reduced their effort

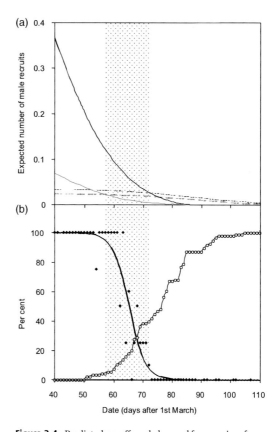

Figure 3.4. Predicted payoffs and observed frequencies of breeding and helping strategies in relation to the date of nest failure. (a) Predicted fitness payoffs, measured in male recruits, from the alternative strategies of renesting (solid lines) and helping (dashed lines) under alternative model assumptions (bold and faint lines); the hatched area indicates the period of the breeding season when individuals are predicted to switch from a strategy of independent breeding to a strategy of helping. (b) Observed probabilities of renesting (closed symbols) and the cumulative total of helpers (open symbols) in relation to date of the breeding season. From MacColl and Hatchwell (2002).

when helped, but found that at typical large brood sizes, male breeders reduced their provisioning rate more than did females. This differential reduction in effort when helped was reflected in a relatively high survival rate for males with larger brood sizes (male survival probability increased by 19% at the modal brood size), while there was no such increase in female breeders' survival. Individual fitness of both sexes is positively correlated with lifespan (MacColl and Hatchwell 2004), so a marginal effect of helpers on male breeder survival enhances their lifetime reproductive success.

Of course, any effect of helpers on adult survival may not result from the load-lightening per se but may instead be the consequence of a group size effect, assuming that members of larger groups have lower predation risk during the winter. We believe this is unlikely; flocks are not simply families plus helpers, but often comprise multiple families and immigrants, so there is no direct relationship between the presence of helpers during breeding and subsequent flock size. Furthermore, a group size effect would not predict the observed sexual asymmetry in survival, whereas the load-lightening interpretation does.

This asymmetry in load-lightening, with a benefit accrued by males but not females, is intriguing in another respect. Most helpers are related to male breeders, so indirect fitness benefits will be gained primarily from increased male survival. Therefore, male-biased load-lightening is best for helpers, and it is unclear why female breeders do not also take advantage of the same opportunity to reduce their reproductive costs in the presence of helpers.

In the course of this study, detection of a positive effect of load-lightening on long-tailed tit breeder survival proved elusive, whereas the effect of helpers on productivity was quickly apparent. In general, a marginal effect of reduced reproductive costs on parental survival requires much more extensive data, especially given the likely confounding effect of group size in most species. Nevertheless, parents reduce their effort when helped in many cooperative breeders (Hatchwell 1999); so, although fitness benefits of load-lightening have rarely been demonstrated, I suspect that the effect we have found in long-tailed tits is underestimated in the cooperative breeding literature.

Direct fitness benefits

Long-tailed tits are characterized by their flocking behavior, and given the apparent importance of winter flocks and communal roosting, earlier studies naturally suggested that a likely benefit of helping was to "buy" membership of a winter flock and access to the direct benefits they offer (Glen and Perrins 1988). If help is payment for flock membership, then helpers should have higher survival rates than nonhelpers. Other potential direct benefits from helping include increased productivity through direct reproduction in the helped brood, acquisition of reproductive skills (the "skills" hypothesis), and reciprocal help from breeders or offspring at a helper's future breeding attempts.

Some of these potential direct benefits can be easily dismissed. We observed very few cases of cobreeding or brood parasitism by females over 21 years, and extra-pair paternity (EPP) is relatively low ($< 7\%$ of nestlings in 24% of broods; Hatchwell et al. 2002). Moreover, when EPP does occur, a helper has rarely been the assigned father. (Some degree of helper EPP is expected to occur by chance simply because some neighboring potential extra-pair males will be relatives that will subsequently become helpers.) A low rate of helper reproduction in helped broods is also consistent with the fact that helpers are not associated with the breeding pair during the female's fertile period. Similarly, we have no evidence for an increase in productivity with age or experience, either as a breeder or as a helper (Meade and Hatchwell 2010). An earlier analysis of nest placement and predation (Hatchwell et al. 1999b) suggested that helpers choose better nest sites and are more successful than nonhelpers in later years, but this finding has not been substantiated in subsequent analyses.

A direct survival benefit of helping is suggested by the fact that failed breeders that help have higher over-winter survival than failed breeders that do not help (59% vs. 45%, respectively), with successful breeders having intermediate survival (51%; Meade and Hatchwell 2010). This apparent survival benefit does not withstand closer scrutiny, however. The effect appears to be a consequence of a biased sample of failed breeders who are in good condition choosing to become helpers. A proportion of failed breeders with close kin available to help choose not to become helpers and these birds had very poor survival (24%). These two samples of helpers and nonhelpers, all of which had the opportunity to help, also differed in condition. Therefore, the suggested effect of help on survival is probably an artifact of individual quality or condition influencing helping decisions. Of course, the ultimate test for direct benefits is to ask whether helpers have higher future productivity than nonhelpers. Meade and Hatchwell (2010) detected no such benefit of being a helper in year n on the likelihood of being a successful breeder in either year $n + 1$ or year $n + 2$.

Closer examination of the process of flock formation and interactions within flocks makes the absence of a direct benefit of helping unsurprising. Unlike the stable family groups of most cooperative species, the nonbreeding flocks of long-tailed tits are not simply nuclear families plus helpers. Instead, membership of flocks is relatively fluid and includes immigrants that by the end of the winter comprise approximately 40% of flock membership. Furthermore, McGowan et al. (2007) found membership of flocks was not conditional on help the previous breeding season; there was no significant difference in flock size or composition for birds that had bred successfully, helped, or not helped. Therefore, helping cannot be explained by the "payment of rent" hypothesis (Gaston 1978; Kokko et al. 2002).

We have also investigated whether more subtle interactions within flocks could result in fitness benefits accruing to helpers, perhaps through nepotistic interactions determining status within dominance hierarchies or position within communal roosts. Field observation of dominance interactions in large, dynamic winter flocks is difficult, and communal roosts are even harder to study because they form in dense vegetation where individual identification is impossible. Therefore, to investigate within-flock interactions, we studied 18 captive winter flocks housed in outdoor aviaries for 7–10 days.

Each night, during roost formation, birds compete for central positions within the roost, attempting to avoid being one of the two birds at either end of the linear huddles (McGowan et al. 2006). The reason for this competition is that birds lose about 9% of body mass each night at ambient winter temperatures, those in outer positions losing significantly more weight than those occupying inner positions (Hatchwell et al. 2009). Therefore, the benefits of communal roosting vary with position, but what determines which birds gets access to the preferred inner positions?

McGowan et al. (2006) found that birds of low status usually ended up in the outer positions. Furthermore, Napper et al. (2013) showed that the main predictor of status and roost position is sex, females generally being subordinate to males so that they are forced to occupy outer positions, especially if they are young. Reproductive status in the previous season was unknown for most of the captive birds, but there was no effect of relatedness to the rest of the flock on dominance status, and for males there appeared to be a low risk of being forced into disadvantageous roost positions. Consequently, access to preferred roost positions provides little incentive to help.

Direct and indirect components of inclusive fitness

We have shown that there are indirect fitness benefits, but no direct fitness benefits from helping in long-tailed tits, indicating that their cooperative breeding system is a product of kin selection. Several early studies of cooperative breeders evaluated the relative importance of direct and indirect fitness in the evolution of cooperative behavior using the kinship index (Vehrencamp 1979; Emlen 1991). Such calculations are difficult for complex social systems where life history events and fitness returns are age-structured, and in long-lived species they must usually be applied to cross-sectional data. Long-tailed tits are eminently suitable for an alternative, longitudinal approach, being short-lived and having a simple helping system in which birds switch back and forth between breeding and helping throughout their lives. MacColl and Hatchwell (2004) used data on the number of recruits as an index of lifetime reproductive success (LRS) to determine each bird's inclusive fitness, taking into account genetic parentage and the effect of helpers on productivity. This process, deceptively easy to describe but difficult to apply, involves calculating direct fitness by stripping from each bird the component of annual reproductive success attributable to helpers. This indirect fitness component was then divided among helpers according to their relatedness, and these fractions added to direct fitness to calculate each bird's inclusive fitness (Hamilton 1964; Oli 2003). Inclusive fitness and

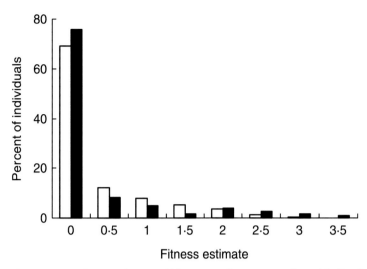

Figure 3.5. Distributions of estimated lifetime reproductive success (x 0.5, filled bars) and inclusive fitness (open bars) for 228 long-tailed tits that attempted to breed. From MacColl and Hatchwell (2004).

LRS were correlated with each other and with the production of grand-offspring.

In our sample of 228 birds, only 70 (31%) had non-zero inclusive fitness, so a large proportion (69%) of adults that recruited into the breeding population failed to achieve any inclusive fitness in their lifetime (Figure 3.5). The mean proportion of inclusive fitness gained indirectly was 22%, but this was not evenly distributed among individuals. Of the 70 birds with non-zero inclusive fitness, 15 (21%, 13 of them males) had zero LRS; that is, they achieved no direct fitness, and accrued fitness only through helping kin. Interestingly, only 2 (3%) of the birds with nonzero inclusive fitness gained both direct and indirect fitness. This reveals the importance of helping as an alternative source of fitness for birds that achieved zero direct fitness from breeding and that may have achieved zero inclusive fitness had they not adopted a helping strategy.

Fitness costs of helping

From the breeders' perspective, there appears to be no cost of having helpers. Long-tailed tits are not territorial, so breeders do not have to share a finite resource base with "extra" birds, nor risk future loss of territory.

There also appears to be weak inter- or intra-sexual competition for mates; there is an even sex ratio and all adults usually breed, and the low rate of extra-pair paternity, weak size dimorphism, and lack of ornamentation suggests weak sexual selection. Therefore, the presence of male helpers does not appear to be a threat to pair bonds that in any case are short-lived due to high mortality and divorce rates (Hatchwell et al. 2000).

From the helpers' perspective, there is no opportunity cost of helping. Helpers do not forego breeding, helping only when they have failed to breed successfully and when there is little prospect of future successful breeding that year (Figure 3.4). Helpers could incur a cost if their help increases local population density and their over-winter survival was density dependent. Within the range of population densities observed in the Rivelin Valley, however, we have found no evidence for density dependence in adult survival (Gullett et al. 2013b). On the other hand, helpers work almost as hard as parents for the period that they help and so would be expected to incur a survival cost from this alloparental investment. Indeed, the observation that some failed breeders that are in relatively poor condition spurn the opportunity to help kin suggests that it is costly (Meade and Hatchwell 2010).

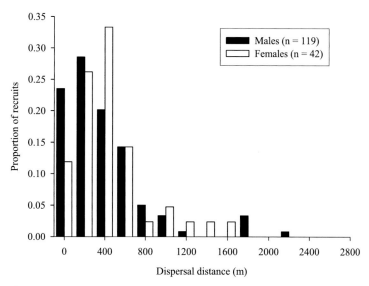

Figure 3.6. Distributions of proportions of natal dispersal distances for male (closed bars) and female (open bars) long-tailed tits that were born and recruited into the study population. From Sharp et al. (2008a).

We have recently concluded that helpers do indeed incur a survival cost from their helping behavior. Helpers' survival was estimated as 23% lower than equivalent birds that did not help, indicating that helping is altruistic because of this direct fitness cost. Despite the fairly low relatedness between helpers and recipients in long-tailed tits, this cost is outweighed by the combined indirect fitness benefits of increased productivity of helped broods and the increased survivorship of male breeders that are described above. Thus, helping behavior is consistent with Hamilton's rule for the evolution of altruism (Hatchwell et al. 2014).

Factors generating the conditions for kin-selected helping

The usual explanation for family formation, focusing on offspring dispersal decisions, dates back 50 years to the habitat saturation hypothesis (Selander 1964). This idea was later formalized as part of Emlen's (1982) ecological constraints hypothesis in which dispersal is constrained and some individuals help in their natal group before eventually inheriting the territory or dispersing to breed

independently. Long-tailed tits do not conform to this typical pattern, because natal dispersal occurs in juveniles' first winter and virtually all adults attempt to breed each year. This pattern of dispersal is very similar to many noncooperative species in the United Kingdom, a point readily illustrated by inter-specific comparisons of recapture data from national banding schemes (Paradis et al. 1998; Russell 1999). In addition, detailed comparison of the natal dispersal distances of long-tailed tits with several noncooperative species reveals similar patterns of dispersal (Hatchwell 2009; Figure 3.6).

So, how does the kin structure that facilitates kin-directed helping arise? Three processes are likely to be important. First, although dispersal occurs in the first winter, preceding breeding and helping, many birds, and especially males (the predominant helping sex), do not disperse far. Second, natal dispersal does not necessarily dilute relatedness if coalitions of relatives disperse together (Heinsohn et al. 2000; Koenig et al. 2000). In long-tailed tits there is a strong tendency for groups of siblings, especially of the same sex, to disperse a similar distance and direction even when controlling for sampling bias caused by the finite study area and discontinuous habitat (Sharp et al. 2008a).

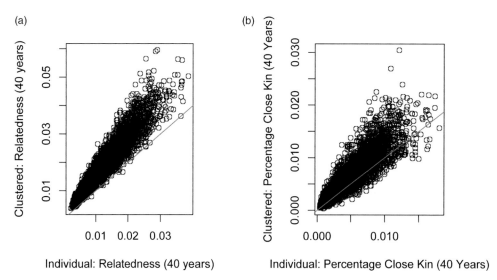

Figure 3.7. Results of simulation models of the effect on population relatedness under alternative predation regimes: "clustered" predation targeted at whole broods and "individual" predation targeted at individual offspring. Figures show the effect of predation regime (all other demographic factors held equal) on: (a) the mean relatedness of simulated populations, and (b) the proportion of individuals having a first-order relative in the simulated proportion. If predation regime had no effect, simulations would fall along the 1:1 line. From Beckerman et al. (2011).

This family signal in dispersal behavior may indicate a genetic component to dispersal (Pasinelli et al. 2004; Matthysen et al. 2005) that would be worth further exploration, but it is clear that whatever process is involved, recruitment of same-sex relatives in kin neighborhoods is common.

Genetic analysis of immigrants into our study population confirmed this phenomenon of coordinated dispersal of kin. The majority of immigrants into our study population (53%, $N = 203$) belonged to sibships of 2–7 individuals (mean size = 2.9 siblings; Sharp et al. 2008b). Importantly, when the opportunity arose, members of these sibships often helped a relative with which they had dispersed into our population, and none of them helped a confirmed nonrelative. Thus, dispersers retain functional family ties that are used in future helping decisions.

The third process generating kin structured populations in long-tailed tits is their atypical demography. The high rate of nest predation results in strongly skewed reproductive success and hence a small effective population size. Each year, only about one-third of pairs

reproduce successfully, but each successful pair produces a mean brood size of over eight fledglings. Relative to cavity-nesting or multi-brooded species, each fledgling's probability of recruitment is high, with 14–27% of ringed fledglings recruiting locally (Sharp et al. 2011). Because these recruits are drawn from a small number of successful families, siblings, and especially brothers, are likely to recruit into the same breeding population. All else being equal, this unusual life history, which is driven largely by nest predation, has a profound effect on kin structure (Figure 3.7). Importantly, kin-structure emerges in simulated populations without any positive feedback from having kin in the same population. In other words, the effect of helpers on productivity is excluded from these models, but would be expected to enhance the likelihood of kin-structure.

Proximate factors promoting the expression of helping behavior

Kin selection plays a fundamental role in the cooperative breeding system of long-tailed tits. But what proximate factors promote cooperation? One approach to tackling this question is to manipulate key resources, such as nest cavities (Du Plessis 1992; Walters et al. 1992), food (Covas et al. 2004) or territory vacancies (Pruett-Jones and Lewis 1990) and determine the effect of relaxed constraints on cooperative behavior. An alternative approach is to use correlational studies in which the prevalence of helping is compared either across populations that differ ecologically, or across years using the same population.

We took the latter approach, examining measures of cooperative behavior in the Rivelin Valley population across a 17-year period (Hatchwell et al. 2013). The occurrence of helping was related to two ecological factors. First, nest predation rate was an important predictor of the prevalence of helping (Figure 3.8a). When predation rates were low there were few failed breeders and hence few potential helpers, while at high nest predation rates there were few nests available to be helped, so the prevalence of helping peaked at intermediate predation rates. The other significant factor was the length of the breeding season, where the predicted relationship followed a similar logic. In short breeding seasons, failed pairs have little opportunity to renest, whereas in long breeding seasons multiple breeding attempts are possible. Again, the observed pattern of helping matched this prediction, being negatively correlated with breeding season length (Figure 3.8b).

The length of the breeding season is a function of environmental factors. In the Rivelin Valley, the start of laying is closely correlated with early spring (March) temperatures, while termination of breeding is a function of late spring (April) temperatures, presumably through environmental effects on the development rates of insect prey (Gullett et al. 2013a). Thus, the proximate driver of helping is variation in spring temperatures and its effect on the length of the breeding season.

Given the kin-selected cooperative breeding system of long-tailed tits, we were surprised to find no correlation between annual measures of helping behavior and population-level relatedness (Hatchwell et al. 2013). The latter varies considerably across years and we expected it to determine the availability of kin for failed breeders to help. This finding may be attributable to population-level relatedness being a crude measure of

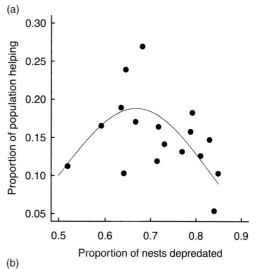

(a)

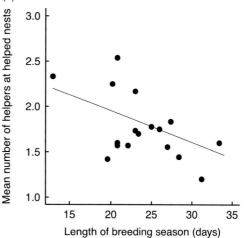

(b)

Figure 3.8. The relationship between measures of cooperative behavior and ecological traits across 17 years: (a) the proportion of breeders that became helpers in relation to the proportion of all nests depredated; (b) the mean number of helpers at helped nests in relation to the length of the breeding season. Each point represents one year, lines show predictions from models with all other parameters set to their median values. From Hatchwell et al. (2013).

an individual's helping options. Population-level relatedness does not equate to social associations, which are obviously critical in helping decisions (Sharp et al. 2005). In addition, not all birds are equally likely to help even when kin with active nests are available, either because of their condition or sex.

This final point is illustrated by Sharp et al.'s (2011) study of recruitment, kinship, and helping in two populations with contrasting demography: the Rivelin Valley (RV) and Melton Wood (MW), an isolated woodland. The two populations had similar productivity, but local recruitment in the isolated population was higher (RV 14%: MW 27%), especially for females (RV 9%; MW 27%), so that both sexes had a higher probability of having close kin in the population. But, despite this difference in genetic structure, there was no difference in the prevalence of helping between the populations.

There are probably two reasons for this result. First, females are less helpful than males, so levels of helping may not be correlated with variation in female kin structure. Second, even though local recruitment, and hence kinship, is higher in the isolated population, the social organization may be similar, so that although close kin are present in the population they are not necessarily in the same social groups and so are not available to help or be helped. Therefore, although intraspecific comparisons among populations are a useful means of testing ecological hypotheses for the evolution of cooperative breeding (Reyer 1990), they should also be treated with caution because other factors that influence individual-level decision-making may not be accounted for.

Conclusions

The long-tailed tit has a simple cooperative breeding system that has facilitated quantification of the fitness benefits of helping and experimental analysis of the mechanisms involved in decision-making. We have also been able to identify the ecological, demographic, and life history factors that generate kin structure and allow kin selection to operate on helping behavior. Nevertheless, there are still several unanswered questions.

First, a full understanding of the evolutionary dynamics of social behavior requires that the genetic and environmental influences on behavioral and life history traits be determined. We are currently extending

the quantitative genetic approach of MacColl and Hatchwell (2003b) to investigate the genetic and environmental basis for variation in cooperative behavior (Adams et al. 2015) and to determine the relationship between phenotypic traits and the direct and indirect components of fitness.

Second, about one-fifth of helpers are unrelated to the brood they provision, and thus gain no fitness from helping. It is possible that we have overlooked some direct fitness benefit for these helpers, but we believe this is unlikely. Alternatively, this apparently maladaptive behavior may be a consequence of selection for helpers to be generous with their help. Recognition systems are rarely perfect, so recognition cues are likely to overlap between desirable and undesirable recipients, with position of the acceptance threshold being a function of the relative costs of recognition errors and benefits of correct recognition (Reeve 1989; Sherman et al. 1997). If helping in long-tailed tits is cheap, and the potential fitness benefits of helping kin are substantial, failed breeders should have a low threshold for acceptance of another individual as kin (Hatchwell et al. 2014). This idea is supported by the positive correlation between helper effort and relatedness, suggesting that helpers hedge their bets and invest less when kinship is less certain (Nam et al. 2010). We are currently investigating the social, environmental, and genetic factors influencing an individual's decision to help, including the similarity of calls between helpers and recipients.

Third, an ultimate goal of research in the field of cooperative breeding is to explain why sociality has evolved in some lineages but not others. Detailed studies of single species have been extremely successful in providing species-specific solutions to the general problem, and they serve an important function in identifying key factors in the evolution of animal societies. Across species, the answer is likely to involve a combination of ecology, life history, and phylogeny, but while interspecific analyses at a global scale have made significant progress (Cockburn 2006; Jetz and Rubenstein 2011), a comprehensive understanding of the factors promoting social evolution remains elusive. One reason for this is the tendency to treat cooperative breeding as a single phenomenon, rather than recognizing the diversity of social systems represented. For example, it would be interesting to determine whether the ecological and demographic factors that promote the expression of helping in long-tailed tits may also apply to other species with redirected helping. Such analyses may provide valuable insights into one of the major evolutionary transitions in the history of life on earth.

Acknowledgments

A long-term study is the fruit of many people's labor, and one of the great pleasures of this project has been the opportunity to work with many outstanding scientists. I would particularly like to thank, in roughly chronological order: Andy Russell, Martin Fowlie, Douglas Ross, Andrew MacColl, Andy McGowan, Stuart Sharp, Michelle Simeoni, Jess Meade, Beth Woodward, Ki-Baek Nam, Jin-Won Lee, Pip Gullett, Clare Napper, Jamie Hutchison, and Mark Adams. I am also grateful to the landowners in the Rivelin Valley who have allowed me access to their land, especially Sheffield City Council, Hallamshire Golf Club, Yorkshire Water, and Blackbrook Farm. Sorby Breck Ringing Group, especially Geoff Mawson, has been particularly supportive over the years. Colleagues deserving particular mention are Terry Burke and members of the NERC Biomolecular Analysis Facility in Sheffield, Andrew Beckerman, and Matt Robinson for their various contributions to the study. Most of our work has been funded by the Natural Environment Research Council. Additional funding has come from the University of Sheffield, Nuffield Foundation, Association for the Study of Animal Behaviour, and the Leverhulme Trust. Finally, my thanks to Walt Koenig and Janis Dickinson for their helpful comments on an earlier draft of this chapter.

REFERENCES

Adams, M. J., Robinson, M. R., Mannarelli, M. E., and Hatchwell, B. J. (2015). Social genetic and social environment effects on parental and helper care in a cooperatively breeding bird. *Proc. R. Soc. London B*, 282, 20150689.

Beckerman, A. P., Sharp, S. P., and Hatchwell, B. J. (2011). Predation, demography and the emergence of kin structured populations: implications for the evolution of cooperation. *Behav. Ecol.*, 22, 1294–1303.

Brown, J. L. (1987). *Helping and Communal Breeding in Birds*. Princeton, New Jersey: Princeton University Press.

Cockburn, A. (2006). Prevalence of different modes of parental care in birds. *Proc. R. Soc. London B*, 273, 1375–1383.

Cornwallis, C. K., West, S. A., and Griffin, A. S. (2009). Routes to indirect fitness in cooperatively breeding vertebrates: kin discrimination and limited dispersal. *J. Evol. Biol.*, 22, 2445–2467.

Covas, R., Doutrelant, C., and Du Plessis, M. A. (2004). Experimental evidence of a link between breeding conditions and the decision to breed or to help in a colonial cooperative breeder. *Proc. R. Soc. London B*, 271, 827–831.

Cramp, S. and Perrins, C. M. (1993). *The Birds of the Western Palearctic. Volume VII: Flycatchers to Shrikes*. Oxford: Oxford University Press.

Crick, H. Q. P. (1992). Load-lightening in cooperatively breeding birds and the cost of reproduction. *Ibis*, 134, 56–61.

del Hoyo, J., Elliott, A., and Christie, D. A. (2008). *Handbook of the Birds of the World*, vol. 13. Barcelona: Lynx Edicions.

Dickinson, J. L., Koenig, W. D., and Pitelka, F. A. (1996). The fitness consequences of helping behavior in the western bluebird. *Behav. Ecol.*, 7, 168–177.

Du Plessis, M. A. (1992). Obligate cavity-roosting as a constraint on the dispersal of green woodhoopoes: consequences for philopatry and the likelihood of inbreeding. *Oecologia*, 90, 205–211.

Emlen, S. T. (1982). The evolution of helping. I. An ecological constraints model. *Am. Nat.*, 119, 29–39.

Emlen, S. T. (1991). Evolution of cooperative breeding in birds and mammals. In: *Behavioural Ecology: An Evolutionary Approach*, ed. J. R. Krebs and N. B. Davies. Oxford: Blackwell, pp. 301–335.

Emlen, S. T. and Wrege, P. H. (1988). The role of kinship in helping decisions among white-fronted bee-eaters. *Behav. Ecol. Sociobiol.*, 23, 305–316.

Emlen, S. T., Emlen J. M., and Levin S. A. (1986). Sex-ratio selection in species with helpers-at-the-nest. *Am. Nat.*, 127, 1–8.

Gaston, A. J. (1973). The ecology and behaviour of the long-tailed tit. *Ibis*, 115, 330–351.

Gaston, A. J. (1978). The evolution of group territorial behaviour and cooperative breeding. *Am. Nat.*, 112, 1091–1100.

Glen, N. W. and Perrins, C. M. (1988). Cooperative breeding by long-tailed tits. *Brit. Birds*, 81, 630–641.

Gullett, P. R., Hatchwell, B. J., Robinson, R. A., and Evans, K. L. (2013a). Phenological indices of avian reproduction: cryptic shifts in phenology and prediction across large spatial and temporal scales. *Ecol. Evol.*, 3, 1864–1877.

Gullett, P. R., Evans, K. L., Robinson, R. A., and Hatchwell, B. J. (2013b). Climate and adult survival in a temperate passerine: partitioning seasonal effects and predicting future patterns. *Oikos*, 123, 389–404.

Hamilton, W. D. (1964). The genetical evolution of social behaviour, I and II. J. *Theor. Biol.*, 7, 1–52.

Hatchwell, B. J. (1999). Investment strategies of breeders in avian cooperative breeding systems. *Am. Nat.*, 154, 205–219.

Hatchwell, B. J. (2009). The evolution of cooperative breeding in birds: kinship, dispersal and life history. *Phil. Trans. R. Soc. London B*, 364, 3217–3227.

Hatchwell, B. J. and Russell, A. F. (1996). Provisioning rules in cooperatively breeding long-tailed tits *Aegithalos caudatus*: an experimental study. *Proc. R. Soc. London B*, 263, 83–88.

Hatchwell, B. J., Fowlie, M. K., Ross, D. J., and Russell, A. F. (1999a). Incubation behaviour of long-tailed tits: why do males provision incubating females? *Condor*, 101, 681–686.

Hatchwell, B. J., Russell, A. F., Fowlie, M. K., and Ross, D. J. (1999b). Reproductive success and nest-site selection in a cooperative breeder: the effect of experience and a direct benefit of helping. *Auk*, 116, 355–363.

Hatchwell, B. J., Russell, A. F., Ross, D. J., and Fowlie, M. K. (2000). Divorce in cooperatively breeding long-tailed tits: a consequence of inbreeding avoidance? *Proc. R. Soc. London B*, 267, 813–819.

Hatchwell, B. J., Anderson, C., Ross, D. J., Fowlie, M. K., and Blackwell, P. G. (2001a). Social organisation in cooperatively breeding long-tailed tits: kinship and spatial dynamics. *J. Anim. Ecol.*, 70, 820–830.

Hatchwell, B. J., Ross, D. J., Fowlie, M. K., and McGowan, A. (2001b). Kin discrimination in cooperatively breeding long-tailed tits. *Proc. R. Soc. London B*, 268, 885–890.

Hatchwell, B. J., Ross, D. J., Chaline, N., Fowlie, M. K., and Burke, T. (2002). Parentage in cooperatively breeding long-tailed tits. *Anim. Behav.*, 64, 55–63.

Hatchwell, B. J., Russell, A. F., MacColl A. D. C., Ross, D. J., Fowlie, M. K., et al. (2004). Helpers increase long-term but not short-term productivity in cooperatively breeding long-tailed tits. *Behav. Ecol.*, 15, 1–10.

Hatchwell, B. J., Sharp, S. P., Simeoni, M., and McGowan, A. (2009). Factors influencing overnight loss of body mass in the communal roosts of a social bird. *Func. Ecol.*, 23, 367–372.

Hatchwell, B. J., Sharp, S. P., Beckerman, A. P., and Meade, J. (2013). Ecological and demographic correlates of helping behaviour in a cooperatively breeding bird. *J. Anim. Ecol.*, 82, 486–494.

Hatchwell, B. J., Gullett, P. R., and Adams, M. J. (2014). Helping in cooperatively breeding long-tailed tits: a test of Hamilton's rule. *Phil. Trans. R. Soc. London B*, 369, 20130565.

Heinsohn, R. G., Dunn, P., Legge, S., and Double, M. C. (2000). Coalitions of relatives and reproductive skew in cooperatively breeding white-winged chough. *Proc. R. Soc. London B*, 267, 243–249.

Jetz, W. and Rubenstein, D. R. (2011). Environmental uncertainty and the global biogeography of cooperative breeding in birds. *Curr. Biol.*, 21, 72–78.

Koenig, W. D., Hooge, P. N., Stanback, M. T., and Haydock, J. (2000). Natal dispersal in the cooperatively breeding acorn woodpecker. *Condor*, 102, 492–502.

Kokko, H., Johnstone, R. A., and Wright, J. (2002). The evolution of parental and alloparental effort in cooperatively breeding groups: when should helpers pay to stay? *Behav. Ecol.*, 13, 291–300.

Lack, D. and Lack, E. (1958). The nesting of the long-tailed tit. *Bird Study*, 5, 1–19.

Lessells, C. M. (1990). Helping at the nest in European bee-eaters: who helps and why? In: *Population Biology of Passerine Birds: An Integrated Approach*, ed. J. Blondel, A. Gosler, J. D. Lebreton and R. H. McCleery. Berlin: Springer, pp. 357–368.

Ligon, J. D. and Burt, D. B. (2004). Evolutionary origins. In: *Ecology and Evolution of Cooperative Breeding in Birds*, ed. W. D. Koenig and J. L. Dickinson. Cambridge: Cambridge University Press, pp. 5–34.

Matthysen, E., Van de Casteele, T., and Adriaensen, F. (2005). Do sibling tits (*Parus major, P. caeruleus*) disperse over similar distances and in similar directions? *Oecologia*, 143, 301–307.

MacColl, A. D. C. and Hatchwell, B. J. (2002). Temporal variation in fitness pay-offs promotes cooperative breeding in long-tailed tits *Aegithalos caudatus*. *Am. Nat.*, 160, 186–194.

MacColl, A. D. C. and Hatchwell, B. J. (2003a). Sharing of caring: nestling provisioning behaviour of long-tailed tit (*Aegithalos caudatus*) parents and helpers. *Anim. Behav.*, 66, 955–964.

MacColl, A. D. C. and Hatchwell, B. J. (2003b). Heritability of parental care in a passerine bird. *Evolution*, 57, 2191–2195.

MacColl, A. D. C. and Hatchwell, B. J. (2004). Determinants of lifetime fitness in a cooperative breeder, the long-tailed tit *Aegithalos caudatus*. *J. Anim. Ecol.*, 73, 1137–1148.

McGowan, A., Sharp, S. P., and Hatchwell, B. J. (2004). The structure and function of nests of long-tailed tits *Aegithalos caudatus*. *Func. Ecol.*, 18, 578–583.

McGowan, A., Sharp, S. P., Simeoni, M., and Hatchwell, B. J. (2006). Competing for position in the communal roosts of long-tailed tits. *Anim. Behav.*, 72, 1035–1043.

McGowan, A., Fowlie, M. K., Ross, D. J., and Hatchwell, B. J. (2007). Social organization of cooperatively breeding long-tailed tits: flock composition and kinship. *Ibis*, 149, 170–174.

Meade, J. and Hatchwell, B. J. (2010). No direct fitness benefits of helping in a cooperative breeder despite higher survival of helpers. *Behav. Ecol.*, 21, 1186–1194.

Meade, J., Nam, K. B., Beckerman, A. P., and Hatchwell, B. J. (2010). Consequences of load-lightening for future indirect fitness gains by helpers in a cooperatively breeding bird. *J. Anim. Ecol.*, 79, 529–537.

Nam, K. B., Simeoni, M., Sharp, S. P., and Hatchwell, B. J. (2010). Kinship affects investment by helpers in a cooperatively breeding bird. *Proc. R. Soc. London B*, 277, 3299–3306.

Nam, K. B., Meade, J., and Hatchwell, B. J. (2011). Brood sex ratio variation in a cooperatively breeding bird. *J. Evol. Biol.*, 24, 904–913.

Napper, C., Sharp, S. P., McGowan, A., Simeoni, M., and Hatchwell, B. J. (2013). Dominance, not kinship, determines individual position within the communal roosts of a cooperatively breeding bird. *Behav. Ecol. Sociobiol.*, 67, 2029–2039.

Oli, M. K. (2003). Hamilton goes empirical: estimation of inclusive fitness from life-history data. *Proc. R. Soc. London B*, 270, 307–311.

Paradis, E., Baillie, S. R., Sutherland, W. J., and Gregory, R. D. (1998). Patterns of natal and breeding dispersal in birds. *J. Anim. Ecol.*, 67, 518–536.

Pasinelli, G., Schiegg, K., and Walters, J. R. (2004). Genetic and environmental influences on natal dispersal distance in a resident bird species. *Am. Nat.*, 164, 660–669.

Pruett-Jones, S. G. and Lewis, M. J. (1990). Sex ratio and habitat limitation promote delayed dispersal in superb fairy-wrens. *Nature*, 348, 541–542.

Reeve, H. K. (1989). The evolution of conspecific acceptance thresholds. *Am. Nat.*, 133, 407–435.

Reyer, H. U. (1990). Pied kingfishers: ecological causes and reproductive consequences of cooperative breeding. In: *Cooperative Breeding in Birds: Long-term Studies of Ecology and Behavior*, ed. P. B. Stacey and W. D. Koenig. Cambridge: Cambridge University Press, pp. 529–557.

Riehm, H. (1970). Okologie und verhalten der schwanzmeise (*Aegithalos caudatus*). *Zool. Jahr. Syst.*, 97, 338–400.

Russell, A. F. (1999). Ecological constraints and the cooperative breeding system of the long-tailed tit *Aegithalos caudatus*. Ph.D. thesis, University of Sheffield, Sheffield, U.K.

Russell, A. F. and Hatchwell, B. J. (2001). Experimental evidence for kin-biased helping in a cooperatively breeding vertebrate. *Proc. R. Soc. London B*, 268, 2169–2174.

Selander, R. K. (1964). Speciation in wrens of the genus *Campylorhynchus*. *Univ. Calif. Publ. Zool.*, 74, 1–224.

Sharp, S. P. and Hatchwell, B. J. (2005). Individuality in the contact calls of cooperatively breeding long-tailed tits. *Behaviour*, 142, 1559–1575.

Sharp, S. P. and Hatchwell, B. J. (2006). Development of family-specific contact calls in the long-tailed tit *Aegithalos caudatus*. *Ibis*, 148, 649–656.

Sharp, S. P., McGowan, A., Wood, M. J., and Hatchwell, B. J. (2005). Learned kin recognition cues in a social bird. *Nature*, 434, 1127–1130.

Sharp, S. P., Hadfield, J., Baker, M. B., Simeoni, M., and Hatchwell, B. J. (2008a). Natal dispersal and recruitment in a social bird. *Oikos*, 117, 1371–1379.

Sharp, S. P., Simeoni, M., and Hatchwell, B. J. (2008b). Dispersal of sibling coalitions promotes helping among immigrants in a cooperatively breeding bird. *Proc. R. Soc. London B*, 275, 2125–2130.

Sharp, S. P., Simeoni, M., McGowan, A., Nam, K. B., and Hatchwell, B. J. (2011). Patterns of recruitment, relatedness and cooperative breeding in two populations of long-tailed tits. *Anim. Behav.*, 81, 843–849.

Sherman, P. W., Reeve, H. K., and Pfennig, D. W. (1997). Recognition systems. In: *Behavioural Ecology: An Evolutionary Approach*, ed. J. R. Krebs and N. B. Davies. Oxford: Blackwell, pp. 69–96.

Simeoni, M. (2011). Inbreeding and inbreeding avoidance in the long-tailed tit *Aegithalos caudatus*. Ph.D. thesis, University of Sheffield, Sheffield, U.K.

Simeoni, M., Dawson, D. A., Ross, D. J., Chaline, N., Burke, T. A., et al. (2007). Characterization of 20 microsatellite loci in the long-tailed tit *Aegithalos caudatus* (Aegithalidae: AVES). *Mol. Ecol. Notes*, 7, 1319–1322.

Vehrencamp, S. L. (1979). The roles of individual, kin and group selection in the evolution of sociality. In: *Handbook of Behavioural Neurobiology*, ed. P. Marler and J. G. Vandenbergh. New York: Plenum Press, pp. 351–394.

Walters, J. R., Copeyon, C. K., and Carter, J. H. (1992). Test of the ecological basis of cooperative breeding in red-cockaded woodpeckers. *Auk*, 109, 90–97.

4

Red-cockaded woodpeckers: Alternative pathways to breeding success

Jeffrey R. Walters and Victoria Garcia

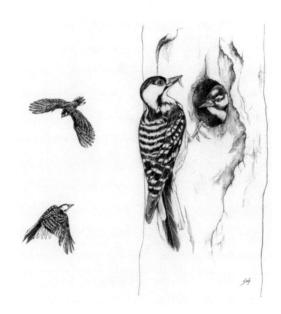

Introduction

The red-cockaded woodpecker (*Picoides borealis*) is the only cooperative breeder within its genus, and it is clear that its seemingly simple, helper-at-the-nest system arose relatively recently from noncooperative ancestors (Ligon and Burt 2004). Our work has focused on examining the lifetime fitness consequences for individuals choosing alternative life-history pathways, including different modes of dispersal and different trajectories to breeding. Hence, studies of this species have been especially useful in addressing fundamental questions related to the origins of cooperative breeding.

A fortuitous consequence of the unusual ecology of the red-cockaded woodpecker is that it is tractable to monitor large numbers of groups. As a result, our long-term studies of this species have generated uniquely comprehensive demographic data sets that have been fertile ground for addressing questions related to the demography of cooperative breeding.

Cooperative Breeding in Vertebrates: Studies of Ecology, Evolution, and Behavior, eds W. D. Koenig and J. L. Dickinson.
Published by Cambridge University Press. © Cambridge University Press 2016.

The red-cockaded woodpecker has been designated a federally endangered species within the United States (USFWS 2003). Its status, along with its large area requirements, renders it a major driver of forest management and conservation over a large portion of the southeastern United States, to which it is endemic. Insights gained from our work have resulted in a new management paradigm that has been highly successful in increasing populations (Walters 1991). Thus, this species provides an especially clear example of the relevance of basic research generally, and of understanding cooperative breeding systems specifically, to species management and biodiversity conservation.

The attention its endangered status has brought the species has resulted in a vast literature encompassing four symposia volumes (Thompson 1971; Wood 1983; Kulhavy et al. 1995; Costa and Daniels 2004), more than a thousand journal articles and a substantial gray literature. Although much of this literature focuses on management and monitoring, it also provides an abundance of demographic and population data over significant periods of time from several sites across the range of the species. In this chapter we rely primarily on our own long-term work, but also draw on the extensive body of knowledge provided by these parallel studies.

Natural history

The red-cockaded woodpecker was once abundant in the coastal plain and Piedmont of the southeastern United States, ranging north to New Jersey, west to Texas and Oklahoma, and inland to Kentucky, Tennessee, and Missouri (Jackson 1971). It has been extirpated north of North Carolina except for one small population in southeastern Virginia, and from all interior states except Arkansas and Oklahoma. Where it still occurs it is no longer broadly distributed, but rather exists in isolated populations (USFWS 2003). It is a cooperative breeder throughout its range, but exhibits geographic variation in demography with higher survival and lower fecundity in coastal and southern populations compared to inland and northern ones (Conner et al. 2001).

The most unusual feature of the ecology of the red-cockaded woodpecker is that it excavates its cavities exclusively in living pines. Within its territory a group has a set of cavity trees, termed the cavity tree cluster. Each group member has its own roost cavity, and the roost cavity of the breeding male, or occasionally the breeding female, is used for nesting. The cluster often contains additional completed cavities beyond those currently being used by group members, plus several incomplete excavations, termed cavity starts, in various stages of completion.

A completed cavity consists of a horizontal entrance tunnel excavated through the sapwood and into the heartwood of the tree, and a vertical cavity chamber within the heartwood. To be suitable for cavity excavation a tree must contain a sufficient diameter of heartwood to house the cavity chamber; otherwise resin from the sapwood leaks into the cavity. Heartwood diameter is a function of tree age, and thus red-cockaded woodpeckers require old pines a minimum of 80–120 years old, depending on the species, for cavity excavation.

Whereas most woodpeckers can excavate a cavity in dead wood in a matter of days or weeks, red-cockaded woodpeckers excavating in living pines require years to complete their cavities. Conner and Rudolph (1995) estimated excavation times in a Texas population to be over 6 years in longleaf pine (*Pinus palustris*) and about 2 years in loblolly (*P. taeda*) and shortleaf pine (*P. echinata*). Using larger samples and techniques that enabled inclusion of incomplete cavities, Harding and Walters (2004) estimated excavation times to be 9–13 years in longleaf pine, and 4–9 years in loblolly pine in three North Carolina populations. Although excavation in living heartwood poses challenges, excavation of the entrance tunnel through sapwood is the most time consuming and is typically done intermittently over many years. Intermittent excavation of sapwood appears to be a means to avoid exposure to actively flowing resin, since birds are sometimes killed due to becoming stuck in pools of resin that form in the entrance tunnel (Conner et al. 2001).

The same resin that poses such a danger to red-cockaded woodpeckers during cavity excavation serves to protect them once the cavity is complete. The birds chip daily into the sapwood above and

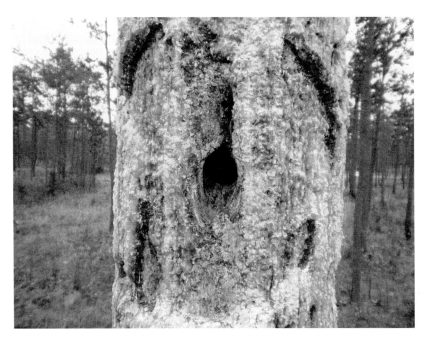

Figure 4.1. A red-cockaded woodpecker cavity, protected by a barrier of pine resin. Photo by Michelle Jusino. See plate section for color figure.

below the cavity around the entire circumference of the tree, stimulating copious resin flow that results in a protective barrier against rat snakes (*Elaphe obsoleta* and *E. guttata*), the major predators of cavity-dwelling birds in their habitat (Figure 4.1). The resin fouls the ventral scales the snakes use to grip the tree, rendering them incapable of climbing and causing them to fall to the ground (Rudolph et al. 1990). The birds maintain resin wells around the cavities in which they are roosting and nesting, thereby protecting themselves and their eggs and young. The birds also scale bark from their cavity trees, creating a smooth surface that impedes climbing snakes from gripping the tree.

Red-cockaded woodpeckers prefer longleaf pine over other species for cavity excavation, most likely because of the resin barrier. Although excavation times are longer in longleaf pine, once completed cavities in longleaf are used twice as long on average as cavities in other pine species (Harding 1997; Conner and Rudolph 1995), averaging roughly a decade of use and in extreme cases up to 30 years (Conner et al. 2001). Apparently

the superior capability of longleaf pine to produce resin (Conner et al. 1998) favors the birds continuing to use a longleaf cavity until it suffers structural damage such as enlargement by other woodpecker species, or the tree dies, whereas they sometimes abandon intact cavities excavated in other pine species (Harding and Walters 2002).

Further evidence of the importance of the association between this bird and longleaf pine is the geographic range of the bird, which is largely coincident with that of the longleaf pine ecosystem. This ecosystem is more savanna than forest, characterized by an open canopy of scattered large, old pines, a sparse midstory consisting primarily of several species of small oaks (*Quercus* spp.) and regenerating pine, and a rich, highly diverse, herbaceous groundcover (Figure 4.2). The birds prefer habitat with these features and groups are larger and more productive within such habitat (James et al. 1997; 2001; Walters et al. 2002; USFWS 2003). Historically, habitat was maintained in preferred condition by frequent, low intensity fires at 1–5 year intervals, many of

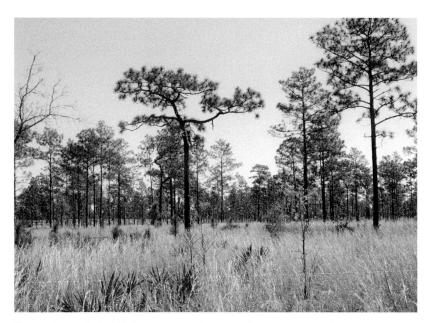

Figure 4.2. Longleaf pine habitat on our study area at Eglin Air Force Base, Florida. Photo by Lori Blanc.

which occurred in spring and summer and were ignited by lightning strikes.

Red-cockaded woodpecker territories are exceptionally large for a bird of its size (McFarlane 1992), 50–150 ha depending on the population (Conner et al. 2001; USFWS 2003). Variation in territory size is due to habitat type and habitat condition, and in some instances to lack of availability of cavity trees, which causes population density to be lower than it potentially could be. Within their large territories family groups travel and forage together, departing from their cavity trees just after dawn and returning just before dusk. The daily routine consists of periods of active foraging, during which the group moves frequently and communicates constantly with contact calls, and quiescent periods during which the group settles in an area to rest and preen. The birds forage almost exclusively on pines, from which they scale bark to reveal arthropods underneath. They also excavate in dead and dying trees and branches, and on green cones, and have occasionally been observed engaging in a multitude of other foraging behaviors such as eating fruit, foraging on hardwoods, gleaning arthropods

from foliage, and visiting bird feeders (Conner et al. 2001; USFWS 2003). Outside of the breeding season, foraging red-cockaded woodpeckers regularly travel with the large mixed-species foraging flocks characteristic of southern pine habitats (Rodewald et al. 2013), within which they may function as a nuclear species (Conner et al. 2001).

Red-cockaded woodpeckers exhibit a pronounced sexual dimorphism in foraging behavior. The limbs and twigs are the domain of males, which excavate more than females, and the lower trunk below the first limbs is the domain of females, which rely more on scaling (Ligon 1968). Both sexes forage on the upper trunk. There may be some separation between breeding and helper males as well, with the latter foraging more on lateral branches than the former (Rudolph et al. 2007). Morphological differences between the sexes based on birds captured in the field are consistent with these foraging differences: males, which often hang from twigs and limbs, have longer tarsi and bills, whereas females, which spend more time hitching up and down the trunk, have longer tails (Pizzoni-Ardemani 1990).

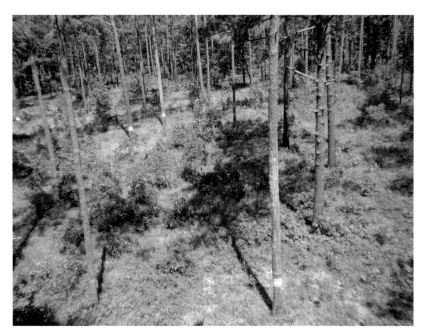

Figure 4.3. Cavity trees of red-cockaded woodpeckers are conspicuous due to the whitish coat of dried resin and the reddish appearance of fresh resin and scaled bark. Photo by Michelle Jusino. See plate section for color figure.

Study areas

We are conducting long-term studies of red-cockaded woodpeckers at three locations, the Sandhills region in south-central North Carolina (1980 – present), Marine Corps Base Camp Lejeune (MCBCL) on the central coast of North Carolina (1986 – present), and Eglin Air Force Base on the Gulf Coast in the western panhandle of Florida (1996 – present). Our monitoring methods are much the same at all three sites and are described in detail in Walters et al. (1988). Locating and monitoring all of the groups in a study area is facilitated by the resin-coated cavity trees, which are a highly conspicuous indicator of their presence and easily visible at long distances (Figure 4.3), and the long-term stability of territories. That each bird has an individual roost cavity makes targeting a particular bird for capture simple. We have taken advantage of these features in emphasizing complete sampling of large study populations of marked birds (e.g., > 250 groups in the Sandhills) rather than intensive sampling of a smaller number of

groups, such as characterizes many of the other studies described in this volume.

The social system

Territories

Because the cavity tree cluster within a territory is a highly valuable resource that can be passed from one generation to the next, territories are highly stable. Many of the groups we monitor currently are the same family groups in the same locations as when our long-term studies began 35 years ago. All group members participate in territory defense. Unpaired males defend territories but unpaired females do not, although they will roost in otherwise unoccupied territories. Territories are abandoned when all the cavity trees are lost (Doerr et al. 1989) or when the habitat becomes so degraded, most commonly due to fire suppression, that it can no longer support red-cockaded woodpeckers. New territories

Table 4.1. Proportion of fledglings achieving a given status at age one

	N	Dead	Natal Helper	Natal Breeder	Dispersed Breeder	Floater	Unrelated Helper
MCBCL male	942	43%	43%	2%	5%	6%	2%
Sandhills male	4773	54%	33%	2%	6%	4%	1%
Estimated SH male	4773	49%	33%	2%	9%	6%	1%
MCBCL female	985	53%	10%	0.3%	17%	18%	1%
Sandhills female	4832	67%	2%	1%	23%	7%	1%
Estimated SH female	4832	60%	2%	1%	28%	8%	1%

Estimated values for the Sandhills (Estimated SH) include corrections of observed data (Sandhills) based on estimated dispersal out of the study area (Walters 1990). Dispersal from the MCBCL study area is negligible.

are formed either by budding, the dividing of one territory and its cavity tree cluster into two, or pioneering, the creation of a new territory and new cavity tree cluster in formerly unoccupied habitat (Hooper 1983). The rate at which these processes occur is low, producing an annual population growth rate of only 1–2%, with budding accounting for the majority of new territories. The rarity of pioneering attests to the importance of existing cavity trees to territory viability.

For the past 25 years the majority of new territories have not formed through these natural processes, but rather in response to creation of clusters of artificial cavities, termed recruitment clusters, in unoccupied habitat (Copeyon et al. 1991). Deployment of recruitment clusters has significantly increased the rate of population growth and helped to bring this species back from the brink of extinction.

Group size and composition

Red-cockaded woodpecker groups consist of a single breeding pair and up to five nonbreeding helpers. Most helpers are previous offspring retained on the natal territory, the majority of which are male. Many individuals of both sexes disperse from the natal territory in their first year rather than remaining as helpers, however. These individuals may acquire breeding positions at age one, but many instead become floaters, and some join other groups as unrelated helpers.

Breeding positions become available less frequently at MCBCL than in the Sandhills because breeder

survival rates are higher in the former population (males 82%; females 79%) than the latter (males 76%; females 70%). In the more socially competitive environment of MCBCL, more fledglings of both sexes remain as natal helpers at age one and fledgling survival to age one is correspondingly higher (Table 4.1). Mortality rates of breeders have not changed over the duration of our studies at either site despite improvements in habitat. However, the proportion of male fledglings remaining as helpers in the Sandhills has increased since the early years of our study (33% compared to 28%; Walters 1990), suggesting that habitat quality influences whether juveniles elect to disperse or remain on the natal territory.

Excluding unpaired males, average group sizes in our study populations have ranged from just over two to just over three birds depending on the year and the population. Group sizes have increased over time, and are higher at MCBCL than in the Sandhills, a difference expected given differences in survival and frequency of natal helpers (Table 4.2). Shifts toward higher group sizes are characterized by increases in large (4–7 adults) groups and decreases in unassisted pairs. The increases in group size observed correspond to improvements in habitat quality, which began earlier at MCBCL (early 1990s) than in the Sandhills (late 1990s) (Table 4.2).

In the early years of our studies, unpaired males were observed regularly, accounting for over 10% of the occupied territories in some years in both the Sandhills (Walters 1990) and MCBCL. Solitary males were considered an indicator of poor habitat quality as the

Table 4.2. Mean, distribution, and changes over time of group size in the Sandhills and MCBCL study areas

	N	Two	Three	Four	5–7	Mean
Sandhills 1980–1999	3975	60%	32%	7%	1%	2.47
Sandhills 2000–2013	3554	50%	33%	13%	4%	2.71
MCBCL 1986–1991	173	55%	34%	9%	1%	2.83
MCBCL 1992–2013	1392	42%	35%	18%	5%	2.88

territories on which they occurred typically were abandoned rather than occupied by other birds when the resident male died (Walters 1991). Now that the habitat degradation due to fire suppression that led to territory abandonment in these early years has been remedied, solitary males are much less frequent, representing only 1–5% of occupied territories, and are no longer associated with poor quality territories, but rather with new territories created through recruitment cluster construction. These typically are young males that have occupied the new territory but not yet attracted a mate (Walters et al. 2004), whereas in the early years of our work solitary males were often older birds that had previously had mates and helpers.

Mating system

Red-cockaded woodpeckers are monogamous. Copulations by the breeding pair are highly conspicuous, noisy, prolonged, and occur on a seemingly daily basis throughout the year, suggesting they have a display as well as reproductive function. In contrast, copulations involving helpers have never been observed, nor have extra-pair copulations with individuals outside the group. Genetic analyses found no instances of extra-pair fertilization in one study (Haig et al. 1993) and a rate of 1% in a second study with a larger sample (Haig et al. 1994). The single case of extra-pair paternity revealed by these studies involved a male outside the group rather than a helper, confirming that groups include a single breeder of each sex.

Red-cockaded woodpeckers recognize kin based on familiarity, and avoid mating with individuals identified as kin. Individuals do not pair with brood mates or with birds that helped raise them, even when offspring

and helper are not genetically related, as occurs when birds join groups as unrelated helpers. When a helper male inherits the breeding position on a territory following the death of his father, the current breeding female will emigrate, apparently of her own volition, if she is the male's mother. However, females unrelated to the helper (e.g., stepmothers) almost always remain and pair with the former helper. This incest avoidance mechanism precludes females, in contrast to males, from inheriting their natal territories except rarely. When a breeding female dies or departs, the breeding male remains and if he is a relative of the natal helper female, as is almost always the case, he will pair with a new emigrant female rather than the helper female. Our data contain exceptions to these patterns of incest avoidance in which the putative breeders are familiar relatives, but these are cases in which a former breeder recently died and was not replaced during the breeding season. In these cases the group does not nest, and the expected breeder replacement occurs by the next breeding season.

There is no evidence that red-cockaded woodpeckers can recognize genetic relatives with which they are unfamiliar (Daniels and Walters 2000a). Unfamiliar kin who disperse from the natal territory in different years pair as frequently as one would expect based on dispersal patterns of the two sexes and random mating with respect to kinship. Mating between close kin results in inbreeding depression in the form of reduced hatching success and reduced survival and recruitment of offspring produced. Also, when female offspring of inbred pairs are recruited into the breeding population, they appear to be unable to adjust their egg-laying dates in response to climate change as are other individuals – a putative case of the reduced capacity of inbred individuals to respond to environmental challenges (Schiegg et al. 2002). Despite these negative impacts, inbreeding avoidance does not appear to be an important selective force affecting dispersal beyond the natal territory. Genetic population structure is such that females could avoid pairing with close kin by dispersing more than three territories away from the natal site, but the majority of females do not disperse this far (Daniels and Walters 2000a).

Dominance relationships

Dominance relationships within family groups govern the social system. With only rare exceptions, males are dominant to females as nestlings and remain so as fledglings (Ragheb and Walters 2011). Dominance of males over females, expressed through incest avoidance, excludes females from inheriting breeding status on the natal territory – the life-history pathway that appears to have the highest fitness payoff (see "Alternative life-history pathways").

Ranks among male helpers are strictly governed by age, resulting in stable age queues that determine territory inheritance. Male helpers are invariably different ages, as only rarely do two males from the same brood remain as helpers, and when they do, almost always one is gone by the second year, suggesting it was a bird whose (early) dispersal was delayed by a few months rather than one behaving as a natal helper. Among same-sex broodmates, larger birds dominate smaller birds, and they maintain their size advantage well beyond nutritional independence. It is the dominant male that remains as a helper (Pasinelli and Walters 2002); subordinate males often overwinter with their natal group, but only remain as a helper subsequently if their dominant brother perishes (Ragheb and Walters 2011). Thus dominance among broodmates governs the life-history pathways followed by juvenile males.

Whereas aggression among adults is rare, aggression among fledglings is frequent. The few observations made inside the cavity reveal that high rates of aggression, some of it violent, characterize the nestling stage as well (DeLotelle et al. 2004). Once out of the cavity, fledglings squabble for weeks on end, manifested primarily as dominant birds attacking and displacing

subordinates that are being fed or are following foraging adults. Thus, just as kin cooperation involving helpers is an important characteristic of the social system of the red-cockaded woodpecker, so too is kin competition.

Sex ratio

Young red-cockaded woodpeckers can be sexed beginning at about 14 days of age based on the presence of a red crown patch in males that persists until the fall molt. In contrast, the crowns of females are black. Most mortality of nestlings occurs in the first few days following hatching (LaBranche and Walters 1994; DeLotelle et al. 2004) before nestlings can be sexed, but sex ratios do not differ between broods that have suffered some partial brood loss and those that have not (LaBranche 1992). Thus, we can assume that there are no sex differences in nestling mortality and treat reported sex ratios among fledglings as equivalent to sex ratios at hatching.

Gowaty and Lennartz (1985) reported a male-biased sex ratio in a South Carolina population. They related this finding to the local resource enhancement model of Clark (1978), which predicts a bias toward the philopatric sex when that sex contributes to parental survival and reproductive success, as do male helpers (see "Helper effects on breeder survival and reproduction"), because these positive effects reduce the cost of producing the philopatric sex. Emlen et al. (1986) and Lessells and Avery (1987) developed this application of the local resource enhancement concept to cooperative breeders in what has been called the "repayment model." Koenig and Walters (1999) applied the repayment model to our Sandhills and MCBCL populations and found that the model predicted precisely the same male-biased sex ratio observed by Gowaty and Lennartz (1985) (0.59, $N = 166$ fledglings) for both populations. The actual sex ratios (Sandhills: 0.50, $N = 4{,}029$; MCBCL: 0.49, $N = 518$) in these populations, however, differed significantly from the predicted sex ratios, and were not significantly different from 50:50. Thus, it is not clear that there is any bias in offspring sex ratios in red-cockaded woodpeckers. The sex ratio among adults is, in contrast, male-biased due to higher female mortality associated with the sex differences in philopatry that characterize the social system.

Helpers

With the exception of their exclusion from mating, red-cockaded woodpecker helpers participate fully in every aspect of group life, including territory defense, construction and maintenance of cavities, and care of eggs and young. They participate in incubation beginning with the laying of the first egg, developing brood patches prior to egg-laying just as breeders do. Male helpers vary in their contributions to nesting, but the relatedness of helpers to the breeding female and male does not affect helping behavior. For example, the contributions and behavior of immigrant helpers unrelated to the breeders are indistinguishable from those of natal helpers assisting both parents (Conner et al. 2001). Contributions of the less common female helpers are less well documented than those of male helpers, but it appears that some female helpers actively contribute to incubation and offspring care whereas others contribute little if at all. The basis of this variation is unknown, but relatedness to the breeders is likely a factor given some of the distinctions between the natal helper and immigrant helper life-history pathways among females.

Consistent with their seemingly indistinguishable parental behavior, the hormonal profiles of helper and breeder males are identical. Both have low testosterone prior to breeding, peak levels during the copulation period, and low levels during the incubation and nestling phases (Khan et al. 2001). In both, prolactin levels increase through the copulation and incubation periods and decline during the nestling stage (Khan et al. 2001). Baseline and maximal levels of plasma corticosterone do not differ between male breeders and helpers, with maximal levels peaking during the nestling stage (Malueg et al. 2009).

Although the hormonal profiles of helper males provide a proximate explanation of their involvement in care of eggs and young, they pose a quandary for their lack of mating activity, since helpers are not excluded from activities during the mating period and their hormonal profiles indicate they are fully capable of breeding. Indeed, helper males can immediately take over the breeding position and father offspring upon the death of the former breeding male. What prevents helper males from fathering offspring under normal circumstances? Mate guarding is not the answer (Lape 1990), but the mechanism likely is behavioral. The unusual copulatory behavior of the species, which evidently has display function, may provide a clue.

Helper effects on breeder survival and reproduction

Red-cockaded woodpecker helpers have positive effects on both the survival and productivity of the breeders they assist. Productivity increases with the addition of the first and second helper, but additional helpers provide no further increments in reproductive success (Figure 4.4). The correlation between group size and productivity arises from effects of both helpers and territory quality. Higher quality territories are more productive, and higher productivity results in more male offspring that might remain as helpers, promoting larger group sizes. Heppell et al. (1994) controlled for territory quality by analyzing productivity of breeding pairs that were assisted by varying numbers of helpers during their breeding years and estimated that in the Sandhills, the first helper increases productivity by 0.39 fledglings per year and the second helper by an additional 0.36 fledglings per year. Based on these estimates, the helper's effect accounts for 62% of the increment in productivity in groups of three compared to pairs, and 76% of the additional increment in groups of four compared to groups of three.

The pattern of nestling mortality in red-cockaded woodpeckers suggests brood reduction, that is, adaptive adjustment of brood size after hatching to match environmental conditions (O'Connor 1978): eggs hatch asynchronously and most nestling death occurs during the first few days after hatching (LaBranche and Walters 1994; DeLotelle et al. 2004). One might expect that the positive effect of helpers on reproductive success would be manifested in a reduction in partial brood loss, but this is not the case. Consistent with this finding, provisioning rates are not significantly higher in larger groups, but rather the workload of each group member, including the breeders, is reduced (Khan and Walters 2002). Helpers do reduce whole brood loss (Lennartz et al. 1987; Conner et al. 2001), however, suggesting that they improve protection of nests against

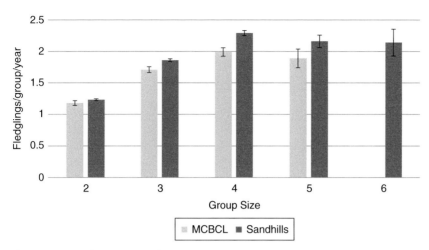

Figure 4.4. Mean (± standard error) of number of fledglings produced per group per year as a function of group size for the MCBCL and Sandhills populations. For MCBCL, "5" represents group sizes of 5–7; for the Sandhills, "6" represents group sizes of 6–7. Sample sizes in group-years for MCBCL and Sandhills respectively are 2: 680, 4166; 3: 544, 2438; 4: 271, 737; 5: 70, 152; 6: 36.

predators, cavity usurpers, or intruding conspecifics that might destroy nests. Clutch size and the probability of nesting increase with group size (Conner et al. 2001), suggesting that helpers increase the group's capacity to raise young. However, the extent to which these correlations between group size and components of reproduction (i.e., whole brood loss, clutch size, probability of nesting) are driven by territory quality, helper effects, or both is unknown.

Fitness is enhanced not only by increased mean productivity but also by reduced variance in productivity (Gillespie 1977; Lacey et al. 1983). Helpers might reduce variance in breeder productivity through impacts on whole brood loss or probability of nesting. The latter component of reproduction exhibits considerable annual variation in red-cockaded woodpeckers, with up to 25% of family groups foregoing nesting in some years, and none in others (Conner et al. 2001). Young breeders are especially likely to refrain from nesting, and helpers increase the likelihood of nesting among young as well as old breeders (Reed and Walters 1996). Despite these impacts of helpers, Reed and Walters (1996) found no effect of helpers on the variation in productivity of the breeders they assist. Thus, the impacts of helpers on reproduction are limited to effects on

mean productivity, in contrast to those described for superb starlings (*Lamprotornis superbus*) (Chapter 11).

Territory quality has a large impact on breeder survival, but there is an additional, sizeable, independent effect of the presence of helpers (Khan and Walters 2002). In the Sandhills, each helper reduces the mortality rate of male (21%) and female (15%) breeders by comparable amounts, whereas at MCBCL there is a marked effect on male breeders (a 42% reduction) but no effect on female breeders. Helpers also augment breeder survival indirectly through the increased production of fledglings attributable to their presence (Khan and Walters 2002). In the Sandhills, each juvenile reduces the estimated mortality rate of male (16%) and female (26%) breeders by amounts comparable to the direct effects of helpers. The effects are much stronger at MCBCL, and in contrast to direct effects of helpers, apply to both female (42%) and male (42%) breeders.

The effect of juveniles is likely due to benefits of larger group size related to predation, and the effect of helpers may be as well. The reduced workload during nesting that breeders enjoy when helpers are present might also contribute to their increased survival (Khan and Walters 2002), although this does not account for the difference between the sexes.

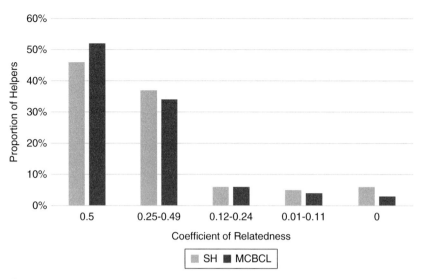

Figure 4.5. Proportion of male helpers with different coefficients of relatedness to the offspring they help raise, ranging from full siblings ($r = 0.5$) to unrelated helpers ($r = 0$) for the Sandhills (SH, $N = 3,979$ helper-years) and MCBCL ($N = 1,076$ helper-years) populations.

Benefits of helping

Delaying dispersal and remaining on the natal territory as a helper is an effective means of acquiring a breeding position. This benefit appears to be sufficient to explain why helpers stay (Walters et al. 1992a). The additional question of why they help (Emlen 1991) cannot yet be answered completely. The majority of helpers are indeed related to the breeders they assist, most of them as full or half-siblings (Figure 4.5), and thus male helpers gain indirect fitness benefits in most cases. Whether indirect benefits exceed the costs of helping and thus are sufficient to explain helping is more difficult to answer. The cost of helping is the difference in fitness between nonbreeding group members that help and those that do not, but because all male helpers help, costs cannot be estimated directly. In any case, helpers unrelated to the breeders that cannot derive any indirect fitness benefits from helping do not differ in their provisioning from related helpers (Conner et al. 2001).

Although unrelated helpers are rare (3–6% of helpers, Figure 4.5), their behavior suggests that direct benefits of helping exist. Given the lack of extra-pair paternity,

helpers gain no direct benefits from fathering offspring. Pseudoreciprocity – assisting in raising young that will later assist the helper when it becomes a breeder – occurs in two forms, but both are too infrequent to be a significant benefit of helping. Joint dispersal, in which a helper is assisted in competing for and acquiring a breeding position by younger males they helped raise, occurs but is exceedingly rare (Conner et al. 2001). Helpers are more likely to be assisted by younger males they helped raise if they inherit the breeding position on the territory on which they served as a helper, but again this is rare (probability of reciprocation 1–8% depending on the population and relatedness; Khan and Walters 2000). Nor do the young that the helper helps raise enhance its survival: in contrast to the positive effects of group size on breeder survival, helper survival decreases with increasing group size (Conner et al. 2001).

Neither do male helpers appear to gain experience through helping that is of value when they become breeders. Productivity of breeding males increases through age four, and at any given age experienced breeders are more productive than individuals breeding for the first time (Conner et al. 2001). However, naïve breeders with helping experience are no more productive than those that previously were floaters or lived in groups that did not nest and thus had never helped raise young (Khan and Walters 1997).

Most of the other direct benefits of helping that have been proposed have similarly been eliminated as possibilities for the red-cockaded woodpecker (Conner et al. 2001). The one exception is the pay-to-stay hypothesis (Gaston 1978), which stipulates that helpers assist with reproduction to repay the cost breeders bear in sharing their territory with helpers; this hypothesis has yet to be tested in this species.

As for female helpers, differences among populations in the frequency of natal helpers suggest that benefits related to acquisition of breeding positions explain why helpers stay, but little can be said about why female helpers help. Females that are unrelated to either breeder account for a relatively large proportion (13–30%) of female helpers. Whether contributions of female helpers to nesting, which are more variable than those of male helpers, differ between unrelated and natal female helpers is unknown. Female helpers tend to disperse to neighboring territories more and remain on the natal territory less compared to male helpers, so there is reason to suspect that their contributions may differ from those of males.

Although the conceptual evolutionary framework developed for male helpers is applicable to natal female helpers, unrelated female helpers need to be examined within a broader framework that also includes other associations of females with nonnatal groups. There is a continuum of relationships of females to nonnatal groups ranging from antagonistic floaters that disrupt nesting and eventually displace the breeding female to females that are accepted by the group, help tend the nest, and eventually inherit the breeding position or in rare instances become cobreeders with the resident female. It is likely that the impact of these unrelated birds on resident breeders range from positive to negative, in association with variation in their behavior. The nature of these relationships, including the reproductive competition and cooperation involved, represents the most important gap in our understanding of the social system of this species.

Alternative life-history pathways

One of the remarkable aspects of the social system of the red-cockaded woodpecker is the variety of life-history pathways available to young birds. Although some pathways may have higher fitness payoffs than others, all offer some probability of success. Different pathways are characterized by different dispersal behavior. The same pathways occur in both sexes but at different frequencies, reflecting differences between the sexes in their fitness payoffs.

Males

Among males, the choice to stay as a helper rather than disperse as a juvenile is facultative (Pasinelli and Walters 2002), but this pathway is open only to the dominant surviving juvenile within a brood, supporting the assertion that it is the preferred pathway (Walters et al. 1992a). The natal helper pathway is associated with not only delayed dispersal, but also reduced dispersal distance. Many natal helpers inherit the breeding position on their natal territory, and most of those that disperse move to adjacent territories. Virtually none disperse farther than three territories (about 3 km) from their natal site. Not all males that have the option to stay do so, and this choice appears to be based on an assessment of local conditions, specifically that of the local neighborhood: males are more likely to stay when there are more high quality territories within 1 km (but not 3.5 km) of the natal site (Pasinelli and Walters 2002).

For those males dispersing as juveniles rather than remaining as natal helpers, acquiring a breeding position is not the only outcome, and perhaps is not even the outcome yielding the highest fitness. Some males acquire a breeding position at age one, but others join nonnatal groups as unrelated helpers and many become floaters. The behavior of "unaffiliated" floaters matches the traditional concept of floating: these individuals show little or no association with any particular territory, are often seen alone rather than in the vicinity of a resident group, and evoke aggression from resident groups when detected. Unaffiliated floaters may eventually fill a breeding vacancy on a territory where they

Table 4.3. Fitness payoffs of alternative life-history pathways followed by male red-cockaded woodpeckers at MCBCL, divided into pathways where males remain on their natal territory at age one (Stay) and those where they disperse during their first year (Depart)

Pathway	P (Breed)	Years	Fledglings	Annual production	Fitness	N
Stay						
Helper Inherit	53%*	4.1	6.6	1.60	3.5	98
Helper Disperse	53%*	4.5	6.1	1.41	3.2	88
Juvenile Inherit	100%	5.9	8.3	1.38	8.3	19
Depart						
Breeder	100%	4.0	4.6	1.14	4.6	44
Helper	38%	3.7	3.7	1.25	1.4	15
Floater	60%	4.6	6.2	1.42	3.7	51

Measures include the probability of becoming a breeder (P (Breed)), the average number of years spent as a breeder (Years), the average number of fledglings produced over the breeding lifetime (Fledglings), the average number of fledglings produced per year (Annual Production), and the average number of fledglings produced per individual (including those that died before becoming breeders) (Fitness). Sample sizes are the number of breeding individuals in each category, except for Depart: Helper and Depart: Floater, which are the total number of individuals following that pathway including those that died before becoming breeders.

* Calculated jointly based on the proportion of helpers that died prior to becoming breeders.

were previously observed, but they may also become breeders elsewhere. In contrast, "affiliated" floaters are consistently observed on a particular territory, usually in close proximity to the resident group, with which they engage in highly antagonist interactions. Male affiliated floaters often eventually become breeders in the neighborhood of the territory with which they are associated, sometimes through budding. More rarely, male affiliated floaters replace the resident breeder or join the group as an unrelated helper.

The factors influencing the choices of dispersing juvenile males to become breeders, unrelated helpers, or floaters are unknown, but the fitness payoffs of these pathways offer some clues. Our data indicate that remaining on the natal territory is indeed an effective means to acquire a high quality territory, as (1) annual productivity of natal helpers that become breeders is high, and (2) among individuals that become breeders at age one, those breeding on their natal territory are more productive than those breeding on nonnatal territories (Table 4.3). Departing the natal territory in the first year to become an unrelated helper has a particularly low payoff, as many such individuals die before

becoming a breeder, and those that do breed are not very productive. This, and the fact that males can only join groups lacking other male helpers (Walters 1990), suggests that unrelated helpers occur on relatively low-quality territories.

An alternative interpretation of these patterns is that the dominant males that remain on their natal territory outperform subordinate males that depart due to inherent differences between dominants and subordinates. The high productivity of males that become breeders through floating belies this interpretation. Early discussions of the evolution of cooperative breeding postulated that the inviability of floating was one of the factors that promoted retention of offspring on the natal territory (Koenig and Pitelka 1981). In red-cockaded woodpeckers, however, floating appears to be an effective means for subordinate males to attain breeding status on high-quality territories.

The fitness payoffs presented in Table 4.3 apply to males that have survived to age one. Dominant males have a survival advantage over subordinate males during the first year (Ragheb and Walters 2011) that is sufficient, when combined with the greater productivity of males that become breeders through natal helping, to more than compensate for the fact that not all natal helpers become breeders. Consequently, staying as a helper has a higher fitness payoff than dispersing as a juvenile (Walters et al. 1992a). Among males dispersing as juveniles, the payoffs of floating and breeding on a nonnatal territory at age one are very close (Table 4.3), confirming that floating is a viable pathway to becoming a breeder for subordinate males. Relative to the latter, the former involves delaying breeding in order to acquire a higher quality territory, analogous to the contrast between natal helpers and dispersing juveniles. Becoming an unrelated helper appears to be "making the best of a bad job."

Females

In contrast to males, females rarely inherit breeding status on the natal territory, either in their first year or after helping, as it requires the death of all male relatives living on the territory (Table 4.1). Besides being fewer, female natal helpers do not remain as long as male natal helpers: on MCBCL only 6% of natal female helpers are age three or older, compared to 31% of male helpers. Female mortality is not sufficiently high to account for this difference, suggesting that female helpers are more actively trying to disperse than male helpers.

Most females disperse from the natal territory as juveniles, and at age one, like males, they may be breeders, unrelated helpers, unaffiliated floaters, or affiliated floaters. Juvenile females engage in foraying prior to dispersing, and most disperse within foraying range, which is approximately twice the range of helper dispersal (Kesler et al. 2010). There is an additional long tail in the distribution of female dispersal distances that is accounted for by "jumpers," individuals that, having forayed from their natal territory for several months, make a sudden (i.e., typically accomplished in a single day) long-distance movement to a location well beyond their previous foraying range. The timing of jumping, and the finding that fitness is inversely related to dispersal distance (Pasinelli et al. 2004) suggests that jumping may be a less preferred strategy followed by juveniles that were unable to disperse through foraying.

In any case, the dispersal distance distribution of males has the same three components as that of females – a short-distance distribution associated with natal helpers, an intermediate-distance distribution associated with juveniles, and a long tail associated with juveniles – suggesting that male dispersal behavior is similar to that documented in females.

The same differences in degree of association and aggression with resident groups distinguish unrelated helpers, unaffiliated floaters, and affiliated floaters for both one-year-old females and males. In contrast to males, the subsequent fates of these three types of individuals are very similar among females. There are some differences, however. Juvenile females sometimes displace resident breeders, as opposed to replacing a breeder that has perished (Daniels and Walters 2000b), and this appears to be the bailiwick of affiliated floaters. The rare instances of cobreeding, which takes the form of two females laying in the same nest, involve females that joined groups as unrelated helpers and participated in nesting with the resident female after several years of helping.

The fitness consequences associated with the various pathways open to females follow the same pattern as in males, but are not complicated by differences in age or dominance rank. Remaining on the natal territory as a helper appears to be an effective way to acquire a high-quality territory, despite the fact the inheriting the natal territory is not an option (Table 4.4). As with males, it appears that unrelated helpers are associated with low-quality territories, that floating is an effective means to acquire a high-quality territory, and that the unrelated helper pathway has the lowest fitness payoff. Floaters and natal helpers are less common in the Sandhills than at MCBCL, where competition for breeding positions is more intense (Table 4.1). This suggests that acquiring a breeding position at age one is the best pathway for females when sufficient numbers of breeding positions are available, but that natal helping and floating are good options that focus on high-quality territories when breeding opportunities are more scarce. In general, however, we know little about how the capabilities of the individual and the social dynamics of the resident groups interact to influence the pathways followed by dispersing juveniles.

Table 4.4. Fitness payoffs of alternative life-history pathways followed by female red-cockaded woodpeckers at MCBCL, divided into pathways where females remain on their natal territory at age one (Stay) and those where they disperse during their first year (Depart)

Pathway	P (Breed)	Years	Fledglings	Annual production	Fitness	N
Stay						
Helper Disperse	50%	3.8	6.2	1.61	3.1	92
Depart						
Breeder	100%	3.4	4.8	1.46	4.8	173
Helper	77%	2.5	3.1	1.28	2.4	14
Floater	58%	3.7	5.7	1.55	3.3	171

Measures include the probability of becoming a breeder (P (Breed)), the average number of years spent as a breeder (Years), the average number of fledglings produced over the breeding lifetime (Fledglings), the average number of fledglings produced per year (Annual Production), and the average number of fledglings produced per individual (including those that died before becoming breeders) (Fitness). Sample sizes are the total number of individuals following that pathway including those that died before becoming breeders.

Unraveling the complexities of these dynamics is the next challenge in understanding the social system of the red-cockaded woodpecker.

Conservation

Twenty-five years ago we drilled artificial cavities in live pine trees to test the hypothesis that variation in habitat quality, specifically presence or absence of their unique clusters of cavities, explained the evolution of cooperative breeding in red-cockaded woodpeckers. We interpreted this experiment as a test of the benefits of philopatry and habitat saturation hypotheses (Walters et al. 1992b). The experiment worked, with 18 of 20 (90%) experimental territories occupied within two years compared to 0 of 20 control territories in similar unoccupied habitat without drilled cavities. The results had clear management implications, as the experiment resulted in the addition of 18 groups, representing an unprecedented population increase (Copeyon et al. 1991) at a time when many populations were declining toward likely extirpation (Conner et al. 2001).

That experiment, although motivated by a desire to test a key hypothesis regarding the evolution of cooperative breeding, provided critical information for species conservation. It led to a new management paradigm

that focused on managing territory quality rather than habitat per se, or predators and competitors, as had the previous management strategy (Walters 1991). The new paradigm included constructing recruitment clusters to stimulate population increases and protection of existing cavities through prescribed fire to prevent encroachment by vegetation. This new paradigm eventually became codified in a revised Recovery Plan (USFWS 2003) and is now employed throughout the range of the species. The paradigm works: all three of our formerly declining study populations have increased under its application (Figure 4.6), and two (Sandhills, Eglin) have been formally declared recovered. Dramatic population increases have occurred elsewhere as well, to such an extent that fears of extinction have been replaced with hopes that the species may be removed from the endangered species list in the near future.

The case of the red-cockaded woodpecker thus illustrates the value of basic research and the relevance of behavioral ecology to conservation. Applied research seldom results in paradigm shifts; rather, these result from new knowledge gained through basic research. This is especially true where failure of current management suggests that understanding of the biology of the species is incomplete, as was the case with red-cockaded woodpeckers. Caro and Sherman (2010)

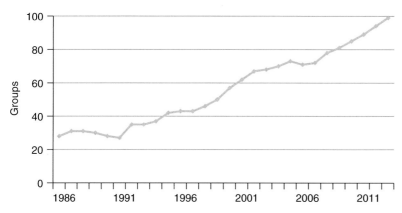

Figure 4.6. The number of family groups of red-cockaded woodpeckers on MCBCL, 1986–2013. The new management paradigm was applied beginning in 1991.

argue that behavioral ecologists cannot be content to limit themselves to answering basic scientific questions if they wish their work to be relevant to conservation, but must also convey the implications of their work to the management and applied conservation communities. Conservation of red-cockaded woodpeckers exemplifies the interaction between behavioral ecologists and managers that Caro and Sherman (2010) advocate. We were provided opportunities to demonstrate the effectiveness of the new management paradigm at MCBCL (Figure 4.6) and Eglin. Both demonstration projects involved a close collaboration of our research group with base biologists and natural resource managers to fully implement the management paradigm and measure the results.

Conclusions

Young red-cockaded woodpeckers behave as they do because remaining on the natal territory as a helper is an effective way to compete for limited, high quality breeding positions. In this case a critical resource, the unique cavity trees, creates the basic limitation in breeding positions by separating high-quality (with existing cavities) from low-quality (no cavities) habitat (although the birds also appear to assess variation within high-quality habitat). Thus the fundamental

concept expressed in the habitat saturation and benefits of philopatry models of the evolution of cooperative breeding, and the general hypothesis that high levels of spatial variation combined with high temporal autocorrelation select for philopatry (Bowler and Benton 2005), work for the red-cockaded woodpecker. Although this concept clearly does not explain all cases of cooperative breeding, we believe that it applies to species characterized by a heritable critical resource, such as the unusually stable, extensive burrow systems of pine voles (*Microtus pinetorum*) and naked mole rats (*Heterocephalus glaber*; Chapter 19), and the granary trees of acorn woodpeckers (*Melanerpes formicivorus*; Chapter 13), as well as the cavity trees of red-cockaded woodpeckers. Old ideas live on when it comes to explaining why helpers help in red-cockaded woodpeckers as well. Most direct benefits of helping have been ruled out, whereas the conditions necessary for helpers to receive indirect benefits through kin selection have been shown to hold.

Many questions remain, however. Is male dispersal behavior similar to that documented in females? Why is floating such an effective strategy, and what determines whether a one-year-old juvenile becomes a floater instead of a breeder? Is there a hierarchy among these choices, such that individuals float only because they failed to become a breeder, or do some elect to float from the outset? Are becoming an unrelated helper and jumping options of last resort, or are they favored options of inferior individuals unable to compete by other means? Do juvenile females detect weaknesses in resident breeding females on high quality territories, or assess receptivity from the breeder and/or helper males, and does this influence whether they choose to become an affiliated floater rather than searching further for breeding opportunities? After more than 30 years of research that began as an attempt to explain the behavior of helping and has taken us deep into the fields of population biology and conservation, we are back where we started, trying to explain social behavior.

Acknowledgments

For funding we thank the U.S. Department of Defense, including Marine Corps Base Camp Lejeune, Department of the Army, Fort Bragg, and Eglin Air Force Base; the National Science Foundation (BSR-8307090, BSR-8717683); and the Harold H. Bailey Fund at Virginia Tech. We thank all past and current field staff and graduate students at Virginia Tech and North Carolina State University for their contributions to the red-cockaded woodpecker long-term demographic data sets. We are particularly indebted in the Sandhills to J. H. Carter III, P. Doerr, and the staff of the Sandhills Ecological Institute: K. Brust, S. Anchor, V. Genovese, and J. Maynard; at MCBCL to K. Rose, B. Simmons, J. Goodson, K. Brust, C. Nycum, R. Meekins, C. Clarkson, and J. Hammond; and at Eglin Air Force Base to L. Blanc, S. Goodman, K. Jones, V. Genovese, A. Butler, J. Tomcho, and K. Gault. We also thank the natural resource staff with which we have worked for their assistance and support: in the Sandhills, U.S. Army Fort Bragg Endangered Species Branch, J. Britcher and J. Schillaci, and the North Carolina Sandhills Gamelands and Wildlife Resources Commission, B. Beck; at MCBCL, C. Tenbrink, G. Haught, J. Townson, and W. Rogers; at Eglin Air Force Base, B. Hagedorn, K. Gault, and C. Petrick. The chapter benefited greatly from comments from the editors, W. Koenig and J. Dickinson.

REFERENCES

Bowler, D. E. and Benton, T. G. (2005). Causes and consequences of animal dispersal strategies: relating individual behavior to spatial dynamics. *Biol. Rev.*, 80, 205–225.

Caro, T. and Sherman, P. W. (2010). Endangered species and a threatened discipline: behavioural ecology. *Trends Ecol. Evol.*, 26, 111–118.

Clark, A. B. (1978). Sex ratio and local resource competition in a prosimian primate. *Science*, 201, 163–165.

Conner, R. N. and Rudolph, D. C. (1995). Excavation dynamics and use patterns of red-cockaded woodpecker cavities: relationships with cooperative breeding. In: *Red-cockaded Woodpecker: Road to Recovery*, ed. R. Costa and S. J. Daniels. Blaine, Washington: Hancock House Publishing, pp. 343–352.

Conner, R. N., Saenz, D., Rudolph, D. C., Ross, W. G., and Kulhavy, D. L. (1998). Red-cockaded woodpecker nest-cavity selection: relationships with cavity age and resin production. *Auk*, 115, 447–454.

Conner, R. N., Rudolph, D. C., and Walters, J. R. (2001). *The Red-cockaded Woodpecker: Surviving in a Fire-maintained Ecosystem*. Austin: University of Texas Press.

Copeyon, C. K., Walters, J. R., and Carter, J. H., III. (1991). Induction of red-cockaded woodpecker group formation by artificial cavity construction. *J. Wildl. Manage.*, 55, 549–556.

Costa, R. and Daniels, S. J., eds. (2004). *Red-cockaded Woodpecker: Road to Recovery*. Blaine, Washington: Hancock House Publishing.

Daniels, S. J. and Walters, J. R. (2000a). Inbreeding depression and its effects on natal dispersal in red-cockaded woodpeckers. *Condor*, 102, 482–491.

Daniels, S. J. and Walters, J. R. (2000b). Between-year breeding dispersal in red-cockaded woodpeckers: multiple causes and estimated cost. *Ecology*, 81, 2473–2484.

DeLotelle, R. S., Leonard, D. L., Jr., and Epting, R. J. (2004). Hatch failure and brood reduction in three central Florida red-cockaded woodpecker populations. In: *Red-cockaded Woodpecker: Road to Recovery*, ed. R. Costa and S. J. Daniels. Blaine, Washington: Hancock House Publishing, pp. 616–623.

Doerr, P. D., Walters, J. R., and Carter, J. H., III. (1989). Reoccupation of abandoned clusters of cavity trees (colonies) by red-cockaded woodpeckers. *Proc. Annu. Conf. Southeast. Assoc. Fish Wildl. Agencies*, 43, 326–336.

Emlen, S. T. (1991). Evolution of cooperative breeding in birds and mammals. In: *Behavioural Ecology: An Evolutionary Approach*, 3rd edn, ed. J. R. Krebs and N. B. Davies, Oxford: Blackwell, pp. 301–337.

Emlen, S. T., Emlen, J. M., and Levin, S. A. (1986). Sex-ratio selection in species with helpers-at-the-nest. *Am. Nat.*, 127, 1–8.

Gaston, A. J. (1978). The evolution of group territorial behavior and cooperative breeding. *Am. Nat.*, 112, 1091–1100.

Gillespie, J. (1977). Natural selection for variances in offspring numbers: a new evolutionary principle. *Am. Nat.*, 111, 1010–1014.

Gowaty, P. A. and Lennartz, M. R. (1985). Sex ratios of nestling and fledgling red-cockaded woodpeckers (*Picoides borealis*) favor males. *Am. Nat.*, 126, 347–353.

Haig, S. M., Belthoff, J. R., and Allen, D. H. (1993). Examination of population structure in red-cockaded woodpeckers using DNA profiles. *Evol.*, 47, 185–194.

Haig, S. M., Walters, J. R., and Plissner, J. H. (1994). Genetic evidence for monogamy in the cooperatively breeding red-cockaded woodpecker. *Behav. Ecol. Sociobiol.*, 34, 295–303.

Harding, S. R. (1997). The dynamics of cavity excavation and use by the red-cockaded woodpecker (*Picoides borealis*). M.Sc. thesis, Virginia Tech, Blacksburg, Virginia.

Harding, S. R. and Walters, J. R. (2002). Processes regulating the population dynamics of red-cockaded woodpecker cavities. *J. Wildl. Manage.*, 66, 1083–1095.

Harding, S. R. and Walters, J. R. (2004). Dynamics of cavity excavation by red-cockaded woodpeckers. In: *Red-cockaded Woodpecker: Road to Recovery*, ed. R. Costa and S. J. Daniels. Blaine, Washington: Hancock House Publishing, pp. 412–422.

Heppell, S. S., Walters, J. R., and Crowder, L. B. (1994). Evaluating management alternatives for red-cockaded woodpeckers: a modeling approach. *J. Wildl. Manage.*, 58, 479–487.

Hooper, R. G. (1983). Colony formation by red-cockaded woodpeckers: hypotheses and management implications. In: *Red-cockaded Woodpecker Symposium II*, ed. D. A. Wood. Atlanta, Georgia: Florida Game and Freshwater Fisheries Commission and U.S. Fish and Wildlife Service, pp. 72–77.

Jackson, J. A. (1971). The evolution, taxonomy, distribution, past populations and current status of the red-cockaded woodpecker. In: *The Ecology and Management of the Red-cockaded Woodpecker*. Tallahassee, Florida: Bureau of Sport Fisheries and Wildlife, and Tall Timbers Research Station, pp. 4–29.

James, F. C., Hess, C. A., and Kufrin, D. (1997). Species-centered environmental analysis: indirect effects of fire history on red-cockaded woodpeckers. *Ecol. Appl.*, 7, 118–129.

James, F. C., Hess, C. A., Kicklighter, B. C., and Thum, R. A. (2001). Ecosystem management and the niche gestalt of the red-cockaded woodpecker in longleaf pine forests. *Ecol. Appl.*, 11, 854–870.

Kesler, D. C., Walters, J. R., and Kappes, J. J., Jr. (2010). Social influences on dispersal and the fat-tailed dispersal distribution in red-cockaded woodpeckers. *Behav. Ecol.*, 21, 1337–1343.

Khan, M. Z. and Walters, J. R. (1997). Is helping a beneficial learning experience for red-cockaded woodpecker (*Picoides borealis*) helpers? *Behav. Ecol. Sociobiol.*, 41, 69–73.

Khan, M. Z. and Walters, J. R. (2000). An analysis of reciprocal exchange of helping behavior in the red-cockaded woodpecker. *Behav. Ecol. Sociobiol.*, 47, 376–381.

Khan, M. Z. and Walters, J. R. (2002). Effects of helpers on breeder survival in the red-cockaded woodpecker (*Picoides borealis*). *Behav. Ecol. Sociobiol.*, 51, 336–344.

Khan, M. Z., McNabb, F. M. A., Walters, J. R., and Sharp, P. J. (2001). Patterns of testosterone and prolactin concentrations and reproductive behavior of helpers and breeders in the cooperatively breeding red-cockaded woodpecker (*Picoides borealis*). *Horm. Behav.*, 40, 1–13.

Koenig, W. D. and Pitelka, F. A. (1981). Ecological factors and kin selection in the evolution of cooperative breeding in birds. In: *Natural Selection and Social Behavior: Recent Research and New Theory*, ed. R. D. Alexander and D. W. Tinkle. New York: Chiron Press, pp. 261–280.

Koenig, W. D. and Walters, J. R. (1999). Sex-ratio selection in species with helpers at the nest: the repayment model revisited. *Am. Nat.*, 153, 124–130.

Kulhavy, D. L., Hooper, R. G., and Costa, R., eds. (1995). *Red-cockaded Woodpecker: Recovery, Ecology and Management*. Nacogdoches, Texas: Center for Applied Studies in Forestry, College of Forestry, Stephen F. Austin State University.

LaBranche, M. S. (1992). Asynchronous hatching, brood reduction and sex ratio biases in red-cockaded woodpeckers. Ph.D. thesis, North Carolina State University, Raleigh.

LaBranche, M. S. and Walters, J. R. (1994). Patterns of mortality in nests of red-cockaded woodpeckers in the Sandhills of southcentral North Carolina. *Wilson Bull.*, 106, 258–271.

Lacey, E. P., Real, L., Antonovics, J., and Heckel, D. G. (1983). Variance models in the study of life histories. *Am. Nat.*, 122, 114–131.

Lape, J. J. (1990). Mate guarding in the red-cockaded woodpecker. M.S. thesis, North Carolina State University, Raleigh.

Lennartz, M. R., Hooper, R. G., and Harlow, R. F. (1987). Sociality and cooperative breeding of red-cockaded woodpeckers, *Picoides borealis*. *Behav. Ecol. Sociobiol.*, 20, 77–88.

Lessells, C. M. and Avery, M. I. (1987). Sex-ratio selection in species with helpers at the nest: some extensions of the repayment model. *Am. Nat.*, 129, 610–620.

Ligon, J. D. (1968). Sexual differences in foraging behavior in two species of *Dendrocopus* woodpeckers. *Auk*, 85, 203–215.

Ligon, J. D. and Burt, D. B. (2004). Evolutionary origins. In: *Ecology and Evolution of Cooperative Breeding in Birds*, ed. W. D. Koenig and J. L. Dickinson. Cambridge: Cambridge University Press, pp. 5–34.

Malueg, A. L., Walters, J. R., and Moore, I. T. (2009). Do stress hormones suppress helper reproduction in the cooperatively breeding red-cockaded woodpecker (*Picoides borealis*)? *Behav. Ecol. Sociobiol.*, 63, 687–698.

McFarlane, R. W. (1992). *A Stillness in the Pines*. New York: W. W. Norton.

O'Connor, R. J. (1978). Brood reduction in birds: selection for fratricide, infanticide, and suicide? *Anim. Behav.*, 26, 79–96.

Pasinelli, G. and Walters, J. R. (2002). Social and environmental factors affect natal dispersal and philopatry of male red-cockaded woodpeckers. *Ecology*, 83, 2229–2239.

Pasinelli, G., Schiegg, K., and Walters, J. R. (2004). Genetic and environmental influences on natal dispersal distance in a resident bird species. *Am. Nat.*, 164, 660–669.

Pizzoni-Ardemani, A. (1990). Sexual dimorphism and geographic variation in the red-cockaded woodpecker (*Picoides borealis*). M.S. thesis, North Carolina State University, Raleigh.

Ragheb, E. L. H. and Walters, J. R. (2011). Favouritism or intrabrood competition? Access to food and the benefits of philopatry for red-cockaded woodpeckers. *Anim. Behav.*, 82, 329–338.

Reed, J. M. and Walters, J. R. (1996). Helper effects on variance components of fitness in the cooperatively breeding red-cockaded woodpecker. *Auk*, 113, 608–616.

Rodewald, P. G., Withgott, J. H., and Smith, K. G. (2013). Pine warbler (*Setophaga pinus*). In: *The Birds of North America Online*, ed. A. Poole. Ithaca, New York: Cornell Lab of Ornithology, doi: 10.2173/bna.438.

Rudolph, D. C., Kyle, H., and Conner, R. N. (1990). Red-cockaded woodpeckers vs. rat snakes: the effectiveness of the resin barrier. *Wilson Bull.*, 102, 14–22.

Rudolph, D. C., Conner, R. N., Schaefer, R. R., and Koerth, N. E. (2007). Red-cockaded woodpecker foraging behavior. *Wilson J. Ornithol.*, 119, 170–180.

Schiegg, K., Pasinelli, G., Walters, J. R., and Daniels, S. J. (2002). Inbreeding and experience affect response to climate change by endangered woodpeckers. *Proc. R. Soc. London B*, 269, 1153–1159.

Thompson, R. L., ed. (1971). *The Ecology and Management of the Red-cockaded Woodpecker*. Tallahassee, Florida: Bureau of Sport Fisheries and Wildlife and Tall Timbers Research Station.

U.S. Fish and Wildlife Service (USFWS). (2003). Recovery plan for the red-cockaded woodpecker (*Picoides borealis*). Atlanta, Georgia: U.S. Fish and Wildlife Service.

Walters, J. R. (1990). Red-cockaded woodpeckers: a "primitive" cooperative breeder. In: *Cooperative Breeding in Birds: Long-term Studies of Ecology and Behavior*, ed. P. B. Stacey and W. D. Koenig. Cambridge: Cambridge University Press, pp. 67–102.

Walters, J. R. (1991). Application of ecological principles to the management of endangered species: the case of the red-cockaded woodpecker. *Annu. Rev. Ecol. Syst.*, 22, 505–523.

Walters, J. R., Doerr, P. D., and Carter, J. H., III. (1988). The cooperative breeding system of the red-cockaded woodpecker. *Ethology*, 78, 275–305.

Walters, J. R., Doerr, P. D., and Carter, J. H., III. (1992a). Delayed dispersal and reproduction as a life history tactic in cooperative breeders: fitness calculations from red-cockaded woodpeckers. *Am. Natur.*, 139, 623–643.

Walters, J. R., Copeyon, C. K., and Carter, J. H., III. (1992b). Test of the ecological basis of cooperative breeding in red-cockaded woodpeckers. *Auk*, 109, 90–97.

Walters, J. R., Daniels, S. J., Carter, J. H., III, and Doerr, P. D. (2002). Defining quality of red-cockaded woodpecker foraging habitat based on habitat use and fitness. *J. Wildl. Manage.*, 66, 1064–1082.

Walters, J. R., Gault, K. E., Hagedorn, B. W., Petrick, C. J., Phillips, L. F., Jr., et al. (2004). Effectiveness of recruitment clusters and intrapopulation translocation in promoting growth of the red-cockaded woodpecker population on Eglin Air Force Base, Florida. In: *Red-cockaded Woodpecker: Road to Recovery*, ed. R. Costa and S. J. Daniels. Blaine, Washington: Hancock House Publishing, pp. 325–334.

Wood, D. A., ed. (1983). *Red-cockaded woodpecker Symposium II*. Atlanta, Georgia: Florida Game and Freshwater Fisheries Commission and U.S. Fish and Wildlife Service.

5

Florida scrub-jays: Oversized territories and group defense in a fire-maintained habitat

John W. Fitzpatrick and Reed Bowman

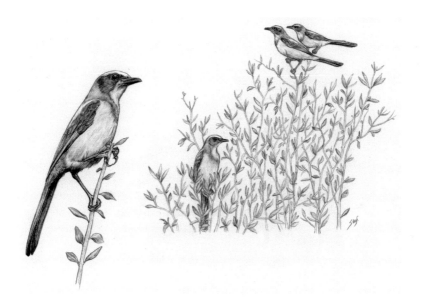

Introduction

Long-term study of Florida scrub-jays (*Aphelocoma coerulescens*) at Archbold Biological Station began in 1969 when Glen E. Woolfenden noticed extra jays at a nest, and color-banded birds in seven territories. Aware of growing interest in helpers-at-the-nest and the evolution of cooperation, Glen correctly guessed that he had found an informative species for examining the population biology of a group-living bird. By 1972, when John Fitzpatrick first joined him as a college intern, Woolfenden's study tract had expanded to 18 territories and we witnessed our first example of "territorial budding" (Woolfenden and Fitzpatrick 1978). In 1991, Reed Bowman joined the team and expanded the study to include two nearby populations, one in suburban and the other in fragmented habitat; by 2003 we were studying Florida scrub-jays in over 150 territories. Here, we focus on data from the ongoing study in the original "demography tract" at Archbold (currently 75 to 85 territories), drawing also on insights gained from the other populations.

The Florida scrub-jay presents an exceptional model for studying a comparatively simple cooperative breeding system. The species lives in naturally low-stature scrub on two-dimensional terrain, facilitating detailed observation and monitoring of both behavior and nesting. Every jay born into our population is color-banded and genetically sampled on a standardized post-hatch day (day 11), and immigrants are captured and banded readily. The Florida scrub-jay easily habituates to humans, and even learns to approach us if occasionally rewarded with peanut bits. Consequently, we have been able to census the study population exhaustively every month since April 1971, yielding an extraordinarily detailed record of survivorship, reproduction, and dispersal. Territories are vigorously defended year-round along narrow and clear-cut boundaries, permitting us to map precisely the tightly packed spatial configuration of the population each year. Because the Florida scrub-jay is nonmigratory, highly philopatric, and socially and genetically monogamous, we have accumulated a 14-generation pedigree of known-age, known-parentage individuals whose lifespans and breeding outputs we measured precisely.

Moreover, the Florida scrub-jay is a singular-nesting species in which pre-breeding offspring typically remain in the natal territory for a minimum of one year, living as a cooperative family group with their parents or stepparents. These features make the Florida scrub-jay "blessedly simple" as a model species exhibiting an early stage along what we presume to be an evolutionary track toward more complex cooperative-breeding social systems (Fitzpatrick and Woolfenden 1986). Adding to the fortuitous beauty of this model is the fact that its sister complex of scrub-jay taxa in western North America and Mexico (western scrub-jay, *A. californica* and island scrub-jay, *A. insularis*) do not exhibit cooperative breeding except at the extreme southern end of the former's range (Oaxaca, Mexico; Burt and Peterson 1993), while a closely related congener – the Mexican jay (*A. wollweberi*) – exhibits large group sizes and plural nesting within territories that are about the same size as in the singular-breeding Florida scrub-jay. So, for purposes of this chapter, three questions serve as our focus: (1) Why does a scrub-jay cooperate in Florida, and not in western North America? (2) Given

cooperation, why not nest plurally? (3) Given singular nesting, why defend such large territories? The answers to these questions are best provided in reverse order.

Geographical ecology

The only bird species endemic to Florida, the Florida scrub-jay has one of the most narrowly restricted ranges of any North American bird. Confined to distinctive fire-maintained, xeric oak scrub on patches of well-drained sandy soils, the species probably once numbered well over 100,000 family groups across the Florida peninsula (Woolfenden and Fitzpatrick 1996). Genetic sampling across the species' range has revealed 14 genetically distinct subpopulations (Coulon et al. 2008), suggesting long association with a naturally fragmented landscape of sandy ridges, many of which were deposited as beach dunes during Pleistocene marine inundations. The Florida scrub-jay has been isolated and genetically diverging from western scrub-jay populations since the late Miocene or early Pliocene (Emslie 1996; McCormack et al. 2010).

During the twentieth century, habitat loss resulting from widespread agricultural conversion, residential and commercial development, and fire suppression caused extensive population fragmentation and local extirpation. A thorough survey in 1992–1993 documented that the population had declined by more than 90% in 100 years, and 25% in the previous decade alone. At that time, the total population size consisted of about 10,000 individuals living in ~3,000 family groups (Fitzpatrick et al. 1994; Stith et al. 1996).

The study population at Archbold Biological Station is located near the southern end of a central Florida sand ridge (Lake Wales Ridge), on which a north–south oriented network of preserves currently protects about 500 family groups (Turner et al. 2006). For numerous reasons, Florida scrub-jay populations on unprotected habitat are demographically unstable and continue to decline across their dwindling range. However, by 2010, even Florida scrub-jays on protected lands had declined by an additional 25%, and the total population was estimated to be about 6,000 individuals in about 2,400 family groups (Boughton and Bowman 2011).

Natural history

Life on a precarious resource base

Within contiguous habitat, Florida scrub-jays live in a tight mosaic of permanently defended territories varying in size from 4–15 ha (mean = 10 ha), which is extremely large for a corvid of its body size (70–85 g; Shank 1986). Territories are occupied only where proper habitat exists: a rare, distinctive, fire-prone mix of stunted woody perennials growing on sandy, nutrient-starved soils. Florida scrub is dominated by five species of clonal oaks (*Quercus* spp.), two species of palmetto (*Serenoa repens and Sabal etonia*), ericaceous shrubs, and patches of bare sand. Tree cover in optimal habitat is sparse (<15% canopy cover), mainly slash pine (*Pinus elliotii*) and sand pine (*P. clausa*) (Breininger et al. 2006). Fires are frequent unless suppressed by humans, with natural return intervals of 7–15 years (Menges 2007). As detailed in the "All important fire cycle" section, Florida scrub-jays show strong preference for recently burned scrub and rapidly disappear from fire-suppressed habitat, which in turn becomes occupied by a more arboreal competitor/predator, the blue jay (*Cyanocitta cristata*).

Florida scrub-jays forage on or near the ground by searching and probing leaves for arthropods (mainly orthoptera, lepidoptera, and arachnids) and small vertebrates (tree frogs, anoles, and small snakes). Acorns – the fruit of oaks – constitute a crucial resource during fall and especially during the winter dry season, when animal food is especially scarce. Each individual jay harvests 6,000 to 8,000 acorns each fall, caches them singly in open sand areas throughout the territory, and recovers and consumes them during winter months (DeGange et al. 1989). Even in optimal habitat, both animal and acorn resources are seasonally variable and thinly distributed across the oak scrub, so Florida scrub-jays spend up to half their time foraging (DeGange 1976). Territory means everything to the birds, as it guarantees access to scarce and difficult-to-find resources in a comparatively unproductive biotic environment.

Each territory is defended by a permanently mated, monogamous pair (fewer than 3% of pair-bonds end in divorce; Marzluff et al. 1996), and these territory-holding pairs are the only jays to build nests and sire offspring. In any given year about half the territories also contain 1–4 nonbreeding helpers, mainly comprised of surviving offspring from preceding breeding seasons (Woolfenden and Fitzpatrick 1984).

Pairs or family groups move about the territory together. During much of the day, at least one of the group members perches on a high snag, watching for predators and conspecific territorial intruders, constituting a well-coordinated sentinel system (McGowan and Woolfenden 1989). All group members participate in territory defense, which occurs year-round and consists of ritualized flight displays, distinctive loud vocalizations (including an elaborate, female-specific *hiccup* display), and chases. Outright physical fights between rival males at territorial boundaries are rare and brief.

Breeding is synchronous (mid-March through early June). With rare exceptions only a single brood is produced, but pairs renest several times if early attempts fail (almost always owing to predation). Clutch size varies from 2–5 and most clutches are 3–4 eggs. In most years about a third of pairs fail to produce any fledglings. Nest success improves with group size up to four helpers, after which it declines (Woolfenden and Fitzpatrick 1984; Mumme 1992).

Survival and reproduction are highly variable from year to year. In good habitat, survival of both male and female breeders averages 81%, and survival of fledglings to age one year averages 35%. On average, production of offspring surviving to age one exceeds the appearance of breeding vacancies caused by death of breeding adults by more than 50% (Figure 5.1). Yearling jays are physiologically capable of breeding, but almost always remain in their natal territory as nonbreeding helpers. Ninety percent of helpers reside with at least one of their parents, and 55% reside with both (Woolfenden and Fitzpatrick 1984). Beginning mainly after reaching age one, female nonbreeders engage in dispersal forays in which they visit territories up to several kilometers from home, usually returning to the natal territory by late afternoon. Male nonbreeders are more philopatric, and during nesting season they are more attentive to nestlings and dependent fledglings than are females (Stallcup and Woolfenden 1978;

Table 5.1. Ages at first breeding for Florida scrub-jays in long-term demographic study tract at Archbold Biological Station, 1969–2014

	Age (percent of total for each sex)							Total
	1	2	3	4	5	6	7	
Males	16 (4.1)	199 (51.6)	116 (30.1)	35 (9.1)	14 (3.6)	4 (1.0)	2 (0.5)	386
Females	20 (6.3)	163 (51.3)	112 (35.2)	20 (6.3)	2 (0.6)	0	1 (0.3)	318

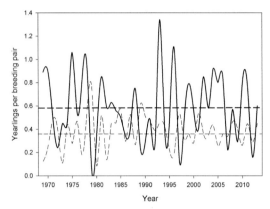

Figure 5.1. Annual production of Florida scrub-jay yearlings per pair observed in the study tract, 1969 to 2013 (bold lines) compared to the number of yearlings required to replace lost breeders (= twice the yearly mortality of breeders in the tract; dashed lines). For both parameters, annual data are splined and straight lines are long-term means. In 35 of 45 years, more yearlings were produced (mean = 0.582 per pair) than breeding vacancies appeared (mean = 0.347 per pair).

pair and successfully defend a new territory well away from the natal territory of either. Importantly, such "de novo" pairing is most frequent in areas where fire has converted a large patch of previously unsuitable habitat into optimal, but unoccupied scrub.

Breeding vacancies caused by death of a breeder immediately result in active, multiple-day competitions for the widow – and his/her territory – among members of the appropriate sex. In addition to courtship feeding, during which the breeder male feeds the breeder female, initial pairing behavior is characterized by extensive, repeated, and coordinated territorial displays. The male performs exaggerated undulating flights accompanied by repeated loud calls, and the female follows, perches near the male, and delivers vigorous *hiccup* displays. Pairing is an individual affair for both males and females. Same-sex siblings may compete for the same breeding vacancy, and coalitions play no obvious role in conferring an advantage to the winner.

McGowan and Woolfenden 1990). Helpers of both sexes actively defend territory boundaries, participate in sentinel duties, and mob predators. Male helpers, especially older ones, are almost as vigorous in territory defense as the male breeder.

Modal age at first breeding is two years for both sexes (Table 5.1), and two-thirds of new breeders do so by pairing with a widowed jay in an already-established territory (breeder replacement). Replacement males that pair with a neighboring widow sometimes retain a portion of their natal territory (bud-replacement). About a quarter of male breeders do so by territorial budding or direct inheritance. Only rarely do two jays

Among- and within-group competition

Exclusive ownership of a significant parcel of high quality oak scrub habitat is the essential commodity governing fitness in this species. Every aspect of the Florida scrub-jay social system relates to the overriding importance of competing for, and successfully defending, a large territory.

By definition, in a system where territory ownership is everything, among-group competition rules. Florida scrub-jay territories grow and shrink as a function of group size (Woolfenden and Fitzpatrick 1984). Successful breeding begets helpers, which participate in territory defense and help the family retain and gain ground. Breeders that fail to produce young for a year or two are at a competitive disadvantage, and their territories shrink. Novice pairs struggle for space, sometimes for years. The importance of owning as large a territory as the neighborhood will allow cannot be overstated.

Within family groups, conventional dominance hierarchies exist, but except in the vicinity of the nest, dominance is expressed only subtly and infrequently through jabs and supplants, especially over food. Males dominate females, breeders dominate helpers, and older sibs dominate younger ones (Woolfenden and Fitzpatrick 1977). Dominant jays also occasionally recover and steal acorns cached by subordinates.

Monogamy and reproductive skew

Among socially monogamous bird species, the Florida scrub-jay anchors near absolute genetic monogamy. An extensive parentage analysis (Townsend et al. 2011) compared our three ecologically distinct populations (native, suburban, and fragmented) over a 3-year span. Among 279 fully genotyped broods, only 2 of 771 offspring (0.26%; one each in two different nests) had been sired by a male other than the social father. Even the many groups in which nonbreeding auxiliaries were unrelated to the opposite-sex breeder (resulting from mate replacement) yielded no cases of within-group extra-pair siring. We interpret absence of extra-pair parentage as a consequence of an extremely competitive territorial environment: long-lived breeders defend super-large territories in a severely limited habitat. The comparatively few individuals that become territory owners have demonstrated their quality, so females lack incentive to invite extra-territorial males to sire their offspring. Moreover, division of labor is strong within the pair, and reproductive success increases with pair-bond duration (Marzluff et al. 1996), so breeders of both sexes have significant incentive to invest in the survival of their mate. Togetherness prevails.

Lacking opportunity for helpers to sire offspring within the group, it would seem that reproductive skew is absolute in this species, even when presence of step-parents removes incest avoidance as an issue. Indeed, male breeders routinely dominate their sons and stepsons near the nest until well after the eggs hatch.

Begging the question of skew, however, is the fact that many male helpers do ultimately gain breeding status through territorial budding on a portion of their parents' territory. The breeding pair may inhibit budding by dominating and chasing prospecting females, but just as often they actually assist in the budding process by aggressively expanding territorial boundaries in the region where a son is beginning to pair (Woolfenden and Fitzpatrick 1984). The questions of which males bud and why many do not remain unresolved but, as discussed in the "Territorial budding: not for the faint of heart" section, may reflect individual differences in quality.

Incest taboo and sex ratio

As a rule, group members do not pair with one another, so close incest (sib-sib or parent-offspring matings) is rare. Of 4,248 known-parentage nestlings, only 27 (0.6%) were the product of parent-offspring pairs ($N = 6$ pairs, none lasting more than one year, and 10 offspring) or sib-sib pairs ($N = 1$ pair that produced 17 offspring over four years). More distant inbreeding (including cousin-cousin, nephew-aunt, and grandparent-grandoffspring) occurs infrequently, an incidental outcome of short-dispersal distances. We have detected no evidence of kin recognition or kin avoidance beyond the taboo against breeding with a member of the immediate family group. Lifetime reproductive success of inbred offspring is significantly lower than that of noninbred offspring, indicating strong selection on incest avoidance (N. Chen, unpubl. data).

The sex ratio of nestlings is even (of 2,373 nestlings with sex documented genetically at day 11 post-hatch, 1,167 [49.2%] were males and 1,206 [50.8%] were females). In most years the nonbreeding population is modestly skewed toward males, because the more dispersive female nonbreeders experience elevated mortality while male nonbreeders mainly remain at home and "accumulate" as older helpers (Woolfenden and Fitzpatrick 1984). However, this modest bias does not result in differential breeding opportunities, because breeder mortality (i.e., the appearance of breeding vacancies) is exactly equal between the sexes (males: 81.0%, $N = 2,071$ bird-years; females: 81.2%,

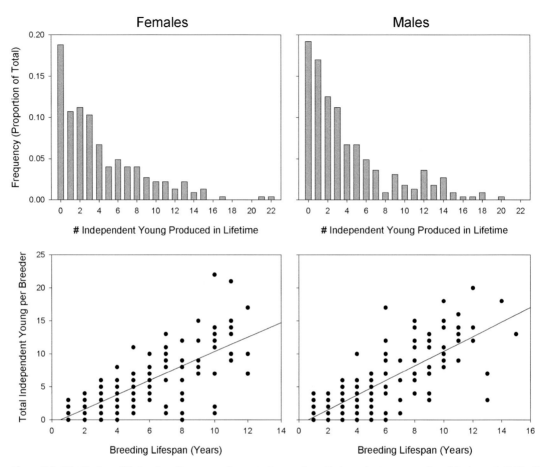

Figure 5.2. Distribution of lifetime breeding success (presented as number of independent young produced during an individual's full breeding life) and its relation to breeding lifespan. Patterns are identical for females ($N = 265$) and males ($N = 307$). Samples are restricted to breeders whose entire reproductive histories are known and whose breeding cohorts are all dead.

$N = 2{,}101$ bird-years). Given strict monogamy, the sexes experience symmetrical breeding opportunities and identical distributions of lifetime reproductive success (Figure 5.2).

Kinship and fitness benefits of helping

Because most helpers live with their surviving parents, the Florida scrub-jay cooperative unit is a kin group and helpers contribute to rearing and defending the territory of close relatives. Moreover, reproductive success increases significantly with group size, up to 4 helpers

(Figure 5.3), so nonbreeders gain fractional indirect fitness benefits by helping. Specifically, mean production of yearlings increases by about 0.1–0.2 yearlings per helper, and while these "extra" fractional yearlings are not always full-sibs, clearly they represent indirect benefits that reinforce any direct selective advantages of helping.

Several lines of evidence suggest that indirect benefits do not by themselves explain the origin and maintenance of the Florida scrub-jay cooperative-breeding system. First, incremental increases in mean reproductive success with helper number are slight compared to

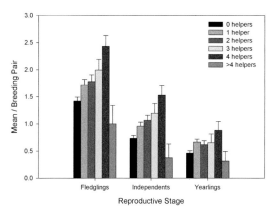

Figure 5.3. Mean annual reproductive success for three offspring stages relative to Florida scrub-jay group size. Offspring production is significantly higher for groups with helpers (1 helper, $N = 456$; 2 helpers, $N = 264$; 3 helpers, $N = 150$, 4 helpers, $N = 51$, >4 helpers, $N = 24$) than without ($N = 1,038$), but the increase clearly drops with >4 helpers.

the fitness benefits of independent breeding (Fitzpatrick and Woolfenden 1989). Second, increased production of yearlings among larger groups is less clear-cut than for production of fledglings (Figure 5.3), suggesting that increased group size actually negatively influences offspring survival. As discussed later, this negative impact is most apparent for groups inhabiting smaller territories, and it ultimately dampens the indirect fitness gains for each individual helper among larger groups. Nevertheless, we see no evidence of jays dispersing earlier, or declining opportunities to help, when born into larger groups, as we might expect if indirect benefits alone drive pre-breeding behavior.

Third, through various circumstances, some individuals reside with unrelated breeders, and while frequency of provisioning at the nest declines with relatedness to the nestlings being fed (Mumme 1992), unrelated helpers are otherwise fully engaged as members of the cooperative group. Fourth, helpers are more likely to disperse when a same-sex stepparent pairs with a widowed parent than when an opposite-sex stepparent does so (Goldstein et al. 1998), yet the indirect fitness benefits of helping would be identical in either case. Behavioral observations suggest that this pattern results from aggression by the stepparent to an

individual perceived as a same-sex rival for the privilege of breeding. We conclude that fractionally positive kinship benefits add an indirect component to inclusive fitness, reinforcing a behavioral syndrome among pre-breeders (delayed dispersal, cooperative territory defense, coordinated sentinel system, and feeding of dependent young) that is selectively favored in an intensely competitive territorial environment primarily as a strategy for directly improving the odds of entering the breeding population.

Endocrine factors and cooperative breeding

Studies of reproductive hormones indicate that helpers, even yearlings, are physiologically competent to breed. Male Florida scrub-jay nonbreeders have similar levels of luteinizing hormone (LH) as breeders and exhibit similar increases in LH following a gonadotropic-releasing hormone (cGnRH) challenge, suggesting that the hypothalamo-pituitary-gonadal endocrine axis is functional in nonbreeders. Nonbreeders have lower testosterone (T) levels and smaller testes than breeders during the breeding season, but their seasonal changes in T-levels parallel those of breeders and their testes are much larger than regressed testes (Schoech et al. 1996a). Male nonbreeders exposed to females with experimentally elevated estradiol (E) exhibit higher T-levels than control nonbreeders. Female nonbreeders have similar levels of E and LH as breeders, and have similar responses to a cGnRH challenge. Thus, nonbreeders are physiologically primed for breeding, and probably just lack necessary extrinsic stimuli such as within-pair interactions that accompany acquiring a mate and territory. This interpretation is supported by the increased frequency of breeding among yearlings when constraints on independent breeding are relaxed, such as in suburban populations.

Breeding behavior also can be modulated by the hypothalamo-pituitary-adrenal axis, through the production of corticosterone (CORT), produced in response to a wide range of stressors. Since breeding Florida scrub-jays socially dominate within-group nonbreeders, agonistic interactions could keep CORT levels in nonbreeders elevated and thus suppress breeding, producing the lower T-levels observed in nonbreeders. However, neither baseline nor stress responses differed between breeders and nonbreeders, so it seems unlikely that nonbreeders are reproductively suppressed via CORT (Schoech et al. 1997).

Florida scrub-jay helpers sire no offspring, even though physiologically capable of doing so. However, they do exhibit parental care, feeding both nestlings and fledglings of the territorial pair. In many vertebrates, increases in prolactin and progesterone are associated with parental care, and in birds these hormones peak during incubation and nestling periods. In Florida scrub-jays, females have higher prolactin levels than males, breeders have higher levels than nonbreeders, and nonbreeders that feed young have higher levels than those that do not. For both breeders and nonbreeders, nestling feeding rates vary with prolactin levels, supporting the hypothesis that nestling-feeding by nonbreeders is mediated by prolactin (Schoech et al. 1996b).

Early corticosterone levels may influence fitness

Increasing evidence exists that exposure to early developmental stress has profound effects throughout an animal's life (Schoech et al. 2012). Early levels of CORT may set the stress responses of individuals later in life, even shaping suites of correlated behavioral traits in adults. In Florida scrub-jays, maternal nest attentiveness and paternal provisioning influence nestling CORT levels, with increased parental care resulting in lower CORT levels (Rensel et al. 2010). Parental care may vary with individual quality, but it is also mediated by environmental conditions, such as predation risk and food availability. In suburbs, where predictable food leads to efficient foraging, breeders increase both provisioning rates and nest attentiveness (Aldredge et al. 2012; Niederhauser and Bowman 2014), both of which reduce nestling CORT levels. Nestling baseline and stress-induced CORT levels are repeatable at older ages (Rensel and Schoech 2011), and indeed, baseline CORT levels of suburban adults are much lower than those from wildlands (Schoech et al. 2007).

Experimental food supplementation can reduce CORT levels of wildland adults, but not to the extent observed in the suburbs (Reynolds et al. 2003).

Nestling mass is correlated with feeding rates, and is an important predictor of subsequent fitness (Mumme et al. 2015), so some correlation between early CORT exposure and fitness probably exists. This leads to a surprising paradox among suburban birds, which fledge at lighter mass (which predicts poorer fitness) but with low baseline CORT levels. This paradox could lead to surprising differences in fitness patterns across populations in different landscape contexts (Tringali and Bowman 2015). Early exposure to CORT may have other effects, leading to individual variation in traits that could have profound fitness effects, such as dispersal distance (Ferguson et al. 2014), antipredator behavior (Jones et al. 2014), and learning flexibility (Bebus et al. 2014).

Suburban habitat provides resource-base comparisons

Conversion of native Florida scrub into suburban residential communities significantly reduces arthropod prey of Florida scrub-jays (Shawkey et al. 2004), but also results in spatially and temporally predictable sources of high-nutrient foods such as peanuts, bird seed, and dog food that can be efficiently gathered with minimal search time (Fleischer et al. 2003). Likely in response to abundant food, suburban jays defend smaller territories, begin breeding earlier in the spring, and lay larger clutches compared to jays in nearby wildland habitats (Bowman 1998; Schoech et al. 2004). In addition, in suburban jays mean age at first breeding is lower with more birds breeding rather than helping at age one compared to jays in wildlands. Similar patterns have been observed under enhanced environmental conditions in other cooperative breeders (Covas et al. 2004).

Despite the surplus of human-provided foods, scarcity of arthropods creates a foraging paradox during the nestling period. Wildland jays feed nestlings exclusively arthropods (Stallcup and Woolfenden 1978), but 15–30% of suburban nestlings' diet is comprised of human-provided foods, mostly of plant origin (Sauter et al. 2006). Optimal foraging rules may influence diet choices of suburban Florida scrub-jays: when given a choice between lepidoptera larva and peanuts for provisioning young, suburban jays exclusively chose lepidoptera, but when handling time for lepidoptera was slightly increased, providers switched to peanuts. Suburban nestlings reared on human-provided food grow more slowly, are more prone to brood reduction, and fledge at smaller body mass, which in turn reduces postfledging survival (Bowman 1998; Sauter 2005). Significantly reduced capacity of breeders to produce offspring that survive to age one is a primary cause of decline among suburban Florida scrub-jay populations over much of their modern range, and underscores the importance for this species of having sufficient, high-quality resources within the territory.

Predictors of recruitment

Age, dominance, group size, and territory size

Beginning before age one, nonbreeders explore their neighborhood, exhibiting particular interest in noisy boundary disputes that accompany competitions over breeding vacancies. Yearlings in native habitat rarely become breeders because both ecological and social conditions constrain breeding opportunities (Table 5.1). Older nonbreeders prevail in pairing with widows. When two or more male nonbreeders coexist in a family, the older is first to become a breeder, whether via direct inheritance, budding, or mate-replacement nearby; if they are the same age, the dominant individual is first to breed (Woolfenden and Fitzpatrick 1984). Older male helpers that have one or more siblings have a higher probability of breeding the following year than do singleton helpers (Fitzpatrick and Woolfenden 1986). In suburban jay populations, changes in both ecological and social conditions reduce the constraints on independent breeding, leading to much higher rates of breeding among yearlings (Bowman 1998). Specifically, compared to Florida scrub-jays in pristine habitat, suburban breeders have higher mortality and reduced offspring survival, hence fewer suburban breeders have helpers and those that

do have fewer. All these differences produce a more relaxed competitive environment in suburban habitats, leading to earlier age-at-first breeding including more yearling breeders and a greater frequency of *de novo* territory formation.

Group size positively affects fledgling body mass, which in turn positively correlates with probability of becoming a breeder (Mumme et al. 2015). However, for fledglings raised in smaller territories, group size negatively affects juvenile survivorship, such that individuals raised in larger territories have a significantly higher probability of eventually becoming breeders. This important relationship suggests that competition for resources within family groups is especially deleterious for groups occupying smaller territories. Groups able to defend larger areas of oak scrub have the highest probability of producing offspring that survive and recruit into the breeding ranks.

Fitness benefits of short-distance dispersal

Although females disperse earlier and farther than males, for both sexes modal age at first breeding is two years (Table 5.1) and modal dispersal distance is within two territories of the natal territory (Coulon et al. 2010). Data on lifetime reproductive success in relation to dispersal distance provide evidence that short-distance dispersal confers a surprisingly large selective advantage over long-distance dispersal (Fitzpatrick et al. 1999). For both sexes, individuals that become breeders within two territories of home exhibit longer lifespans, and produce more offspring, than do those that become breeders farther away (Table 5.2).

The 20–30% fitness advantage to breeding within the home neighborhood does not result from differences in annual fecundity, but rather from differences in mean lifespan that manifest very early postdispersal. Males breeding within two territories of home have a significantly higher chance of surviving to their third breeding year than longer-distance dispersers (67% vs. 54%, $N = 150$ and 84, respectively; $P < 0.01$); a similar pattern holds for females (78% vs. 54%, $N = 85$ and 144, respectively; $P < 0.01$).

The reasons for elevated postdispersal mortality among longer-distance dispersers remain unclear.

Table 5.2. Mean breeding lifespan and mean lifetime reproductive success versus natal dispersal among known-age breeder cohorts in study tract, 1971–2001

Dispersal type or distance	N	Breeding years	Fledglings	Independent offspring	Yearlings
Males					
Inherited	10	5.5	10.9	7.6	4.2
Budded	47	4.5	8.2	4.6	2.4
1 territory	69	4.2	7.2	4.6	2.6
2 territories	24	5.2	9.4	6.2	4.3
3 territories	16	4.3	8.1	4.9	2.6
4–19 territories	15	3.6	5.4	3.4	1.9
Immigrant from off the study area	53	3.7	6.4	4.0	2.1
Females					
Inherited or 1 territory	52	5.0	8.5	5.4	3.3
2 territories	33	4.5	8.5	5.4	3.2
3–5 territories	34	4.1	7.8	4.4	2.6
4–19 territories	21	2.6	4.1	2.6	1.2
Immigrant from off the study area	89	4.3	7.0	4.5	2.6

Similar annual reproductive performances between short- versus long-distance dispersers suggest that their survival differences do not reflect differences in average quality (McDonald et al. 1996). Cross-boundary leniency – nepotism – between family members familiar with one another could contribute, as new breeders occasionally visit their natal territories after pairing, especially if they share a boundary with both parents. This effect is temporary, however, as most boundaries are defended vigorously irrespective of relatedness within a year or two after pairing. We suspect that the survival advantage of breeding close to home stems mainly from close familiarity with the physical and social features of their breeding neighborhood among the shorter-distance dispersers.

Territorial budding: not for the faint of heart

About a quarter of breeding males recruit via territorial budding, defined as pairing with a dispersing or widowed jay on a portion of the natal territory or on immediately adjacent space aggressively acquired through territorial expansion during pairing (Woolfenden and Fitzpatrick 1978, 1984). Not all budding attempts succeed. Every spring, a few male and female pre-breeders

begin to act as pairs by attempting to defend ground together, but then struggle to gain exclusive ownership because of dominance by established territory owners. Pairs that fail to establish at least ~4 ha of exclusively held scrub during their first breeding season together usually fail to rear offspring, even foregoing nesting altogether, and frequently separate. Newly budded pairs that do stay together spend the rest of the year working hard to enlarge their territory. Significant territorial expansion is aided by the death of a neighboring breeder, which leaves the surviving widow vulnerable to losing space until he or she acquires a new mate.

Budding appears to be as risky as long-distance dispersal during the first two years after pairing. Males that became breeders via budding experienced reduced survival during their first year as a breeder (72.3%, $N = 47$), compared to males that inherited their territory outright (90%, $N = 10$) or that paired with widowed jays on territories within two territories of their natal territory (82.8%, $N = 93$). Males that paired three or more territories from home experienced the lowest survival during their first year as a breeder (67.9%, $N = 84$). Surprisingly, survivorship of males that budded increases so dramatically after the second breeding

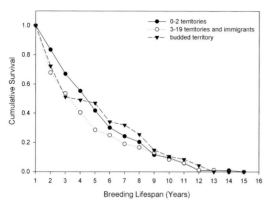

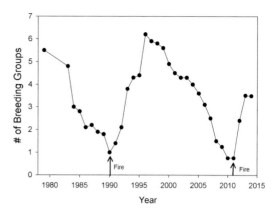

Figure 5.4. Cumulative survival for Florida scrub-jay breeding males of three dispersal types. Birds that dispersed >2 territories from their natal territory (*N* = 84, including long-distance immigrants) experienced significantly higher mortality during their first two years as breeders than those that dispersed within the natal neighborhood (0–2 territories; *N* = 103). Males that budded territories (*N* = 47) experienced high mortality equal to long-distance dispersers during the first two years of breeding, then their survival exceeded the other two categories. Data are uncensored: samples are restricted to jays with fully documented breeding histories that first bred in the study tract from 1971 to 2001, all of which are now dead.

Figure 5.5. Density of Florida scrub-jay breeding pairs within a 55 ha habitat tract at Archbold Biological Station subjected to prescribed fires in 1990 and 2010. Fire had been suppressed for at least 20 years prior to 1990, and was excluded from the tract between 1990 and 2010. Pairs were scored as contributing to density, from 0 to 100%, based on the proportion of their territory inside the tract each year.

year (Figure 5.4) that their lifetime reproductive success is similar to that of the remaining pool of males that inherited or became breeders within two territories of home (Table 5.2). Extraordinarily high survivorship among males that budded *and lived to their third breeding year* suggests that the budding strategy pays off mainly for high-quality males, as lower-quality budders tend to be culled early while trying to expand their territory.

The all-important fire cycle

Intense convective thunderstorms are frequent during the Florida summer (June through September), and the peninsula experiences the highest lightning-strike frequency in North America. Lightning-generated wildfires are common in native scrub, which consequently is dominated by fire-adapted clonal oaks,

palmettos, and ericaceous shrubs. Fire blackens or eliminates above-ground vegetation, but fresh new growth emerges from underground rhizomes within days after the fire. Rapid postfire succession results in fully mature scrub structure and composition within just a few years (Abrahamson 1984). Vital for the Florida scrub-jay, oak shrubs begin producing copious acorn crops 2–3 years after burning (Ostertag and Menges 1994; Abrahamson and Layne 2002).

Survival and reproductive success of Florida scrub-jays in habitat that undergoes periodic burning is significantly higher than in patches where fire has been suppressed (Fitzpatrick and Woolfenden 1986). To document the fire-cycle explicitly, in 1990 we subjected a 55 ha tract of overgrown, fire-suppressed scrub to a thorough prescribed burn, then suppressed all fire in this tract for the ensuing 20 years while monitoring the Florida scrub-jay population response. What had been a steeply declining population in the unburned scrub began recovering immediately after the fire and reached peak density after about 6 years. About 10 years postfire, the population began declining again, eventually replicating its preburn trajectory almost precisely (Figure 5.5).

Table 5.3. Key Florida scrub-jay demographic responses during immediate postfire recovery period (1990–1999) compared with unburned successional conditions (1983–1989 and 2000–2009, pooled) on a 55 ha experimental tract intensively burned via prescribed fire in March 1990

	0–9 years postfire (N = 54)	10+ years postfire (N = 76)
Fledglings	1.26/pair	1.63/pair
Yearlings	0.63/pair	0.49/pair
Juvenile survival	0.50	0.30**
Breeder replacement	0.88	0.71
De novo territories	6	1

Sample sizes (N) are pooled pair-years.

** $P < 0.01$ (χ^2 test).

Paradoxical demographics of postfire populations

Our multidecadal fire-cycle experiment highlighted two crucial demographic features of population increases during the 10 years immediately after a fire as the scrub habitat regenerated. First, survival of fledglings to age one (50%) was significantly higher during the early postfire period than during the two periods when the scrub was overgrown (Table 5.3), and considerably exceeded average juvenile survival for our population as a whole (35%; Woolfenden and Fitzpatrick 1984). Second, immigration of new breeders into the burned tract spiked during the postfire period, with nearly two-thirds of these coming from relatively long distances away, including more than half that were unbanded immigrants into the study tract. Probability of a widow gaining a mate in situ, rather than moving away to pair elsewhere, was higher in the early successional scrub (0.88 vs. 0.71), and many immigrants established *de novo* territories in early successional scrub that had been unoccupied prior to the fire (Table 5.3). These results are consistent with postfire demographic patterns documented for Florida scrub-jays elsewhere in Florida (Breininger and Oddy 2004; Franzreb and Zarnoch 2011), and we hypothesize that they reflect a unifying feature of Florida scrub-jay behavioral ecology: dispersing jays are attracted to postfire successional habitat specifically because the probability of producing

surviving offspring is substantially elevated in this early seral stage.

Scrub habitat undergoing postfire succession provides conditions favoring postfledging survival all the way to their recruitment as breeders, the ultimate currency of fitness. Across our population as a whole over the 45-year course of our study, pairs defending territories in which less than 25% of the oak scrub had burned at least once during the preceding 9 years produced 33% fewer offspring that eventually became breeders compared to those pairs defending higher proportions of early successional postfire habitat (Figure 5.6).

Paradoxically, fires are not universally beneficial to Florida scrub-jay family groups. Pairs or groups whose territories are extensively and intensely burned are at risk of having few or no acorns within their preburn territory boundaries during the subsequent fall, as scrub oaks devote several years to regenerating non-acorn-bearing woody growth (Ostertag and Menges 1994; Abrahamson and Layne 2002). Groups facing this situation engage in frequent boundary disputes during the late summer and fall acorn-harvest season to gain ownership of acorn-bearing scrub at the expense of neighboring families. These prolonged skirmishes often succeed, but they also have dire consequences. Mortality of breeders whose territories are extensively burned increases during the autumn months, which coincide with migration of Accipiters and falcons, the most dangerous predators of adult jays. At the population level, exceptionally large and

Table 5.4. Mortality of Florida scrub-jay breeders during the first year following three extensive fires affecting the study tract at Archbold Biological Station

Year	Territory >70% burned		Territory <70% burned	
	Percent mortality	N	Percent mortality	N
1984	35.7	28	25.0	48
1989	55.6	18	33.3	108
2001	31.0	42	18.2	176
Combined	37.5	88	24.1	332

Difference between the combined burned categories is significant ($\chi^2 = 6.4$, df = 1, P < 0.02).

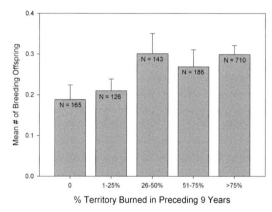

Figure 5.6. Mean number of breeding offspring produced pair^{-1} year^{-1} in relation to the proportion of the territory burned within the preceding 9 years. Territories containing more than 25% early successional scrub ($N = 1,039$ pair-years) produced significantly more breeders than those nearly or entirely lacking successional scrub (0–25% burned, $N = 291$; GLM ANOVA, $P = 0.02$).

thorough fires lead to significant elevations in breeder mortality among those territories most extensively burned (Table 5.4).

Large territories provide triple insurance

The Florida scrub-jay occupies a distinctive, two-dimensional habitat in which natural fire-return intervals are shorter than the lifespan of many individual jays, and in which the essential food resources of arthropods, small vertebrates, and acorns are thinly

and evenly dispersed. Persistence in such a habitat is difficult and precarious, requiring perpetual territorial vigilance. In at least three respects, pursuing the strategy of always defending the largest territory allowed by the immediate social neighborhood represents an essential "insurance policy."

First, fires reset the successional clock, regenerating productive habitat conditions and – most important – significantly reducing predation on juvenile jays for several years after the fire. Jays show unambiguous behavioral preferences for early postfire habitat, and territorial pairs are most successful if they own some habitat that was recently burned. Natural wildfires are unpredictably patchy, and when a fire occurs the probability that a jay territory is at least partially burned will vary with territory size. Larger territories are more likely to experience the demographic advantages of postfire successional conditions, and to experience these more frequently, than smaller territories.

Second, every territory faces the risk of being extensively or completely blackened when a fire roars through. Florida scrub-jays living in territories that are extensively burned pay a major price in increased energetic demands and higher mortality as they work to secure unburned, acorn-bearing resources in the fall and unburned scrub for nesting safely in the spring. Small territories are most vulnerable to being burned completely, while larger territories are more likely to retain unburned patches postfire.

Third, juveniles reared in larger territories have higher body mass at fledging and higher probability of becoming breeders compared to those reared in smaller territories (Mumme et al. 2015). Intragroup competition for resources appears to be a limiting factor within smaller territories, whereas it is reduced or functionally eliminated within larger territories regardless of group size.

All three of these factors combine to produce an overwhelming advantage for defending the largest territory possible. Because this advantage compounds the level of intergroup competition, and success at defending large territories is a function of group size, we suspect that this advantage is paramount in selecting for group living and cooperative breeding in the Florida scrub-jay.

Fitness consequences

Why delay dispersal?

The Florida scrub-jay is a Pliocene relic that persists in Florida only in sharply delimited patches of a xeric scrub ecosystem in which five species of low-growing clonal oaks produce a reliable annual acorn crop. Acorns cached individually in the sand supply the essential food during dry winter months when the jays' primary food supplies – arthropods and small vertebrates – are at their lowest levels. Reliance upon thinly dispersed animal foods and cached acorns distributed across a two-dimensional habitat selects for a year-round territorial social system. Juvenile Florida scrub-jays rely on acorns that they personally cached in order to survive their first winter, so remaining in their natal territory at least until the following spring is mandatory. At that point, opportunities to disperse and breed at age one are extremely limited, both because suitable oak scrub habitat is saturated with vigorously territorial pairs, and because the neighborhood is already crowded with older nonbreeders who prevail in the scrambles to fill breeding vacancies caused by breeder deaths. Yearlings join the ranks of nonbreeders competing for outright territory ownership – the required currency for breeding – and the natal territory provides the safest place from which to compete.

We emphasize that remaining home is not simply a consequence of extended parental care or making the best of a bad job: helpers contribute actively to growing the family group and to enlarging their territory, thereby directly improving their chances of breeding the following year. In a system characterized by perpetually heightened competition for space, the behavior of Florida scrub-jay nonbreeders is entirely consistent with doing everything possible to become a breeder while minimizing the risk of dying before breeding.

Territory size matters, a lot

Helpers actively contribute to establishment and maintenance of territorial boundaries throughout the year, and groups can defend larger territories than lone pairs. Larger family groups can control more area, including key acorn-bearing oak patches, and can more successfully expand their territories into desirable recently burned scrub than can pairs or smaller groups.

Pairs occupying larger territories are more likely than those in smaller territories to retain acorn-bearing resources after a fire, and more likely to produce fledglings that survive to become breeders. Large groups in large territories produce the largest fledglings, which in turn have the highest survival probabilities. Everything points to a system in which the optimal strategy for both breeders and nonbreeders is to live and work in a group that defends as large a territory as possible. Ultimately, territory size is limited only by the pressures exerted against it by neighboring groups, all of which are pursuing the same strategy. Florida scrub-jays are the ultimate despots (*sensu* Fretwell and Calver 1969), occupying and defending against other conspecifics to own absolutely as much space as they can. Indeed, pairs without helpers often appear to be defending far more resources than they need just for themselves, as if they are "banking" resources to accommodate a larger group in the future. Consistent with this interpretation, during initial translocations of Florida scrub-jays into a large, newly restored, optimal scrub capable of supporting more birds than initially translocated, the few pairs that formed immediately defended enormous territories, even exceeding 50 ha, which ultimately impeded translocation of additional birds into the site (R. Bowman unpubl. data).

Singular nesting ensures sufficiency of resources

Florida scrub-jay breeders actively prohibit immigration into their group and dominate their offspring, effectively controlling the number of jays that have access to their territory's resources. Reproductive success declines for group sizes larger than six jays (i.e., groups with four helpers), suggesting that plural nesting in this species would result in too large a group size to be accommodated by the defendable resources. Territorial budding may be regarded as a transitional stage toward plural nesting (Fitzpatrick and Woolfenden 1986), but it is tolerated and ultimately successful only if the new pair actively gains control over new resources at the expense of neighboring groups. Budding is a successful strategy for offspring recruitment only for larger territories or when it can be accompanied by territorial expansion. For this reason, budding is a risky dispersal strategy that works best for high-quality males. We hypothesize that Mexican jays exhibit plural nesting because larger group sizes confer competitive advantages in defending highly concentrated resources along their mostly linearly oriented riparian habitats.

Conservation

Although still formally listed only as *Threatened* by the U. S. Fish and Wildlife Service and *Vulnerable* by BirdLife International and IUCN, in reality the Florida scrub-jay is severely endangered today. Reduced to a few thousand groups, the species has disappeared across vast areas of its former range and is declining dramatically within every one of its extant metapopulations. Two ecological and behavioral features contributing to this decline merit emphasis in the context of the present chapter.

First, this species is tightly specialized on an oak scrub habitat which, while always patchy and well-defined, originally was extensive across the peninsula. The same factors that led Florida scrub-jays to be *socially* sedentary and philopatric also made them *ecologically* so. Individual jays are so remarkably unwilling to disperse across even tiny habitat gaps that they are genetically isolated and differentiating today across nonscrub

gaps as little as 5 km apart (Coulon et al. 2012). As twentieth-century human settlement fragmented the Florida scrub into today's tiny remnants, the habitat's flagship jay populations became isolated from one another and small, the latter effect being exacerbated by their unusually large territory sizes. Not only are these small populations now blinking out because of standard island-biogeographic effects, but recolonization is effectively nil because of the above-mentioned reluctance to cross habitat gaps (Stith et al. 1996). Short of large-scale and perpetual human-assisted rescue operations, the overriding long-term conservation solution is to ensure that extant metapopulations are protected via networks of preserves separated from one another by minimal habitat gaps (preferably, less than 5 km).

Second, the pervasive importance of the natural fire cycle in shaping Florida scrub-jay social behavior places them at odds with modern-day human occupation of the Florida peninsula. Literally for millions of years, fires swept regularly across these scrub landscapes. Florida scrub-jays adapted to these recurring ecological reset-events, with strong attraction to postfire successional patches and a social system built to compete for oversized territories containing already-burned or about-to-burn scrub. Fire suppression by humans has caused scrub habitat to become unsuitable for Florida scrub-jays in essentially every region where they still occur, with the sole exception being lands under informed and progressive conservation management. Long-term preservation of Florida scrub-jay populations absolutely requires human-managed burning regimes prescribed to mimic the natural conditions and fire-return intervals to which this species is so exquisitely adapted.

Why don't scrub-jays cooperate in western North America?

Cooperative breeding is a common behavioral trait among New World jays (Brown 1987; Edwards and Naeem 1993), and presumably is a primitive trait within the genus *Aphelocoma* (Peterson and Burt 1992). Nevertheless, except in southern Mexico (Burt and Peterson 1993) cooperative breeding is absent in western North America. Even the island scrub-jay – a sister species of the western scrub-jay – does not breed cooperatively despite being restricted to a single 250 km² island functionally saturated with jay territories (Sillett et al. 2012). Rates of survival and annual reproduction among western scrub-jays are similar to those in Florida (Carmen 2004; Caldwell et al. 2013), so the difference in social systems between the western and Florida scrub-jay species cannot be explained by demography alone.

We hypothesize that two mutually reinforcing factors explain the absence of cooperation in the Western United States. First, and probably most important, populations of scrub-jays across arid and semiarid regions of western North America face conspicuously fewer habitat constraints than do those in Florida. In sharp contrast to Florida scrub-jays, the range of habitat types occupied by both western and island scrub-jays is extraordinarily broad, and resource-bearing habitats that can be occupied at least temporarily by non-breeding jays are even more variable and widespread (Peterson and Vargas 1993; Curry et al. 2002; Carmen 2004; Langin et al. 2015). Consequently, pairing and attempted breeding at age one are common, albeit often in suboptimal habitats that are peripheral to those bearing higher densities of breeding territories (Carmen 2004; Caldwell et al. 2013). Having the capacity to overwinter and breed in a multitude of habitat types of varying quality, yearling scrub-jays in the West experience little pressure to delay attempting reproduction.

Second, most scrub-jay populations in the West rely on fruits of oaks (acorns) or pinyon pines (pine nuts), both of which are notorious for undergoing bumper crops some years and irregularly occurring total mast failures in others (Koenig and Knops 2000, 2002). For jays in these habitats, an essential resource supply varies year to year from superabundance to total absence. Such extreme variability means that in some years or some places, resources favor first-year breeding even in peripherally usable habitat, while in other years all jays – young and old – are forced to abandon their territories and move large distances in order to locate resources (Carmen 2004). Abundance of western

scrub-jays across California varies generally with oak species diversity, and also locally with acorn production during the previous year (Koenig et al. 2009). Wide annual and spatial variation in resource abundance favors a more flexible and mobile life history than scrub-jays adopt in the Florida oak scrub, where acorn production is more stable and mast failures do not occur (Abrahamson and Layne 2003). In the West, variable resources, ample opportunity to breed at age one, and occasional necessity to move long distances all reduce or eliminate the competitive advantages of investing in lifelong, year round, group-aided territorial defense that is so characteristic of Florida scrub-jays.

The challenge remains to explain apparent cooperative breeding in the scrub-jays of Oaxaca, Mexico (Burt and Peterson 1993), where mean territory size (1.5 ha) is similar to noncooperative western scrub-jays farther north. We concur with the possibility posed by those authors that "cooperative breeding in this population [may not be] adaptive under current conditions, instead reflecting selection in ancestral populations under very different ecological situations" (Peterson and Burt 1992). Specifically, jays in the Oaxaca study occupied severely human-altered habitats that varied widely in structure and, presumably, in resource abundance and distribution. Brood reduction was the rule (from 3-egg clutches to a maximum of one surviving fledgling per pair), suggesting that the population may not be demographically stable. We find exactly this situation where Florida scrub-jays occupy grossly altered suburban habitats (Shawkey et al. 2004), cooperation breaks down, and breeding at age one, rather than helping, is far more common than in intact native scrub. Clearly, for purposes of clarifying what may be multiple ecoevolutionary routes to cooperation among *Aphelocoma* jays, the scrub-jays of Oaxaca merit detailed study, especially in areas where they occupy native habitats not yet altered by humans.

Conclusions

We regard cooperative breeding by scrub-jays in Florida as an adaptive response to a suite of biotic and abiotic features of the relictual, nutrient-poor habitat to which these jays are limited. Florida scrub-jays survive and reproduce only in open-growing scrub oak patches that are confined to sharply-defined sandy soil deposits. This habitat provides seasonally reliable resources, including acorns of five scrub oak species that do not undergo mast failures. Both acorn and animal resources are thinly dispersed, however, and access to them requires substantial year-round energy investment in the form of territorial defense.

Owing to Florida's spectacularly high lightning frequency, the jays' scrub habitat is characterized by a wildfire cycle having relatively short (7–15 year) return intervals. Thin resources and frequent fires in a sharply delimited habitat selectively favor defense of extremely large territories and active competition for habitat patches of highest quality. Jays breeding in larger territories produce more surviving offspring than those in smaller ones, and offspring in these territories have a competitive advantage for becoming breeders. These ecological features set up an intensely competitive social milieu, which favors delayed breeding and group defense in order to establish and hold territories, and to gain ground while enjoying the survival benefits of a coordinated sentinel system. Helping to raise sibs and half-sibs within their natal territory adds incrementally to nonbreeders' inclusive fitness, but more importantly it also helps increase group size, territory size, and subsequent probability of recruitment. Recruits that disperse and become breeders within their natal neighborhood achieve significantly higher lifetime reproductive success than those breeding farther away, which compounds the selective advantages of delaying dispersal and competing locally from the safety of the natal territory.

Viewed in this way, delayed dispersal and helping by Florida scrub-jays is not "making the best of a bad job" (*sensu* Koenig et al. 1992). Rather, it represents an active strategy for gaining a competitive social advantage in the scramble for access to breeding, where a fitness premium (elevated survival, hence longer breeding lifespan) is conferred on individuals that become breeders within their natal neighborhood. Florida scrub-jay helpers cooperate as nonbreeders within a group because this suite of actions maximizes their chances to become a breeder where their chances of success are highest, in an intensely and persistently competitive social environment.

Acknowledgments

We remain deeply indebted to the Archbold Biological Station and its dedicated staff for protecting, managing, enhancing, and progressively enlarging the native habitat preserve within which our study has been nested since 1969, and for providing significant institutional support over the decades. Additional significant funding for work based at Archbold has been provided by the National Science Foundation, the Cornell Lab of Ornithology, and the U. S. Fish and Wildlife Service. We thank Raoul Boughton, Nancy Chen, Shane Pruett, Ron Mumme, and the annual teams of interns at Archbold for their help with data gathering and analysis related to this chapter. We appreciate fruitful discussions about cooperative breeding with Walt Koenig and Janis Dickinson, as well as their helpful comments on this chapter. Finally, both authors share lifelong gratitude to the late Glen E. Woolfenden (1930–2007) for his foresight in launching this long-term study, and for his mentorship and unique friendship with us over the decades. We dedicate this chapter to Glen and Jan.

REFERENCES

Abrahamson, W. G. (1984). Post-fire recovery of Florida Lake Wales ridge vegetation. *Am. J. Bot.*, 7, 9–21.

Abrahamson, W. G. and Layne, J. N. (2002). Post-fire recovery of acorn production by four oak species in southern ridge sandhill association in south-central Florida. *Amer. J. Bot.*, 89, 119–123.

Abrahamson, W. G. and Layne, J. N. (2003). Long-term patterns of acorn production for five oak species in xeric Florida uplands. *Ecology*, 84, 2476–2492.

Aldredge, R. A., LeClair, S. C., and Bowman, R. (2012). Declining egg viability explains higher hatching failure in a suburban population of the threatened Florida scrub-jay *Aphelocoma coerulescens*. *J. Avian. Biol.*, 43, 369–375.

Bebus, S. E., Jones, B. C., and Schoech, S. J. (2014). Stress-response, experience, and neophobia in free-living Florida scrub-jays (*Aphelocoma coerulescens*). *Integr. Comp. Biol.*, 54 (Suppl. 1), E14.

Boughton, R. and Bowman, R. (2011). State wide assessment of Florida Scrub-Jay on managed areas: A comparison of current populations to the results of the 1992–93 survey. Report to USFWS, 37 pp.

Bowman, R. (1998). Population dynamics, demography, and contributions to metapopulation dynamics by suburban populations of the Florida scrub-jay, *Aphelocoma coerulescens*. Nongame Wildlife Program Final Report. Tallahassee, Florida, Florida Game and Freshwater Fish Commission, pp. iii-137.

Breininger, D. R. and Oddy, D. M. (2004). Do habitat potential, population density, and fires influence scrub-jay source-sink dynamics? *Ecol. Appl.*, 14, 1079–1089.

Breininger, D. R., Toland, B., Oddy, D. M., and Legare, M. L. (2006). Landcover characterizations and Florida scrub-jay (*Aphelocoma coerulescens*) population dynamics. *Biol. Conserv.*, 128, 169–181.

Brown, J. L. 1987. *Helping and Communal Breeding in Birds: Ecology and Evolution.* Princeton, NJ: Princeton University Press.

Burt, D. B. and Peterson, A. T. (1993). Biology of cooperative breeding scrub-jays (*Aphelocoma coerulescens*) of Oaxaca, Mexico. *Auk*, 110, 207–214.

Caldwell, L., Bakker, V. J., Sillett, T. S., Desrosiers, M. A., Morrison, S. A., and Ingeloni, L. M. (2013). Reproductive ecology of the Island Scrub-Jay. *Condor*, 115, 603–613.

Carmen, W. J. (2004). Noncooperative breeding in the California scrub-jay. *Stud. Avian Biol.*, 28, 1–100.

Coulon, A., Fitzpatrick, J. W., Bowman, R., Stith, B. M., Makarewich, C. A., et al. (2008). Congruent population structure inferred from dispersal behaviour and intensive genetic surveys of the threatened Florida scrub-jay (*Aphelocoma coerulescens*). *Mol. Ecol.*, 17, 1685–1701.

Coulon, A., Fitzpatrick, J. W., Bowman, R., and Lovette, I. J. (2010). Effects of habitat fragmentation on effective dispersal of Florida scrub-jays. *Conserv. Biol.*, 24, 1080–1088.

Coulon, A., Fitzpatrick, J. W., Bowman, R., and Lovette, I. J. (2012). Mind the gap: genetic distance increases with habitat gap size in Florida scrub jays. *Biol. Lett.*, 8, 582–585.

Covas, R., Doutrelant, C., and Du Plessis, M. A. (2004). Experimental evidence of a link between breeding conditions and the decision to breed or to help in a colonial cooperative bird. *Proc. R. Soc. London B*, 271, 827–832.

Curry, R. L., Peterson, A. T., and Langen, T. A. (2002). Western scrub-jay (*Aphelocoma californica*). In: *The Birds of North America Online*, ed. A. Poole. Ithaca, NY: Cornell Lab of Ornithology. Retrieved from The Birds of North America Online: http://bna.birds.cornell.edu/bna/species/712

DeGange, A. R. (1976). The daily and annual time budget of the Florida scrub-jay. M.S. thesis, University of South Florida, Tampa, FL.

DeGange, A. R., Fitzpatrick, J. W., Layne, J. N., and Woolfenden, G. E. (1989). Acorn harvesting by Florida scrub-jays. *Ecology*, 70, 348–356.

Edwards, S. V. and Naeem, S. (1993). The phylogenetic component of cooperative breeding in perching birds. *Am. Nat.*, 141, 754–789.

Emslie, S. D. (1996). A fossil scrub-jay supports a recent systematic decision. *Condor*, 98, 675–680.

Ferguson, S. M., Small, T. W., and Schoech, S. J. (2014). We gotta get out of this place: relationships between corticosterone and dispersal distance in the Florida scrub-jay (*Aphelocoma coerulescens*). *Integr. Comp. Biol.*, 54 *(Suppl. 1)*, E63.

Fitzpatrick, J. W. and Woolfenden, G. E. (1986). Demographic routes to cooperative breeding in some New World jays. In: *Evolution of Animal Behavior: Paleontological and Field Approaches*, ed. M. N. Nitecki and J. A. Kitchell. Chicago, IL: University of Chicago Press, pp. 137–160.

Fitzpatrick, J. W. and Woolfenden, G. E. (1989). Florida scrub-jay. In: *Lifetime Reproduction in Birds*, ed. I. Newton. London: Academic Press, pp. 201–218.

Fitzpatrick, J. W., Pranty, W., and Stith, B. (1994). *Florida Scrub-Jay Statewide Map, 1992–1993.* Report to U. S. Fish and Wildlife. Archbold Biological Station, Lake Placid, FL.

Fitzpatrick, J. W., Woolfenden, G. E., and Bowman, R. (1999). Dispersal distance and its demographic consequences in the Florida scrub-jay. *Proc. Int. Ornithol. Congr.*, 22, 2465–2479.

Fleischer, A. L. Jr., Bowman, R., and Woolfenden, G. E. (2003). Variation in foraging behavior, diet, and time of breeding of Florida scrub-jays in suburban and wildland habitats. *Condor*, 105, 515–527.

Franzreb, K. E. and Zarnoch, S. J. (2011). Factors affecting Florida scrub-jay nest survival on Ocala National Forest, Florida. *J. Wildl. Manage.*, 75, 1040–1050.

Fretwell, S. D. and Calver, J. S. (1969). On territorial behavior and other factors influencing habitat distribution in birds. *Acta Biotheor.*, 19, 37–44.

Goldstein, J. M., Woolfenden, G. E., and Hailman, J. P. (1998). A same-sex stepparent shortens a prebreeder's duration on the natal territory: tests of two hypotheses in Florida scrub-jays. *Behav. Ecol. Sociobiol.*, 44, 15–22.

Jones, B. C., Bebus, S., and Schoech, S. J. (2014). Learned anti-predator behavior is impaired by exogenous corticosterone in free-living Florida scrub-jays (*Aphelocoma coerulescens*). *Integr. Comp. Biol.*, 54 (Suppl. 1), E103.

Koenig, W. D. and Knops, J. M. H. (2000). Patterns of annual seed production by northern hemisphere trees: a global perspective. *Am. Nat.* 155, 59–69.

Koenig, W. D. and Knops, J. M. H. (2002). The behavioral ecology of masting in oaks. In: *Oak Forest Ecosystems*, ed. W. J. McShea and W. M. Healy. Baltimore, MD: Johns Hopkins University Press, pp. 129–148.

Koenig, W. D., Krakauer, A. H., Monahan, W. B., Haydock, J. Knops, J. M. H., et al. (2009). Mast-producing trees and the geographical ecology of western scrub-jays. *Ecography* 32: 561–570.

Koenig, W. D., Pitelka, F., Carmen W. J., Mumme, R. L., and Stanback, M. T. (1992). The evolution of delayed dispersal in cooperative breeders. *Q. Rev. Biol.*, 67, 111–150.

Langin, K. M., Sillett, T. S., Funk, W. C., Morrison, S. A., Desrosiers, M. A., et al. (2015). Islands within an island:repeated adaptive divergence in a single population. *Evolution*, 69, 653–665.

Marzluff, J. M., Woolfenden, G. E., Fitzpatrick, J. W., and Balda, R. P. (1996). Breeding partnerships of two New World jays. In: *Partnerships in Birds: The Study of Monogamy*, ed. J. M. Black. Oxford: Oxford University Press, pp. 138–161.

McCormack, J. E., Heled, J., Delaney, K. S., Peterson, A. T., and Knowles, L. L. (2010). Calibrating divergence times on species trees versus gene trees: implications for speciation history of *Aphelocoma* jays. *Evolution*, 65, 184–202.

McDonald, D., Woolfenden, G. E., and Fitzpatrick, J. W. (1996). Actuarial senescence and demographic heterogeneity in the Florida Scrub Jay. *Ecology*, 77, 2373–2381.

McGowan, K. J. and Woolfenden, G. E. (1989). A sentinel system in the Florida scrub jay. *Anim. Behav.*, 37, 1000–1006.

McGowan, K. J. and Woolfenden, G. E. (1990). Contributions to fledgling feeding in the Florida scrub jay. *J. Anim. Ecol.*, 59, 691–707.

Menges, E. (2007) Integrating demography and fire management: an example from Florida scrub. *Aust. J. Biol.*, 55, 261–272.

Mumme, R. L. (1992). Do helpers increase reproductive success? An experimental analysis in the Florida scrub jay. *Behav. Ecol. Sociobiol.*, 31, 319–328.

Mumme, R., Bowman, R, Pruett, M. S., and Fitzpatrick, J. W. (2015). Natal territory size, group size, and body mass affect lifetime fitness in the cooperatively breeding Florida scrub-jay. *Auk: Ornithol. Advances*, 132, 634–646.

Niederhauser, J. M. and Bowman, R. (2014). Testing sources of variation in nestling-stage nest success of Florida scrub-jays in suburban and wildland habitats. *J. Field Ornithol.*, 85, 180–195.

Ostertag, R. and Menges, E. S. (1994). Patterns of reproductive effort with time since last fire in Florida scrub plants. *J. Veg. Sci.*, 5, 303–310.

Peterson, A. T. and Burt, D. B. (1992). Phylogenetic history of social evolution and habitat use in the *Aphelocoma* jays. *Anim. Behav.*, 44, 859–866.

Peterson, A. T. and N. Vargas B. (1993). Ecological diversity in scrub jays (*Aphelocoma coerulescens*). In: *The Biological Diversity of Mexico*, eds. T. P. Ramamoorthy, R. Bye, A. Lot and J. Fa. Oxford, U.K.: Oxford University Press, pp. 309–317.

Rensel, M. A. and Schoech, S. J. (2011). Repeatability of baseline and stress-induced corticosterone levels across early life stages in the Florida scrub-jay (*Aphelocoma coerulescens*). *Horm. Behav.*, 59, 497–502.

Rensel, M. A., Wilcoxen, T. E., and Schoech, S. J. (2010). The influence of nest attendance and provisioning on nestling stress physiology in the Florida scrub-jay. *Horm. Behav.*, 57, 162–168.

Reynolds, S. J., Schoech, S. J., and Bowman, R. (2003). Nutritional quality of prebreeding diet influences breeding performance of the Florida scrub-jay. *Oecologia*, 134, 308–316.

Sauter, A. (2005). Shall we feed suburban Florida scrub-jays *Aphelocoma coerulescens*? The importance of human-provided foods on parental food choice, nestling growth and survival. Ph.D. thesis, University of Zurich, Zurich, Switzerland.

Sauter, A., Bowman, R., Schoech, S. J., and Pasinelli, G. (2006). Does optimal foraging theory explain why suburban Florida scrub-jays (*Aphelocoma coerulescens*) feed their young human-provided food? *Behav. Ecol. Sociobiol.*, 60, 465–474.

Schoech, S. J., Mumme, R. L., and Wingfield, J. C. (1996a). Delayed breeding in the cooperatively breeding Florida scrub-jay (*Aphelocoma coerulescens*): inhibition or the absence of stimulation? *Behav. Ecol. Sociobiol.*, 39, 77–90.

Schoech, S. J., Mumme, R. L., and Wingfield, J. C. (1996b). Prolactin and helping behaviour in the cooperatively breeding Florida scrub-jay, *Aphelocoma coerulescens*. *Anim. Behav.*, 52, 445–456.

Schoech, S. J., Mumme, R. L., and Wingfield, J. C. (1997). Corticosterone, reproductive status, and body mass in a cooperative breeder, the Florida scrub-jay (*Aphelocoma coerulescens*). *Physiol. Zool.*, 70, 68–73.

Schoech, S. J., Bowman, R., and Reynolds, S. J. (2004). Food supplementation and possible mechanisms underlying early breeding in the Florida scrub-jay (*Aphelocoma coerulescens*). *Horm. Behav.*, 46, 565–573.

Schoech, S. J., Bowman, R., Bridge, E. S., and Boughton, R. K. (2007). Baseline and acute levels of corticosterone in Florida scrub-jays (*Aphelocoma coerulescens*): effects of food supplementation, suburban habitat, and year. *Gen. Comp. Endocrin.*, 154, 150–160.

Schoech, S. J., Rensel, M. A., and Wilcoxen, T. E. (2012). Here today, not gone tomorrow: long-term effects of corticosterone. *J. Ornithol.*, 153, 217–226.

Shank, C. C. (1986). Territory size, energetics, and breeding strategy in the Corvidae. *Am. Nat.*, 128, 642–652.

Shawkey, M. D., Bowman, R., and Woolfenden, G. E. (2004). Why is brood reduction in Florida scrub-jays higher in suburban than in wildland habitats? *Can. J. Zool.*, 82, 1427–1435.

Sillett, T. S., Chandler, R. B., Royle, J. A., Kéry, M., and Morrison, S. A. (2012). Hierarchical distance-sampling models to estimate population size and habitat-specific abundance of an island endemic. *Ecol. Appl.*, 22, 1997–2006.

Stallcup, J. A. and Woolfenden, G. E. (1978). Family status and contributions to breeding by Florida scrub-jays. *Anim. Behav.*, 26, 1144–1156.

Stith, B. M., Fitzpatrick, J. W., Woolfenden, G. E., and Pranty, B. (1996). Classification and conservation of metapopulations: a case study of the Florida scrub-jay. In: *Metapopulations and Wildlife Conservation*, ed. D. R. McCullough. Washington D.C.: Island Press, pp. 187–215.

Townsend, A. K., Bowman, R., Fitzpatrick, J. W., Dent, M., and Lovette, I. J. (2011). Genetic monogamy across variable demographic landscapes in cooperatively breeding Florida scrub-jays. *Behav. Ecol.*, 22, 464–470.

Tringali, A. and Bowman, R. (2015). Suburban immigrants to wildlands disrupt honest signaling in ultra-violet plumage. *Avian Cons. Ecol.*, 10(1), 9.

Turner, W. R., Wilcove, D. S., and Swain, H. M. (2006). Assessing the effectiveness of reserve acquisition programs in protecting rare and threatened species. *Cons. Biol.*, 20, 1657–1669.

Woolfenden, G. E. and Fitzpatrick, J. W. (1977). Dominance in the Florida scrub jay. *Condor*, 79, 1–12.

Woolfenden, G. E. and Fitzpatrick, J. W. (1978). Inheritance of territory in group-breeding birds. *BioScience*, 28, 104–108.

Woolfenden, G. E. and Fitzpatrick, J. W. (1984). *The Florida Scrub Jay: Demography of a Cooperative-breeding Bird.* Princeton, NJ: Princeton University Press.

Woolfenden, G. E. and Fitzpatrick, J. W. (1996). Florida scrub-jay (*Aphelocoma coerulescens*). In: *Birds of North America*, no. 228, ed. A. Polle and F. Gill. Philadelphia, PA and Washington, D.C.: The Academy of Natural Sciences and The American Ornithologists' Union, pp. 1–28.

6

Carrion crows: Family living and helping in a flexible social system

Vittorio Baglione and Daniela Canestrari

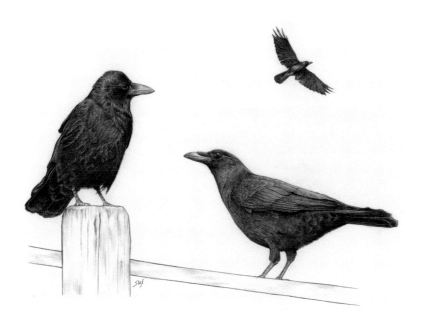

Introduction

Although until late 1990s Carrion crows *Corvus (corone) corone* were thought to breed in socially monogamous pairs (Cramp and Perrins 1994) with examples of cooperative breeding being rare, we discovered a truly cooperatively breeding population of carrion crows in northern Spain in 1995. In this population, approximately 75% of territories are held year-round by groups of up to nine individuals that share in chick provisioning as well as other parental duties (Baglione et al. 2002b). Discovery of such striking geographical variation of the social organization was the starting point of our long-term research project. As our study progressed, we uncovered the complexity of the crow society, which proved to be suitable for testing the adaptive value of helping at the nest and the role of kin selection in the evolution and maintenance of cooperative breeding.

Table 6.1. Geographic variability of the cooperative social system among European populations of carrion/hooded crows

Study site	Phenotype	Occurrence of coop. breed.	References
Northern Spain	*Corvus corone*	73.3%	Baglione et al. 2002b
Northern Italy	*Corvus c. cornix*	0%[a]	Baglione et al. 2005
Switzerland, rural area	*Corvus corone*	0%	Richner 1990
Switzerland, urban area	*Corvus corone*	6%	Richner 1990
Southern Sweden	*Corvus c. cornix*	0%[a]	Loman 1985
Scotland	both	0%	Charles 1972
Germany	*Corvus corone*	0%	Wittenberg 1988

The occurrence of cooperative breeding is reported as proportion of breeding territories with helpers at nest.

[a] Anecdotal cases of "third bird" in territories sampled during the breeding season. Helping role unclear.

Crows are challenging birds for ornithologists: a long history of human persecution has made them wary and intolerant of humans such that catching and banding them requires many hours in the field. Behavioral observations must be done almost exclusively by automatic video recording. Uncovering their fascinating social life has, however, repaid all the effort that our team has put into this research. Today carrion crows provide a model system for investigating the ecological correlates of cooperative breeding, including insights gathered from comparing populations instead of species, which overcomes the confounding effects of phylogeny and differences in life history, and had allowed for novel field experiments that shed light on the role of the environment in family formation and cooperation.

Phylogeny, phylogeography, and natural history

There is considerable debate regarding the taxonomy of the carrion crow, *Corvus (corone) corone,* and the hooded crow, *Corvus (corone) cornix,* which differ in coloration but exhibit near absence of genetic differentiation (Haas et al. 2009; Poelstra et al. 2013, 2014). In this chapter we regard carrion/hooded crows as "phenotypes" because hybridization occurs and produces

viable descendants. Although our study focuses mostly on carrion crows, we will also use data on hooded crow populations for some comparisons. Regardless of the phenotype, early studies of several European populations always reported the crows as breeding in socially monogamous pairs whose offspring leave home as soon as they are independent at approximately two months of age (Cramp and Perrins 1994). Rare exceptions of three birds holding a territory were reported both in Sweden (Loman 1985) and northern Italy (Baglione et al. 2002b), whereas in an urban area of Switzerland one helper-at-the-nest was found in 3 of 33 territories (crows in rural Switzerland are invariably socially monogamous, Richner 1990; Table 6.1).

Carrion/hooded crows are distributed throughout Eurasia, including Japan, and inhabit a large variety of habitats from farmland, open woodland, and coastal areas to mountains as high as 3600 m in central Asia (Madge and Burn 1999). The western and eastern populations of black crows, *Corvus (corone) corone,* are separated by a central area occupied by the hooded crows and the two phenotypes meet in 50–150 km wide hybrid zones in central Europe and East Asia. Crows are sedentary in the central-south part of their geographic range and are partially migratory in the north (Cramp and Perrins 1994). At the beginning of the spring in late March and early April females lay 2–7 eggs that they alone incubate in a conspicuous open nest (Canestrari et al. 2008b). Upon nest failure at egg or hatching stages, crows may renest up to three times in a breeding season, but only one successful brood is raised per year.

As indicated above, the singularity of this species is the geographical plasticity of the social organization. In most European populations, both carrion and hooded crows form socially monogamous pairs that alone raise a brood of 1–5 nestlings. Territorial behavior in spring varies across populations according to environmental factors. When nest sites are limited and population density high, crows can form loose colonies with nests as close as 50 m apart and pairs can share their feeding home range with neighbors, although they always appear to defend a small area around their nest. In contrast, in populations where nest sites are less limiting and population densities are low, breeding territories are well defended and exclusive (Baglione et al. 2005). About 4–5 weeks after fledging, offspring leave the natal territory and join a flock of nonbreeders until they can fill a territory vacancy, typically several years later. In most populations, adult breeders also join a flock after the breeding season to exploit temporally abundant food resources that arise outside their breeding home range. In late autumn and winter, they reoccupy breeding territories, but continue spending time on communal feeding areas and join large flocks for roosting (Wittenberg 1988).

The most remarkable documented exception to the patterns described above is our study population of carrion crows in northern Spain (42°37' N, 5°26' W). Here crows form cooperatively breeding groups of up to nine individuals (mean groups size ± standard error [S.E.] = 3.7 ± 0.1, Figure 6.1) that defend all-purpose territories year-round (Baglione et al. 2002b). Unassisted pairs inhabit approximately 25% of territories and the rest live in groups of 3–9 birds. In winter, group members roost communally and temporarily visit communal feeding spots, and often collect food that they carry back to the territory for caching. Most of the time, however, they stay and forage in their own territory throughout the year, although a minority of nonbreeders form permanent flocks like those that are found in pair-living populations (Baglione et al. 2005).

In northern Spain, groups are enlarged families that comprise a resident breeding pair, retained offspring

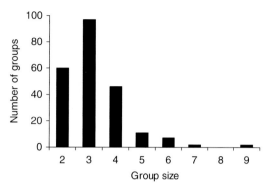

Figure 6.1. Breeding group size in the Spanish population of carrion crows in 105 territories sampled over five years. From Baglione et al. (2002b).

from previous broods, and immigrants, mostly males, that are related to the same-sex resident breeder (Baglione et al. 2003). Groups thus form via two different mechanisms – juvenile delayed dispersal and immigration.

Delayed natal dispersal: the role of the environment

Juvenile crows in Spain delay natal dispersal up to four years, during which time they can assist their parents in raising new broods. Delayed dispersal is male-biased, with sons being twice as likely to stay at home as daughters (Baglione et al. 2002b). The variability of juvenile dispersal behavior across carrion crow populations set the stage for a unique field experiment testing the role of the environment in driving family living. In spring of 2002, we collected eggs from a pair-living crow population in rural Switzerland and transferred them to Spain, leaving half of each donor clutch in its original nest as a control (Baglione et al. 2002a). After artificial incubation, we transferred the Swiss hatchlings into Spanish foster nests. Nine and five nests produced young in Switzerland and Spain respectively, with no significant difference in the number of fledglings between areas.

The results were clear. Of six transferred Swiss fledglings that survived until the following year in Spain, five delayed dispersal and were still living with their foster

Table 6.2. Territory turnover, population sex ratio, and number of competitors per breeding vacancy in Spain and Italy during the study period

	Year	Turnover (%) (N individuals)		Sex ratio population	Number of competitors per vacancy	
		♂♂	♀♀	♂♂ : ♀♀	♂♂	♀♀
Spain	2000	20.0 (10)	28.6 (7)	1 : 0.67	4.7	1.3
	2001	20.0 (15)	45.5 (11)		5.0	0.9
	2002	18.2 (11)	16.7 (6)		4.8	2.3
Italy	2001	22.2 (9)	37.5 (8)	1 : 0.61	8.1	2.0
	2002	30.8 (13)	37.5 (16)		6.5	2.2

parents at the beginning of the new breeding season, and one eventually helped at the nest. Conversely, none of their siblings raised in Switzerland did so; rather, all joined flocks of nonbreeders soon after independence. By showing that crows born from pair-living parents were capable of delaying dispersal and helping at the nest, the experiment proved that the rearing environment plays a key role in shaping crow social organization. The next question was what exactly in the environment determines the choice between staying at home and leaving?

A widely accepted explanation for this question is that offspring delay dispersal when the environment limits the opportunity for finding a suitable vacant territory to reproduce in, leading to the conclusion that staying at home and waiting is making "the best of a bad job." The environment can constrain dispersal through saturation of breeding territories, a shortage of mates, or low probability of survival during natal dispersal (Emlen 1991). Despite the low predictive power of the "ecological constraints hypothesis" (Cockburn 1998), evidence that most family-living bird species indeed suffer some kind of constraint has long been considered evidence in support of it. Comparison between our cooperatively breeding crows in Spain and the pair-living population in northern Italy offered an opportunity to test this hypothesis more rigorously than is possible for within-populations studies. The ecological constraints hypothesis predicts that crows should live in families where the habitat is more saturated, more dangerous, or where potential mates are scarcer. Juveniles delayed

dispersal in the less competitive environment of Spain where population density was lower, vacant territories more common, and potential mates were more abundant, led us to conclude that the ecological constraints hypothesis does not explain intraspecific variation of dispersal strategies in crows (Table 6.2, Figure 6.2; Baglione et al. 2005).

An alternative explanation is that in Spain, juveniles that prolong the association with their parents on the natal territory obtain benefits that are not available to their conspecifics in central Europe. We suggest that year-round territoriality of adult crows in northern Spain (Figure 6.3) is the key factor that makes the natal territory a "safe haven" for young, largely because retained young enjoy free access to defended resources only if they stay with their parents (Ekman et al. 2001; Kokko and Ekman 2002; Chiarati et al. 2011). Conversely, elsewhere in Europe adult crows do not defend a territory outside the breeding season, but join flocks on constantly changing communal foraging areas that are temporally very productive, but where parents cannot defend resources to share exclusively with their offspring. Consequently young crows cannot gain benefits by staying at home and maintaining social bonds with their parents.

If young crows make dispersal decisions according to these benefits of philopatry, we would predict that increasing "parents' wealth" will facilitate delayed dispersal in populations where family formation occurs. Because the timing of natal dispersal varies from a few months up to four years of age, we were able to

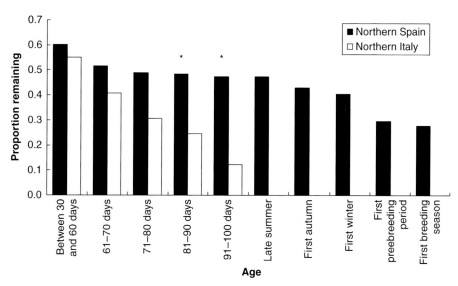

Figure 6.2. Proportion of banded offspring remaining on their natal territory throughout their first year in Italy and Spain. Asterisks indicate significant differences (after correction for multiple comparisons). From Baglione et al. (2002b).

experimentally test this prediction. When we increased the value of territories by supplementing with food (canned dog food that is very palatable for crows), juvenile crows significantly delayed dispersal and increased philopatry compared to same-age conspecifics living on unfed territories that were not supplemented (Figure 6.4). As adults do not adjust their tolerance toward offspring according to resource availability (Chiarati et al. 2011), the experiment demonstrates that young respond to the value of their natal territory, with individuals living on wealthy territories exhibiting stronger tendency to stay.

Other benefits of living with parents have been documented in several species, including the Siberian jay (*Perisoreus infaustus*), where retained offspring enjoy parents' protection against predators on the natal territory (Chapter 1). Our ongoing research is trying to elucidate whether this is also the case in crows. Inheritance of the natal territory is hypothesized to drive natal philopatry (Cockburn 1998), but this does not apply to the long-lived crows, where young typically disperse before a suitable breeding vacancy occurs at home. Thus, at the moment, it appears that the main benefit that crow parents provide to their young is access to

defended food resources. Indeed, dominant breeder males are more tolerant toward their offspring than to less related immigrant group members (Chiarati et al. 2011), and they also facilitate the access to novel and potentially dangerous food sources with their bold exploratory behavior, which helps shy, neophobic juveniles to become more exploratory (Chiarati et al. 2012). Overall, these benefits provide strong incentive for young to stay at home and represent the most plausible explanation for the observed intraspecific variability of natal dispersal patterns in this species.

Alliances and the role of kinship in crow society

Delayed dispersal is not the only route to group formation in crows. Immigrants – mostly males – can also permanently join an established family group and provision the nestlings during the breeding season. Based on microsatellite analyses, we found that immigrant males are related to the dominant resident breeding males that they join and help (mean relatedness $[r] \pm$ S.E. = 0.23 $\pm$ 0.07, Figure 6.5), whereas they are unrelated to the

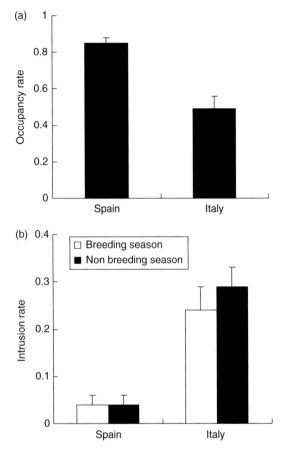

Figure 6.3. (a) Mean (± S.E.) territory occupancy rate (number of times territory owners were found "at home" divided by the total number of surveys) during the nonbreeding period in northern Spain where carrion crows are cooperative breeders and northern Italy where hooded crows are not cooperative breeders; (b) Mean (± S.E.) rate of intrusion into territories (number of times a conspecific intruder was found foraging on a given territory divided by the total number of surveys) during the breeding and nonbreeding season in the two populations. From Baglione et al. (2005).

breeding female (mean $r = 0.06 \pm 0.06$). Therefore, immigration into a territory by individuals born elsewhere does not disrupt the kin structure of cooperative groups, which are extended families (Baglione et al. 2003).

Population viscosity, whereby males disperse over shorter distances than females and tend to settle close

to their natal place, could explain these genetic patterns. The key prediction of this hypothesis, however, is that the population exhibits a genetic structure in which pairwise estimates of relatedness between males are negatively correlated with the distance between their territories (Queller 1992). In contrast to this prediction, we found no such correlation (Figure 6.6), suggesting that crows actively choose to join family members. Resident territory holders are effective at evicting intruders and thus the fact that they form alliances only with relatives indicates a selective tolerance of kin. In contrast, it is unclear whether immigrants also deliberately choose to help relatives or if they merely prospect territories at random and settle where they are tolerated. In any case, the genetic patterns we found support the hypothesis that kinship is key to the formation of cooperative alliances in crows.

Cooperation and competition in a complex society

We observe two mechanisms of group formation in crows – offspring delay dispersal and young birds (usually males) immigrate into cooperative groups. These two mechanisms drive both variability in the degree of kinship among group members and differences in opportunities for mating within the groups, the latter being higher for immigrants than for retained offspring. This implies that dominants may be selective in sharing the resources of the territory, for example by favoring retained offspring over more distantly related immigrants, and that immigrants may gain different benefits from group membership and provisioning at the nest than offspring. Variability in group composition thus has important implications for social interactions, including dominance hierarchies, mating behavior, and helping behavior of carrion crows.

Dominance hierarchy and nepotism

Negotiation over resources is crucial for group-living animals because conflicts may disrupt the stability of the group and ultimately hinder cooperation. By analyzing dyadic interactions at food sources we found

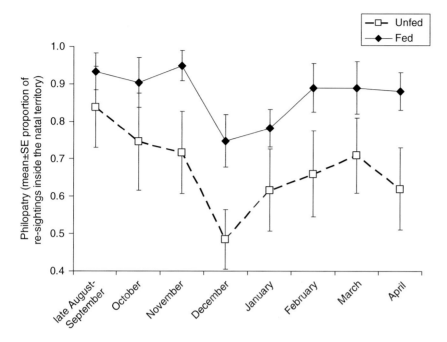

Figure 6.4. Philopatry, measured as the mean (± S.E.) proportion of resightings inside the natal territory, among fed (filled circles) and unfed (open circles) radio-tagged juvenile crows throughout the study period. From Baglione et al. (2006).

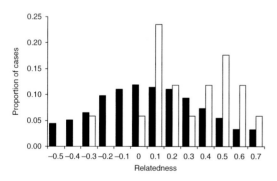

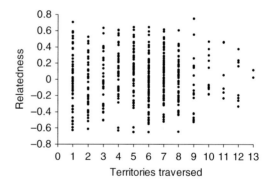

Figure 6.5. Distribution of pairwise relatedness (r) estimates in the population (filled bars) and in the sample of same-sex immigrant and resident crows cooperating on a territory (white bars). From Baglione et al. (2003).

Figure 6.6. Estimates of genetic relatedness between pairs of males plotted against the distance (in territories traversed) between the territories where they settled. From Baglione et al. (2003).

that group members form stable linear dominance hierarchies that are stronger for males than for females (Chiarati et al. 2010). The resident breeding male occupies the alpha position followed by immigrant males,

retained male offspring, and, at the bottom of the hierarchy, all the females (Figure 6.7). Therefore, one consequence of alpha males' forming alliances with immigrants is that their own offspring are relegated to

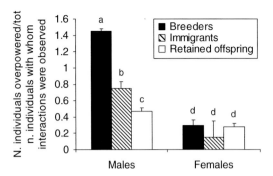

Figure 6.7. Mean (± S.E.) normalized DIdom index (number of animals dominated by an individual/the number of animals with which that individual interacted; Lamprecht 1986) of members of crow groups. A different letter (a, b, c, d) indicates a significant difference (*P* < 0.05) between social categories. From Chiarati et al. (2010).

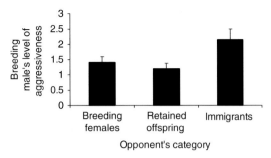

Figure 6.8. Mean (± S.E.) aggressiveness of breeding males toward different categories of opponents. From Chiarati et al. (2011).

lower positions of the hierarchy, which potentially determines access to food.

Alpha males overcome this disadvantage by behaving nepotistically, associating and sharing food more frequently with their offspring than with immigrants, and behaving more aggressively toward the latter (Figure 6.8). As a result, both sons and daughters spend more time feeding on an experimental food source than do immigrants, despite their lower dominance rank. After this interaction between dominance and nepotism is accounted for, the presence of immigrants in the family group ultimately does not reduce the preferential access to food that offspring derive from remaining with their parents on the natal territory.

Mating system

Microsatellite parentage analysis confirmed a high frequency of polyandry, with resident males and male immigrants sharing reproduction and siring offspring in the same brood or in consecutive years (Baglione et al. 2002c). Conversely, communal nesting by multiple females is rare, probably because enlarged clutches have little chance of being raised successfully. The fact that extra-pair mating was found only in groups with immigrants but never in nuclear families (parents + retained offspring) or in unassisted pairs, and that the genotype of extra-pair chicks was always compatible with one of the adult males of the group, indicates that extra-group parentage is rare in this population.

The genetic data therefore confirm that immigrant males can gain immediate or deferred direct fitness benefits from joining an established group, unlike retained offspring for which no within-group parentage was found, most likely because it would generally entail incest. Conversely, indirect fitness benefits remain available to all subordinates because cobreeders are relatives and therefore the average degree of relatedness between the helpers and the chicks they contribute to raise remains high despite frequent polyandry.

Individual contribution to chick care

Due to the various routes to group membership and to the complexity of the mating system, groups may contain a sole female breeder that is unrelated to the breeder males and up to three additional types of group members: (1) male breeders, either territory residents or immigrants, that contribute genetically to the current brood, (2) birds that have potential mates in the group and that could breed nonincestuously, but do not. Although these are potential breeders, we consider them helpers according to their function within the group, (3) sexually immature immigrants or retained offspring, which are unequivocally nonbreeding helpers. With the exception of incubation and brooding, which are carried out exclusively by breeding females, both breeders and helpers participate in activities related to reproduction including nest building, chick provisioning, nest sanitation, and territory defense. Nevertheless, the workload is not shared evenly among group members. Several lines of evidence indicate that trade-offs between investment in the current brood and future reproduction differ in relation to sex and reproductive status.

The costs of chick provisioning

Nestling provisioning is a conspicuous task that is easy to measure in video-recorded observations at nests. Carrion crows carry food in their crops, and during a nest visit, they regurgitate the food into a nestling's open gape, repeating the act with the same nestling or several others in what we consider a "feed." The number of feeds made by an adult in each nest visit is positively correlated with the volume of its crop swelling, providing a good estimate of the amount of food brought to the nest (Canestrari et al. 2005).

Chick provisioning is costly in crows, and caregivers lose an average of 5.4% of their body weight during the breeding season (Canestrari et al. 2007). Mass loss is proportional to individual workload irrespective of age, sex, or breeding status (Figure 6.9). To test whether weight loss reflects an energetic cost of nestling care rather than an adaptive strategy to increase flight ability during a period when individuals make frequent trips to the nest (Moreno 1989), we supplemented territories with food during the breeding season. Food supplementation eliminated the relationship between individual workload and body weight loss, and individuals on supplemented territories lost significantly less weight (only 1.4%) than unfed ones, supporting the hypothesis that provisioning is costly (Canestrari et al. 2007). Similar costs in terms of weight loss have been reported in white-winged choughs *Corcorax melanorhamphos* (Heinsohn and Cockburn 1994) and meerkats *Suricata suricatta* (Chapter 17), while in other biparental species reproduction reduces fertility, survival or the efficiency of the immune system (Clutton-Brock 1991).

While the energetic costs of nestling provisioning do not vary greatly among individuals, different group members obtain different benefits from allofeeding,

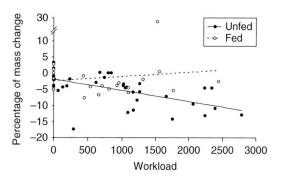

Figure 6.9. Percentage mass change plotted against estimate of workload (number of feeds per hour × hours of chick provisioning per day × number of days of provisioning) for unfed and fed crows. Negative values indicate mass loss, while positive values indicate mass gain. From Canestrari et al. (2007).

which in turn drives variation in individual contributions to chick care. Several lines of evidence indicate that future reproductive success is also highly valued, however, and thus the trade-off between current and future benefits also affects investment decisions in both breeders and helpers.

Distribution of workload among group members

Molecular data on parentage and relatedness within groups combined with video-recorded observations at the nest reveal that genetic mothers and fathers provision chicks at the highest rates, with no significant difference between them (Figure 6.10). Breeding males do not, however, adjust their effort to their actual share of parentage (Canestrari et al. 2005).

On average, helper contribution to brood provisioning is about two-thirds that of breeders, with unsuccessful potential breeders and nonbreeders feeding the chicks at similar frequencies (Canestrari et al. 2005). Relatedness with the nestlings is not correlated with individual variation in helping effort in both categories (unsuccessful potential breeders and nonbreeders), probably because, as consequence of the genetic structure of the cooperative groups, the average degree of relatedness among helpers and nestlings is always high (Baglione et al. 2003).

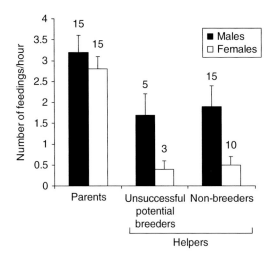

Figure 6.10. Number of feedings per hour by male and female parents, unsuccessful potential breeders, and nonbreeders. Sample sizes are given above bars. From Canestrari et al. (2005).

Among helpers, males provide significantly more food than females (Figure 6.10), which often refrain from visiting the nest altogether. The sex bias in helping behavior is likely to be due to differences in reproductive value between nonbreeding males and females. Theory suggests that helpers should reduce costly investment in nondescendant young when the probability of future reproduction increases (Cant and Field 2001). Crows fit this prediction. In the study population, turnover of breeding females is higher than that of males, resulting in a higher probability for young females obtaining a dominant breeding position when they reach sexual maturity and disperse. In contrast, males stay on the natal territory for longer and, when they disperse, they often have to queue in a new group before reaching the alpha breeding position (Baglione et al. 2005).

The trade-off between current and future reproduction: breeders' and helpers' strategies in variable conditions

The costs of chick care and the different potentials for future reproduction among group members determine important differences in investment strategies between breeders and helpers. Even though breeders work harder to feed and care for young in the current brood, breeders (especially females) also reduce their current reproductive effort when they have sufficient help, saving resources for future breeding attempts. For example, breeders reduce their workload when assisted by more than one helper, whereas nonbreeders do not vary their effort with the number of caregivers (Canestrari et al. 2007). Second, when territories are experimentally supplemented during the breeding season, breeders invest additional resources in self-maintenance, reducing mass loss instead of increasing chick provisioning. They do this despite the fact that chick starvation is frequent in this population and augmenting nestling feeding rate would likely increase nestling survival.

Third, breeders (especially females) fine-tune their provisioning effort by evaluating chick hunger during each nest visit and deciding whether to deliver the food item to the brood or to consuming all or part it themselves, sometimes even retrieving their own or another bird's prey from a chicks' gape (Canestrari et al. 2004, 2010). Such "false-feeding" occurs in about 16% of nest visits and is exhibited mainly by breeding females, indicating that it is unlikely to have evolved as a deceptive strategy in which helpers increase their perceived helping effort in the eyes of dominants (Boland et al. 1997).

Indeed, false-feeding occurs in the presence of onlookers as frequently as when individuals are alone at the nest and, when detected, provokes no visible reaction by other group members. Instead, experiments indicate that false-feeding results from a trade-off between chicks' needs and adult condition during nest visits (Canestrari et al. 2010). When chicks were experimentally fed in the nest, they reduced begging intensity and the frequency of false feeding increased among breeders. Similarly, breeders, but not helpers, augmented false feeding when their condition was experimentally worsened by clipping two primary feathers of each wing, which increased the costs of flying. These patterns contrast with a deceptive function of false-feeding and indicate that adults fine-tune their investment in the brood at every nest visit.

Although breeders invest heavily in chick provisioning, our data indicate that they value future reproduction and conserve resources whenever possible. This makes sense in a long-lived species like the crows, where current breeders have the highest probability of breeding in subsequent breeding seasons. Conversely, nonbreeders have little chance of achieving a breeding position in the near future and do not seem to work at the top of their abilities when they help, since regardless of age, their provisioning rate at nests is significantly less than that of breeders. Nonbreeders may therefore be more likely to increase investment in the current brood in response to environmental change. Indeed, when food was experimentally supplemented year-round, helpers, but not breeders, increased their provisioning rates and decreased their frequency of false feeding (Canestrari et al. 2008a, 2010).

Helpers also showed higher plasticity than breeders in an experiment where a group member that fed the nestlings at high frequency was temporarily handicapped by clipping two primary feathers, thus decreasing its provisioning rate. Helpers, unlike breeders, increased their effort after the manipulation and fully compensated for the lower contribution of the impaired group member (Baglione et al. 2010). Interestingly, those nonbreeders that initially made the lowest contribution to chick care, including those that were never observed at the nest before the treatment, were the ones that compensated most for the reduced provisioning by the handicapped groupmate, indicating that "lazy" group members are tolerated in the group because they represent a substitute workforce that can be mobilized when needed.

Even though helpers contribute less than breeders and breeders decrease their contribution when aided by several helpers, the presence of several care-givers has an additive effect on the total provisioning rate of a group, such that within the first ten days of life, individual chicks receive significantly more food as group size increases, an effect that disappears among older broods 15–20 days of age (Canestrari et al. 2008b). The consequences of these provisioning patterns on nestling survival and fledgling quality are discussed in the "Benefits of cooperation" section.

Other kinds of assistance: nest sanitation and vigilance

Unlike other cooperatively breeding species such as naked mole-rats (Burda et al. 2000; Chapter 19) and eusocial insects, a clear division of labor does not occur in crow groups. Besides nestling provisioning, our analyses of individual contributions of group members to nest sanitation and vigilance during foraging indicate that helpers do not compensate for their lower effort in chick feeding with a higher investment in other duties.

With the exception of fecal sac removal, which is performed by any adult present at the nest at the moment of excretion, other nest sanitation activities, including nest and chick cleaning and fluffing-up of the inner nest layer, are carried out mainly by breeding females, revealing a certain degree of specialization in cleaning tasks. Helpers contribute very little to these duties. Because a clean nest is crucial for successful reproduction in most birds, sanitation activities probably increase brood survival by reducing parasites and bacterial infections, and therefore benefit all group members.

Why do breeding females alone carry out most of the cleaning duties? We believe the answer is that they gain more by cleaning, because they carry out all incubation and brooding and are therefore more exposed than other group members to the risks of an unhygienic nest. This hypothesis is supported by the fact that adult females that are experimentally fed during the breeding season, and are presumably better able to fight against parasites, reduce the time they spend in sanitation activities without augmenting their provisioning rates (Bolopo et al. 2014).

Adults are also significantly more vigilant during foraging than are young helpers (Vera 2010). The frequency and duration of vigilance activities are significantly higher in adults than in yearlings. Adult group members decrease the time allocated to vigilance as the number of group members increases, consistent with the theory of "many eyes" (Pulliam 1973; Powell 1974). However, they adjust their vigilance rate only to the number of adult group members, ignoring young individuals. As a consequence, the presence of inexperienced group members does not decrease the per capita time dedicated to vigilance by adults, and young birds therefore benefit from the proximity to adults in term of antipredatory defense.

Standardized data on territory defense and mobbing behavior against predators are not yet available. However, field observations indicate that adults are more likely than juveniles to engage in territorial disputes and mobbing, and they also occupy more prominent positions during aerial fights (Baglione et al. 2002b).

The benefits of cooperation

Both direct and indirect fitness benefits of cooperation are likely to be important for the evolution and maintenance of cooperative breeding. As shown earlier, groups are strongly kin-structured, so that nonbreeders increase their indirect fitness by aiding relatives, while birds that can breed nonincestuously within the group additionally obtain often a share of reproduction and so increase their direct fitness. Breeders, on the other hand, may increase their current reproductive success thanks to the aid of several caregivers, and they may also augment the number of lifetime reproductive events if help allows them to lighten their investment in current reproductive attempts. These ideas are supported by the positive effect of group size on annual fledgling production and the load-lightening effect of "helpful" helpers on breeders.

Our analyses, based on a 10-year dataset, have revealed that the presence of extra-birds other than the breeding pair significantly increases fledgling production after controlling for a potential confounding effect of territory quality (Canestrari et al. 2008b). Throughout the study period, reproductive success in the population varied annually between 0.65 and 1.24 fledglings per breeding group, with the proportion of territories successfully fledging at least one chick ranging between 27% and 55%. Trios, however, produce 0.10 fledglings more than pairs and quartets 0.2 chicks more than trios, with fledging success leveling off in larger groups (Figure 6.11a).

The increased annual production of cooperative groups is due to a positive effect of group size on different stages of reproduction. Crows lay an average (± S.E.) of 4.6 ± 0.1 eggs (range 1–7) in the first breeding attempt

of each season. If the nest fails at the egg or hatching stage, crows can renest up to two, and occasionally three times, laying smaller clutches in replacement nests. Group size does not affect clutch size or hatching success, but larger groups have significantly higher probabilities of renesting after failure. Furthermore, group size increases the probability of nest success and, among successful nests, augments the number of fledglings produced.

Helpers not only increase the number of fledglings but their quality as well. We found that the number of male helpers, which are more helpful than females in provisioning the brood, is positively correlated with fledgling body mass (Figure 6.11b). Offspring weight at fledging is an important component of adult reproductive success because postfledging survival is greater for heavier young. Our data therefore show that helpers increase the reproductive output of breeders in multiple ways, setting the stage for kin selection to shape cooperative behavior.

Maternal strategies in relation to helping behavior

Besides increasing the number and quality of chicks fledged, helpers lighten the workload of breeders and compensate for a sudden decrease in the provisioning effort of group mates, as discussed earlier. Furthermore, we have evidence for "concealed helper effects" with helpers compensating for reduced investment in egg volume by breeding females in groups containing male helpers where, despite originating from smaller eggs, fledglings are eventually heavier than in groups without male helpers (Canestrari et al. 2011). Egg production is a costly process (Monaghan et al. 1998; Visser and Lessells 2001) and breeding female crows can lay up to 21 eggs during a single breeding season (Canestrari et al. 2008b, 2011). In cooperative groups, breeding females reduce egg size by 2.2% with each additional subordinate male (Figure 6.11c). This is unlikely to be a nonadaptive consequence tied to maternal condition, because egg volume was correlated with the number of male subordinates, but not with total group size. Instead, reduced egg size apparently represents an adaptive strategy that allows breeding females to

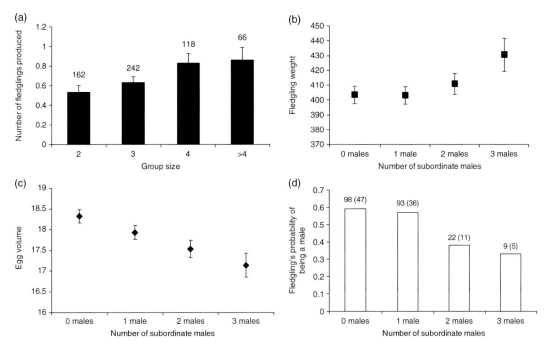

Figure 6.11. (a) Mean (± S.E.) fledglings produced per year by groups of 2, 3, 4, and >4 members in 1995–2004. Sample sizes are given above bars. (b) Effect of the number of male subordinates on fledgling weight based on a linear mixed model (LMM). (c) Effect of the number of male subordinates on egg volume based on a LMM. (d) Effect of the number of male subordinate group members on fledgling sex. Number of chicks (broods in brackets) given above bars. From Canestrari et al. (2008b, 2011, 2012).

conserve resources for future breeding attempts in the presence of "helpful" helpers, which overcome the effects of producing smaller eggs in the current brood. Similar effects of helpers on egg size have been documented in two other species (Russell et al. 2007; Paquet et al. 2012) and may be widespread, although apparently not universal among cooperative breeders (Koenig et al. 2009). To the extent that it occurs, however, it needs to be accounted for in estimates of the fitness consequences of helping.

The importance of male help shapes adjustment of the sex ratio of the brood with group composition (Canestrari et al. 2012). In our population, the brood sex ratio at fledging is biased toward males in groups lacking male subordinates. Conversely, in groups with working helpers, the sex ratio is biased toward females. These patterns appear to arise through a combination of manipulation of primary offspring sex ratio at the

egg stage and secondary adjustments after hatching. Both the primary and secondary sex ratio exhibit a prevalence of males in groups with less than two subordinate males (Figure 6.11d), although the trend is not significant at hatching. Furthermore, the primary sex ratio changes with the hatching sequence, with sons being positioned early in the hatching sequence in the first clutch and daughters being positioned early in later clutches. This indicates that breeding females are able to manipulate egg sex in a way that favors fledging by the more costly males in the first attempt and, in cases of renesting after failure, "cheaper" females in subsequent attempts. Subsequent changes in sex ratio during the nestling period indicate that post-hatching adjustments through preferential provisioning also take place. It is still unclear whether both breeders and helpers participate in such secondary adjustment of brood sex, or how it is achieved.

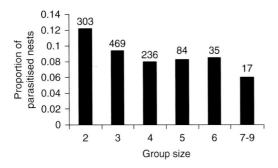

Figure 6.12. Proportion of crow nests that were parasitized in relation to group size. Sample sizes are given above bars. From Canestrari et al. (2009).

The relationship between cooperative crows and a brood parasite

Carrion crows are the secondary hosts of the great spotted cuckoo (*Clamator glandarius*), a brood parasite specialized on corvids that does not evict host eggs/chicks and is therefore raised alongside host nest mates. In our population of carrion crows, the percentage of nests with cuckoo eggs fluctuates annually between 1.2% and 70% (Canestrari et al. 2009) and parasitized nests contain on average 1.5 cuckoo eggs (range 1–3).

The relationship between a brood parasite and a cooperatively breeding host can be complex (Rowley and Russell 1990; Poiani and Elgar 1994). Theory suggests that increased activity at nests of cooperative breeders makes them more conspicuous to adult brood parasites or larger groups may be better defended against brood parasites. Furthermore, the nests with helpers may be preferred by parasites if increased provisioning efficiency augments parasite fledging success. Data on cooperatively breeding carrion crows show that parasitism rates decrease with group size (Figure 6.12), with unassisted pairs being the most frequently targeted breeding units despite consisting of only 25% of groups. This is unlikely to be due to the parasite's active choice of the "optimal" foster parents, because unassisted pairs are in general the least successful breeders (Canestrari et al. 2008b) and do not confer higher reproductive success to cuckoos compared to larger groups (Canestrari et al. 2009).

The lack of a correlation between group size and cuckoo reproductive success is due to two counterbalancing effects of group size. On the one hand, egg-laying by female cuckoos is better synchronized with the host in nests of unassisted pairs, providing cuckoo chicks with a larger age advantage over host nestmates. On the other hand, groups with helpers are more efficient in provisioning the brood and thus late-hatched cuckoos are able to make up for their initial age disadvantage, ending up with the same rate of survival as for chicks raised by pairs. As a result, cuckoo chick survival is unrelated to crow group size.

Because cuckoo females do not choose the best foster parents and do not lay their eggs according to the availability of host group size, the lower parasitism rate of groups with helpers – the most abundant breeding units – is probably due to a defensive effect of supernumerary group members. This does not appear to be a consequence of active nest defense against adult cuckoos, however, as crows do not mob adult parasites and do not eject alien eggs from the nest (Soler et al. 2001; Canestrari et al. 2009). Instead, it appears to be an indirect consequence of decreased laying opportunities for female cuckoos, which rarely find nests of large groups unattended. In cooperative groups, incubating females are fed at the nest by the other group members, so that the presence of helpers increases the proportion of time females incubate. These results suggest that cooperative species may have an indirect advantage in the fight against brood parasites even when they lack specific defensive behaviors.

Whether the indirect defense against great spotted cuckoos is indeed an advantage for cooperative crows is unclear, however. While the presence of a cuckoo chick reduces the number of crow fledglings in successful nests, cuckoo chicks seem to protect the nest against predators with a repellent secretion produced under threat. Thus nests containing a cuckoo chick are less likely to fail than unparasitized nests, a surprising result that we have demonstrated using chick translocation between parasitized and nonparasitized nests. This provides an unexpected benefit to crow parents that may counterbalance the negative effect on the number of chicks produced. Indeed, when nest predation is frequent, parasitized nests produce more crow fledglings than nonparasitized ones, while the pattern is reversed when predation is infrequent (Canestrari et al. 2014). Therefore, the net effect of parasitism in cooperative crows fluctuates between parasitism and mutualism according to environmental conditions, primarily predator density.

Conclusions

Geographic variation in the social organization of crows sheds light on the ecology of family living. Shortages of breeding vacancies and/or mates are ubiquitous, but delayed dispersal by offspring occurs where conditions are more favorable for young to remain on their natal territory, contrary to the predictions of the ecological constraints hypothesis. Specifically, the key factor promoting stable families is the benefit that young derive from the association with their parents and this arises only where adults occupy and defend a territory year-round and can provide their offspring a "safe haven" with preferential access to food, protection, and resources.

Indirect fitness benefits are important in shaping provisioning behavior, as indicated by the fact that cooperative alliances between territory residents and immigrants of the same sex arise only among relatives and that helpers increase the reproductive output of breeders, both in terms of the quantity and quality of fledglings produced. Direct fitness benefits also play a role, however, as immigrant males often sire some offspring within the brood, partly eroding the parentage of the dominant male and the indirect fitness gains of retained offspring that are functioning as helpers.

In this complex society, where individuals within the group pursue different benefits and have contrasting interests, high relatedness among group members is crucial for maintaining group stability and cooperation. Our ongoing research is focused on confirming this hypothesis by quantifying the pay-offs of helping for each group member. This can be difficult because helpers in crows confer "hidden" effects on breeders' reproduction and survival that can be easily overlooked, such as allowing breeder females to produce smaller eggs without reproductive consequences.

Corvids (crows, jays, magpies, and allied groups) originated from a branch of the oscine parvorder Corvida that currently inhabits the Australo-Papuan region and comprises several cooperatively breeding lineages (Russell 1989; Cockburn 1996). During their radiation from the Southern Hemisphere, corvids have gained and lost cooperative breeding several times, making the identification of their ancestral state difficult. These multiple transitions suggest that cooperative breeding is highly plastic in this clade (Ekman and Ericson 2006), consistent with the intraspecific variability found in the carrion crows where, as we have shown, individuals of noncooperative populations retain the capability to delay dispersal and help in response to environmental or social change. Corvids in general have proven to be a suitable group for testing the phylogenetic basis of cooperative breeding, and further study of the many poorly known species in this group is likely to provide new insights into the evolution of family living and helping in birds.

Considerable research has recently focused on the remarkable cognitive abilities of corvids, the so called "feathered apes" (Clayton 2012), investigating how these abilities are used in the context of cooperative tasks. Integrating studies of social cognition with understanding of behaviors associated with cooperative breeding is a particularly promising approach for the future.

Unlike studies of cooperation in general, cooperative breeding research has devoted relatively little attention to the proximate mechanisms that regulate helping (Bergmüller et al. 2007). We believe that a closer focus on how individuals communicate and respond to each other's behavior will allow a better understanding of the dynamics of cooperation at the nest and, ultimately, its function. Crows are well suited for this approach, which is one of the challenges of our future research.

Acknowledgments

We are grateful to J. L. Dickinson and W. D. Koenig for reviewing this chapter and providing most valuable insights. We thank our coworkers José Manuel Marcos, Elisa Chiarati, Rubén Vera, Diana Bolopo, Michael

Griesser, Jan Ekman, Marta Vila, Giuseppe Bogliani, Guido Andreotti, and Cristiana Bardini for their effort in collecting and analyzing much of the data summarized in this chapter. Gloria Robles, Rudy Valfiorito, Matthias Loretto, and Gianluca Roncalli helped in the field. During these years, many referees, most of them anonymous, provided valuable insights and suggestions that greatly improved our work. We are also grateful to Hugo Robles for countless inspiring discussions and help with statistics. This study has been funded by the Spanish Ministry for Science (grants CGL2005-02083/BOS, SEJ2007-29836-E in the framework of the EU program ESF-EUROCORES, CGL2008-01829BOS and CGL2011-27260), the Junta and Castilla y León (grants VA001A05 and VA059A11), the Gates Cambridge trust (to DC), and the Association for the Study of Animal Behaviour – ASAB (to DC).

REFERENCES

Baglione, V., Canestrari, D., Marcos J. M., Griesser, M., and Ekman, J. (2002a). History, environment and social behaviour: experimentally induced cooperative breeding in the carrion crow. *Proc. R. Soc. London B*, 269, 1247-1251.

Baglione, V., Marcos, J. M., and Canestrari, D. (2002b). Cooperatively breeding groups of Carrion Crow (*Corvus corone corone*) in northern Spain. *Auk*, 119, 790-799.

Baglione, V., Marcos J. M., Canestrari, D., and Ekman, J. (2002c). Direct fitness benefits of group living in a complex cooperative society of carrion crows, *Corvus corone corone*. *Anim. Behav.*, 64, 887-893.

Baglione, V., Canestrari, D., Marcos, J. M., and Ekman, J. (2003). Kin selection in cooperative alliances of carrion crows. *Science*, 300, 1947-1949.

Baglione, V., Marcos, J. M., Canestrari, D., Griesser, M., Andreotti, G., et al. (2005). Does year-round territoriality rather than habitat saturation explain delayed natal dispersal and cooperative breeding in the carrion crow? *J. Anim. Ecol.*, 74, 842-851.

Baglione, V., Canestrari, D., Marcos J. M., and Ekman, J. (2006). Experimentally increased food resources in the natal territory promote offspring philopatry and helping in cooperatively breeding carrion crows. *Proc. R. Soc. London B*, 273, 1529-1535.

Baglione, V., Canestrari, D., Chiarati, E., Vera, R., and Marcos, J. M. (2010). Lazy group members are substitute helpers in carrion crows. *Proc. R. Soc. London B*, 277, 3275-3282.

Bergmüller, R., Johnstone, R. A., Russell, A. F., and Bshary, R. (2007). Integrating cooperative breeding into theoretical concepts of cooperation. *Behav. Proc.*, 76, 61-72.

Boland, C. R. J., Heinsohn, R., and Cockburn, A. (1997). Deception by helpers in cooperatively breeding white-winged choughs and its experimental manipulation. *Behav. Ecol. Sociobiol.*, 41, 251-256.

Burda, H., Honeycutt, R. L., Begall, S., Locker-Grutjen, O., and Scharff, A. (2000). Are naked and common mole-rats eusocial and if so, why? *Behav. Ecol. Sociobiol.*, 47, 293-303.

Canestrari, D., Marcos, J. M., and Baglione, V. (2004). False feedings at the nests of carrion crows *Corvus corone corone*. *Behav. Ecol. Sociobiol.*, 55, 477-483.

Canestrari, D., Marcos, J. M., and Baglione, V. (2005). Effect of parentage and relatedness on the individual contribution to cooperative chick care in carrion crows. *Behav. Ecol. Sociobiol.*, 52, 422-428.

Canestrari, D., Marcos, J. M., and Baglione, V. (2007). Costs of chick provisioning in cooperatively breeding carrion crows: an experimental study. *Anim. Behav.*, 73, 349-357.

Canestrari, D., Chiarati, E., Marcos, J. M., Ekman, J., and Baglione V. (2008a). Helpers but not breeders adjust provisioning effort to year-round territory resource availability in carrion crows. *Anim. Behav.*, 76, 943-949.

Canestrari, D., Marcos, J. M., and Baglione, V. (2008b). Reproductive success increases with group size in cooperative carrion crows *Corvus corone corone*. *Anim. Behav.*, 75, 403-416.

Canestrari, D., Marcos, J. M., and Baglione, V. (2009). Cooperative breeding in carrion crows reduces the rate of brood parasitism by great spotted cuckoos. *Anim. Behav.*, 77, 1337-1344.

Canestrari, D., Vera, R., Chiarati, E., Marcos, J. M., Vila, M., et al. (2010). False feeding: the trade-off between chick hunger and caregivers needs in cooperative crows. *Behav. Ecol.*, 21, 233-241.

Canestrari, D., Marcos, J. M., and Baglione, V. (2011). Helpers at the nest compensate for reduced maternal investment in egg size in carrion crows. *J. Evol. Biol.*, 24, 1870-1878.

Canestrari, D., Vila, M., Marcos, J. M., and Baglione, V. (2012). Cooperatively breeding carrion crows adjust offspring sex ratio according to group composition. *Behav. Ecol. Sociobiol.*, 66, 1225-1235.

Canestrari, D., Bolopo, D., Turlings, T. C. J., Röder, G., Marcos, J. M., and Baglione, V. (2014). From parasitism to mutualism: unexpected interactions between a cuckoo and its host. *Science*, 343, 11350-1352.

Cant, M. A. and Field, J. (2001). Helping effort and future fitness in cooperative animal societies. *Proc. R. Soc. London B*, 268, 1959-1964.

Charles, J. K. (1972). Territorial behaviour and the limitations of population size in cros, *Corvus corone* and *C. cornix*. Ph.D. thesis, University of Aberdeen, Aberdeen, Scotland.

Chiarati, E., Canestrari, D., Vera, R., Marcos, J. M., and Baglione, V. (2010). Linear and stable dominance hierarchies in cooperative carrion crows. *Ethology*, 316, 346–356.

Chiarati, E., Canestrari, D., Vila, M., Vera, R., and Baglione, V. (2011). Nepotistic access to food resources in cooperatively breeding carrion crows. *Behav. Ecol. Sociobiol.*, 65, 1791–1800.

Chiarati, E., Canestrari, D., Vera, R., and Baglione, V. (2012). Subordinates benefit from exploratory dominants: response to novel food in cooperatively breeding carrion crows. *Anim. Behav.*, 83, 103–109.

Clayton, N. (2012). Corvid cognition: feathered apes. *Nature*, 484, 453–454.

Clutton-Brock, T. H. (1991). *The Evolution of Parental Care*. Princeton, NJ: Princeton University Press.

Cockburn, A. (1996). Why do so many Australian birds cooperate: social evolution in the Corvida? In: *Frontiers of Population Ecology*, ed. R. B. Floyd, A. W. Sheppard, and P. J. de Barro. Melbourne: CSIRO Publishing, pp. 451–472.

Cockburn, A. (1998). Evolution of helping behavior in cooperatively breeding birds. *Annu. Rev. Ecol. Syst.*, 29, 141–177.

Cramp, S. and Perrins C. M. (1994). *The Birds of the Western Palearctic. Vol VIII. Crows to Finches*. Oxford: Oxford University Press.

Ekman, J. and Ericson, P. G. P. (2006). Out of Gondwanaland; the evolutionary history of cooperative breeding and social behaviour among crows, magpies, jays and allies. *Proc. R. Soc. London B*, 273, 1117–1125.

Ekman, J., Baglione, V., Eggers, S., and Griesser, M. (2001). Delayed dispersal: living under the reign of nepotistic parents. *Auk*, 118, 1–10.

Emlen, S. T. (1991). Evolution of cooperative breeding in birds and mammals. In: *Behavioural Ecology: An Evolutionary Approach*, 3rd edn, ed. J. R. Krebs and N. B. Davies. Oxford: Blackwell, pp. 301–335.

Haas, F., Pointer, M. A., Saino, N., Brodin, A., Mundy, N. I., et al. (2009). An analysis of population genetic differentiation and genotype–phenotype association across the hybrid zone of carrion and hooded crows using microsatellites and MC1R. *Mol. Ecol.*, 18, 294–305.

Heinsohn, R. and Cockburn, A. (1994). Helping is costly to young birds in cooperatively breeding white-winged choughs. *Proc. R. Soc. London B*, 256, 293–298.

Koenig, W. D., Walters, E. L., and Haydock, J. (2009). Helpers and egg investment in the cooperatively breeding acorn woodpecker: testing the concealed helper effects hypothesis. *Behav. Ecol. Sociobiol.*, 63, 1659–1665.

Kokko H. and Ekman, J. (2002). Delayed dispersal as a route to breeding: territorial inheritance, safe havens, and ecological constraints. *Am. Nat.*, 160, 468–484.

Loman, J. (1985). Social organization in a population of the hooded crow. *Ardea*, 73, 61–75.

Madge, R. D. and Burn, H. (1999). *Crows and Jays*. London: Christopher Helm.

Monaghan, P., Nager, R. G., and Houston, D. C. (1998). The price of eggs: increased investment in egg production reduces the offspring rearing capacity of parents. *Proc. R. Soc. London B*, 265, 1731–1735.

Moreno, J. (1989). Strategies of mass change in breeding birds. *Biol. J. Linn. Soc.*, 37, 297–310.

Paquet, M., Covas, R., Chastel, O., Parenteau, C., and Doutrelant, C. (2012). Maternal effects in relation to helper presence in the cooperatively breeding sociable weaver. *PLoS One*, 8, e59336.

Poelstra, J. W., Ellegren, H., and Wolf, J. B. (2013). An extensive candidate gene approach to speciation: diversity, divergence and linkage disequilibrium in candidate pigmentation genes across the European crow hybrid zone. *Heredity*, 111, 467–473.

Poelstra, J. W., Vijay, N., Bossu, C. M., Lantz, H., Ryll, B., et al. (2014). The genomic landscape underlying phenotypic integrity in the face of gene flow in crows. *Science*, 344, 1410–1414.

Poiani, A. and Elgar, M. A. (1994). Cooperative breeding in the Australian avifauna and brood parasitism by cuckoos (Cuculidae). *Anim. Behav.*, 47, 697–706.

Powell, G. V. N. (1974). Experimental analysis of the social value of flocking by starlings (*Sturnus vulgaris*) in relation to predation and foraging. *Anim. Behav.*, 22, 501–505.

Pulliam, H. R. (1973). On the advantages of flocking. *J. Theor. Biol.*, 38, 419–422.

Queller, D. C. (1992). Does population viscosity promote kin selection? *Trends Ecol. Evol.*, 7, 322–324.

Richner, H. (1990). Helpers-at-the-nest in carrion crows *Corvus corone corone*. *Ibis*, 132, 105–108.

Russell, E. M. (1989). Co-operative breeding – a Gondwanan perspective. *Emu*, 89, 61–62.

Rowley, I. and Russell, E. M. (1990). Splendid fairy-wrens: demonstrating the importance of longevity. In: *Cooperative Breeding in Birds: Long-term Studies of Ecology and Behavior*, ed. P. B. Stacey and W. D. Koenig, Cambridge: Cambridge University Press, pp. 1–30.

Russell, A. F., Langmore, N. E., Cockburn, A., Astheimer, L. B., and Kilner, R. M. (2007). Reduced egg investment can conceal helper effects in cooperatively breeding birds. *Science*, 317, 941–944.

Soler, M., Soler, J., Perez-Contreras, T., and Martinez, J. (2001). Differential reproductive success of great spotted cuckoos *Clamator glandarius* parasitising magpies *Pica pica* and carrion crows *Corvus corone*: the importance of parasitism costs and host defences. *Avian Sci.*, 1, 1–9.

Vera, R. (2010). Grupos sociales cooperativos de corneja negra: agregaciones no territoriales, comportamiento de vigilancia y compromiso entre las necesidades de pollos y adultos en el aprovisionamiento al nido. Ph.D. thesis, Universidad de Valladolid, Palencia, Spain.

Visser, M. E. and Lessells, C. M. (2001). The costs of egg production and incubation in great tits (*Parus major*). *Proc. R. Soc. London B*, 268, 1271–1277.

Wittenberg, J. (1988). Langfristige Entwicklung einer Population der Rabenkrähe (*Corvus c. corone*) bei Braunschweig, ihre Zusammensetzung und ihr Einfluss auf andere Arten. *Beiheft Veröffentlichungen Naturschutz Landschaftspflege Baden-Württemberg*, 53, 2111–2223.

7

Southern pied babblers: The dynamics of conflict and cooperation in a group-living society

Amanda R. Ridley

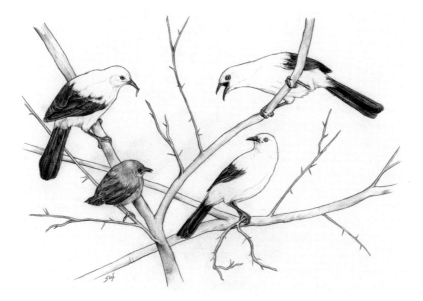

Introduction

The 30 species of *Turdoides* babblers range from communal to cooperative, most displaying some degree of social behavior. Distributed across much of the African continent and through the Middle East to India, they are an easily identifiable, highly vocal, and ubiquitous feature of many bird communities. Only a few members of the genus have been studied in sufficient detail to determine the exact level of sociality. However, based

on observations of the Arabian babbler (*T. squamiceps*, Zahavi 1990), Indian or jungle babbler (*T. striatus*, Gaston 1977) and southern pied babbler (*T. bicolor*, the focus of this chapter), cooperative breeding is likely to be widespread among members of the genus.

The southern pied babbler, which is easily distinguished by its distinctive black and white plumage and harsh chattering call, has a geographic range centered on the Kalahari desert biome (Hockey et al. 2005). Groups are common along the dry riverbeds and open

Cooperative Breeding in Vertebrates: Studies of Ecology, Evolution, and Behavior, eds W. D. Koenig and J. L. Dickinson.
Published by Cambridge University Press. © Cambridge University Press 2016.

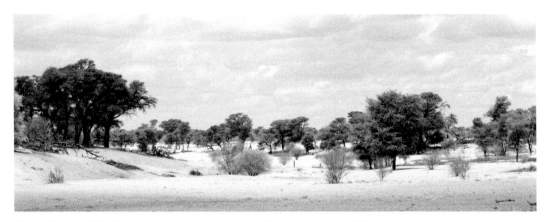

Figure 7.1. Typical babbler habitat: A dry riverbed dominated by large *Acacia erioloba*. Photo by Elizabeth Wiley.

acacia woodlands of the semi-arid Kalahari and sur-rounding areas (Figure 7.1). Pied babblers are rarely seen alone, indicating a high degree of sociality. This attribute, combined with their highly vocal behavior and habit of foraging in open woodland, makes them easily observable and thus an ideal species on which to conduct investigations into the causes and conse-quences of cooperative breeding behavior.

As with most other members of the genus *Turdoides,* pied babblers are characterized by a pot-bellied body shape and long tail. They are sexually monomorphic, with differences in breeding and calling behavior the primary way to distinguish the sexes. Genetic tests, however, are the only truly reliable way to sex adults in the absence of breeding activity. Fledglings have completely brown plumage, gradually changing to a mottled brown and white plumage by three months post-hatching, until full black-and-white adult plumage is achieved by one year of age. The transition of plum-age from brown to full adult plumage is highly variable among juveniles, and appears to be based upon devel-opmental triggers. Small, injured or disabled fledglings tend to retain their brown plumage for longer periods compared to broodmates that do not face such devel-opmental hurdles.

Pied babblers primarily forage for food by glean-ing or digging in the substrate for subterranean food items. They are largely insectivorous, with Coleopteran, Lepidopteran, and Orthopteran prey items comprising

the bulk of their diet. Larger prey items, such as scorpi-ons, lizards, frogs, and pygmy snakes are occasionally taken, as are seasonal fruits.

The pied babbler research project

Long-term monitoring of cooperative behaviors in pied babblers has been conducted in the southern Kalahari since 2003. Since project establishment, my colleagues and I have been monitoring significant life history events for each individual in the population on a reg-ular basis. We carefully document significant events throughout an individual's life, including dominance status, dispersal, eviction, reproduction, divorce, pre-dation, overt aggression, and prospecting behavior (defined as a temporary foray by an individual or coa-lition of individuals from their current group to other groups) in an attempt to gain insight into the costs and benefits of cooperative group-living behavior.

An important step into gaining these insights was habituating the babblers to human presence. In a pro-cess similar to that achieved at the Arabian babbler study site by Amotz and Avishag Zahavi, and at the meer-kat study site by Tim Clutton-Brock (Chapter 17), my colleague Nichola Raihani and I habituated ten groups of wild pied babblers. This allowed us to observe indi-viduals at a distance of 2–5 m without causing the birds any distress or noticeable change in natural behaviors

(Ridley and Raihani 2007a). We used a small amount of food on a top-pan balance to entice each individual to jump on and be weighed at dawn each day before any foraging had begun. This weighing was, and remains, an important aspect of our research, allowing us to gain insights into the body condition of each individual and how it changes according to significant life history events (Ridley and Raihani 2007b). After establishing the study population, we were joined over the years by a number of researchers and increased the number of habituated groups we followed; active research continues at the present time. The following thus represents the collaborative effort of many researchers working on the project over the years.

Social system

Pied babblers are highly cooperative and it is rare to find only a pair holding a territory. Group size ranges between 3 and 15 adults, with most groups having 5–6 adults comprising a dominant breeding pair and a variable number of subordinate helpers, usually offspring of the dominant pair. Pied babblers display high reproductive skew, and there is only one dominant male and female in each group that monopolize access to reproductive activity (Nelson-Flower et al. 2011).

Reproduction by subordinates is rare, occurring in newly formed groups where a clear hierarchy is not yet established, or following the death of one member of a dominant pair. When a new, unrelated individual immigrates into the group to fill a breeding vacancy, subordinates of the opposite sex are freed from inbreeding avoidance and may attempt to breed with the new dominant individual. Although subordinates may attempt to mate with a new opposite-sex dominant, even when the same-sex dominant is still present, they are hardly ever successful. Genetic analyses spanning over 200 group-years and 500 breeding attempts have revealed that in complex groups where subordinates have an opportunity to breed with opposite-sex dominants less than 10% of breeding events involve a subordinate successfully gaining reproduction (Nelson-Flower et al. 2011).

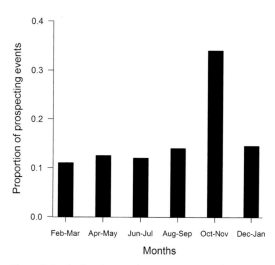

Figure 7.2. The distribution of prospecting events (where individuals search surrounding groups for dispersal opportunities) throughout the year. October–November is the period immediately prior to breeding. Rainfall causes the onset of the breeding season to change slightly each year, but all groups are usually engaged in courtship displays during October and November.

The reason that subordinates rarely achieve parentage is not for lack of trying, but rather because fights for dominance usually occur prior to a clutch being laid. Therefore, genetic analyses of parentage can be misleading, and do not represent true levels of competition for reproductive access. Our research has revealed that females fight fiercely for access to the dominant position, including eating each other's eggs (Nelson-Flower et al. 2013), engaging in physical conflicts, and attempting to evict each other (Raihani et al. 2010).

Reproductive competition, dispersal attempts, and prospecting for reproductive opportunities are behaviors observed primarily in the few months leading up to the breeding season (Figure 7.2). In 19% of dispersal attempts individuals disperse together in a coalition, similar to the behavior observed in the closely related Arabian babbler. Females are more likely to disperse in a coalition than males, and, again similar to Arabian babblers, coalitions are more likely to succeed in overthrowing a resident competitor than if they dispersed alone (Ridley 2012).

Once individuals have dispersed into a new group, a hierarchy is established between coalition members; two individuals of the same sex in the same group do not share dominant breeding positions. Dominance is a relatively easy behavior to observe. Although physical fighting is rare, dominant individuals display threat behaviors to subordinate group members. These behaviors include wing-splays, chest-puffing, pecks, and "jumps," where the dominant may jump on the subordinate's back or wrestle the subordinate so that it is lying on the ground with its legs in the air in a submissive posture.

Pied babblers can live for more than ten years in the wild, and some individuals that were dominant when I started the study in 2003 are still alive as of 2014. Dominant female turnover is slightly higher than that of dominant males, because females can be depredated during nocturnal incubation of eggs or brooding of nestlings. Attempts to found new groups are not uncommon, but rarely succeed. Usually a founding attempt occurs when a male is evicted from his group by a competing or dominant male, and establishes a territory to which females are attracted through repeated male calling behavior. Large males tend to be more successful at attracting females to a new territory, suggesting that there is information in the male call that reveals body condition to prospective female mates. Our research on the relationship between male calling behavior, body mass, and attractiveness to females is currently underway.

Breeding behavior

Breeding is a prolonged process, beginning with a courtship display by the male involving the presentation of sticks to the female, midair chasing, and an exaggerated "display walk" with wing and tail feathers splayed out while walking repeatedly past the female. This courtship phase may last several days, after which the dominant pair begins to nest-build together.

Pied babbler nests are an open cup built of thick twigs, with fine grasses lining the cup. The female lays one egg per day with a clutch size of up to four (modal clutch size = 3 eggs). Only the dominant female

incubates at night, but during the day all group members take turns to incubate, and the nest is rarely left unattended (Ridley and van den Heuvel 2012).

Incubation lasts for 13–15 days. After hatching, the nestlings are fed by all group members, with no observed cases of an adult group member not contributing to provisioning young. The timing of fledging varies widely and is strongly related to group size (Raihani and Ridley 2007a). Small groups, which are less able to defend the nest against predators, fledge their young earlier (around 13–15 days) than large groups (around 16–18 days post-hatching). Presumably this is because as the nestlings grow older, their begging becomes louder, such that predation rates increase dramatically toward the end of the nestling period (Ridley and van den Heuvel 2012).

Postfledging, young cannot fly and instead run after the group between foraging sites. They must climb up the tree to reach the rest of the group when they roost, and often fall out of the trees or end up roosting alone on the ground or low-lying vegetation for the first few days postfledging (Raihani and Ridley 2007b). After about one week, young begin to be able to fly short distances, but do not become accomplished flyers until approximately three weeks postfledging.

Similar to some other cooperatively breeding bird species (Langen 2000), pied babbler fledglings have an extended period of care. During this time they are highly reliant on adults to provision them, and most fledglings do not become independent foragers for several months postfledging (Ridley and Raihani 2007b).

Groups are highly territorial and defend a territory year-round (Golabek et al. 2012). Groups aggressively exclude extra-group individuals (which can include smaller groups, pairs, or lone individuals) from prime foraging habitat, which may be a major reason why pairs are so rare in the population. All adult group members help to participate in territory defense, and juveniles will begin to join in some territorial displays at about six months of age. Territorial border displays are common, occurring almost daily. In most cases, these displays are highly ritualized and commonly involve members lining up together on the same branch or a series of neighboring branches and giving a communal, raucous chorus. The vocal display is usually

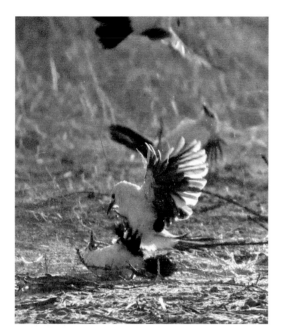

Figure 7.3. Two dominant females from neighboring groups engaged in a physical fight during an intergroup interaction. Although intergroup interactions are common, such physical aggression is relatively rare. Photo by Amanda Ridley. See plate section for color figure.

of over 400 border interactions has revealed that individuals are less likely to invest in territorial displays on borders that they share with kin. This result suggests both kin recognition and greater tolerance of kin than nonkin on territory borders (Humphries et al. 2015).

The costs of dispersal and the trade-off between helping and dispersing

Unlike most birds, there is no sex-biased dispersal in pied babblers. Females disperse slightly more often than males, but after accounting for the slight female-bias in the sex ratio, this higher rate is not significant (Nelson-Flower et al. 2012). Both males and females remain with their natal group as helpers for several years on average, and contribute to raising subsequent broods produced by the dominant pair. Helping behavior includes incubation and brooding of young, provisioning, teaching, escorting young, cooperative predator-mobbing, territory defense, and sentinel behavior. Given that pied babblers have no sex-biased dispersal, it is not surprising that there is no detectable difference in provisioning rates between the sexes (Figure 7.4).

The probability of dispersal can be reliably predicted from provisioning rates. This is because dispersal is a costly activity that results in a considerable loss of body mass (Ridley et al. 2008) and therefore dispersing individuals try to gain as much mass as they can prior to a prospecting foray or dispersal attempt. By comparing the helping rate of individuals toward same-aged broods during periods when no dispersal occurred and just prior to prospecting or dispersal taking place, there was a clear pattern of reduced investment and increased weight gain prior to dispersal (Figure 7.5).

Dispersal may be voluntary or forced. Voluntary dispersal occurs when an individual leaves the group to prospect at groups elsewhere, whereas forced dispersal is when an individual is physically attacked, forcibly evicted, and not allowed to return. In almost all cases, eviction occurs among same-sex individuals, and eviction is far less common than voluntary dispersal (Raihani et al. 2010). The most common form of eviction is between same-sex broodmates, or when

accompanied by a rapid pumping up and down of the wings, and piloerection of the head and breast feathers. There are distinctive male and female calls within the chorus, and these may provide opposing groups with information about group composition as well as the existence of breeding vacancies (Golabek 2010).

On rare occasions (< 10% of interactions), these ritualized displays turn into physical aggression, where members of opposing groups fly to the ground, peck at, and try to pin each other down (Figure 7.3). This sometimes leads to injury, but usually only results in the loss of feathers for the victim. Violent territorial interactions usually result from one group strongly incurring onto the territory of another group.

Territorial displays range widely in investment, from a vocal exchange of less than a minute to extended interactions lasting up to 30 minutes. Territorial displays can be costly to group members and result in considerable loss of body mass. Interestingly, an analysis

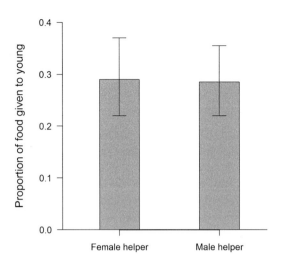

Figure 7.4. The proportion of food captured that individual female and male helpers subsequently gave to young as opposed to the total biomass given away in order to account for differences in foraging ability. There is no difference between the sexes in the level of contribution to young. Data based on foraging contributions by more than 200 helpers over an 11-year period.

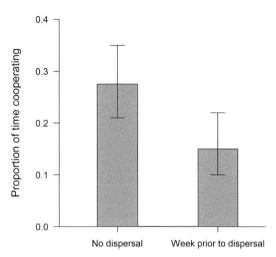

Figure 7.5. The relationship between dispersal and helping behavior. The proportion of focal observation time spent contributing to cooperative activities (including incubating, provisioning young, sentinel behavior, and predator mobbing) for individuals during a week when they did not subsequently attempt to disperse compared to the same individuals during the week prior to attempted dispersal. To account for the potential confound of age, data were paired for broods within the same breeding season, for groups that had the same brood size and same group size for each breeding event considered. $N = 11$ paired comparisons.

coalition members disperse into a breeding position together. Coalitions tend to be unstable and one partner may eventually evict or subordinate the other, resulting in only a single dominant individual of each sex. Voluntary dispersal typically only occurs once individuals become adults, with the average age of first dispersal being 2 years of age post-hatching (range 1–6). There is no difference between the sexes in the average age of dispersal, and older individuals are more likely to successfully disperse (Raihani et al. 2010).

Dispersal patterns are strongly affected by relatedness: individuals disperse farther from their natal territory than nonnatal territories, presumably because neighboring groups tend to contain close relatives (Nelson-Flower et al. 2012). In addition, individuals generally do not attempt to disperse into groups where the opposite-sex dominant is a close relative that they have had prior experience with, indicating inbreeding avoidance (Nelson-Flower et al. 2012).

Since dispersal is costly, using the natal territory as a "safe haven" while waiting for opportunities for dispersal could be highly beneficial (Ekman and Griesser

2002; Kokko and Ekman 2002). Failed dispersers or evicted individuals with no fixed territory "float" in the population looking for foraging sites and opportunities to join a group. Floating behavior is likely to be costly, and may provide a reasonable explanation for delayed dispersal in many cooperative species (Koenig et al. 1992). To determine the cost of floating, we compared the time-activity budget and body mass of individuals when they were in a group compared to when they were floating and found that floaters spend significantly more time being vigilant for predators and less time foraging, with a steady decline in body mass over time (Ridley et al. 2008).

Floating can therefore have both long- and short-term consequences. In the short-term, an individual suffers lower foraging efficiency, greater exposure to predators, and mass loss. In the long-term, a continual decline in body mass can affect the probability of an individual successfully fighting for a position in a new group (Ridley et al. 2008).

When we compared the dispersal success of individuals that used the natal territory as a safe haven between breeding events compared to those that floated within the population, we found that the former, with a higher body mass, were more likely to successfully disperse and to gain the dominant breeding position in a new group (Ridley et al. 2008). Therefore dispersal is not only costly, but the dispersal *strategy* is important; in particular staying on the natal territory and making prospecting forays, similar to that described for other cooperative-breeding species (Double and Cockburn 2000; Young and Monfort 2009; Mares et al. 2012), is less costly than being a floater. Our findings therefore support previous research suggesting that using the natal territory as a "safe haven" can be highly beneficial.

The balance of competition and cooperation

Pairs comprise less than 5% of groups, and unless a pair is successful at recruiting helpers they are generally ephemeral, with a high likelihood of dissolution within a few months of formation. Of 14 instances of pairs forming in the population, we have observed only two cases where a pair successfully raised young to adulthood and the group persisted beyond a single breeding season. This is in contrast to groups of more than two, of which 87% successfully raised young to independence each year and group persistence into the next breeding season was above 70%.

The challenges facing a pair are significant: they must share the effort of raising a brood among only two adults, and they must successfully defend their territory from neighboring groups. By conducting time–activity watches to determine how much time each individual apportions to finding food to feed young, we found that pairs need to work harder than individuals in groups (Figure 7.6). By investing so much time into foraging for young, pairs had less time to be vigilant for predators and forage for themselves, resulting in significantly higher mass loss during the breeding period compared to individuals in groups (Figure 7.7). This effect was most pronounced in drought years, when food

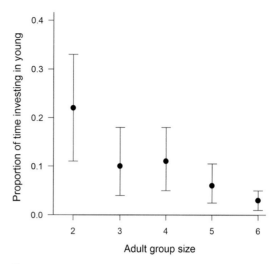

Figure 7.6. The effect of group size on workload during chick-rearing. Pairs spend a greater proportion of their time foraging for food to provision young, as well as incubating and brooding young. $N = 943$ focal watches of 77 individuals in 14 groups during the chick-rearing period. Data were restricted to focal watches conducted on the same day post-hatching in nests with the same broodsize.

availability was particularly limiting. In fact, mass loss was so high for some pairs as to be unsustainable, and likely explains why we observed such high chick mortality in the nests of pairs.

These results suggest that cooperative breeding has an important influence on reproductive success in the pied babblers. While pairs can on occasion breed successfully, and thus the species cannot strictly be considered an obligate cooperative breeder, the likelihood of success is much lower, and the physical toll on the adults in terms of mass loss is significantly greater.

The benefits of cooperation are borne out in developmental differences in young birds. Young that are raised in large groups receive care from adults for a longer period of time, are heavier, and have higher foraging proficiency at independence. In addition, such birds are more likely to successfully disperse into a dominant breeding position, and therefore start to gain access to reproductive opportunities at a younger age than those that receive shorter periods of care (Figure 7.8).

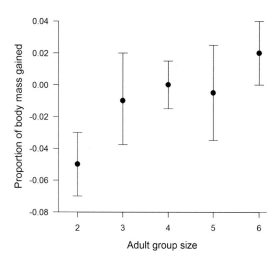

Figure 7.7. The relationship between group size and the proportion of prebreeding body mass gained over the duration of the chick-rearing period. Data restricted to groups rearing broods of the same size at the same age post-hatching. Pairs suffer a greater proportion of body mass loss than group members.

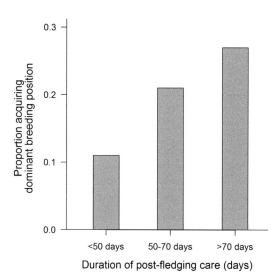

Figure 7.8. The relationship between the duration of postfledging care that individuals received and whether or not they attained a dominant breeding position by two years of age. $N = 110$ individuals that were observed from hatching until they were more than two years of age. From Ridley and Raihani (2007b).

Similar developmental benefits have been observed previously in noncooperative-breeding species, where the influencing factor is parental quality rather than helper investment (Lindström 1999), but there has been limited evidence for a developmental benefit in early life influencing individual fitness in cooperative breeders. The results from our life-history monitoring raise the possibility that group size can influence the lifetime fitness of young raised in such groups. Given their long lifespan, however, we may have to wait many more years in order to fully quantify the fitness benefits of group-living and cooperative behavior.

Although the "helper effect" during reproduction is a commonly studied and well-recognized benefit of cooperative breeding behavior (Dickinson and Hatchwell 2004), another less studied effect is the importance of territory defense. Babblers constantly quarrel at their territory borders, and good habitat is rarely left empty. Indeed, we have observed smaller groups being "pushed out" of prime foraging areas by larger, more aggressive groups. This can result in disastrous consequences for the small group, including dispersal of subordinate helpers to more suitable habitat

and the inability to reach suitable breeding condition, thus resulting in delays in reproductive activity.

Large babbler groups can display a division of labor among group members where some stay behind to defend the nest area from predators and feed young while the rest of the group defends the territory border (Ridley and Raihani 2008). Smaller groups cannot divide labor in such a way, leaving the nest exposed to predators, and nestlings hungry for extended periods during territory defense. This is likely to be, at least in part, the reason for the significantly higher rates of nest predation that we observe in small groups.

Group size is therefore important for group persistence, reproductive success, helper retention, and successful territory defense. Not only do groups have a significant reproductive advantage over pairs, but group size itself has an important influence on reproductive success. We quantified this by determining the number of young that survived to adulthood. Using this measure, we found that an optimal group size exists in pied babblers, peaking at around 5–6 adults (Figure 7.9).

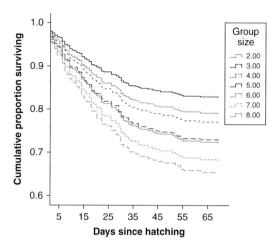

Figure 7.9. The relationship between survival and group size represented through Kaplan-Meier survival curves. These curves were generated for 11 breeding seasons of reproductive success data, representing 273 broods where eggs produced nestlings.

This represents a very important aspect of cooperative breeding behavior: there is a trade-off between the benefits of group size such as enhanced predator detection, increased reproductive success, load-lightening benefits, and territory defense, and the costs of group size such as reproductive and resource competition.

As an example of these costs, reproductive competition among females greatly depressed group reproductive output (Nelson-Flower et al. 2013). Video cameras revealed that this was because competing females committed oophagy – eating one another's eggs – and repeatedly abandoned nesting attempts. As a result, groups with competing females suffered significantly lower annual reproductive success.

Benefits of group size

One consequence of the group size effect on reproductive success found in pied babblers is that small groups, suffering from low chick recruitment, face a significant risk of extinction. Extinction represents a significant cost to group members, because although adults can disperse to groups elsewhere, prospecting for vacancies

can be highly costly (Ridley 2008; Young and Monfort 2009; Mares et al. 2012) and it may take some individuals an extended period of time to find a group that they will be accepted into.

Recruitment of young is the primary way that groups can increase in size. A less common route, however, is through the recruitment of unrelated individuals. Although kin selection has long been considered to be important to cooperative behavior, direct benefits are also likely to play a role in the evolution of cooperation (Nowak 2006; Leimar and Hammerstein 2010). Under some circumstances it would be potentially beneficial to recruit unrelated individuals, even if they may become reproductive competitors in the future, than to lose a chance to breed altogether when facing imminent group extinction.

Recruitment patterns in pied babblers support this hypothesis. Large groups, which presumably do not need the extra "help" that such individuals offer, actively repel prospecting individuals. In contrast, aggression toward prospectors is lower in small groups, and a greater proportion of these prospectors are accepted as group members (Figure 7.10). It is possible that the costs of defense against prospectors in small groups are simply too high to prevent prospectors from joining. Although we cannot exclude this possibility, the highly affiliative behavior that individuals of small groups display toward prospectors suggest that the potential high cost of defense is not the primary reason for greater rates of adult immigration into smaller groups.

Annual extinction rates reveal the importance of such recruitment: groups that failed to raise any young during the breeding season or to recruit any helpers from outside the group went extinct 52% of the time. In contrast, no group that recruited at least two or more individuals went extinct within a breeding season.

The group size effect on extinction rates is so pronounced that it is the likely explanation for the particularly striking behavior of kidnapping, defined here as the physical removal of a bird from its group while its parents and other group members are still alive and providing care for it, thus distinguishing it from adoption, which occurs when young are abandoned or orphaned. Kidnapping has now been observed in the study population 14 times. Although this may not seem

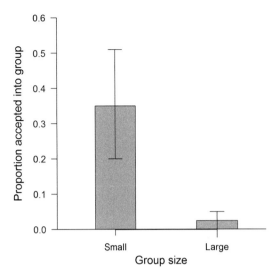

Figure 7.10. The relationship between group size and the likelihood of prospectors being nonaggressively accepted into an established group. Small group sizes are those containing four or fewer adults, large groups are those containing more than four adults. Data from 563 observed prospecting events, but including only those situations where individuals were attempting to join a group that did not have a current breeding vacancy; that is, individuals attempting to join as a subordinate helper.

like a lot, these rare events occur in a highly predictable way. The kidnapping group initiates a border interaction with the victim's group by calling on their territory border. This usually results in the victim's group responding by flying to their border to display. Young are usually left behind in the safety of thick vegetation, except in larger groups where one or two adults remain behind with the young, apparently as protection, while the rest of the group goes to the border.

After the kidnapping group engages the victim's group at the territorial border, one member of the kidnapping group leaves the display and searches for young birds from the defending group by giving quiet "food calls" with a piece of food. Young are highly responsive to these calls and indiscriminately pursue adults giving them (Raihani and Ridley 2007b, 2008). The kidnapper uses the food as a "bribe": as young approach, begging for food, the kidnapper backs away and gives the call again, encouraging young to approach once more

(Figure 7.11). By doing this repeatedly, young follow the kidnapping bird all the way into the latter's territory. Once a kidnapping has occurred, other members of the kidnapping group will join in feeding and moving the kidnapped young further into the territory.

Kidnapped young continue to be provisioned, brooded, and preened by the adult members of their new group at similar rates to their natal group. In several cases we have observed kidnapped young develop into adults and help to raise young produced by their kidnappers in subsequent broods. Therefore, kidnapping is one means by which helpers are successfully recruited into a group.

The occurrence of kidnapping raises a number of questions. Why would groups be willing to bear the cost of kidnapping, which may involve fighting with adults from the victim's group? And why would they invest in unrelated young given that raising young can be costly (Ridley and Raihani 2007b)?

A closer look at the pattern of kidnapping reveals demographic explanations for this unusual behavior. Only groups that repeatedly attempted but failed to raise their own young engaged in kidnapping behavior. Kidnapping therefore primarily occurs at the end of the breeding season, when the kidnapping group no longer has time to initiate another breeding attempt. Such groups therefore face the risk of extinction or the loss of significant amounts of territory to neighboring groups that have successfully fledged young.

When faced with such costs, it may be more beneficial to steal young from neighboring groups than face the costs of small relative group size. This benefit is confirmed by the findings that kidnapping groups were less likely to go extinct or lose territory size than groups that failed to breed but did not kidnap young, and that kidnapped young delayed dispersal and acted as helpers, thus providing benefits to their kidnappers.

All observed kidnapping attempts were directed at young less than three months of age. Thus, despite the apparent demographic advantages, it is unclear why kidnappers target dependent rather than independent young, which would not require the kidnappers to invest in raising them. A potential answer to this pattern may be that young do not develop social recognition of group members until after three months of age

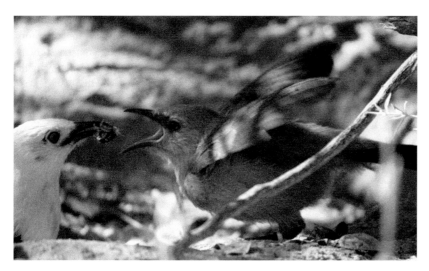

Figure 7.11. An adult feeding a young fledgling. Adults typically give a "food call" when about to feed young, and young will indiscriminately run up and beg from any adult giving this call. Kidnappers use this call and a food "bribe" to get fledglings to follow the kidnapper out of their territory and into the kidnapper's own territory. Photo by Alex Thompson. See plate section for color figure.

(Humphries 2013). Consequently, kidnapping occurs when young cannot discriminate among adults and are unlikely to display aggressive behavior toward kidnapping individuals.

Kin recognition and discrimination

The ability to recognize kin from nonkin is thought to be an important force driving the evolution of social behavior (Penn and Frommen 2010). Hamilton (1964) suggested that when individuals will gain the greatest benefits from helping kin, then the ability to discriminate kin from nonkin should also evolve. Recent work by Cornwallis et al. (2009) provide support for this idea, but point out that kin discrimination should be more likely in species where there is high variation in relatedness among group members. In group-living species where the same individuals interact repeatedly, stable cooperation may require the ability of individuals to monitor the contributions made by other group members (Nowak and Sigmund 1998; Brosnan et al. 2010). Remembering the outcomes of previous encounters may therefore be critical to regulating group dynamics,

as well as intergroup interactions such as mate selection and inbreeding avoidance following dispersal.

Nonetheless, there is currently limited evidence for kin recognition in cooperatively breeding species (McDonald 2012; Akçay et al. 2013). One of the first to provide such evidence was a study of long-tailed tits (*Aegithalos caudatus*) (Chapter 3) demonstrating that individuals were able to discriminate relatives from nonrelatives based on behavioral response to playbacks (Sharp et al. 2005). While it is relatively easy to determine whether offspring tend to help putative kin, which they can do with some accuracy based on spatial cues alone, the mechanism of kin recognition can constrain or enable fine degrees of discrimination, such that determining whether and how animals recognize kin is an essential aspect of understanding the behavioral patterns observed in cooperative-breeding societies.

Unlike long-tailed tits, where failed breeders revert to becoming helpers at the nests of other individuals, pied babblers do not have a fluid group composition, and the only time individuals move between groups is during dispersal or prospecting events (Raihani et al. 2010). Pied babblers are relatively long-lived, however, and there is considerable movement of individuals between groups over time. Therefore, simple family groups are not the predominant group type in our study population, and the presence of unrelated helpers within a group is not uncommon (Nelson-Flower 2010). Hence, pied babblers might be expected to develop some level of kin recognition (Cornwallis et al. 2009).

Supporting this conjecture, our experimental research has unveiled considerable evidence for recognition at the individual level based on several of the most commonly given calls. Detailed sound analysis has shown that individuals produce individually distinct calls, and playbacks have revealed that individuals can discriminate familiar kin from nonkin, but cannot discriminate unfamiliar nonkin (Humphries 2013). Therefore, recognition occurs through prior association rather than phenotype-matching based on inheritance of vocal signatures. This can result in occasional inbreeding among relatives that have never met before, several cases of which have been confirmed by our genetic analyses (Nelson-Flower et al. 2012).

The fact that individuals in cooperative breeding species can discriminate kin from nonkin becomes evolutionarily interesting when it affects cooperative behaviors, dispersal patterns, and group movements. We have been monitoring contributions to helping behavior in the population (including all feeding, incubation, and brooding events) for many years, and have found no evidence that unrelated individuals provide less help to young than related individuals (Nelson-Flower 2010). There are other reasons why unrelated individuals help to raise young, however, that are not related to the ability to discriminate kin from nonkin, including direct fitness benefits such as pay-to-stay, acquisition of skills, coalition formation, and social prestige (McDonald 2014; Chapter 10). We therefore examined other cooperative behaviors to determine whether there were behavioral trends that may indicate kin discrimination was occurring. Several of the behaviors we investigated suggested that kin discrimination was occurring. For example, we found that individuals invest less in costly territorial displays with neighboring groups that contain close relatives, and are less likely to display for mates next to groups that contain close relatives (Humphries 2013). In addition, individuals tend

neither to prospect at, nor disperse into, the dominant breeding position at groups where the opposite-sex dominant is a close relative (Nelson-Flower et al. 2012). Therefore, pied babblers are not only capable of kin recognition, but kinship influences their dispersal, calling, and territorial behavior.

Vocal communication

Communication and the coordination of cooperation

Vocal communication plays an important role in survival and reproduction and is therefore of central importance in the lives of many species (Fichtel and Manser 2010; Bradbury and Vehrencamp 2011). In stable cooperative groups, where there are additional individuals involved in interactions, vocal communication can become both complex and an important aspect of group stability. Our work on pied babblers indicates that vocal communication plays an important role in the regulation of cooperative activities and interactions both within and between groups. Pied babblers are highly vocal, and groups are often located by their calls before they are seen. Their vocal repertoire includes a series of alarm calls, several "loud calls" that broadcast over long distances of up to one kilometer, foraging contact calls, group choruses, a sentinel call and food discovery call, teaching calls, begging calls, and aggressive screams given during physical fighting or predator mobbing.

The influence of calling rates on foraging behavior and group spacing

The foraging or *chuck* call is given constantly by foraging individuals, but is only rarely given in other contexts, such as perching, preening, roosting, and brooding. In addition, evicted or lone individual floaters rarely give *chuck* calls, suggesting that this call has a function in intragroup foraging communication. By conducting playback experiments on *chuck* call rate, we found that individuals use these calls to maintain spacing among group members. They not only gave *chuck* calls more frequently when their neighbors were closer to them, they maintained greater distance from playbacks of *chuck* calls than control calls (Radford and Ridley 2008).

Individuals also use *chuck* calls to gain information about the need to invest in vigilance behavior. In particular, when several surrounding individuals are giving *chuck* calls, focal individuals are less likely to invest in personal vigilance behavior (Radford and Ridley 2007), presumably because of a dilution effect (Rosenzweig et al. 1997). In addition, individuals that only heard playbacks from one direction, thus suggesting that they were on the edge of a foraging group, were more likely to invest in vigilance than those that were surrounded by *chuck* calls (Radford and Ridley 2007). Thus, *chuck* calls play an important role in group cohesion and may act to minimize aggressive encounters in competition for resources.

Information exchange during sentinel activity

Sentinels are individuals that place themselves in prominent positions above a foraging group and are constantly vigilant. The presumed purpose of sentinel behavior is for efficient predator detection: sentinels are more likely to detect predators than are foraging group members, and they reliably give alarm calls (Manser 1999; Ridley et al. 2010). While there has been considerable debate about whether sentinel activity is a cooperative or selfish behavior, recent research on pied babblers and meerkats (*Suricata suricatta*) supports the former (Ridley et al. 2013; Santema and Clutton-Brock 2013). This is because sentinels are more at risk of predator attack than are foragers, contrary to previous research (Clutton-Brock et al. 1999; Wright et al. 2001), and group members both benefit from the detection of danger and share the workload of acting as a sentinel (Ridley et al. 2013).

In pied babblers, sentinels give a constant soft vocalization, described as the "watchman's song," which informs other group members that a sentinel is active (Radford et al. 2009). This allows the rest of the group to invest more time in foraging behavior and less time in vigilance. Through experimental manipulation of the height and frequency of the sentinel call, we showed

that group members responded strongly to the presence of a sentinel. Not only did group members forage further from cover when a sentinel was present, thus allowing them to utilize a greater variety of foraging patches, but they also foraged more intensively, achieving greater foraging success compared to when no sentinel was present (Hollén et al. 2008). Thus, the presence of a sentinel is a cooperative behavior that provides group members with measurable foraging and vigilance benefits. Individuals within the group communicate constantly with each other regarding sentinel presence, and sentinel behavior appears coordinated, with usually only one individual on sentinel at a time.

Effects of environmental conditions

Pied babblers inhabit an area of climatic unpredictability. The Kalahari biome can experience extended periods of drought resulting in widespread germination failure for the annual plant species that many emerging insects rely on for food, shelter, and breeding. The average annual rainfall experienced in the Kalahari biome is between 210 and 260 mm per year. However, this can vary widely, with less than 100 mm recorded in some years. Combined with the sandy soils and intense midsummer heat, drought can result in extreme resource scarcity for many Kalahari animals.

Unlike the large ungulates that travel hundreds of miles during droughts to reach more suitable foraging areas, migration is not an option for pied babblers, which are highly territorial and relatively poor fliers. Not only are summer temperatures high (in excess of 40°C), but winter temperatures can fall to less than −10°C in midwinter. Consequently environmental conditions can have a severe impact on body condition, survival, and potentially group size and stability.

Records of the timing and outcome of reproductive attempts indicate a strong influence of rainfall on reproductive success. Large groups seem better able to buffer this effect than small groups (Figure 7.12), but overall reproductive success is severely depressed compared to nondrought years. When groups fail to recruit young, a marked behavioral shift occurs in the population. As described earlier, there is an optimal group size in pied

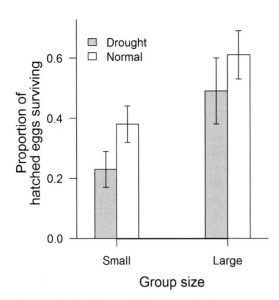

Figure 7.12. The effect of rainfall on reproductive success varies according to group size: large groups tend to be able to buffer the effects of drought on chick survival better than small groups. Small groups are those containing four adults or less.

babblers groups, below which groups are at increased risk of going extinct. This leads to unusual behaviors such as kidnapping and the nonaggressive acceptance of unrelated birds in small groups.

An equally unusual behavior occurs during extreme drought: that of group-merging events. This is where two or more groups join to become one larger group that collectively defends a territory. This behavior is extraordinary in a highly territorial species in which usually only one individual of each sex within the group breeds: some individuals are willing to give up their dominant breeding position to join another group when conditions become too harsh. These merged groups are highly unstable, and there is considerable aggressive jostling for dominance until a hierarchy is established. Stability is then maintained until the rains arrive and ecological constraints are lowered, at which point the joint-group fragments into its smaller component groups once more.

Group merging is a temporary strategy but highly interesting for the insights it offers into grouping behavior. First, merging occurs when ecological constraints

are high; second, group merging is highly unstable; and third, merging indicates that individuals are willing to facultatively adjust levels of cooperation and social grouping as a result of constraints on independent breeding. Groups merge when there is limited food on the current territory and thus constraints on dispersal are especially great. Individuals are also less willing to invest in costly territory defense when conditions are poor, making larger groups more advantageous (Golabek et al. 2012). Finally, body condition and foraging efficiency are depressed during drought conditions, and larger groups are more able to defend prime foraging habitat.

Current climate models predict that the Kalahari biome will get substantially hotter over the next half century (Parry et al. 2007). If hotter climates make it more physically costly to raise young, we may expect to see larger group sizes, higher reproductive skew at the population level, and a critical trade-off point reached where adults trade-off investment in raising young against their own body condition and survival. In support of this idea, recent research on the cooperatively breeding western Australian magpie (*Cracticus tibicen dorsalis*) found a sharp decline in investment in young during high temperatures (Edwards 2014). Initial research into the potential effect of climate change on pied babblers has revealed that they are very sensitive to high temperatures. Above a critical temperature of 35°C, individuals partition their time between heat dissipation and foraging. As a consequence, individuals suffer lower biomass intake on hot days, and a subsequent lower body mass, losing body mass on days hotter than 38°C (Du Plessis et al. 2012). The increasing regularity of very hot days and heat-waves during the breeding season may therefore severely depress reproductive success.

If the ability of adults to invest in young is depressed by climatic conditions, then the dynamics of cooperation may be directly impacted. For example, if larger groups can buffer environmental impacts better because there are more individuals to contribute to raising young, then larger group sizes may become more prevalent. In some cases, pairs may no longer be able to raise young, thus switching from facultative to obligate cooperation. In addition, if ecological constraints are high, then the decision of when to disperse and the size of groups that individuals may attempt to disperse to, may change.

Conclusion

Cooperative breeding is a behavior that occurs as a consequence of some individuals delaying their own opportunities to disperse and breed in order to help others raise young. Therefore the key questions in cooperative breeding research come down to understanding why individuals delay dispersal and delay breeding. In addition, it is important to understand why those that delay dispersal invest in helping behavior, since staying and helping do not always go together.

In pied babblers, individuals delay dispersal for several years on average. This seems to occur for a numbers of reasons:

(1) Living alone is costly, and individuals do better by staying on the natal territory and opportunistically prospecting for dispersal opportunities rather than leaving and floating in the population until breeding opportunities arise (Ridley 2008; Raihani et al. 2010).

(2) Pairs suffer low breeding success and a higher physical cost of parental investment than groups (Ridley and Raihani 2008; Ridley and van den Heuvel 2012). It may therefore be more beneficial for individuals to delay dispersal until a vacancy arises in a group rather than joining a new mate with no helpers. The inclusive fitness benefits of staying and helping compared to breeding in a pair for individuals of the same age remains to be determined, however.

(3) Small groups are more prone to instability and extinction and less likely to recruit young.

Pied babblers also delay breeding opportunities for a number of years, apparently because of the following factors:

(1) Groups are kin-structured and inbreeding is avoided. Therefore birds that delay dispersal must delay reproduction as well in order to avoid incest.

(2) Groups are highly territorial, and physical fighting can ensue if individuals encroach on territories. Therefore opportunities for extra-group matings are limited, and genetic analyses confirm that extra-group mating does not occur.

(3) When subordinates do attempt to reproduce, reproductive competition is costly, resulting in nest abandonment, oophagy, and significant delays in breeding. Individuals may therefore achieve greater direct and/or indirect fitness benefits by delaying reproduction and helping to raise young of the dominant pair rather than attempting to breed themselves.

All adult pied babblers help to provision the young produced within their group. In no cases have we observed a "freeloader" that does not contribute to cooperative activities. Since helping is costly, why do pied babblers invest in helping behavior? Our research has suggested the following reasons:

(1) Given high within-group relatedness, helpers can gain indirect fitness benefits. The amount of help young receive during early development results in long-term reproductive advantages for offspring, and therefore individuals gain significant indirect fitness benefits by provisioning young rather than simply using the territory as a safe haven.

(2) If provisioning by helpers enhances the survival of young, individuals may gain direct fitness benefits by investing in helping behavior. For example, young raised in the group may become coalition partners during dispersal, increasing the chance of successfully gaining a breeding position in a new group (Ridley 2012). Young may also help to raise subsequent broods, and they can defend the territory during border interactions. Above a certain number of helpers, the fitness benefits that each helper receives from their investment in helping is likely to decline, and this may explain why we see an optimal group size effect in our population. Above this optimal group size, reproductive success starts to decline due to conflict among reproductive individuals, while in small groups below the optimal group size, we see a decline in reproductive success, territory size, and adult survival.

Our detailed observations over many years has led to an understanding of patterns of reproductive skew and dispersal, group membership, and the costs of living alone. Our studies are ongoing, with the hope that the accumulation of long-term data over many years will help us to understand the difference in life-history trajectories between individuals, and the long-term causes and consequences of helping behavior. It is evident from our observations thus far that helping behavior and group membership is highly dynamic and changes according to prevailing social and demographic conditions. While our investigations into the social lives of the southern pied babblers have unveiled some interesting patterns related to the benefits of cooperation, we still have much yet to uncover before we truly understand the factors promoting cooperative breeding behavior in this fascinating African bird.

Acknowledgments

I would like to thank the numerous hard-working, dedicated, and inspiring individuals that have helped out along the way. First and most importantly, thanks to Nichola Raihani, who came as my assistant in the very first year and helped me to habituate the population. The study population has benefited from many amazing research students over the years, including Nichola Raihani, Krystyna Golabek, David Humphries, Elizabeth Wiley, Martha Nelson-Flower, Alex Thompson, James Westrip, Sabrina Engesser, Matt Child, and Kate Du Plessis. Thanks also to the many research assistants that have helped over the years: Fiona Finch, Rute Mendonca, Liz Davies, Bec Rose, Helen Wade, Erin Love, John Forecast, Lexy Russell, Fraser Niven, Lucy Browning, Rachel Smith, Phoebe Cooke, and Adam Britton for the tireless hours spent in the field. Thanks also to my research colleagues Nicola Raihani, Simon Townsend, Matt Bell, Andrew Radford, Tom Flower, and Linda Hollén. The constant interaction with the enthusiastic and talented volunteers, assistants, and researchers of the Kalahari Meerkat Project has been inspiring and important, as well as the many other researchers that regularly visit the study site. Thanks to Tim Clutton-Brock for suggesting that I research pied babblers in the first place, and to Marta Manser for her constant support and encouragement over the years. Morné Du Plessis and Phil Hockey were constant sources of encouragement and support. This research has received funding from many sources over the years including the University of Cape Town, NRF Centre of Excellence, Newnham College (Cambridge University), the Association for the Study of Animal Behaviour, National Geographic, the Australian Research Council, Macquarie University and the University of Western Australia.

REFERENCES

Akçay, C., Swift, R. J., Reed, V. A., and Dickinson, J. L. (2013). Vocal kin recognition in kin neighborhoods of western bluebirds. *Behav. Ecol.*, 24, 898–905.

Bradbury, J. W. and Vehrencamp, S. L. (2011). *Principles of Animal Communication, 2nd ed.*, Sunderland, MA: Sinauer Associates.

Brosnan, S. F., Salwiczek, L., and Bshary, R. (2010). The interplay of cognition and cooperation. *Phil. Trans. R. Soc. London B*, 365, 2699–2710.

Clutton-Brock, T. H., O'Riain, M. J., Brotherton, P. N. M., Daynor, D., Kansky, R., et al. (1999). Selfish sentinels in cooperative mammals. *Science*, 284, 1640–1644.

Cornwallis, C. K., West, S. A., and Griffin, A. S. (2009). Routes to indirect fitness in cooperatively breeding vertebrates: kin discrimination and limited dispersal. *J. Evol. Biol.*, 22, 2445–2457.

Dickinson, J. L. and Hatchwell, B. J. (2004). Fitness consequences of helping. In: *Ecology and Evolution of Cooperative Breeding in Birds*, ed. W. D. Koenig and J. L. Dickinson. Cambridge: Cambridge University Press, pp. 48–66.

Double, M. and Cockburn, A. (2000). Pre-dawn infidelity: females control extra-pair mating in superb fairy-wrens. *Proc. R. Soc. London B*, 267, 465–470.

Du Plessis, K. L., Martin, R. O., Hockey, P. A. R., Cunningham, S. J., and Ridley, A. R. (2012). The costs of keeping cool in a warming world: implications of high temperatures for foraging, thermoregulation and body condition of an arid-zone bird. *Global Change Biol.*, 18, 3063–3070.

Edwards, E. (2014). The impacts of heat on foraging effort and reproductive behaviour in Australian magpies (*Cracticus tibicen dorsalis*). Honours thesis, University of Western Australia, Crawley, Western Australia.

Ekman, J. and Griesser, M. (2002). Why offspring delay dispersal: experimental evidence for a role of parental tolerance. *Proc. R. Soc. London B*, 269, 1709–1713.

Fichtel, C. and Manser, M. B. (2010). Vocal communication in social groups. In: *Animal Behaviour: Evolution and Mechanisms*, ed. P. M. Kappeler. Berlin: Springer, pp. 29–54.

Gaston, A. J. (1977). Social behaviour within groups of jungle babblers (*Turdoides striatus*). *Anim. Behav.* 25, 828–848.

Golabek, K. A. (2010). Vocal communication and the facilitation of social behaviour in the southern pied babbler (*Turdoides bicolor*). Ph.D. thesis, Bristol University, Bristol, U.K.

Golabek, K. A., Ridley, A. R., and Radford, A. N. (2012). Food availability affects strength of seasonal territorial behaviour in a cooperatively breeding bird. *Anim. Behav.*, 83, 613–619.

Hamilton, W. D. (1964). The genetical evolution of social behaviour. I. *J. Theor. Biol.*, 7, 1–16.

Hockey, P. A. R., Dean, W. R. J., and Ryan, P. G. (2005). *Robert's Birds of Southern Africa, 7th ed.* Cape Town, South Africa: Trustees of the John Voeckler Bird Club.

Hollén, L. I., Bell, M. B. V., and Radford, A. N. (2008). Cooperative sentinel calling? Foragers gain increased biomass intake. *Curr. Biol.*, 18, 576–9.

Humphries, D. J. (2013). The mechanisms and function of social recognition in the cooperatively breeding southern pied babbler *(Turdoides bicolor)*. Ph.D. thesis, Macquarie University, Sydney, Australia.

Humphries, D. J., Finch, F. M., Bell, M. B. V., and Ridley, A. R. (2015). Calling where it counts: subordinate pied babblers target the audience of their vocal advertisements. *PLoS One*, 10 (7), e0130795.

Koenig, W. D., Pitelka, F. A., Carmen, W. J., Mumme, R. L., and Stanback, M. T. (1992). The evolution of delayed dispersal in cooperative breeders. *Q. Rev. Biol.*, 67, 111–150.

Kokko, H. and Ekman, J. (2002). Delayed dispersal as a route to breeding: territorial inheritance, safe havens, and ecological constraints. *Am. Nat.* 160, 468–484.

Langen, T. A. (2000). Prolonged offspring dependence and cooperative breeding in birds. *Behav. Ecol.*, 11, 367–377.

Leimar, O. and Hammerstein, P. (2010). Cooperation for direct fitness benefits. *Phil. Trans. R. Soc. London B*, 365, 2619–2626.

Lindström, J. (1999). Early development and fitness in birds and mammals. *Trends. Ecol. Evol.*, 14, 343–348.

Manser, M. B. (1999). Response of foraging group members to sentinel calls in suricates, *Suricata suricatta. Proc. R. Soc. London B*, 266, 1013–1019.

Mares, R., Young, A. J., and Clutton-Brock, T. H. (2012). Individual contributions to territory defence in a cooperative breeder: weighing up the benefits and costs. *Proc. R. Soc. London B*, 279, 3989–3995.

McDonald, P.G. (2012). Cooperative bird differentiates between the calls of different individuals, even when vocalizations were from completely unfamiliar individuals. *Biol. Lett.*, 8, 365–368.

McDonald, P. G. (2014). Cooperative breeding beyond kinship: why else do helpers help? *Emu*, 114, 91–96.

Nelson-Flower, M. J. (2010). Kinship and its consequences in the cooperatively breeding southern pied babbler *Turdoides bicolor*. Ph.D. thesis, University of Cape Town, Cape Town, South Africa.

Nelson-Flower, M. J., Hockey, P. A. R., O'Ryan, C., Raihani, N. J., Du Plessis, M. A., et al. (2011). Monogamous dominant pairs monopolize reproduction in the cooperatively breeding pied babbler. *Behav. Ecol.*, 22, 559–565.

Nelson-Flower, M. J., Hockey, P. A. R., O'Ryan, C., and Ridley, A. R. (2012). Inbreeding avoidance mechanisms: dispersal dynamics in cooperatively breeding southern pied babblers. *J. Anim. Ecol.*, 81, 876–883.

Nelson-Flower, M. J., Hockey, P. A. R., O'Ryan, C., English, S., Thompson, A.M., et al. (2013). Costly reproductive competition between females in a monogamous cooperatively breeding bird. *Proc. R. Soc. London B*, 280, 20130728.

Nowak, M. A. (2006). Five rules for the evolution of cooperation. *Science*, 314, 1560–1563.

Nowak, M. A. and Sigmund, K. (1998). Evolution of indirect reciprocity by image scoring. *Nature*, 393, 573–577.

Parry, M. L., Canziani, J., Palutikof, J. P., van der Linden, P. J., and Hanson, C. E. (2007). IPCC, 2007: Summary for Policymakers. In: *Climate Change 2007: impacts, Adaptation and Vulnerability. Contribution of Working Group II to the Fourth Assessment Report of the Intergovernmental Panel on Climate Change*, pp. 7–22.

Penn, D. J. and Frommen, J. G. (2010). Kin recognition: an overview of conceptual issues, mechanisms and evolutionary theory. In: *Animal Behaviour: Evolution and Mechanisms*, ed. P. Kappeler. Berlin: Springer, pp. 55–85.

Radford, A. N. and Ridley, A. R. (2007). Individuals in foraging groups may use vocal cues when assessing their need for anti-predator vigilance. *Biol. Lett.*, 3, 249–252.

Radford, A. N. and Ridley, A. R. (2008). Close calling regulates spacing between foraging competitors in the group-living pied babbler. *Anim. Behav.*, 75, 519–527.

Radford, A. N., Hollén, L. I., and Bell, M. B. V. (2009). The higher the better: sentinel height influences foraging success in a social bird. *Proc. R. Soc. London B*, 276, 2437–2442.

Raihani, N. J. and Ridley, A. R. (2007a). Variable fledging age according to group size: trade-offs in a cooperatively breeding bird. *Biol. Lett.*, 3, 624–627.

Raihani, N. J. and Ridley, A. R. (2007b). Adult vocalizations during provisioning: offspring response and postfledging benefits in wild pied babblers. *Anim. Behav.*, 74, 1303–1309.

Raihani, N. J. and Ridley, A. R. (2008). Experimental evidence for teaching in wild pied babblers. *Anim. Behav.*, 75, 3–11.

Raihani, N. J. Nelson-Flower, M. J., Golabek, K. A., and Ridley, A. R. (2010). Routes to breeding in cooperatively breeding pied babblers *Turdoides bicolor. J. Avian Biol*, 41, 681–686.

Ridley, A. R. (2012). Invading together: the benefits of coalition dispersal in a cooperative bird. *Behav. Ecol. Sociobiol.*, 66, 77–83.

Ridley, A. and Raihani, N. (2007a). Facultative response to a kleptoparasite by the cooperatively breeding pied babbler. *Behav. Ecol.*, 18, 324–330.

Ridley, A. R. and Raihani, N. J. (2007b). Variable postfledging care in a cooperative bird: causes and consequences. *Behav. Ecol.*, 18, 994–1000.

Ridley, A. R. and Raihani, N. J. (2008). Task partitioning increases reproductive output in a cooperative bird. *Behav. Ecol.*, 19, 1136–1142.

Ridley, A. R. and van den Heuvel, I. M. (2012). Is there a difference in reproductive performance between cooperative and non-cooperative species? A southern African comparison. *Behaviour*, 149, 821–848.

Ridley, A. R., Raihani, N. J., and Nelson-Flower, M. J. (2008). The cost of being alone: the fate of floaters in a population of cooperatively breeding pied babblers *Turdoides bicolor*. *J. Avian Biol.*, 39, 389–392.

Ridley, A. R., Raihani, N. J., and Bell, M. B. V. (2010). Experimental evidence that sentinel behaviour is affected by risk. *Biol. Lett.*, 6, 445–448.

Ridley, A. R., Nelson-Flower, M. J., and Thompson, A. M. (2013). Is sentinel behaviour safe? An experimental investigation. *Anim. Behav.*, 85, 137–142.

Rosenzweig, M. L., Abramsky, Z., and Subach, A. (1997). Safety in numbers: sophisticated vigilance by Allenby's gerbil. *Proc. Nat. Acad. Sci. (USA)*, 94, 5713–5715.

Santema, P. and Clutton-Brock, T. (2013). Meerkat helpers increase sentinel behaviour and bipedal vigilance in the presence of pups. *Anim. Behav.*, 85, 655–661.

Sharp, S. P., McGowan, A., Wood, M. J., and Hatchwell, B. J. (2005). Learned kin recognition cues in a social bird. *Nature*, 434, 1127–1130.

Wright, J., Berg, E., de Kort, S. R., Khazin, V., and Maklakov, A. A. (2001). Safe selfish sentinels in a cooperative bird. *J. Anim. Ecol.*, 44, 1070–1079.

Young, A. J. and Monfort, S. L. (2009). Stress and the costs of extra-territorial movement in a social carnivore. *Biol Lett.*, 5, 439–441.

Zahavi, A. (1990). Arabian babblers: the quest for social status in a cooperative breeder. In: *Cooperative Breeding in Birds: Long-term Studies of Ecology and Behavior*, ed. P. B. Stacey and W. D. Koenig. Cambridge: Cambridge University Press, pp. 103–130.

8

Superb fairy-wrens: Making the worst of a good job

Andrew Cockburn, Lyanne Brouwer, Nicolas Margraf,
Helen L. Osmond, and Martijn van de Pol

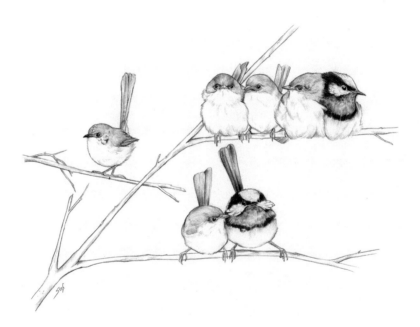

Introduction

Fairy-wrens have always played a pivotal role in the study of cooperative breeding. So far as we are aware, the first recognition that more than two birds could combine to rear a single brood of young comes from John Gould's (1841) depiction of the superb fairy-wren *Malurus cyaneus* in his treatise on the birds of Australia, many decades before Alexander Skutch's explorations of the biology of Neotropical birds (Boland and Cockburn 2002). Indeed, experiments on cooperative breeding were reported for the superb fairy-wren *M. cyaneus* as early as 1910, and in the 1950s this was also the first cooperatively-breeding species to be studied using color-rings to distinguish between individuals (Rowley 1957; Bradley and Bradley 1958). Since then there have been three intensive demographic studies of *Malurus* species lasting more than fifteen years

Cooperative Breeding in Vertebrates: Studies of Ecology, Evolution, and Behavior, eds W. D. Koenig and J. L. Dickinson.
Published by Cambridge University Press. © Cambridge University Press 2016.

(Russell and Rowley 1993, 2000; Cockburn et al. 2008b). Comparative studies between populations also have access to additional data from 13 populations of 7 congeneric species (van de Pol et al. 2013).

It is certain that early detection and sustained interest in cooperative breeding in fairy-wrens reflects the comparative ease with which they can be studied. At least some species are abundant, adapt to the presence of humans, and build nests conveniently close to the ground. In addition, in contrast to many cooperatively breeding species, the sexes are easily distinguished, as adult males are among the most brilliantly-colored of birds, while females and juveniles in most species are much drabber. Species can therefore be instantly identified as cooperative breeders if two males are seen carrying food to the nest (Buchanan and Cockburn 2013).

While early work on fairy-wrens repeatedly informed theory concerning cooperative breeding (Margraf and Cockburn 2013), the current explosion of interest in this group stems from the surprising discovery that most young in most species are not sired by the males that provision and defend them (Brooker et al. 1990; Mulder et al. 1994; Cockburn et al. 2013). Instead, parentage is dominated by extra-group fertilizations initiated by the female. Such rampant infidelity undermines the expectation that helping behavior by subordinate males will be directed toward full-siblings, immediately reducing the potential for indirect fitness benefits at nests with helpers. High levels of infidelity afford an excellent opportunity to investigate the benefits that females obtain from mate choice, because the benefits of acquiring a territory and males to care for the young can be dissociated from possible genetic benefits of mate choice (Cockburn et al. 2008a). However, it raises a second paradox – why do males care for young to which they are often unrelated?

We have been investigating these twin problems of cooperative breeding and sexual selection in an ongoing study of *M. cyaneus* that commenced in 1987, situated in the Australian National Botanic Gardens in Canberra, Australia, where we continuously monitor between 60 and 90 territories. Even by the high standards that have prevailed in long-term studies of cooperatively breeding birds, our study is unusually detailed. We census the entire population every week of the year, and have used genetic methods of parentage determination since the inception of the study. This has allowed us to achieve what is probably the largest genetic pedigree thus far obtained in free-living populations, and unusually detailed data on the timing of key life-history events including dispersal, settlement, pairing, divorce, and death.

Distribution and geographical ecology

The superb fairy-wren is broadly distributed across about 20° of both latitude and longitude in eastern Australia, including Tasmania. It is most common in *Eucalyptus* woodlands and forest, but adapts well to human-modified habitats such as gardens and farmland where blackberry brambles have spread as weeds. In parts of its range it can be the most common small ground bird. While the ocean limits its distribution to the south and east, elsewhere at the edges of its range it is typically replaced by a congener. For example, its sister species the splendid fairy-wren *M. splendens* abuts and overlaps the arid western end of its range.

All members of the Family Maluridae, which occur throughout the Australo-Papuan zoogeographic region – are known or suspected to be cooperative breeders (Rowley and Russell 1997; Cockburn 2006; Margraf and Cockburn 2013). There are species specialized on both canopy and lower strata of rainforests, in tropical grasslands and riparian thickets, in wet and dry *Eucalyptus* forest and woodlands, and in deserts. Across these habitats, they occur in numerous habitat configurations and in local population densities that vary by more than an order of magnitude. It is hence difficult to attribute cooperative breeding to the habitat features affecting any particular species, although at the margins of the range of *M. cyaneus* some populations can lack adult helpers, probably because recruitment is so low that no helpers are ever recruited (Tidemann 1986; Margraf and Cockburn 2013).

Natural history

Superb fairy-wrens live year-round on permanent territories, although in the nonbreeding season they may

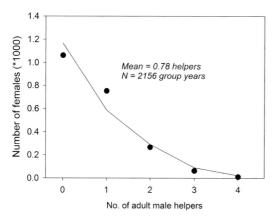

Figure 8.1. The number of females that lived with different numbers of helpers during the course of a breeding season. The continuous line is the Poisson prediction for a mean of 0.78 helpers.

leave their territory each day in order to join feeding flocks that congregate in open habitat. Both females and males contribute to territory defense through song and aggression. They are primarily insectivorous, feeding for the most part on small arthropods found on or close to the ground (Higgins et al. 2001).

In our population females can start nesting as early as late August in the late austral winter. Females are the sole contributors to nest building and incubation. There is just one female on each territory – supernumerary females leave at the start of the breeding season even though they may occasionally help at the first nest of the season. The female forms a strong pair bond with the oldest (and most dominant) male on the territory. In sharp contrast to females, there can also be as many as four helper males, although pairs frequently breed unassisted (Figure 8.1). Dominant and helper males always provision and defend any nestlings and fledglings produced by the female.

Clutch size ranges from 1 to 5 eggs, with a strong mode of three (Figure 8.2a). The breeding season can persist for many months, and in some years the last young are fledged in late March. Over this period females can rear up to three successful broods (Figure 8.2c). Such success is rare, however, as the season can be truncated by unfavorably hot conditions and there are high rates of

nest predation, with pied currawongs (*Strepera graculina*) and eastern brown snakes (*Pseudonaja textilis*) the primary culprits.

Females initiate new nests immediately after nest failure, usually laying the first egg of the new clutch 7 to 8 days later. In birds suffering repeated predation, reproductive investment can be very high (Figure 8.2b). In our most extreme case, a female laid 29 eggs in nine clutches, of which the first eight clutches were depredated. The total investment in eggs in this case was more than three times the body mass of the female, and exceeds the annual productivity of extremely fecund birds such as the well-studied parids living at high northern latitudes. The maximum number of fledglings produced in a season is 11 (Figure 8.2d).

The origins of cooperative breeding in *M. cyaneus* are well-established (Rowley 1965; Pruett-Jones and Lewis 1990; Cockburn et al. 2008b). Male *M. cyaneus* are highly philopatric, more so than any other known year-round territorial bird species. The majority of males – 60% – eventually attain a dominant breeding position on the territory on which they are born, but sometimes need to wait in queues and help for many years (Cockburn et al. 2008b). Males acquire dominance via two main paths. In the first, more common route, they wait on the territory in a passive queue until all older birds have died. In the second route, which is about half as common, they form an alliance with a supernumerary female to fission the territory into two halves (Cockburn et al. 2003, 2008b). When males disperse, 95% of moves are to a neighboring territory where a female has been left unattended by the death of the dominant male (her mate). Pruett-Jones and Lewis (1990) showed experimentally that supernumerary males will not move to a vacant territory, but will disperse immediately if there is a territory with an unmated, unattended female.

In contrast, females never breed on their natal territory and disperse to obtain a breeding vacancy during their first year of their life (Cockburn et al. 2003). This obligate natal dispersal takes place in two discrete phases. Females fledged in the first half of the breeding season disperse toward the end of that breeding season, and although they can occasionally move directly into a breeding vacancy, they are much more likely

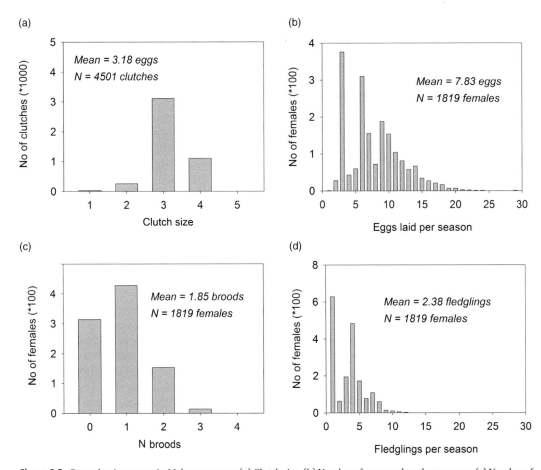

Figure 8.2. Reproductive output in *Malurus cyaneus*. (a) Clutch size. (b) Number of eggs produced per season. (c) Number of broods fledged per season. In the one case where four broods were fledged one of the broods was depredated within 24 hrs of fledging. (d) Number of fledglings per season.

to join a foreign group as a supernumerary and overwinter there. Females fledged in the second half of the breeding season usually overwinter on their natal territory and then disperse.

Supernumerary females on both the foreign and natal territory compete for vacancies during the second dispersal phase, which starts in August as the breeding season approaches and is generally over by mid-November, by which time all females have dispersed and none remain as supernumeraries. After this second period of dispersal, adult females that die are not replaced, and males that lose their mate remain unmated for the remainder of the season (Table 8.1).

Females that have overwintered on a foreign territory have several advantages in territory acquisition: they can inherit the territory if the dominant dies, form an alliance with a helper male and fight to fission the territory into two, and they are also more likely to fill a vacancy that arises on a nearby territory (Cockburn et al. 2003). In contrast, females that have overwintered on their natal territory must disperse in order to fill a breeding vacancy, and usually move at least three territories away to do so. While dominant females become aggressive toward supernumeraries as the breeding season approaches, young females disperse from their natal territory even if there is no

Table 8.1. The structure of *Malurus cyaneus* territorial groups

a. Dominants

Relatedness to hen	No. of group years	% of males paired to a female
Unrelated	1305	96.7%
Paired to mother	44	3.3%
No female	98	
Total paired	1349	

b. Helpers

Helping mother	Helping sire	No. of group years	% of males helping a female
Yes	Yes	113	13.5%
Yes	No	231	27.7%
No	Yes	94	11.3%
No	No	397	47.5%
No female		38	
Total helping mother		344	41.2%
Total helping sire		207	24.8%
Total helping a female		835	

Data are from 19 breeding seasons (1992 to 2010) and take a mid-breeding season (1 December) snapshot of the social organization on each territory.

older female to drive them out, which we suspect is an attempt to reduce the risk of inbreeding.

Dominant males can hold territories for long periods – up to 10 years – and thus in principle the number of helper males that can accumulate on a territory is large. In practice this does not happen, however, and the number of supernumerary males rarely exceeds two (Figure 8.2). One possible reason for this is local negative density-dependence: females who already have helpers are less successful at recruiting further males than those that lack helpers (Cockburn et al. 2003).

The proportion of territories with helpers has fluctuated between breeding seasons during our study from 67% to 29%, with concomitant shift in the mean number of helpers per territory from 1.04 to 0.37. In general there has been a decline in the number of helpers per territory as the study has proceeded associated with drier conditions due to climate change and a reduction in reproductive output (van de Pol et al. 2012).

Some of these dynamics are captured in a population pyramid taken at the start of the breeding season in 2010 toward the end of a nine-year drought, punctuated by a year of average rainfall in 2005 (Figure 8.3).

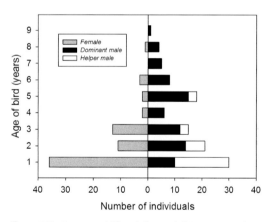

Figure 8.3. Age pyramid for adult superb fairy-wrens at the start of the 2010 breeding season.

The 2005 males, then 5 years old, were heavily recruited, and despite the additional years of attrition, they outnumbered the 2006 and 2007 cohorts in 2010. Indeed, some males from the 2005 cohort were still queuing as helpers in 2010. There is no comparable spike in recruitment for females, as even during drought years there are sufficient dispersing females to replenish any vacancies that become available during the second dispersal phase.

These results also clarify two other features of fairy-wren demography. First, although they can be long-lived, only a small number of females reach advanced age. Survival of females during the non-breeding season can be higher than that of males under some circumstances (Cockburn et al. 2008c), a result discussed in the "Contributions by helpers" section. However, females show greatly elevated mortality relative to males during the breeding season (Cockburn et al. 2008a). Second, while biologists working at high northern latitudes are often surprised by the lifespans of these 9 g birds, the lifespan of *M. cyaneus* sits at the lower end of comparable small insectivorous Australian passerines (Rowley and Russell 1991), including some other species within the genus. For example, one individual of *Malurus elegans* was recorded to live 17 years (Russell et al. 2000), while our maximum is 12 years based on an enormous sample size.

The mating system

Social mating system

The social mating system of fairy-wrens is simple. Each female forms a socially monogamous pair bond with a single male, the oldest male on her territory. Queuing by males to obtain the dominant position is typically completely passive (Cockburn et al. 2008b). Occasionally two same-aged nest-mates reach the senior position at the same time, but even in this case, one appears to adopt the dominant role without overt behavioral conflict. We have observed only three cases where a helper assumes the dominant role when an older male is still present, but this appears to reflect illness or injury to the dominant, and dominance can be reversed if the older bird recovers. One unusual nuance is that males inherit the dominant position even when they are a son of the female to which they pair; about 3% of pairings are between a mother and her son (Table 8.1).

Extra-group parentage

There is probably no bird species where there is a greater disparity between the social mating system and the genetic mating system. The defining feature of fairy-wren reproduction is that extra-group mating by females is rampant (Double and Cockburn 2000; Cockburn et al. 2009). Extra-group fertilizations dominate parentage (61.2% of offspring; 2429/3971), although not to the extent originally reported by Mulder et al. (1994) due to population changes discussed later. We have found four predictors of the extent to which extra-group fertilizations predominate.

First, females paired with their sons do not mate with them, so the extra-group fertilization rate for these females, which comprise 3% of breeding units, is 100%. Second, females paired with unrelated males that also have male helpers (43% of all breeding units) have a much higher rate of extra-group fertilization than do unassisted females of the same pairing type (54% of breeding units) (Mulder et al. 1994; Dunn and Cockburn 1999). We interpret this as indicating that females breeding in pairs increase within-pair fertilizations as a way of inducing their social partners to provide care despite the inevitable, high rate of cuckoldry. This effect of helpers in liberating females to increase their frequency of extra-pair fertilization means that the global rate of extra-pair mating varies with the size of groups and the proportion of territories with helpers.

Third, females with social partners much younger than themselves cuckold them very heavily, even when they do not have helpers or are unrelated to their partner (Dunn and Cockburn 1999). Finally, dominant males whose sperm have a longer flagellum and a relatively smaller head achieved higher within-pair paternity, suggesting that their sperm are better able to compete with those from extra-group males (Calhim et al. 2011).

The behavior underlying extra-group mating in *M. cyaneus* is arguably better known than is true for any other bird species. Radio-tracking has shown that females initiate extra-group mating in the half-hour before dawn, usually on the second and third day prior to the start of egg-laying (Double and Cockburn 2000). They do this by making one or two forays on consecutive mornings three days prior to egg-laying from the bush where they roost with their social group to the song perch of extra-group males, which advertise in the dawn chorus (Dalziell and Cockburn 2008; Cockburn et al. 2009).

Females engaging in extra-group matings show a common preference for males that have been displaying to them for months prior to the breeding season, with the onset of display by males directly associated with the time of year at which he attains full nuptial plumage. There is thus a big advantage to males that are able to molt early, and a few are even able to molt directly from one nuptial plumage to another, although most males retreat into a dull eclipse plumage for all or most of the winter (Dunn and Cockburn 1999; Cockburn et al. 2008a).

This strong preference is potentially undermined by male competition. Helper males sing close to the dominant male, despite high risk of attack by the dominant (Cockburn et al. 2009). They are sometimes successful in this parasitic behavior, and the helpers of attractive early molting males have higher extra-group mating success than most dominants (Double and Cockburn 2003). Low-quality dominants and their helpers also attempt to behave parasitically, singing as close to other, higher-quality dominant males as possible given their territory configuration. Thus, females are confronted with what amounts to a "hidden lek" when she arrives to mate. The resultant confusion allows low-quality males to gain some extra-group reproductive success (Cockburn et al. 2009).

Within-group competition for reproduction

Despite passive queuing and absence of aggressive contests for dominance, within-group interactions between males to mate with females can be extremely aggressive. When the female returns from an extra-group foray, she is immediately joined by the dominant male, who attends her very closely and intently. During this period the dominant attacks his subordinates, sometimes grappling with them on the ground. After a short period < 30 min in length, the female sits on the nest for 5 to 20 min, even though the nest is sometimes incomplete. The dominant then sits very close to the nest until

the female emerges, flies to a nearby perch, and solicits by wing-fluttering. The pair then engage in a single long (5 to 10 second) copulation. Over the next 20 min the male loses interest in the female, and either forages, or departs the territory to display to nearby females. In the event that there is an unrelated helper male (59% of groups), the female often repeats the sequence with the helper. There is no sexual interest by males in the female after that time, and males can spend a long time off territory courting neighbors even when their partner is fertile (Green et al. 1995).

In addition to the fighting before the female initiates matings, we have observed two cases where copulation between the dominant and his social female was disrupted when another male pushed the dominant off the female and then fled. In the case where we determined the identity of the culprit, it was the subordinate that caused the disruption.

Fitness benefits to subordinates initially appear minor, as they sire only 2.4% (96/3971) of nestlings. Where at least one of the helpers is unrelated to the breeding female, however, unrelated helpers gain 23% of the limited paternity obtained by the home males (Cockburn 2004). This is similar to the extent of mate-sharing revealed in the studies of other cooperatively breeding birds in which unrelated males share a mate within a group.

Hence, where the female is assisted by two or more males to which she is unrelated, the within-group mating system is polyandrous, and thus the overall mating system is a form of polyandry with an additional constraint of incest avoidance. Unlike some other avian cooperatively polyandrous systems where there can be many copulations during the fertile period of the female such as in dunnocks (*Prunella modularis*), however, the number of copulations in the fertile period of a female fairy-wren is extremely low. The most likely explanation is that fairy-wrens have evolved a mating system based upon large ejaculates, which may limit the use of copulation frequency to compete for within-group fertilizations. Because the primary axis of competition is between the males living with the female and the extra-group males with which she copulates, males likely compete via ejaculate size and the sheer numbers of sperm transferred to females on the few occasions during which they have the opportunity to mate (Tuttle and Pruett-Jones 2004; Rowe and Pruett-Jones 2011).

Incest and incest avoidance

In our study population there are several features that affect the risk of incest. As we have already seen, most males queue for dominance on their natal territory and progress to the dominant position even if their mother is the breeding female. However, such males never sire young with their mothers. Our observational data suggest that this is behaviorally mediated rather than being due to genetic incompatibility: mothers and sons ignore each other as potential sexual partners. Males living with their mothers show no interest in the female even after she has departed on a foray, and may even depart the territory to court their neighbors before the female returns. Females are also likely to initiate divorce and move to a new vacancy once they are paired to a son, or even when one of their sons has acquired the senior helper position on their territory (Cockburn et al. 2003). This behavior is also consistent with the hypothesis that females move so that any future sons queue for dominance on a new territory. This frees the sons she has already produced for further competition, and allows her sons to start to mate on her territory.

Mother-son pairings are just one of the contexts in which incest might arise. Inadvertent incest can also take place as a result of male philopatry, and extra-group matings by very successful males that then leave descendants throughout entire neighborhoods (Double et al. 2005). In particular, the high frequency of extra-group paternity means that females lack contextual information about their relatedness to the males in their neighborhood. We believe that the risk of incest in the local neighborhood and the absence of contextual information to avoid such incest is the reason that young females always leave the natal territory in order to breed, and usually travel three or more territories away, reducing the probability of mating with close male relatives in their immediate neighborhood (Cockburn et al. 2003).

Sexual selection: female choice

Consistent female preference for the same male phenotype imposes strong sexual selection. There are four apparent effects of female choice on fairy-wren morphology and behavior. The first is striking sexual dichromatism: males are brilliantly colored while females are a dull brown. The second are *furgling* displays where males leave their territory and display to females living as far as seven territories from their own (Mulder 1997; Cockburn et al. 2013). Third, males often augment their own plumage in these displays by carrying a yellow petal or flower. Finally, males display with song. While both sexes use a *chatter* song for territory defense, males have an additional *trill song* that is incorporated unprompted in the dawn chorus when females are making forays to visit extra-group mating partners (Dalziell and Cockburn 2008).

While each of these features plays some role in male display, evidence suggests that the most important trait currently under sexual selection is the time males spend in nuptial plumage. This character is salient to females because males start displaying immediately after they acquire full breeding plumage and, although males tend to molt earlier as they get older, timing of molt is a trait that varies enormously within and between males (Figure 8.4). The ability of males to molt early also depends on environmental conditions; in particular, when conditions preceding the decision to molt early are very dry, only a few males will do so.

The inability of most older males to molt early in dry years impairs the strength of sexual selection. Indeed, during a recent eight-year drought we would not have had the power to detect intersexual selection at all, although data over the full length of the study indicate that the association between the timing of bright plumage acquisition and extra-group mating success is possibly the strongest phenotypic correlation ever recorded in the study of extra-pair mating in birds (Dunn and Cockburn 1999; Cockburn et al. 2008a). These results affirm the importance of long-term perspectives on evolutionary questions and the special role that long-term datasets on cooperatively breeding

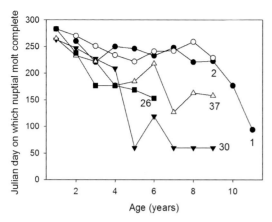

Figure 8.4. Lifetime molt trajectory of five male *M. cyaneus*. The lifetime reproductive success of each male (fertilizations of both extra- and within-group young) is given at the end of their trajectory. The two unsuccessful males both held dominant positions for at least 6 years. The male that produced 30 young molted directly from one nuptial plumage to another, for which we have assigned an arbitrary date of 60.

species have to play in understanding more general questions in evolution and ecology.

It is reasonable to suspect that the long-term trend toward drier conditions currently being experienced in Australia may have led to later timing of plumage acquisition in fairy-wrens. However, the plastic response of males to low rainfall has to some extent been masked by climate-driven demographic changes (van de Pol et al. 2012). In particular, the same low rainfall that restricts early molting by old males hampers offspring recruitment, thereby increasing the average age of males in the population. These effects cancel each other out, and at the population level there has not been a long-term shift in molt date.

Facultative sex-ratio adjustment

There are several ways that facultative sex allocation might prove adaptive in *M. cyaneus*. Notably, early-fledged females gain a huge advantage in recruitment into the local population because of their early dispersal to overwinter with a foreign group and

consequent privileged opportunities to inherit the territory and exploit nearby vacancies (see "Natural history"). Nonetheless, Cockburn and Double (2008) concluded that there was no evidence of facultative variation in the sex ratio in relation to any strand of sex allocation theory, despite large sample size. There was, however, a slight but highly significant tendency to overproduce sons regardless of the social or environmental circumstances faced by the mother (52.6%, or 11 sons for every 10 daughters), for reasons that remain unclear.

Contributions by helpers

All males living with a female contribute to feeding the young, although feeding rates vary by more than an order of magnitude among individuals (Dunn et al. 1995). Either the female, the dominant male, or one of the helpers can be the major contributor to care at a particular nest.

Male provisioning in fairy-wrens is subject to an unusual physiological constraint, because males invest simultaneously in within- and extra-group reproduction over long periods. Male care appears to be crucial for successful rearing of the brood, yet most reproductive success is gained by males via the extra-group pathway. Throughout the breeding season, males devote considerable energy to extra-group courtship through visits to neighboring females and through singing in the dawn chorus. Extra-group advertisement is tightly linked to high testosterone levels, which prevents the expression of parental care in most birds (Peters et al. 2000, 2001). Peters and her coworkers have shown experimentally that testosterone levels are set for each male at a level that allows both behaviors, but that the set point differs among males (Peters 2002; Peters et al. 2002).

The care provided by males is different in one critical respect from that provided by females. Females increase provisioning rates as the chicks grow older, whereas males feed at a constant rate throughout the nestling period (Dunn and Cockburn 1996). This is not because males are incapable of feeding at higher rates; in fact, they can be experimentally induced to do so by playbacks of begging (MacGregor and Cockburn 2002). Instead it appears that in natural circumstances males contribute a fixed amount while females do all the fine-tuning (Margraf and Cockburn 2013). This difference is potentially explained by sexual conflict theory, which predicts that female choice should select for predictable and consistent provisioning from their male partners where the likelihood of male care is jeopardized by the possibility of desertion, so the females can reliably assess the additional effort that they will have to provide in order to ensure that the young thrive (Royle et al. 2010; Schuett et al. 2010).

The presence of helpers in cooperatively breeding birds typically provides two types of assistance to the dominant male and female. In the short term, they can increase immediate reproductive output by increasing food delivery and defending the nest. In the longer term, helpers allow the dominants to lighten their load by reducing their provisioning rate, thus either increasing renesting or enhancing survival.

Demonstrating these benefits is fraught with difficulty because a correlation between the presence of helpers and reproductive output and/or survival provides no indication of causation. It is easy to understand how extra food could enhance productivity, or how load-lightening could affect survival. In societies where cooperative breeding is associated with natal philopatry such as fairy-wrens, however, productive parents or territories are likely to fledge more young and therefore recruit more helpers. Territories that facilitate survival are also likely to allow recruitment of more helpers. Distinguishing these alternatives has been one of the most long-standing and troublesome empirical problems in the study of cooperative breeding (Dickinson and Hatchwell 2004; Cockburn et al. 2008c).

In our study area, there is a strong association between the presence of helpers and the number of young fledged each season. Careful statistical analysis, however, prompts us to conclude that this correlation is driven by a correlation between good parents and high-quality territories rather than being a consequence of positive effects driven by extra provisioning by helpers (Cockburn et al. 2008c). There is no evidence that an effect of help emerges in either favorable or unfavorable environments.

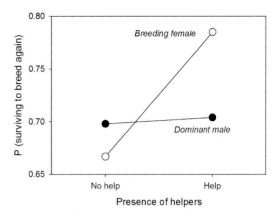

Figure 8.5. Proportion of adult *M. cyaneus* surviving from one breeding season to the next by sex, and whether they were assisted by helpers. From Cockburn (2008).

This lack of an immediate fecundity effect leads to a focus on load-lightening. Both sexes reduce their feeding rates in the presence of helpers, so an effect on survival is plausible. While females are much more likely to survive to breed again when they are assisted by helpers, however, the dominant male gains no advantage (Figure 8.5).

This unexpected result could be explained if males use load-lightening to invest in some other activity rather than enhanced survival. Green et al. (1995) speculated that the ability to increase courtship might be one such an activity. That hypothesis has not been sustained as courtship during the breeding season has no effect on female choice, and is instead dominated by neighbors that are often avoided as potential sires (Green et al. 2000). Furthermore, females appear to have established any preferences for extra-group sires before the start of the breeding season (Cockburn et al. 2009).

The solution to this paradox was discovered when we found that females lay smaller eggs of lower nutritional content when they have helpers (Russell et al. 2007). Any disadvantage they might impose on young is fully compensated as helpers increase combined feeding rates to overcompensate for load-lightening by the dominants, such that the young from small eggs rapidly reach the mass of the chicks reared by pairs from larger eggs.

Direct and indirect benefits of helping

Our understanding of social evolution was transformed by the idea that the behavior of nonreproductives could gain indirect fitness benefits by increasing the productivity of their relatives. Early data from *M. cyaneus* were used in a number of influential textbook accounts to demonstrate the application of Hamilton's rule to predict the occurrence of helping for this reason (Brown 1975; Grafen 1984). We now know those applications were wrong for many reasons (Margraf and Cockburn 2013). Most importantly, extra-pair fertilization undermines the importance of kinship. In our study, the modal condition is for helpers to be helping neither their mother nor their sire (48.5%, Table 8.1). Just 14% of helpers assist both their sire and mother.

The benefits to helpers therefore require further consideration. An obvious possibility is that helpers gain direct fitness benefits while queuing for dominance. Helpers can potentially benefit by mating via both the within-pair and extra-pair routes. In the former case, when they are assisting a female other than their mother (59% of cases), they can compete with the dominant male to fertilize young produced within the group. The value of this pathway is reduced because when females have helpers, they are more likely to mate exclusively with extra-group males. However, helpers gain 2.4% of all parentage via extra-group fertilizations (Figure 8.6). About 8% (47/598) of unrelated helpers gain success via this path at least once while they are subordinates. The majority of such helpers (62% of 47) did not subsequently gain paternity success on the territory, including about a quarter of the males that went on to become a dominant.

Helpers can also gain parasitic extra-group reproductive success, particularly if their dominant male is attractive. This is a much more common path to reproductive success, with 19% (116/598) of helpers gaining some success via this route. Once again, many of these did not subsequently gain success once they became dominants. Remarkably, some of those that did so gained success through carryover effects, which arise when a male preferred by a female dies just at the start of the breeding season, but the female continues to visit the territory of that male, mating with the helper instead (Cockburn et al. 2009).

Direct benefits via the extra-group pathway do not explain why helpers provision at nests. The unintended consequences of Mulder and Langmore's (1993) experiment cast light on this question. They removed helpers for 24 hrs during the nestling period to determine whether dominant males responded to their absence by increasing care to the level expected from unassisted males. Dominants did not adjust their feeding rate when the helper was removed, but violently attacked the helper when he was returned to the territory. By contrast, removal of the helper at other parts of the annual cycle generated much less reaction. This suggests that the dominant male may be using the threat of punishment to coerce helpers to provide care.

Conclusions

The authors contributing to this volume were asked to conclude by addressing a set of standard questions about avian cooperative breeding, such as why delay dispersal, why defer breeding, and why help? The simple answer to these questions is that superb fairy-wrens fit the image of a "typical" cooperative breeder: group-living arises because of natal philopatry; males are the nondispersive and cooperative sex; males do not disperse unless a territory occupied by a breeding vacancy becomes available next door; and all group members provision and defend offspring. These answers provide virtually no insight concerning the extraordinary social system of fairy-wrens, however.

Infidelity

The first difficulty lies in the unusual nature of the mating system. *M. cyaneus* exhibits a highly structured form of polyandry with an additional mating constraint caused by incest avoidance. Subject to the tight constraint that females never mate with their sons, in every fertile period females always mate with at least one extra-group male and shortly thereafter also mate with their social partner, and often with a subordinate helper as well, providing that the helper is not their

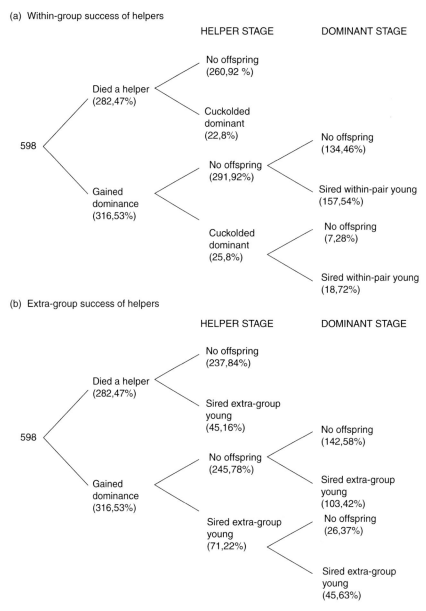

(a) Within-group success of helpers

HELPER STAGE   DOMINANT STAGE

598

Died a helper
(282,47%)

No offspring
(260,92 %)

Cuckolded
dominant
(22,8%)

Gained
dominance
(316,53%)

No offspring
(291,92%)

No offspring
(134,46%)

Sired within-pair young
(157,54%)

Cuckolded
dominant
(25,8%)

No offspring
(7,28%)

Sired within-pair young
(18,72%)

(b) Extra-group success of helpers

HELPER STAGE   DOMINANT STAGE

598

Died a helper
(282,47%)

No offspring
(237,84%)

Sired extra-group
young
(45,16%)

Gained
dominance
(316,53%)

No offspring
(245,78%)

No offspring
(142,58%)

Sired extra-group
young
(103,42%)

Sired extra-group
young
(71,22%)

No offspring
(26,37%)

Sired extra-group
young
(45,63%)

Figure 8.6. The probability that helpers will gain reproductive success at various stages of their lives through (a) the within-group path, and (b) the extra-group path.

son. Parentage is biased toward the extra-group male, particularly when the female has helpers, or when her partner is much younger than her. While females exert strong control over mating opportunities, female choice of extra-group partners is undermined by lower quality males competing with the preferred male in hidden leks, and by effective sperm competition by some dominant males.

With the exception of other species of fairy-wrens besides *M. coronatus* in which extreme levels of infidelity have been lost secondarily (Kingma et al. 2009; Margraf and Cockburn 2013), we are unaware of a comparable cooperative breeding system. The persistence of infidelity and cooperative breeding through multiple speciation events implies evolutionary stability, despite the conflict expected to ensue from persistent cuckoldry of the dominant male.

Females monopolize the benefits from helping

While the mating system is unusual, helping and its consequences add to its complexity. Females gain substantial benefits from the presence of helpers. First, they gain greater freedom to choose the preferred extra-group sires of their offspring without having to concede parentage to their mate. Second, they gain survival benefits from the presence of helpers, which are a reflection of the load-lightening associated with reduced investment in eggs.

Subordinate males also gain benefits, albeit by making the "best-of-a-bad-job." If they are helping their mother, they potentially gain kin-selected benefits. If they are not, they can compete for opportunities to reproduce, which for some males will be equivalent to their lifetime fitness, even if they do eventually gain a dominant position. Finally, both related and unrelated helpers can gain parasitic extra-group fitness, which may be substantial for subordinates helping very attractive males.

Breeding in groups appears to be highly deleterious for the dominant male, however, which almost appears to be making the "worst-of-a-good-job!" Each of the paths through which males can gain reproductive success is jeopardized once helpers are recruited on to the territory. Within-group reproduction is reduced because females with helpers allocate more fertilizations to extra-group males, and because if the helper is unrelated, he is a competitor for reproduction. Attractive dominants gain the most extra-group fertilizations, but they are highly vulnerable to parasitism by their helpers within the hidden leks. We have yet to find any compensating benefits for dominant males. Thus,

in contrast to the conventional framework for assessing the benefits of cooperation, which focuses on why helpers remain philopatric instead of attempting to breed independently, the more difficult question here is: why do dominant males tolerate helper philopatry?

Cockburn (2013) proposed that the *Malurus* system has developed from a history of coevolutionary interactions between males and females involving the following sequence of events:

(1) Because of long life and high population density, there is intense selection on females to find vacancies, so they settle quickly with few opportunities for mate assessment.

(2) Females compensate for lack of mate choice by seeking extra-pair fertilizations, as proposed by Møller (1992).

(3) Males court females seeking these fertilizations and coerce help from subordinates so that they can reduce their provisioning rate (Mulder and Langmore 1993).

(4) Females take advantage of the helpers being forced to feed to increase the cuckoldry rate, tipping the balance of male fitness toward extra-group mating.

(5) Increasingly, it is the ability of males to molt early and display for a long time that becomes the target of selection.

(6) Because display and fertility become dissociated, females need to be able to find the displaying males at a later date, forcing males to defend a territory where they can be found.

(7) Females appease their own mate by copulating with them as well.

(8) Sperm competition between the home male and the extra-group sire leads to a large ejaculate strategy, with consequent limits on sperm replenishment.

(9) Females mate earlier and earlier in the morning to avoid sperm depletion of the extra-group male.

(10) Subordinates (and unattractive males) evolve parasitic strategies to exploit the attractiveness of dominants.

The system remains stable for three reasons. First, extra-group success provides subordinates with an incentive for participation. Second, the asymmetry in reproductive success caused by the success of attractive dominants means that these dominants are the winners that leave most descendants. Third, the same asymmetry means that while most parentage is via extra-group fertilization, most extra-group success is achieved by just a few males. Most males gain no extra-group success, so their best prospects come from fertilizing the female on their own territory, providing an incentive to invest in the offspring that she produces.

Interspecific differences cause problems for cooperative breeding theory

While the model we have proposed allows some understanding of the surprising evolutionary stability of a social system in which the majority of seemingly dominant males are greatly disadvantaged, emerging interspecific comparisons show that considerable diversity can arise within a society based around chronic infidelity.

First, while many populations of other species also exhibit complete or near complete female dispersal, a continuous gradient can be found in the incidence of female philopatry in *Malurus*. In the most extreme case, philopatry by males and females is equally frequent in *M. elegans*. It is of considerable interest that in contrast to the negative evidence for male helpers, there is convincing evidence that female helpers in *M. splendens* enhance productivity (Brooker and Rowley 1995). Brouwer et al. (2014) have uncovered a mechanistic basis for this benefit by showing that although group members load-lighten in response to the presence of male helpers, they ignore the presence of female helpers, so young helped by females receive more food.

One explanation for the failure to load-lighten in the presence of subordinate helper females is that they are less reliable as sources of help, as they are prone to disperse and can initiate their own nest on the territory (Rowley et al. 1989; Russell and Rowley 2000). Females may also be in a stronger position to decline help. In *M. coronatus*, which is unique in having a low rate of extra-group mating, subordinate females feed when they are helping their mother, but not when they are unrelated to the dominant female (Kingma et al. 2011; Margraf and Cockburn 2013). By contrast, in addition to the evidence of coercion of male subordinates, dominant females are extremely sensitive to sudden changes in group size and will not continue to invest in a clutch if a helper is experimentally removed (Dunn and Cockburn 1996).

These observations are united in demonstrating that there is much richer variability surrounding female rather than male help. This variation draws attention to a possible flaw in the research culture that has dominated the study of cooperative breeding, which is exemplified by the long-term studies celebrated in this volume. These studies achieve such intricate detail that they prompt generalization and extrapolation. Sometimes such generalization is unjustified, and focusing on just one species can be misleading.

For example, in one of the classic experiments of cooperative breeding, Pruett-Jones and Lewis (1990) showed that helper males *M. cyaneus* would only disperse to vacant territories if a female was present on the vacant territory. This provides some of the strongest evidence for the idea of ecological constraints as the underpinning of cooperation. In this case, males defer dispersal because there is a shortage of females.

The difficulty with this logic is that in other populations of other *Malurus* species with female helpers this constraint does not exist, yet the incidence of cooperative breeding is much higher than recorded for *M. cyaneus* (Margraf and Cockburn 2013). In addition, the cause of the female shortfall is the high cost of female dispersal, undermining the theoretical argument that high costs of dispersal lead to cooperative breeding (Cockburn 2013).

Interpretations of the *M. cyaneus* mating system suffer a similar problem. The high rate of infidelity was discovered in a population where the incidence of female philopatry was high, leading to rich possibilities for incestuous social pairing. This led Brooker et al. (1990) to propose that infidelity had evolved to avoid incest, an idea that soon collapsed with the demonstration that infidelity was equally high in populations where incestuous pairing was rare (Cockburn et al. 2013). We believe instead that having access to obligate extra-group mating may have allowed incestuous pairing, although once that had happened, more sophisticated inbreeding mechanisms may have evolved to deal with the uncertainty created by mating in conditions when the probability of a neighbor being a close relative is high (Brouwer et al. 2011)

Hence we view the *Malurus* system as having evolved along a complex trajectory that has locked in some features, but created a rich new tapestry on which social evolution can operate. Although the complexity of the *Malurus* system has proved particularly challenging to unravel, we argue that many other avian clades will be best understood once it is recognized that the foundations of cooperative breeding can be very different from the evolutionary forces that shape subsequent evolution. Living in a cooperative society is a potent agent of selection that can force species along evolutionary paths that move them to very different states than the conditions in which cooperation originated (Cockburn 2013).

Acknowledgments

Our long-term research on fairy-wrens has been funded continuously and generously by the Australian Research Council since 1989, and has relied on generosity and help from the Australian National Botanic Gardens since 1986. We are profoundly grateful to both organizations. The study population was established by Raoul Mulder, and our work has benefited from critical contributions from Mike Double, Peter Dunn, David Green, Loeske Kruuk, and Anne Peters, as well as more than 50 seasonal research assistants, students, and colleagues.

REFERENCES

Boland, C. R. J. and Cockburn, A. (2002). Short sketches from the long history of cooperative breeding in Australian birds. *Emu*, 102, 9–17.

Bradley, E. and Bradley, J. (1958). Notes on the behaviours and plumage of colour-ringed blue wrens. *Emu*, 58, 313–326.

Brooker, M. and Rowley, I. (1995). The significance of territory size and quality in the mating strategy of the splendid fairy-wren. *J. Anim. Ecol.*, 64, 614–627.

Brooker, M. G., Rowley, I., Adams, M., and Baverstock, P. R. (1990). Promiscuity: an inbreeding avoidance mechanism in a socially monogamous species? *Behav. Ecol. Sociobiol.*, 26, 191–200.

Brouwer, L., van de Pol, M., Atema, E., and Cockburn, A. (2011). Strategic promiscuity helps avoid inbreeding at multiple levels in a cooperative breeder where both sexes are philopatric. *Mol. Ecol.*, 20, 4796–4807.

Brouwer, L., van de Pol, M., and Cockburn, A. (2014). The role of social environment on parental care: offspring benefit more from the presence of female than male helpers. *J. Anim. Ecol.*, 83, 491–503.

Brown, J. L. (1975). *The Evolution of Behavior*. New York: W. W. Norton.

Buchanan, K. L. and Cockburn, A. (2013). Fairy-wrens and their relatives (Maluridae) as model organisms in evolutionary ecology: the scientific legacy of Ian Rowley and Eleanor Russell. *Emu*, 113, I–VII.

Calhim, S., Double, M. C., Margraf, N., Birkhead, T. R., and Cockburn, A. (2011). Maintenance of sperm variation in a highly promiscuous wild bird. *PLoS One*, 6, e28809.

Cockburn, A. (2004). Mating systems and sexual conflict. In: *Ecology and Evolution of Cooperative Breeding in Birds*, ed. W. D. Koenig and J. L. Dickinson. Cambridge: Cambridge University Press, pp. 81–101.

Cockburn, A. (2006). Prevalence of different modes of parental care in birds. *Proc. R. Soc. London B*, 273, 1375–1383.

Cockburn, A. (2013). Cooperative breeding in birds: towards a richer conceptual framework. In: *Cooperation and its Evolution*, ed. K. Sterelny, R. Joyce, B. Calcott, and B. Fraser. Cambridge, MA: MIT Press, pp. 223–245.

Cockburn, A. and Double, M. C. (2008). Cooperatively breeding superb fairy-wrens show no facultative manipulation of offspring sex ratio despite plausible benefits. *Behav. Ecol. Sociobiol.*, 62, 681–688.

Cockburn, A., Osmond, H. L., Mulder, R. A., Green, D. J., and Double, M. C. (2003). Divorce, dispersal and incest avoidance in the cooperatively breeding superb fairy-wren *Malurus cyaneus*. *J. Anim. Ecol.*, 72, 189–202.

Cockburn, A., Osmond, H. L., and Double, M. C. (2008a). Swingin' in the rain: condition dependence and sexual selection in a capricious world. *Proc. R. Soc. London B*, 275, 605–612.

Cockburn, A., Osmond, H. L., Mulder, R. A., Double, M. C., and Green, D. J. (2008b). Demography of male reproductive queues in cooperatively breeding superb fairy-wrens *Malurus cyaneus*. *J. Anim. Ecol.*, 77, 297–304.

Cockburn, A., Sims, R. A., Osmond, H. L., Green, D. J., Double, M. C., et al. (2008c). Can we measure the benefits of help in cooperatively breeding birds: the case of superb fairy-wrens *Malurus cyaneus*? *J. Anim. Ecol.*, 77, 430–438.

Cockburn, A., Dalziell, A. H., Blackmore, C. J., Double, M. C., Kokko, H., et al. (2009). Superb fairy-wren males aggregate into hidden leks to solicit extragroup fertilizations before dawn. *Behav. Ecol.*, 20, 501–510.

Cockburn, A., Brouwer, L., Double, M., Margraf, N., and van de Pol, M. (2013). Evolutionary origins and persistence of infidelity in *Malurus*: the least faithful birds. *Emu*, 113, 208–217.

Dalziell, A. H. and Cockburn, A. (2008). Dawn song in superb fairy-wrens: a bird that seeks extrapair copulations during the dawn chorus. *Anim. Behav.*, 75, 489–500.

Dickinson, J. L. and Hatchwell, B. J. (2004). Fitness consequences of helping. In: *Ecology and Evolution of Cooperative Breeding in Birds*, ed. W. D. Koenig and J. L. Dickinson. Cambridge: Cambridge University Press, pp. 48–66.

Double, M. and Cockburn, A. (2000). Pre-dawn infidelity: females control extra-pair mating in superb fairy-wrens. *Proc. R. Soc. London B*, 267, 465–470.

Double, M. C. and Cockburn, A. (2003). Subordinate superb fairy-wrens (*Malurus cyaneus*) parasitize the reproductive success of attractive dominant males. *Proc. R. Soc. London B*, 270, 379–384.

Double, M. C., Peakall, R., Beck, N. R., and Cockburn, A. (2005). Dispersal, philopatry, and infidelity: dissecting local genetic structure in superb fairy-wrens (*Malurus cyaneus*). *Evolution*, 59, 625–635.

Dunn, P. O. and Cockburn, A. (1996). Evolution of male parental care in a bird with almost complete cuckoldry. *Evolution*, 50, 2542–2548.

Dunn, P. O. and Cockburn, A. (1999). Extrapair mate choice and honest signaling in cooperatively breeding superb fairy-wrens. *Evolution*, 53, 938–946.

Dunn, P. O., Cockburn, A., and Mulder, R. A. (1995). Fairy-wren helpers often care for young to which they are unrelated. *Proc. R. Soc. London B*, 259, 339–343.

Gould, J. (1841). *The Birds of Australia, Vol. III*. London: Taylor.

Grafen, A. (1984). Natural selection, kin selection and group selection. In: *Behavioural Ecology: an Evolutionary Approach*. 2nd ed., ed. J. R. Krebs and N.B. Davies. Oxford: Blackwell, pp. 62–84.

Green, D. J., Cockburn, A., Hall, M. L., Osmond, H., and Dunn, P. O. (1995). Increased opportunities for cuckoldry may be why dominant male fairy-wrens tolerate helpers. *Proc. R. Soc. London B*, 262, 297–303.

Green, D. J., Osmond, H. L., Double, M. C., and Cockburn, A. (2000). Display rate by male fairy-wrens (*Malurus cyaneus*) during the fertile period of females has little influence on extra-pair mate choice. *Behav. Ecol. Sociobiol.*, 48, 438–446.

Higgins, P. J., Peter, J. M., and Steele, W. K. (eds.) 2001. *Handbook of Australian, New Zealand and Antarctic Birds. Vol. 5. Tyrant-flycatchers to Chats*. Oxford: Oxford University Press.

Kingma, S. A., Hall, M. L., Segelbacher, G., and Peters, A. (2009). Radical loss of an extreme extra-pair mating system. *BMC Ecology*, 9, 1–11.

Kingma, S. A., Hall, M. L., and Peters, A. (2011). Multiple benefits drive helping behavior in a cooperatively breeding bird: an integrated analysis. *Am. Nat.*, 177, 486–495.

MacGregor, N. A. and Cockburn, A. (2002). Sex differences in parental response to begging nestlings in superb fairy-wrens. *Anim. Behav.*, 63, 923–932.

Margraf, N. and Cockburn, A. (2013). Helping behaviour and parental care in fairy-wrens (*Malurus*). *Emu*, 113, 294–301.

Møller, A. P. (1992). Frequency of female copulations with multiple males and sexual selection. *Am. Nat.*, 139, 1089–1101.

Mulder, R. A. (1997). Extra-group courtship displays and other reproductive tactics of superb fairy-wrens. *Aust. J. Zool.*, 45, 131–143.

Mulder, R. A. and Langmore, N. E. (1993). Dominant males punish helpers for temporary defection in superb fairy-wrens. *Anim. Behav.*, 45, 830–833

Mulder, R. A., Dunn, P. O., Cockburn, A., Lazenby-Cohen, K. A., and Howell, M. J. (1994). Helpers liberate female fairy-wrens from constraints on extra-pair mate choice. *Proc. R. Soc. London B*, 255, 223–229.

Peters, A. (2002). Testosterone and the trade-off between mating and paternal effort in extrapair-mating superb fairy-wrens. *Anim. Behav.*, 64, 103–112.

Peters, A., Astheimer, L. B., Boland, C. R. J., and Cockburn, A. (2000). Testosterone is involved in acquisition and maintenance of sexually selected male plumage in superb fairy-wrens, *Malurus cyaneus*. *Behav. Ecol. Sociobiol.*, 47, 438–445.

Peters, A., Astheimer, L. B. and Cockburn, A. (2001). The annual testosterone profile in cooperatively breeding superb fairy-wrens, *Malurus cyaneus*, reflects their extreme infidelity. *Behav. Ecol. Sociobiol.*, 50, 519–527.

Peters, A., Cockburn, A. and Cunningham, R. (2002). Testosterone treatment suppresses paternal care in superb fairy-wrens, *Malurus cyaneus*, despite their concurrent investment in courtship. *Behav. Ecol. Sociobiol.*, 51, 538–547.

Pruett-Jones, S. G. and Lewis, M. J. (1990). Sex ratio and habitat limitation promote delayed dispersal in superb fairy-wrens. *Nature*, 348, 541–42.

Rowe, M. and Pruett-Jones, S. (2011). Sperm competition selects for sperm quantity and quality in the Australian Maluridae. *PLoS One*, 6, e15720.

Rowley, I. (1957). Cooperative feeding of young by superb blue wrens. *Emu*, 57, 356–357.

Rowley, I. (1965). The life history of the superb blue wren. *Emu*, 64, 251–297.

Rowley, I. and Russell, E. (1991). Demography of passerines in the temperate southern hemisphere. In: *Bird Population Studies*, ed. C. M. Perrins, J.-D. Lebreton, and G. J. M. Hirons. Oxford: Oxford University Press, pp. 22–44.

Rowley, I. and Russell, E. (1997). *Fairy-wrens and Grasswrens: Maluridae.* Oxford: Oxford University Press.

Rowley, I., Russell, E., Payne, R. B., and Payne, L. L. (1989). Plural breeding in the splendid fairy-wren, *Malurus splendens* (Aves, Maluridae), a cooperative breeder. *Ethology*, 83, 229–247.

Royle, N. J., Schuett, W., and Dall, S. R. X. (2010). Behavioral consistency and the resolution of sexual conflict over parental investment. *Behav. Ecol.*, 21, 1125–1130.

Russell, A. F., Langmore, N. E., Cockburn, A., Astheimer, L. B., and Kilner, R. M. (2007). Reduced egg investment can conceal helper effects in cooperatively breeding birds. *Science*, 317, 941–944.

Russell, E. M. and Rowley, I. (1993). Demography of the cooperatively breeding splendid fairy-wren, *Malurus splendens* (Maluridae). *Aust. J. Zool.*, 41, 475–505.

Russell, E. and Rowley, I. (2000). Demography and social organisation of the red-winged fairy-wren, *Malurus elegans. Aust. J. Zool.*, 48, 161–200.

Schuett, W., Tregenza, T., and Dall, S. R. X. (2010). Sexual selection and animal personality. *Biol. Rev.*, 85, 217–246.

Tidemann, S. C. (1986). Breeding in 3 species of fairy-wrens (*Malurus*): do helpers really help? *Emu*, 86, 131–138.

Tuttle, E. M. and Pruett-Jones, S. (2004). Estimates of extreme sperm production: morphological and experimental evidence from reproductively promiscuous fairy-wrens (*Malurus*). *Anim. Behav.*, 68, 541–550.

van de Pol, M., Osmond, H. L., and Cockburn, A. (2012). Fluctuations in population composition dampen the impact of phenotypic plasticity on trait dynamics in superb fairy-wrens. *J. Anim. Ecol.*, 81, 411–422.

van de Pol, M., Brouwer, L., Brooker, L. C., Brooker, M. G., Colombelli-Negrel, D., et al. (2013). Problems with using large-scale oceanic climate indices to compare climatic sensitivities across populations and species. *Ecography*, 36, 249–255.

9

Chestnut-crowned babblers: Dealing with climatic adversity and uncertainty in the Australian arid zone

Andrew F. Russell

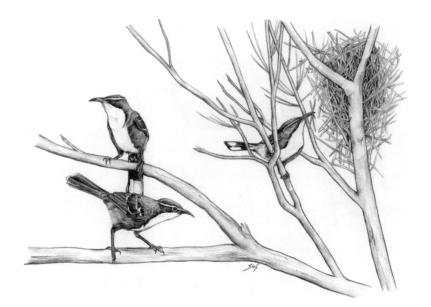

Introduction

Avian cooperative breeders occupy climatically and ecologically diverse habitats. Such diversity will inevitably result in contrasting challenges, and might partly explain their variable social systems. If so, our current appreciation of the key selective forces shaping the form and function of avian cooperative breeding systems is likely to be biased because study sites are distributed nonrandomly across the globe (Introduction,

Figure 1). To derive a more complete understanding, it is imperative that studies encompass the full range of climatic and ecological settings (Cockburn 2003; Cockburn and Russell 2011).

My primary motivation for establishing a long-term study of the 50 g sexually-monomorphic chestnut-crowned babbler (*Pomatostomus ruficeps*) of outback Australia was twofold. First, it offered an investigation of a cooperative breeding system in a novel arid zone environment. Second, nothing was known

Cooperative Breeding in Vertebrates: Studies of Ecology, Evolution, and Behavior, eds W. D. Koenig and J. L. Dickinson.
Published by Cambridge University Press. © Cambridge University Press 2016.

about the social or cooperative system of this species, other than a published remark by an enlightened dog-walker who declared from observing three birds simultaneously bringing food to a nest that, like other Australian babblers, it must be a cooperative breeder (Smith 1992). There are obvious drawbacks to establishing a long-term study on a species that has never been studied before, especially as it turns out, one with such a complicated social system. Nonetheless, I was excited by the prospect, and even a baffled smile from Andrew Cockburn could not deter me.

Phylogeny

The chestnut-crowned babbler is not a true babbler, but one of five extant members of the ancient Australo-Papuan babblers (Pomatostomidae). Recent phylogenetic evidence (Jetz et al. 2012) suggests that this babbler clade branched from the main avian tree ~ 51 million years ago (Ma) along with the family-living but noncooperative Orthonychidae (Australo-Papuan logrunners). Babblers and logrunners diverged 3 million years later, and chestnut-crowned babblers emerged ~ 11 Ma. All five extant Pomatostomid babbler species show cooperative breeding, suggesting this breeding system to be ancestral in the clade. The antiquity of Pomatostomid babblers renders any consideration of the original pressures selecting for cooperative breeding beyond the scope of this chapter, especially since it probably emerged when Australia was covered in forest.

Distribution and ecology

Chestnut-crowned babblers are now found over 10^6 km^2 of arid and semiarid zones in inland southeastern Australia (Higgins and Peter 2002). They primarily frequent open woodland and shrubland habitat, especially in the vicinity of (usually dry) flood plains, salt pans, and creeks. Foraging is chiefly conducted in or on the ground, with digging or overturning stones and dead wood the primary modes, although they also glean from vegetation and uncover or extract prey from living and dead wood. They appear to have a strictly animal-based diet; with spiders, grubs, and caterpillars representing

their favored items, although they also consume a range of other invertebrate and vertebrate prey (e.g., adult insects, centipedes, geckos). Surveys conducted throughout much of their range suggest that the key habitat requirement is abundant, but dispersed, low shrubs that simultaneously offer open ground for foraging and protection from avian predators. Tall shrubs and trees provide additional foraging substrate, and at least some of either are required to position nests, in which babblers both breed and roost (Figure 9.1b).

Study population, habitat, and climate

My fieldsite is located at Fowlers Gap, a University of New South Wales research station on the eastern fringe of the Strzelecki Desert in far western New South Wales (31°05'S, 141°43'E) (Figure 9.1a). The study area increased from 10 km^2 in 2004 to 64 km^2 by 2007. The overall density of breeding units varies annually from 0.5 to 1.5 km^{-2}, totaling some 200–600 birds in adult plumage (i.e., >6 months old). The habitat is dominated by open bluebush/saltbush (chenopod) shrubland habitat. Parallel hill ranges along the length of the fieldsite generate countless narrow creek and drainages, within which the majority of the scant perennial tree and shrub vegetation is found (Figure 9.1a). Unsurprisingly, babblers forage chiefly along drainage zones, where prey availability and cover from predators are more prevalent (Portelli et al. 2009).

The median annual rainfall at Fowlers Gap is 215 mm yr^{-1}, with 63% of years having an annual rainfall below 250 mm yr^{-1} – the cut-off defining arid zones (Figure 9.2a). Among-year variance in annual rainfall is high (coefficient of variation [CV] = 67%). Additionally, in contrast to many other dry regions, there is no seasonal pattern in rainfall, leading to high levels of uncertainty as to whether and when rain will fall in a year (Figure 9.2b). Finally, annual temperature variation is extreme: night temperatures commonly fall to 0°C during winter (mean min. June-July = 5°C) and climb to 45°C during summer days (mean max. December-February = 37°C) (Figure 9.2c). Thus the climate at Fowlers Gap combines adversity with unusually high uncertainty.

(a)

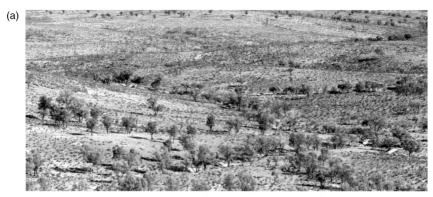

(b)

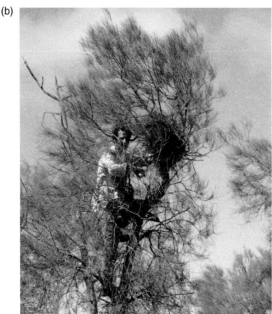

Figure 9.1. (a) Typical open chenopod shrubland habitat at Fowlers Gap; note the scant vegetation is generally limited to short linear stands in drainage lines. (b) A babbler nest in classic position: near the top of a 7 m casuarina. The robust nests are large 30 × 50 cm, single-chambered, and have ~ 6 cm entrance hole. See plate section for color figure.

The social system and group composition

Plural breeding

At Fowlers Gap, the social system of chestnut-crowned babblers is at least two-tiered (Figure 9.3). During nonbreeding, they live in large, stable, and predictable "social groups," but typically, over half of these groups then fragment partially into 2–4 (mode = 2) breeding units for reproduction. Social group fragmentation is primarily determined by the number of immigrant females and winter rainfall, with a quarter of groups fragmenting when rainfall is low, and most doing so when it is high. Breeding units from the same social group, while distinct, are not fully independent; such units forage together a third of the time

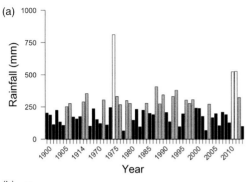

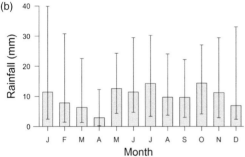

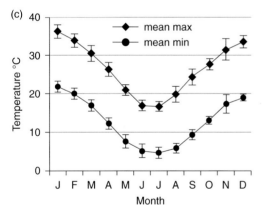

Figure 9.2. Climate at Fowlers Gap. (a) Annual rainfall (mm) for years 1900–1917 and 1967–2013. Note most years are arid (black bars) and almost all others are semiarid (grey bars). (b) Median monthly rainfall over these 60 years showing interquartile ranges. Note the low between-month but high within-month variation. (c) Mean (± standard deviation) daytime maximum and nighttime minimum temperatures for each month (*N* = 5 years).

and overlap spatially by ~ 70% during periods of reproduction (Portelli et al. 2009). The constituent members of breeding units can be predicted by genetic relatedness, but are labile between years due to high breeder turnover. In addition, a minority of nonbreeders that are similarly related or similarly unrelated to breeders at multiple nests in their social group are transient, helping at multiple nests or affiliating in a nonhelping capacity with multiple breeding units, respectively. The latter category mainly involves nonbreeding immigrant females, but philopatric males can also be distantly related to breeders. Finally, breeding units almost always reamalgamate once their respective offspring reach independence with offspring crèching and being protected by the larger social group. Based on the stability of the social group across years, the fluidity of breeding units between years, and affiliation patterns, I consider chestnut-crowned babblers to be plural breeders (Russell et al. 2010).

Size and composition

The number of social groups in the 64 km² fieldsite ranges from 25 to 55 annually, with reduced numbers deriving from drought. Social groups forage over an average of ~ 1 km² and are weakly territorial, vocally or physically interacting with neighbors on 55% of encounters (Sorato et al. 2015). Prior to the onset of breeding, usually from late July (austral winter), social groups number 3–23 (mean = 12) individuals. On average, such groups comprise 16% breeding males and 10% breeding females from the previous year, 34% surviving nonbreeding natal males from previous years, 22% immigrant females, and 18% first-year natal recruits (14% male, 4% female). The sex ratio of social groups averages 64% male (range 25% to 90% male). Overall, 33% of social group members typically breed in the coming breeding season (range = 13–100%).

The number of breeding units ranges from 35 to 85 annually, increasing as a function of the number and size of social groups and the amount of winter rain. Breeding units contain 2–17 birds in adult plumage (mean = 7.5); pairs are rare (~ 6% of breeding units) and only occur as secondary fragments of a larger social group. During breeding, units range over an area

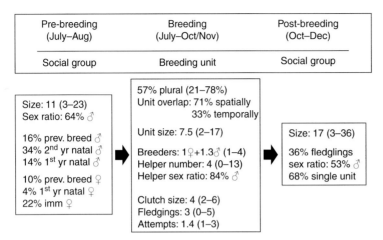

Figure 9.3. Summary of chestnut-crowned babbler socioecology. In 8 of the last 11 years, breeding began during late winter (July) or early spring (August) and finished by late spring-early summer (October-November). In the others it began earlier in autumn or later in midsummer, the latter occurred during back-to-back uniquely wet summers (see Figure 9.2a, years 2010, 2011). Only in 5 of 11 years have breeding units regularly been multibrooded, having up to two (in 4 years) or three (in 1 year) successful attempts. Hence, the months denoting prebreeding, breeding and postbreeding, represent the typical case. This breeding phenology in combination with an incubation phase of 3-4 weeks, a nestling phase of equivalent duration and a month-long postfledging phase, leads to delayed dispersers having the opportunity of helping from the age of 2 months postfledging when their breeding unit is multibrooded, and 9 months when this is not the case. Delayed dispersers only rarely help before they molt into adult plumage at 6 months of age; so most helpers begin at 9 months postfledging.

In all boxes, mean values are presented to the nearest whole number, except where this would be misleading, and ranges are presented in parentheses. In the left-hand box: "size" refers to number of individuals in adult plumage; "prev. breed" shows the percentage of the social group that is comprised of breeders from the previous year; "≥2nd yr natal" refers to the percentage contributed by natal individuals approximating 2 years old or more, while "1st yr natal" refers to natal recruits in their first year of life and "imm." denotes immigrants. In the middle-box, the mean percentage of plural breeding units is provided, along with their spatial and temporal overlap in foraging home-ranges. Unit sizes, reproductive skew, helper numbers, and helper sex ratios, as well as clutch sizes, numbers of fledglings per attempt and the number of successful attempts made in a season are also provided. The right-hand box presents social group sizes inclusive of fledglings, and the percentage representation of fledglings in the group, the sex ratio of fledglings, and the proportion of fledglings derived from a single unit.

of ~ 0.5 km², but nests are not necessarily positioned centrally within their range, and units commonly venture over 1 km from their nest to forage (Sorato et al. 2015). Each breeding unit contains a single reproductive female, 1–4 sires (mode = 1) and 0–13 (mean = 4) nonbreeding helpers which attach to the unit containing the breeder(s) to which they are most related (Browning et al. 2012a). Multiple sires occur in a third of all breeding units, but extra-group paternity is exceptional (<1% of young) (Russell et al. unpubl. data). Co-sires are usually second-order or third-order kin of the primary male. From the perspective of the breeding unit, reproductive skew among females is absolute, while in males it is high, although units can vary from fully polyandrous without nonbreeding helpers to monogamous usually with nonbreeding helpers (Browning et al. unpubl. data).

Annually, clutch sizes average 3–5 eggs, again increasing as a function of winter rain (mean = 4.2; range = 2–6). Although some brood reduction is relatively common, and most units are single-brooded in most years, units can fledge up to nine offspring in a good season (overall mean = 4.5 per unit). Additionally, low nest-predation rates (generally <15%; Russell et al. 2010), in conjunction with plural breeding, can result in up to 17 fledglings being produced in the social group in a favorable season (overall mean = 6.5). Following breeding, social groups number 3–36 individuals (mean = 19).

Between-season dispersal and death

So far we have ringed over 1,300 nestlings and 1,100 free-flying birds. All male offspring remain in their natal social group in the first year and most remain there for life, although a minority join with co-dispersers (usually from other groups) to found new social groups (Rollins et al. 2012). By contrast, few females remain in their natal social group in their first year, and none breeds there. Instead, females typically disperse individually into established social groups following independence, although a minority, like the males, will join with other dispersers of both sexes from other groups to found a new social group.

Overall, an estimated 60% of male fledglings die in their first year of life, and 85% of females in their first year die or disperse, a sex bias that generates most of the observed male-biased sex ratio. Although the survival of nonbreeding immigrant females cannot be determined with confidence due to the confound of further dispersal, ~ 70% of nonbreeding males survive annually from their first year, while the annual survivorship of breeding males and females approximate 80% and 65%, respectively (Russell et al. unpubl. data). Thus, chestnut-crowned babblers are not long-lived, and even if they reach one year of age and remain in their natal group, their average lifespan is only three to four years.

Genetic structure of social groups

Social groups of chestnut-crowned babblers comprise multiple extended families and so are genetically diverse. Females derive from multiple other social groups, and so are predominantly unrelated to each other and are always unrelated to their partner(s). Because immigrant females cannot derive indirect fitness benefits from helping or cobreeding, they are presumably under strong selection to breed separately. Plural breeding, in conjunction with polyandry and relatively high breeder turnover, results in natal

individuals being modally second-order relatives (range in dyadic relatedness = 0–0.5). This high level of variation in relatedness patterns among social group members is expected to generate a strong selection pressure for kin discrimination.

Cooperative breeding

Although nonbreeders cooperate in multiple ways (Table 9.1), the most important and the only one that we have studied in detail is nestling provisioning. In general, individuals do not begin to contribute to cooperation until they are in full adult plumage at around 6 months postfledging. For the majority, helping is initiated in the season following their birth when they are at least 9 months postfledging (Figure 9.3). I term helpers born in season n and helping in season $n + 1$ as yearlings, and all older individuals as adults. I exclude all individuals in juvenile plumage (i.e., <6 m) from definitions of helper number and details of nestling provisioning.

Measuring contributions to nestling provisioning

In 2004, I conducted nest observations from a concealed location approximating 50 m distant from the nest, as trial observations conducted at closer proximity, even with a hide, were clearly invasive. The large number of individuals visiting the nest and their quick movements hampered the quality of the data, and I erroneously concluded that all unit members appear to help (Russell et al. 2010). Following trials in 2005 and 2006, we began using a Passive Integrated Transponder (PIT-tag, also termed RFID) system to monitor individual provisioning rates remotely, and integrated a camera system in a subset of nests. PIT-tags are inserted subcutaneously in the flank, and remain in position throughout the life of the bird. The data presented originates from ~ 2,500 hours of data collected over several full days throughout the 23-day nestling period of 50 breeding units.

The success of this PIT-tag system is facilitated by the domed nest structure of chestnut-crowned babblers

Table 9.1. Candidate cooperative behaviors in chestnut-crowned babblers

Behavior	Cooperative	Explanation	Importance	References
Territoriality	No	Not strong and does not increase for or during reproduction	N/A	Sorato et al. 2015
Sentineling	Yes	Increases when fledglings present (10% to 35% incidences during 3-h focals of foraging groups)	Not yet known, but is positively associated with predation risk and ground foraging.	Sorato et al. 2012
Nest building	Yes	Mainly built by social groups, and secondary units. Most group members contribute	Presumably reduces costs for breeding female, and might explain the abundance of nests (5–25 per social group)	Anecdotal
Nest defense	Yes	Rare, but certainly occurs cooperatively	Predators rarely attempt to penetrate nests, obviating need for defense: foraging occurs far from the nest and attendants never left.	Anecdotal
Female provisioning	Yes	Females call loudly from within nest and routinely fed during incubation and brooding	Preliminary evidence suggests feeding breeding females reduces costs of incubation and brooding	Unpublished data

(Figure 9.1b), which ensures that birds need to pass through an antenna to access their nest. Further, by placing a pen camera into a subset of nests, it was possible to verify the validity of the PIT-tag method (Nomano et al. 2014). The camera system revealed a relatively low rate of nonfeeding (nest visits lacking food) and false-feeding (visits with food but without delivery). Adult and yearling helpers did not feed in 10% and 5% of visits, respectively, and false-fed in 2.5% of visits, with the latter predominantly arising following brood refusal (Young et al. 2013). The camera system also reveals details of prey type, size, and load (Browning et al. 2012b). Because helpers deliver single prey items approximating a babbler bill volume and helpers do not vary prey load size as a function of helper number, provisioning frequency does a good job of approximating the biomass of food delivered by helpers.

Helpers and their provisioning rules

As social groups are genetically diverse, group members commonly have a choice of units to help within their social group. At best, 36% of nonbreeders living in their

natal social group have the opportunity of helping both their parents, 31% have their father only because their mother is dead, 5% have their mother only because their father is dead, while 2% have their parents in separate units, following divorce. The remaining 26% are more distantly related to the current breeders, which include uncles and older half-brothers ($r = 0.25$), half-brothers of uncles and older cousins ($r = 0.125$), second-order cousins ($r = 0.0625$) and nonrelatives. Nonbreeders rarely have the opportunity to help an older full-sib. The evidence presented below suggests that chestnut-crowned babblers have two distinct categories of helper demarked by whether or not they have the opportunity of helping at least one first-order kin breeder (Figure 9.4a; Browning et al. 2012a; Nomano et al. 2015).

Effects of kinship

Over 95% of nonbreeders that have a first-order relative breeding (i.e., at least one parent) in their social group decide to help, and all direct their care toward the most related breeder(s) (Browning et al. 2012a). Differences in prey delivery rates by those helping both parents versus a single parent are apparently

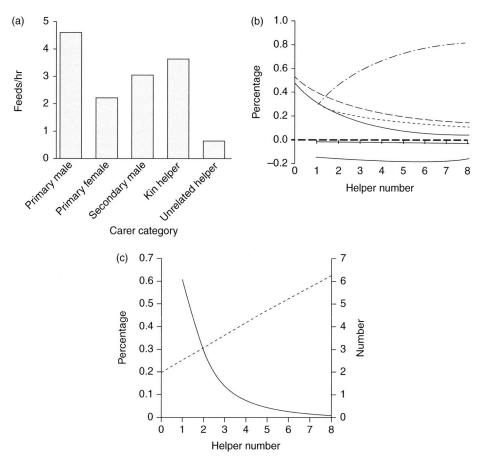

Figure 9.4. Mean helper contributions and consequences. (a) The number of prey items provided hr^{-1} by each carer class modified by the probability that the class contributes to nestling provisioning. Contributions by primary (1°) and secondary (2°) breeders are provided for comparison with nonbreeders providing for offspring of ≥ 1 first-order relative ("kin help") or not ("unrel help"). Note the step-reduction in contributions by the latter. (b) Percentage responses and contributions as a function of increasing helper numbers. The two lines below zero show the percentage response to increasing numbers of helpers (breeding female bold; breeding male dashed). The three declining lines above zero represent the percentage contributions by the breeding female (bold), breeding male (dashed), and each helper (dotted) with increments to helper number. Finally, the increasing line represents the overall percentage of food provided by all helpers combined. (c) Effects of helper number on percentage change to seasonal fledgling production (bold line) and per capita food acquisition rates of nestlings (dotted line). Note the diminishing effect of helpers on productivity despite linearly increasing per capita delivery.

marginal (e.g., 2.7 vs. 2.1 prey items hr^{-1}, based on first-year recruits). It is unlikely that opportunities for paternity confound investment by those that are a first-order relative of the breeding male, but unrelated to the breeding female, because such individuals only rarely gain paternity (Browning et al. unpubl. data). Finally, helpers that are first-order relatives of both breeders, or of the male breeder only, have similar levels of responsiveness to increasing brood age (Nomano et al. 2015).

By contrast, only 30% of those nonbreeders that are second-order or lower relatives of the breeders help and, when they do so, they provision at a level three-to-four-fold lower than more closely related helpers. Combining the probability of helping with the observed rate of helping reveals that on average, such distantly related and unrelated helpers contribute 90% less food hr^{-1} than closely-related helpers. It might be that some of these more distantly-related individuals help for kin-selected benefits, but on the whole their contributions are too low to generate benefits to either parents or offspring and they are not responsive to changes in brood demand (Nomano et al. 2015).

Effects of age, sex, and group size

Helper age has a significant effect on provisioning rates, but there is no effect of helper sex or the number of helpers. First, yearling and adult helpers have similar provisioning rules and deliver prey of similar size and type (Browning et al. 2012b); however, after controlling for differences in relatedness, yearlings contribute food about half as frequently as older adults (Browning et al. 2012a; Nomano et al. 2015). Given that yearlings are typically more related to recipients than are older adults, observed age effects suggest that older adults are superior foragers and/or in better condition than yearlings, but we are unable to verify this currently. Second, although females seldom recruit natally, when they do so, they provision nestlings at rates comparable to natal male recruits. Finally, all helpers are unresponsive to variation in helper number, suggesting that nestlings rarely receive as much food as they can consume across most of the range of helper numbers found.

Brief synthesis

Results described thus far are noteworthy for at least two reasons. First, the effect of kinship on provisioning behavior is unusually strong in chestnut-crowned babblers, rivaling patterns found in redirected care systems (e.g., long-tailed tits *Aegithalos caudatus*; Russell and Hatchwell 2001; Chapter 3); western bluebirds (Chapter 2), and white-fronted bee-eaters (*Merops bullockoides*; Emlen 1990). One explanation for this is that significant genetic diversity creates strong selection to help kin and that plural breeding facilitates kin discrimination (Kramer and Russell 2014). Second, the results suggest that nonbreeding group members are selected to contribute to nestling provisioning when their relatedness to the brood at least approximates that of second-order kin. The precise reason for this apparent relatedness threshold is not yet known, but might relate to the mechanism of kin recognition. It is likely that such threshold effects operate in other systems, but are less obvious because singular breeding and low breeder turnover maintains kinship in excess of the threshold, and/or because dispersal offers a viable alternative for those with below-threshold relatedness.

Helper effects

Helper effects can include: (1) complete load-lightening by breeders such that offspring receive the same amount of food irrespective of helper number; (2) incomplete load-lightening by breeders such that broods receive more food in the presence of helpers (i.e., partially additive care); (3) fully additive care, in which breeders (and other helpers) show little or no load-lightening in response to helper provisioning; or (4) super-additive care, in which breeders increase their contributions in the presence of helpers (Hatchwell 1999; Savage et al. 2013). Here I consider helper effects in groups of up to eight helpers, which includes >90% of nests.

Effects on breeder provisioning

With the average number of four nonbreeding helpers, breeding males and females provision broods at an average rate of 3.9 and 1.5 feeds hr^{-1}, respectively, over the 12 hours of daylight and the 23-day nestling period (Browning et al. 2013b). This difference arises because while breeding males maintain their provisioning rates across the range of helper numbers considered, breeding females reduce theirs by about 15% for every additional helper, leading to an 80% reduction in groups of eight helpers versus pairs (Figure 9.4b).

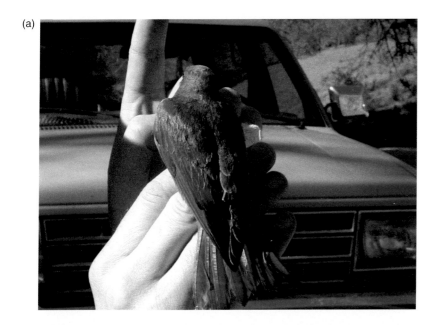

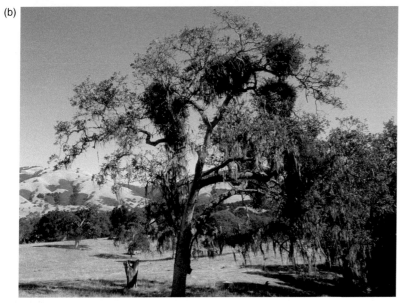

Figure 2.2. Western bluebird male with rufous back patch (left) and blue oak with mistletoe (right).

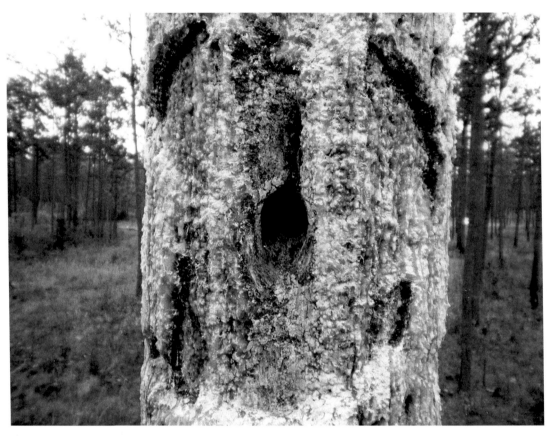

Figure 4.1. A red-cockaded woodpecker cavity, protected by a barrier of pine resin. Photo by Michelle Jusino.

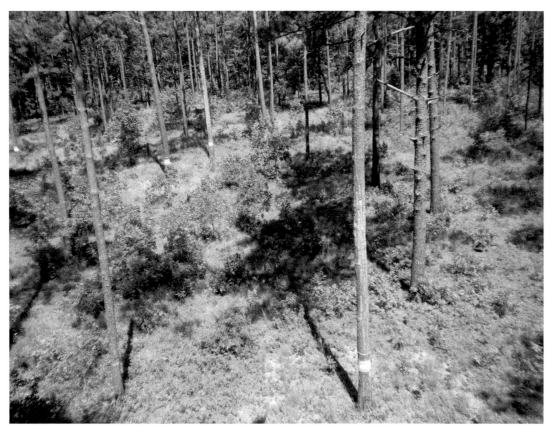

Figure 4.3. Cavity trees of red-cockaded woodpeckers are conspicuous due to the whitish coat of dried resin and the reddish appearance of fresh resin and scaled bark. Photo by Michelle Jusino.

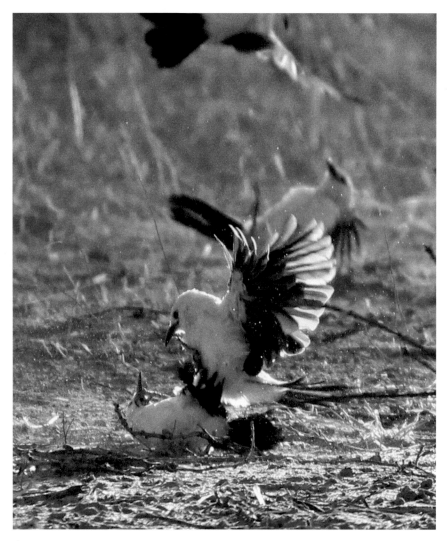

Figure 7.3. Two dominant females from neighboring groups engaged in a physical fight during an intergroup interaction. Although intergroup interactions are common, such physical aggression is relatively rare. Photo by Amanda Ridley.

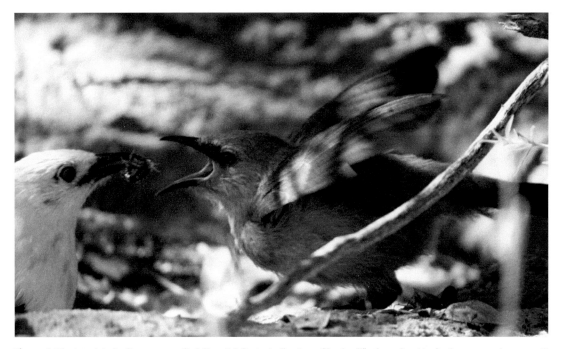

Figure 7.11. An adult feeding a young fledgling. Adults typically give a "food call" when about to feed young, and young will indiscriminately run up and beg from any adult giving this call. Kidnappers use this call and a food "bribe" to get fledglings to follow the kidnapper out of their territory and into the kidnapper's own territory. Photo by Alex Thompson.

(a)

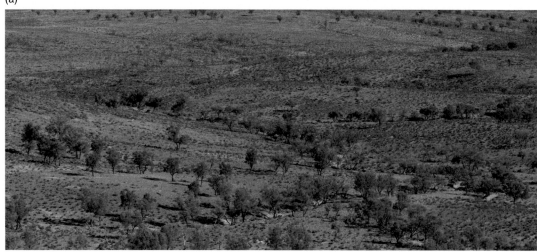

Figure 9.1. (a) Typical open chenopod shrubland habitat at Fowlers Gap; note the scant vegetation is generally limited to short linear stands in drainage lines

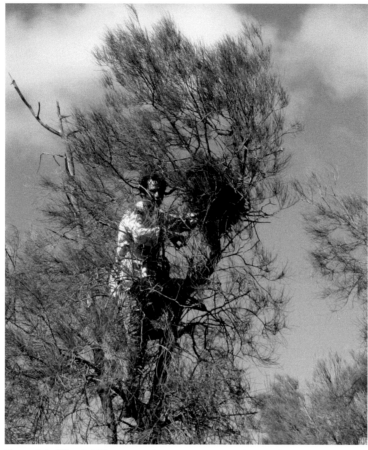

Figure 9.1. (b) A babbler nest in classic position: near the top of a 7 m casuarina. The robust nests are large 30 x 50 cm, single-chambered, and have ~ 6 cm entrance hole.

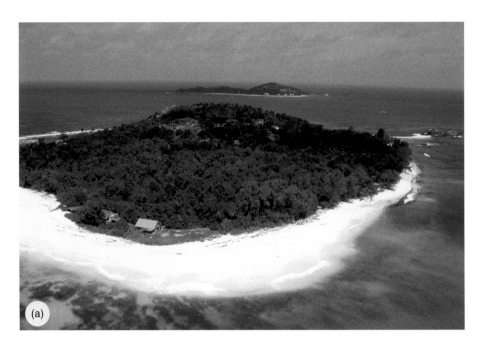

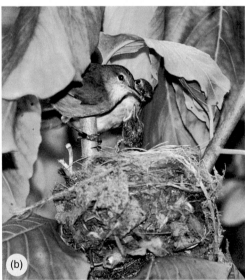

Figure 12.1. (a) Cousin Island, with Cousine Island in the distance. Photograph by David Richardson. (b) Seychelles warblers feeding a nestling. Photograph by Danny Ellinger.

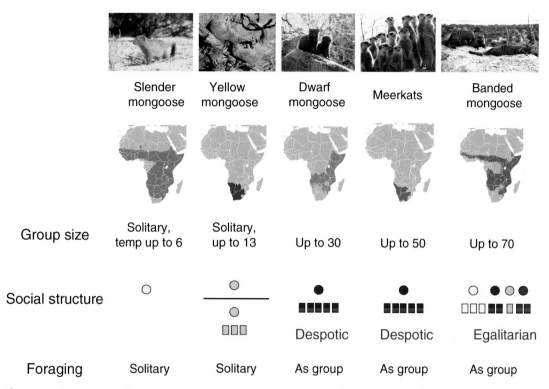

	Slender mongoose	Yellow mongoose	Dwarf mongoose	Meerkats	Banded mongoose
Group size	Solitary, temp up to 6	Solitary, up to 13	Up to 30	Up to 50	Up to 70
Social structure			Despotic	Despotic	Egalitarian
Foraging	Solitary	Solitary	As group	As group	As group

Figure 17.1. Distribution and social structure in five diurnal African mongooses. From Manser et al. (2014).

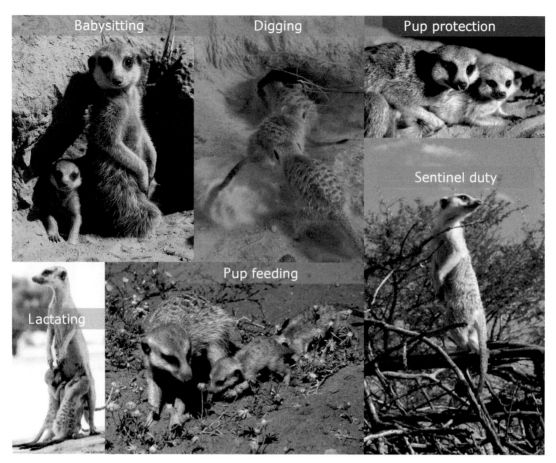

Figure 17.9. All adult helpers contribute to babysitting, pup feeding, burrow renovation, sentinel duty, and the defense of the group's range. Composite photograph by members of the Kalahari Meerkat Project.

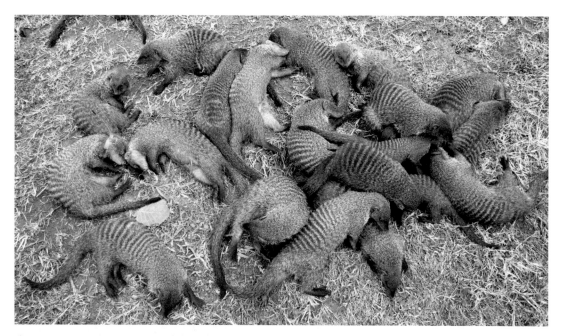

Figure 18.1. A resting group of banded mongooses at our study site in Uganda. Each morning the group leaves the den to forage for 3 or 4 hours before retiring to rest in shade during the hottest part of the day. One individual in each pack wears a radiocollar (note the individual on the far left). Other group members are identified by small fur shavings on the rump. Photo by M. Cant.

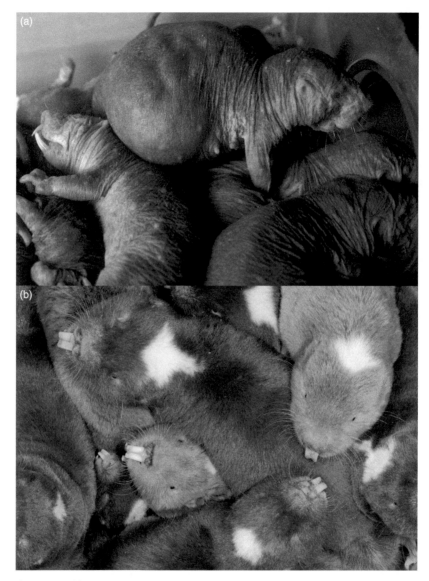

Figure 19.3. (a) Naked mole-rats huddling in a nest chamber. The pregnant queen is on top of the pile of animals, and below her two large animals guard one entrance to the nest. (b) Damaraland mole-rats in a nest chamber. Photographs by C. Faulkes and T. Jackson.

In groups of three, the single helper contributes just under a third of all food, approximately equivalent to that provided by the breeding female. However, in groups of 10, the eight helpers contribute 84% of all the food received by the brood, with the male and female breeder contributing 13% and 3%, respectively. These nestling-feeding patterns generate linear increases in the per capita food received by each nestling; on average, each nestling receives threefold more food in units with eight helpers than in pairs (Figure 9.4c). In other words, because breeding males maintain their provisioning rates across the range of helper numbers and helpers tend to be far more numerous than the single breeding female in each group, her reductions have little impact on the relationship between helper number and total prey delivery. Helper effects on food delivery are largely fully additive, although females do show significant load-lightening, leading to the expectation that helpers will both reduce nestling starvation risk and increase breeding frequency in this system.

Effects on productivity

Helpers have dramatic effects on both within-attempt and within-season productivity. Nestlings have 45% higher survival probability in the presence of eight helpers than in the absence of helpers (Russell et al. 2010), and, following a successful breeding attempt, females without helpers never renest while those with eight helpers do so in 65% of years.

In general, we have found increasing numbers of helpers to be associated with substantial, although strongly diminishing, effects on annual productivity (Browning et al. 2012a). For example, while the presence of two helpers is associated with a 96% increase in seasonal productivity over an absence of helpers, the presence of eight helpers increases productivity by a nonsignificant 1% over the presence of seven (Figure 9.4c). This diminishing productivity–returns relationship, however, ignores any long-term helper effects on offspring success (Hatchwell et al. 2004; Russell et al. 2007), which might help to explain why large groups continue to deliver prey at a high rate.

We tested causality of the overall helper effect on productivity using temporary brood-size manipulation experiments in which natural helper number:brood size ratios were compared with experimentally derived ratios generated by temporarily moving 1–3 offspring between broods (Clutton-Brock et al. 2001; Russell et al. 2008). Effects of experimental changes in helper:brood size ratios on group provisioning rates matched the relationship between natural helper:brood size ratios on productivity, suggesting that helper effects on productivity are causal (Browning et al. 2012a).

Selective mechanisms for nestling provisioning

Five hypotheses have been proposed to account for alloparental investment by nonbreeding helpers. Although kin selection (Hamilton 1964) and group augmentation (Kokko et al. 2001) both predict that helpers have significant effects on some metric of productivity, the former additionally predicts strong kin discrimination where necessary, while the latter predicts discrimination based on group size, because this will impact a helper's current or future survivorship (Kokko et al. 2001) and/or future reproductive success (Kingma et al. 2014).

By contrast, none of the other three hypotheses predicts that helpers influence productivity. Pay-to-stay (Gaston 1978) proposes that group members must provision at a level that offsets the resource-depletion costs of their presence and predicts that distant-kin/nonkin advertise their investment to the dominant member of the philopatric sex to avoid group expulsion (Kokko et al. 2002; Wright 2007). Social prestige is predicated on the idea that by helping, nonbreeding group members advertise their parenting ability, primarily to unrelated opposite-sex breeders, but potentially to same-sex breeders if this improves the probability of their being accepted as cobreeders or co-dispersers (Zahavi 1990). Finally, helping for experience assumes that helpers do not represent a net cost to breeders and predicts that the future breeding success of helpers is greater than for nonhelpers (Komdeur 1996). These latter three hypotheses provide potential candidates for explaining low investment by the unrelated helper category. We have yet to test the experience hypothesis, and do not consider it further, but it offers a possible explanation because breeding tenure lengths are short.

Kin selection versus group augmentation

To test between kin selection and the group augmentation hypotheses, we investigated the roles of kinship versus unit size on which unit in the social group first-year recruits chose to help. Using first-year birds in this analysis avoids confounds associated with prior investment. When asymmetries in kinship arose, decisions of where to help were entirely determined by kinship. In addition, when we compared where yearlings directed care when potential recipient broods were similarly related, helpers neither preferred small units where they could make the greatest impact nor large units where they might gain current survival benefits (Browning et al. 2012a). Presently, therefore, we have no evidence that group augmentation plays a role in governing helping behavior in chestnut-crowned babblers, but significant evidence for a dominant role of kin selection.

Signaling-based hypotheses

Contrary to both signaling hypotheses, we have found no evidence that nonbreeding male helpers attempt to signal their contributions to either of the primary breeders in a given unit (Nomano et al. 2013, 2015). Most compellingly, distantly related male helpers do not attempt to synchronize their nest visits with either the male or female breeders of a unit. In addition, male helpers that are less than first-order kin of both breeders are not responsive to changes in the breeding male's feeding rates, which might be expected if they are selected to increase their visibility to the breeding male. Furthermore, rates of nonfeeding and false-feeding are not influenced by the presence of the breeding female on the nest, and are insufficiently high to change the perception of provisioning rates (Young et al. 2013). Finally, these less-related helpers are not attacked following their temporary removal (Nomano et al. 2015). In short, our available evidence suggests that helping

by those that are unrelated or distantly related to the breeders do not show patterns consistent with signaling, either to influence mating opportunities or to remain as part of the group (facilitating pay-to-stay).

Classic explanations for delayed dispersal

Male chestnut-crowned babblers generally remain philopatric for life, while females seldom delay dispersal from their natal social group, and never do so for more than a year. Understanding the maintenance of cooperative breeding in this system thus requires explaining the pressures selecting for male philopatry. Unfortunately, the relatively invariant sex-specific dispersal patterns observed precludes formal statistical analysis of the various hypotheses posed to explain delayed dispersal. Consequently, I outline the key predictions of the main contender hypotheses and briefly discuss their applicability in accounting for patterns of male philopatry. The conclusions drawn are necessarily speculative, but I believe illuminating, at least in terms of further describing chestnut-crowned babbler socioecology.

Classically, species that show delayed dispersal are suggested to suffer particularly extreme constraints on reproduction mediated through a lack of habitat conducive to successful reproduction and/or a severe lack of mates (Emlen 1982). However, given that non-cooperative species in which offspring refrain from delaying dispersal also face reproductive constraints, additional constraints on floating (Koenig and Pitelka 1981; Koenig et al. 1992) or benefits of remaining at home on certain territories or under certain circumstances are also likely to be required (Stacey and Ligon 1991). None of these hypotheses easily explains universal male philopatry, especially given the highly variable ecology and demography observed over the 11-year study period.

Shortage of territories or mates

In principle, selection on delayed dispersal could operate if territories of suitable quality or mates are lacking in the population.

No lack of territories

Ecological constraints operating through habitat saturation predict dispersal to independent reproductive positions when territories become available (Emlen 1982). Although removal of entire groups has not been conducted to test this hypothesis experimentally, two observations suggest territories are not limiting. First, over the course of the study, the site has gained 11 new social groups in previously unoccupied areas: four arising largely from amalgams of individuals from multiple groups from within the fieldsite and the remaining seven involving groups of unringed individuals often establishing themselves in central locations. Second, in most years a few social groups disperse from the fieldsite and in 2009 we lost 24% of all social groups due to severe drought. These losses were not predicted by group size or prior breeding success. Despite high rainfall in subsequent years (Figure 9.2a), less than a third of these vacant territories have so far been filled. Together, a lack of territories of suitable quality does not appear to constrain dispersal and independent pair-breeding.

Male-biased sex ratios: cause or consequence of delayed dispersal?

The population sex ratio at Fowlers Gap is always male biased, but is never so great that it can explain why all male offspring remain philopatric. For example, in 2007, the population sex ratio was 1.7:1 in favor of males. If delayed dispersal is driven by this bias, all females should have dispersed that year, because they would not lack a mate, and about 40% of males – the proportion expected to gain a mate – should have left their natal group to breed. Neither prediction held: 23% of females and 89–95% of males were delayed dispersers in 2007 (Rollins et al. 2012). Additionally, if the biased sex ratio acted as the sole constraint, we would predict that all females, and an equivalent number of males, would leave their social groups to breed as independent units. In contrast, breeding pairs do not found new social groups. Thus, adult sex-ratio biases alone are unlikely to be an important driver of delayed dispersal independent of some other causal mechanism.

Constraints on floating

Given that breeding habitat appears to be available, it is unlikely that habitat for floaters is constrained. This is especially the case given the large home ranges of social groups and low level of territoriality (Sorato et al. 2015). One possibility, however, is that because chestnut-crowned babblers are obligate nest-roosters, a lack of nests in the environment could act as an impediment to floating, if floating groups of nonrelatives fail to coordinate their construction. However, nests of apparently suitable quality for roosting are incredibly numerous, owing to their common construction and durability, averaging 8 km^{-2} (5–25 per social group). In addition, they are not clumped, but dispersed over several hundred square meters within areas that are (or have been) occupied by babblers. Unsurprisingly, given their abundance and dispersion, they are not defended: social groups and breeding units commonly use the nests built by other groups/units for breeding and roosting. Finally, babblers enter and exit roost nests at dusk and predawn, making it impossible for groups to prevent others from utilizing "their" nests for roosting.

Habitat variance and benefits of philopatry

The variance hypothesis predicts that delayed dispersal is beneficial on high quality territories due to indirect benefits of helping and direct benefits arising via current survival and future reproductive success (Stacey and Ligon 1987; Zack and Stutchbury 1992). In contrast, benefits of philopatry may be important, independently of territory quality, if prolonged nepotism enhances current survival (Ekman et al. 2004). The former is unlikely here because all male offspring delay dispersal irrespective of where they are born. Regarding the latter, chestnut-crowned babblers almost certainly benefit from group living, primarily through reduced predation (Sorato et al. 2012). But as yet we have no evidence to suggest that living with kin is especially important: offspring are fully independent a month postfledging, females typically disperse within their first year, and alarm calls are always uttered upon predator detection and benefit the whole group.

General synthesis: it's a hard life

The key take-home results are that kin selection is the primary route through which helpers accrue fitness and that classic explanations for delayed dispersal do not operate in any obvious fashion. The question, therefore, is: what selects for universal natal philopatry among males in this system? I suggest the answer lies not with enhancements to direct fitness, which are rare, but through the more ubiquitous kin-selected benefits accrued from helping. For example, of those males surviving their first year, 52% will survive into their second when reproduction becomes feasible but only 21% will gain direct fitness in their lifetime. In other words, for the vast majority of individuals, kin-selected benefits represent the only fitness they will ever get and delaying dispersal is integral to the acquisition of such benefits. Thus, for chestnut-crowned babblers, I hypothesize that ecological adversity and uncertainly combine to make "life hard," and that kin-selected benefits of helping currently drives delayed dispersal and the maintenance of kinship ties.

The idea that challenging environmental conditions, cooperative benefits and delayed dispersal could be associated has been offered previously (Emlen 1982, 1990; Dickinson and Hatchwell 2004; Koenig et al. 2011; Rubenstein 2011). For example, Emlen (1982, 1990) proposed that years of poor prey availability could select for breeding restraint, delayed dispersal, and kin-selected cooperative breeding in the same way that a lack of territories could. As such, this "hard life" hypothesis has been viewed simply an extension of the basic ecological constraints hypothesis based on habitat characteristics (Emlen 1990; Koenig et al. 2011). By contrast, I suggest that the habitat-mediated and hard life models are distinct, because in the former, delayed dispersal precedes cooperative breeding, while in the latter it is the (kin-selected) benefits of cooperation that drives selection on delayed dispersal and/or kin recognition. In other words, under a hard life, the two-step process envisaged by the classical form of ecological constraints appears to run in reverse.

A "hard life" will often be evolutionarily derived; as such, it is likely to be most operant in more obligate cooperative breeders for which breeding independently is generally unfeasible and the kin-selected benefits of helping are pervasive. However, the hard life hypothesis might also explain the maintenance of kinship ties in a number of facultative cooperative breeders. For example, long-tailed tit flocks are kin structured during the winter (Chapter 3), but this does not appear to stem from particular constraints on dispersal or benefits of philopatry per se (Russell 1999). Like chestnut-crowned babblers, the majority of long-tailed tit recruits die with indirect fitness only (Hatchwell et al. 2014). Although the reason for the low probability of gaining direct fitness benefits in this case stems from extreme nest predation and a temporally constrained breeding season, it might be that it is the kin-selected benefits of cooperation that drive the maintenance of kin ties (i.e., delayed dispersal) in this system. Similar arguments could be invoked in colonial cooperative breeders, such as white-fronted bee-eaters or sociable weavers (*Philetairus socius*), where again offspring need not disperse to breed, and selective pressures on maintaining kin ties independently of kin-selected benefits of cooperation are not obvious. Perhaps paradoxically, therefore, the hard life hypothesis might similarly pertain to the (near) obligate cooperative breeders as well as the redirected care systems and colonial species.

The relative importance of habitat versus environmentally mediated selection pressures on cooperative breeding is expected to be related to at least two features. First, I expect hard-lifers to be weakly territorial because habitat is not at a premium. Second, I predict that for those in the habitat-mediated camp, inclusive fitness will be primarily composed of direct fitness, but for the hard-lifers indirect fitness benefits will comprise the majority of inclusive fitness for most individuals. Consequently, helper effects on productivity should be relatively weak when habitat-mediated selection pressures are operating on delayed dispersal, but be strong and particularly kin-selected when environmental factors are in force. If upheld, this hypothesis would have significant ramifications for comparative analyses investigating ecological associates of cooperative breeding, because it means that "classic" species in which delayed dispersal leads to cooperative breeding should not be combined with those in which the reverse is true.

Acknowledgments

This study would have been utterly fruitless if it were not for the help of many. Fieldwork has been made possible through the logistical support of Simon Griffith, David Croft, Keith Leggett, the Dowling family, and Zane Turner. Molecular work has been conducted by Simon Griffith, Lee Ann Rollins, Clare Holleley, and Fumi Nomano. For help in the field, I am particularly indebted to my former students: Lucy Browning, Jodie Crane, Fumi Nomano, Dean Portelli; James Savage, Enrico Sorato, Cat Young; and to under-paid and/ or over-worked postdocs: Elena Berg, Maggie Hall, Andrea Liebl, Sam Patrick, Stuart Sharp, Iain Stewart, and Beth Woodward. Funding has been provided by grants from the Australian Research Council, Natural Environment Research Council, and the Royal Society University Research Fellowship scheme. The message of the chapter was greatly clarified by the helpful and very patient Walt and Janis.

REFERENCES

Browning, L. E., Patrick, S. C., Rollins, L. A., Griffith, S. C., and Russell, A. F. (2012a). Kin selection, not group augmentation, predicts helping in an obligate cooperatively breeding bird. *Proc. R. Soc. London B*, 279, 3861–3869.

Browning, L. E., Young, C. M., Savage, J. L., Russell, D. J. F., Barclay, H., et al. (2012b). Carer provisioning rules in an obligate cooperative breeder: prey type, size and delivery rate. *Behav. Ecol. Sociobiol.*, 66, 1639–1649.

Clutton-Brock, T.H., Russell, A.F., Sharpe, L.L., Brotherton, P.N., McIlrath, G.M., et al. (2001). Effects of helpers on juvenile development and survival in meerkats. *Science*, 293, 2446–2449.

Cockburn, A. (2003). Cooperative breeding in oscine passerines: does sociality inhibit speciation? *Proc. R. Soc. London B*, 270, 2207–2214.

Cockburn, A. and Russell, A. F. (2011). Cooperative breeding: a question of climate? *Curr. Biol.* 21, R195–197.

Dickinson, J. L. and Hatchwell, B. J. (2004). Fitness consequences of helping. In: *Ecology and Evolution of Cooperative Breeding in Birds*, ed. W. D. Koenig and J. L. Dickinson. Cambridge: Cambridge University Press, pp. 48–66.

Ekman, J., Dickinson, J. L., Hatchwell, B. J., and Griesser, M. (2004). In: *Ecology and Evolution of Cooperative Breeding in Birds*, ed. W. D. Koenig and J. L. Dickinson. Cambridge: Cambridge University Press, pp. 35–47.

Emlen, S. T. (1982). The evolution of helping. I. An ecological constraints model. *Am. Nat.* 119, 29–39.

Emlen, S. T. (1990). White-fronted bee-eaters: helping in a colonially nesting species. In: *Cooperative Breeding in Birds: Long-term Studies of Ecology and Behavior*, ed. P. B. Stacey and W. D. Koenig. Cambridge: Cambridge University Press, pp. 487–526.

Gaston, A. J. (1978). Evolution of group territorial behavior and cooperative breeding. *Am. Nat.*, 112, 1091–1100.

Hamilton, W. D. (1964). The genetical evolution of social behaviour. *J. Theor. Biol.* 7, 1–52.

Hatchwell, B. J. (1999). Investment strategies of breeders in avian cooperative breeding systems. *Am. Nat.*, 154, 205–219.

Hatchwell, B. J., Russell, A. F., MacColl, A. D. C., Ross, D. J., Fowlie, M. K., et al. (2004). Helpers increase long-term but not short-term productivity in cooperatively breeding long-tailed tits. *Behav. Ecol.*, 15, 1–10.

Hatchwell, B. J., Gullett, P. R., and Adams, M. J. (2014). Helping in cooperatively breeding long-tailed tits: a test of Hamilton's rule. *Phil. Trans. R. Soc. London B*, 369, 20130565.

Higgins, P. J. and Peter, J. M., eds. (2002). Pardalotes to thrushes. In: *Handbook of Australian, New Zealand and Antarctic birds*. Oxford: Oxford University Press, pp. 905–911.

Jetz, W., Thomas, G. H., Joy, J. B., Harmann, K., and Mooers, A. O. (2012). The global diversity of birds in space and time. *Nature*, 491, 444–448.

Kingma, S. A., Santema, P., Taborsky, M., and Komdeur, J. (2014). Group augmentation and the evolution of cooperation. *Trends Ecol. Evol.*, 29, 476–484.

Koenig, W. D. and Pitelka, F. A. (1981). Ecological factors and kin selection in the evolution of cooperative breeding in birds. In: *Natural Selection and Social Behavior: Recent Research and New Theory*, ed. R. D. Alexander and D. W. Tinkle. New York: Chiron, pp. 261–280.

Koenig, W. D., Pitelka, F. A., Carmen, W. J., Mumme, R. L., and Stanback, M. T. (1992). The evolution of delayed dispersal in cooperative breeders. *Q. Rev. Biol.*, 67, 111–150.

Koenig, W. D., Walters, E. L., and Haydock, J. (2011). Variable helpers effects, ecological conditions, and the evolution of cooperative breeding in the acorn woodpecker. *Am. Nat.*, 178, 145–158.

Kokko, H., Johnstone, R. A., and Clutton-Brock, T. H. (2001). The evolution of cooperative breeding through group augmentation. *Proc. R. Soc. London B*, 268, 187–196.

Kokko, H., Johnstone, R. A., and Wright, J. (2002). The evolution of parental and alloparental effort in cooperatively breeding groups: when should helpers pay to stay? *Behav. Ecol.*, 13, 291–300.

Komdeur, J. (1996). Influence of helping and breeding experience on reproductive performance in the Seychelles warbler: a translocation experiment. *Behav. Ecol.*, 7, 326–333.

Kramer, K. L. and A. F. Russell. (2014). Kin-selected cooperation without lifetime monogamy: human insights and animal implications. *Trends Ecol. Evol.*, 29, 600–606.

Nomano, F. Y., Browning, L. E., Rollins, L. A., Nakagawa, S., Griffith, S. C., and Russell, A. F. (2013). Feeding nestlings does not function as a signal of social prestige in cooperatively breeding chestnut-crowned babblers. *Anim. Behav.*, 86, 277–289.

Nomano, F. Y., Browning, L. E., Nakagawa, S., Griffith, S. C., and Russell, A. F. (2014). Validation of an automated data collection method for quantifying social networks in collective behaviours. *Behav. Ecol. Sociobiol.*, 68, 1379–1391.

Nomano, F. Y., Browning, L. E., Savage, J. L., Rollins, L. A., Griffith, S. C., et al. (2015). Unrelated helpers neither signal contributions nor suffer retribution in chestnut-crowed babblers. *Behav. Ecol.*, 26, 986–995.

Portelli, D. J., Barclay, H., Russell, D. J. F., Griffith, S.C., and Russell, A.F. (2009). Social organisation and foraging ecology of the cooperatively breeding chestnut-crowned Babbler (*Pomatostomus ruficeps*). *Emu*, 109, 153–162.

Rollins, L. A., Browning, L. E., Holleley, C. E., Savage, J. L., Russell, A. F., et al. (2012). Building genetic networks using relatedness information: a novel approach for the estimation of dispersal and characterization of group structure in social animals. *Mol. Ecol.*, 21, 1727–1740.

Rubenstein, D. R. (2011). Spatiotemporal environmental variation, risk aversion and the evolution of cooperative breeding in birds. *Proc. Natl. Acad. Sci. (USA)*, 108, 10816–10822.

Russell, A. F. (1999). Ecological constraints and the cooperative breeding system of the long-tailed tit *Aegithalos caudatus*. Ph.D. thesis, University of Sheffield, U.K.

Russell, A. F. and Hatchwell, B. J. (2001). Experimental evidence for kin-biased helping in a cooperatively breeding vertebrate. *Proc. R. Soc. London B*, 268, 2169–2174.

Russell, A. F., Young, A. J., Spong, G., Jordan, N. R., and Clutton-Brock, T. H. (2007). Helpers increase the reproductive potential of offspring in cooperative meerkats. *Proc. R. Soc. London B*, 274, 513–520.

Russell, A. F., Langmore, N. E., Gardner, J. L., and Kilner, R.M. (2008). Maternal investment tactics in superb fairy-wrens. *Proc. R. Soc. London B*, 275, 29–36.

Russell, A. F., Portelli, D. J., Russell, D. J. F., and Barclay, H. (2010). Breeding ecology of the chestnut-crowned babbler: a cooperative breeder in the desert. *Emu*, 110, 324–331.

Savage, J. L., Russell, A. F., and Johnstone, R. A. (2013). Maternal costs in offspring production affect investment rules in joint rearing. *Behav. Ecol.*, 24, 750–758.

Smith, J. (1992). Cooperative breeding in the chestnut-crowned babbler *Pomatostomus ruficeps*. *Australian Birds*, 25, 64–66.

Sorato, E., Gullett, P.R., Griffith, S.C., and Russell, A.F. (2012). Effects of predation risk on foraging behaviour and group size: adaptations in a social cooperative species. *Anim. Behav.*, 84, 823–834.

Sorato, E., Gullett, P. R., Creasey, M. J. S., Griffith, S. C., and Russell, A. F. (2015). Plastic territoriality in group-living chestnut-crowned babblers: roles of resource value, holding potential and predation risk. *Anim. Behav.*, 101, 155–168.

Stacey, P. B. and Ligon, J. D. (1987). Territory quality and dispersal options in the acorn woodpecker, and a challenge to the habitat-saturation model of cooperative breeding. *Am. Nat.* 130, 654–676.

Stacey, P. B. and Ligon, J. D. (1991). The benefits-of-philopatry hypothesis for the evolution of cooperative breeding: variation in territory quality and group size effects. *Am. Nat.*, 137, 831–846.

Wright, J. (2007). Cooperation theory meets cooperative breeding: exposing some ugly truths about social prestige, reciprocity and group augmentation. *Behav. Proc.*, 76, 142–148.

Young, C. M., Browning, L. E., Savage, J. L., Griffith, S. C., and Russell, A.F. (2013). No evidence for deception over allocation to brood care in a cooperative bird. *Behav. Ecol.*, 24, 70–81.

Zack, S. and Stutchbury, B. J. (1992). Delayed breeding in avian social systems: the role of territory quality and "floater" tactics. *Behav.*, 123, 194–219.

Zahavi, A. (1990). Arabian babblers: The quest for social status in a cooperative breeder. In: *Cooperative Breeding in Birds: Long-term Studies of Ecology and Behavior*, ed. P. B. Stacey and W. D. Koenig. Cambridge: Cambridge University Press, pp. 103–130.

10

Bell miners: Kin-selected helping decisions

Jonathan Wright and Paul G. McDonald

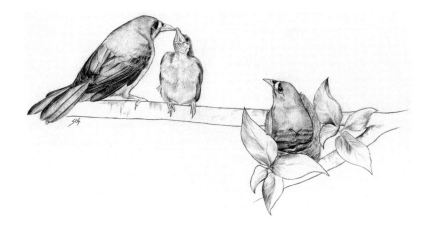

Introduction

Bell miners (*Manorina melanophrys*) inhabit eucalypt woodlands in southeastern Australia. Living exclusively in large colonies that often comprise hundreds of individuals, they actively exclude other insectivorous and nectarivorous bird species from the entire colony area. Colonies contain from one to a number of social units called "coteries," each consisting of several breeding pairs and an attending assemblage of non-breeding helpers (Clarke 1989). Breeding female bell miners aggressively defend small territories from each other, whereas breeding males and helpers are free to move throughout the coterie to forage or help, and throughout the wider colony when defending it from heterospecifics and potential predators (Clarke and Fitz-Gerald 1994). Most helpers are male, and they help while waiting in their natal coterie for a possible breeding vacancy, which it appears the majority of males eventually obtain (94% of 16 male fledglings, Clarke and Fitz-Gerald 1994). In contrast, a lower proportion of helpers are female and this is because most disperse toward the end of their first year to seek breeding positions outside their natal colony, and hence very few females remain as breeders within their natal colony.

The significance of bell miners to our understanding of cooperative breeding is based on this habit of living in large colonies, the complex structure that exists within these colonies, and the large numbers of helpers of both sexes that provision each brood (mean ± standard error

Cooperative Breeding in Vertebrates: Studies of Ecology, Evolution, and Behavior, eds W. D. Koenig and J. L. Dickinson.
Published by Cambridge University Press. © Cambridge University Press 2016.

[S.E.] = 10.7 ± 0.7 helpers per nest; N=23 nests). This complexity is further augmented by observations that helpers and breeding males sometimes help at more than one nest simultaneously, which means that breeding males sometimes also help at nests other than their own. While helpers are often related to the breeding pair that they assist, the near annual turnover of female breeders (Clarke 1989) means that as helpers age they are less related to the broods they aid (Conrad et al. 1998; Painter et al. 2000). The colonial lifestyle of bell miners and their tendency to live in large and socially complex groups makes them an important test case for the evolution of helping behavior. Furthermore, their sex-biased dispersal and the fact that both sexes help at multiple nests of widely varying relatedness provide an unusual opportunity to examine adaptive explanations for within- and between-individual variation in helping behavior.

Our study was conducted between June 2004 and December 2006 on two bell miner colonies located northeast of Melbourne, Australia. The first consisted of only one or two coteries in a colony of 40–45 adult birds at the La Trobe University Wildlife Reserve, Victoria, whereas the second colony involved 120–135 adults and multiple coteries and was situated near Saint Andrews, Victoria (McDonald et al. 2008b). Our results therefore include a total of around 400 individuals and detailed observations of 35 nests. Methods included banding, detailed nest watches, genetic sampling of individuals for genetic relationships, and various experimental playbacks.

A major initial goal of this study was to test two specific hypotheses for potential direct fitness benefits gained by helpers, namely social prestige (Zahavi 1977, 1995; Wright 1999a, 2007) and pay-to-stay (Gaston 1978; Kokko et al. 2002). Under these two hypotheses, helping is seen as either an honest indicator of quality to gain social prestige within the group, or as a way of helpers making themselves useful to dominants and paying "rent" to be allowed to stay within the group. Increased social prestige is suggested to enhance an individual's chances of future breeding or other collaborative opportunities. In contrast, pay-to-stay appeases aggression by dominant group members, making it possible to secure group membership and its associated benefits.

These hypotheses can be thought of as representing two ends of a possible theoretical continuum that includes any number of intermediate possibilities, such as gaining sufficient social prestige to facilitate membership of a cooperative group, or making oneself sufficiently useful in rent payment so as to justify access to mating opportunities, and so on. Despite this lack of theoretical development, social prestige and pay-to-stay are frequently referred to in the cooperative breeding literature as potential explanations for the evolution of helping behavior, although they have rarely been tested in any detail (for exceptions, see Reyer 1990; Mulder and Langmore 1993; Wright 1997, 1998).

Our approach was to concentrate on testing the signaling mechanisms behind these two hypotheses (Wright 1997), because for either social prestige or pay-to-stay to be operating then information concerning helper effort must be signaled between helpers and other group members. This allowed us to focus on the possible existence of behavioral adaptations for the transmission of reliable, or even functionally deceptive, information concerning individual levels of helping, rather than attempting to quantify the more difficult to measure long-term future fitness benefits (Wright 2007). Note that under any signaling hypothesis, helpers gain social benefits by being *perceived* to help irrespective of any actual positive effect their help may or may not have on nestling fitness. We therefore compared all aspects of helping with parental behaviors to see if activities performed by helpers differed in any way from straightforward investment in care according to brood need, and whether provisioning behavior by helpers had similarly positive effects on nestling growth.

Given the speculative nature of such signaling explanations for helping, we also collected data relevant to more traditional investment explanations (Wright 1997). These include indirect fitness benefits from helping genetic relatives (Hamilton 1964) and direct fitness benefits of enhanced future survival or reproduction from group augmentation (Kokko et al. 2001; Clutton-Brock 2002; Wright 2007), because under both these hypotheses helping effort is an adaptive investment aimed at improving helper fitness by enhancing nestling fitness. The bell miner system provides an excellent empirical test of kin selection because it allows assessments of the effects of both kin discrimination and population viscosity (Cornwallis et al. 2009). Bell miners also provide a unique test of the sex differences in helping predicted by group augmentation. Because of the extreme sex-biased dispersal in this system, only male helpers can benefit from augmented group sizes since they are the sex that stays in the group, and only if they help male nestlings that will also be the only offspring to stay and enlarge the group (McDonald et al. 2010; Wright et al. 2010).

Thus, despite the relatively short length of our study, we have been able to critically test predictions for the patterns of behavior and the proximate mechanisms behind almost all current adaptive explanations for helping at the nest by collecting detailed behavioral data on the unusually complex social system of this species. Our work also provides important insights into how to interpret data concerning genetic relatedness when assessing the importance of kin selection to the evolution of helping behavior.

Why helping could be a signal in bell miners, but probably is not

At the beginning of the study there were indications that helping behavior in bell miners might function as a signal. Nests are attended by what appears to be far too many helpers given the modal brood size of two (62 of 78 hatched broods during our study; McDonald et al. 2010), and as a result nestlings seem to beg at relatively low levels and often appear satiated (Clarke 1984). All of this could reflect adaptations to the high risks of nest predation, which is one of the major causes of offspring mortality in bell miners despite their small and relatively cryptic nests. It is also what might be expected if helping evolved as an exaggerated sexual signal for use in a competitive display of individual abilities, as opposed to the collective provisioning by groups of helpers for the sole purpose of offspring nutrition (McDonald et al. 2008a).

There was also circumstantial evidence that groups of male helpers might constitute a lek or breeding queue at each nest to determine the next partner of

the breeding female. Clarke (1989) documented five instances in which breeding males died or disappeared, and on each occasion the widowed female subsequently paired with the unrelated male helper that had provided the greatest assistance in raising her previous brood. The experimental removal of a number of breeding males confirmed this pattern of potential mate choice by widowed females (Jones 1998). While this might simply reflect some age- or quality-related covariance between a male's helping effort and his position in the breeding cue, it could indicate that nonkin male helpers were "showing off" to breeding females in order to enhance their social prestige and chances of future breeding opportunities. The relatively small activity space (~25 m; Clarke and Fitz-Gerald 1994) of breeding females means that this is possible, since the potential audience of the helping signal is always within monitoring distance of the nest. This is particularly important because in most species of cooperative breeding birds the much larger activity space of most birds means that specific individuals are unable to monitor nests to this extent, and hence most helping behavior goes unobserved by those individuals in the group that might potentially make adaptive use of any variation in helping as a signal (Wright 1997, 1999a).

Moreover, adult bell miners produce individually distinctive *mew* calls, not only as they approach to feed nestlings, but also more than half the time as they leave the nest area after a provisioning visit (McDonald et al. 2007a; McDonald and Wright 2008, 2011). This behavior initially appeared encouragingly consistent with a signaling system of helping, particularly as congeners have since been shown to be able to differentiate even unfamiliar individuals based on their calls (McDonald 2012). *Mew* calls therefore offer a means by which key group members, such as breeding females, could keep track of individual helpers' nest visitation rates, even from a distance and in the thick vegetation that often surrounds nests.

There were also reports of "false-feeding" in which helpers arrive without prey or consume the prey themselves instead of feeding it to the nestlings (Clarke 1984) and other potentially deceptive provisioning behaviors such as immature helpers arriving at the nest empty-handed and being subjected to pecking from older individuals (Poiani 1993). We now believe that such reports may reflect unnoticed effects on the birds of observer disturbance at these nests – a potentially serious problem that is rarely recognized or tested for in studies of cooperative breeders, but a confounding effect that we could exclude in the case of our results presented below (Wright, 1997, 1999a; McDonald et al., 2007b). At the beginning of our study, however, such previous observation appeared indicative of helping as a signal in a pay-to-stay or social prestige context (Wright 1997; Boland et al. 1997).

In terms of possible false feeds, McDonald et al. (2007b) examined 7,500 nestling provisioning events and found that only 8.5% were in any way unusual. In 3.7% of these events, food items were not fed to nestlings and were instead eaten by the provisioning individual, either at the nest or elsewhere subsequent to the visit. This could have been indicative of helping being deceptive in these cases, but was better explained by brood begging being unexpectedly low during these visits compared to when the same individual was previously at the nest. Thus, this phenomenon appears to represent a readjustment in the allocation of food between the adult and the nestlings based on updated information concerning their relative nutritional needs.

A further 1.7% of provisioning events included multiple entries of the food item(s) in and out of the nestling's bill, possibly representing an exaggerated behavior designed to amplify the provisioning signal. Instead, these turned out to be caused by sticky food items (i.e., lerp – a sugary secretion of sap sucking Hemiptera) creating transfer errors between the adult bill and the nestling's gape (McDonald et al. 2007b), an effect also observed in the delivery of large and awkward-shaped food items in Arabian babblers *Turdoides squamiceps* (Wright 1997). The remaining 3.1% of unusual provisioning events involved arrivals without food, but instead of being deceptive, they appeared to be primarily inspection visits by neighboring female breeders checking up on the state of the nest.

In addition, none of these patterns of unusual provisioning behavior differed according to the identity of the potential signaler, or of the audience. For example, male helpers that were less related to the nestlings were no more or less likely to be involved in unusual

provisioning events when in the presence of the breeding female at the nest (McDonald et al. 2007b). We therefore conclude that everything we observed in this context equates to normal patterns in avian provisioning rather than supporting the existence of false-feeds under a social prestige or pay-to-stay signaling scenario. Similar results have been found in other systems whenever detailed data have been collected appropriately (Wright 1997; Canestrari et al. 2004; Clutton-Brock et al. 2005). Thus, we believe that little credence can be given to anecdotal reports in the literature of what are often unhelpfully termed "false-feeds" or "deceptive" provisioning. Many of the unusual behaviors and social interactions observed at nests in cooperative breeders are probably part of normal provisioning behavior, and where they are not they are potentially the result of subtle confounding disturbance effects caused by observers or their equipment (Wright 1999a; McDonald et al. 2007b).

We also found little evidence of any of the other types of social interactions around the nest predicted by the hypothesis that helping operates as a signal in bell miners. Specifically, we observed almost no aggressive interactions and there was no evidence of audience effects on helping behaviors (McDonald et al. 2008a). That is, helpers behaved similarly at the nest whether or not they were in the presence of another group member, and there were no effects of helper or audience sex, relatedness, or social status on provisioning behavior. Less-related male helpers did not alter their behavior to coincide with breeding females at the nest, and there was no evidence for the monitoring of unrelated male helpers by breeding females. There was also no effect of the temporary experimental removal of breeding males or females, or of playbacks of their identifying *mew* calls, on individual helping effort or any helper behaviors, and no evidence of any change in aggression toward helpers by removed breeders upon their return (McDonald et al. 2008b). In summary, we could find almost nothing to suggest that helpers were signaling or exhibiting any behaviors around nests that were not linked to simply provisioning the brood.

In fact, after more than 30 years and numerous studies on cooperatively breeding birds, little convincing evidence has emerged for any signaling explanation of the evolution of helping. The only exceptions are certain findings consistent with pay-to-stay from an observational study of different breeding colonies of pied kingfishers *Ceryle rudis* (Reyer 1990) and an experimental removal study on superb fairy-wrens (*Malurus cyaneus*; Mulder and Langmore 1993). Unfortunately, neither of these examples involved the kind of follow-up studies needed to properly confirm (or reject) pay-to-stay, such as evidence for expulsion from the group by dominants of helpers that appeared unwilling to help (Chapter 16). Therefore, unless more convincing evidence comes to light, it seems best to reject such signaling hypotheses as explanations for the evolution of helping behavior in the vast majority of cooperatively breeding bird systems.

We did detect one subtle and rarely reported aspect of provisioning behavior in the bell miner, which was that helpers of both sexes produced more *mew* calls during visits when they coincided at the nest with another helper or the breeding male than when they coincided with the breeding female (McDonald et al. 2008a). This observation can be explained as part of a second finding that helpers and breeding males (but not breeding females) sometimes arrived at the nest at the same time, suggesting that these classes of individuals were to some extent coordinating their provisioning behavior in time. Having found no evidence that this is part of a signaling explanation for helping, we explored other functional reasons for this apparent coordination, hypothesizing that there could be a temporal trade-off between provisioning effort and alternative cooperative activities that only these classes of birds engage in together, such as mobbing predators or chasing away heterospecific competitors from the colony. Such activities would force provisioning into smaller time slots, which would need to be coordinated via mechanisms like the *mew* call vocalizations.

Such coordination in the timing of different behaviors by groups of helpers and breeding males provisioning at the same nest(s) within a coterie could also explain a surprising result obtained during experimental playbacks of begging calls targeted either at the breeding male or a less-related male helper (McDonald et al. 2009). As expected, these begging playbacks caused the targeted individuals to increase their provisioning rates, but they also resulted in increases in provisioning effort by non-targeted helpers and breeding males. This response was not present in the provisioning effort of nontargeted breeding females, which instead decreased their nest visits exactly as might be predicted from the normal situation of uncoordinated cooperative provisioning (Wright and Dingemanse 1999). Hence, only when individuals are apparently cooperating together in activities away from the nest did we see positive responses to experimentally induced increases in collaborator provisioning rates.

These types of differences in behavioral coordination might help explain the variable responses to partner work rates seen across different biparental avian systems. These mostly show the negative compensation reactions to changes in partner work rates that are indicative of uncoordinated pair behavior away from the nest (Harrison et al. 2009). However, the singular biparental example of positive provisioning responses to increases in partner work rates following targeted begging playbacks in great tits *Parus major* (Hinde 2006) mirrors the responses of helpers and breeding males (but not breeding females) that we recorded in bell miners. Our work therefore suggests that this unusual finding in great tits might be explained by coordinated foraging and/or anti-predator behaviors within pairs rather than any use of partner behavior to provide information concerning brood need (*sensu* Johnstone and Hinde 2006).

Helpers help in exactly the same way as do parents

In order to be confident that helping behavior in bell miners does not function as a signal, we compared various aspects of provisioning by helpers with those of parents. Pairs in this species are socially and genetically monogamous, with no divorce or re-pairing prior to the death or disappearance of one of the partners (Clarke 1989). Parental care should therefore have evolved for no other purpose than to promote the fitness of offspring (Wright 1999a). Parental behavior thus provides the ideal benchmark for what helping as an *investment*, rather than as a signal, should look like.

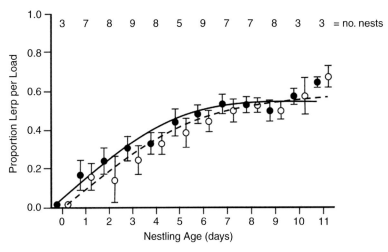

Figure 10.1. The mean (± S.E.) proportion of lerp (a sugary secretion of sapsucking Hemiptera) compared to arthropod prey per load delivered by helpers of different ages after hatching (day 0 to fledging). Helpers are represented by filled circles and the solid line; parents by open circles and the dashed line. The number of nests sampled in each age category is shown at the top. The nonlinear increases in lerp delivery with nestling age did not differ according to helper sex or relatedness, nor between helpers and parents of either sex. Data from te Marvelde et al. (2009).

Bell miners feed nestlings arthropod prey and sugary lerp caps removed from psyllids in roughly equal proportions. Indeed, bell miners have been implicated as a driver of declining forest health as a result of such species-specific foraging behavior that likely promotes or even "farms" parasitic populations of sap sucking psyllids (Haythorpe and McDonald 2010). Perhaps due in part to their aggressive exclusion of other birds from the colony's home range, this apparently leads to much higher densities of psyllids than one would otherwise expect. This high abundance of lerp provides an especially cheap and easily collected food source for bell miners. Foraging experiments have identified that bell miners use their tongue to lick the sugar-rich covering of these psyllids, and more often than other insectivorous birds leave the psyllid intact underneath (Haythorpe and McDonald 2010). Lerp may thus offer opportunities for helpers to cheat by showing off their provisioning at relatively low cost, while providing limited nutritional benefit to the nestlings given that lerp is a carbohydrate-rich diet containing little protein.

Contrary to this hypothesis, the proportion of lerp per provisioning load increases nonlinearly with nestling age in the same way for all sex and relatedness classes of helpers and parents (Figure 10.1). This age effect probably reflects the fact that older nestlings are better able to digest simple sugars, or possibly that lerp with its low water content makes an effective nestling food type (compared to nectar, for example) when nestlings are older and need more energy for growth (te Marvelde et al. 2009). Either way, the types of food delivered appear identical between helpers and the parents at those same nests.

In addition, the biomass of arthropods versus lerp delivered had equally positive effects on nestling growth (Figure 10.2), indicating that the nutritional benefits of lerp and anthropod prey are similar and that both represent similar investment benefits in terms of future offspring fitness (te Marvelde et al. 2009). Although individual parents deliver much larger amounts of food of all types than do individual helpers, the collective efforts of helpers account for more than 60% of the food consumed by nestlings. These findings provide further support for the idea that bell miner helpers really do help in delivering fitness-enhancing nutrients as an investment, rather

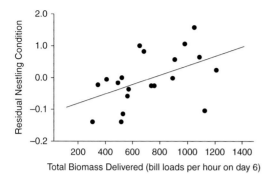

Figure 10.2. The effect of total biomass of food delivered per hour to 6-day-old nestlings on mean residual nestling body condition (mass/head-bill length, controlling for nestling age). The slope of the positive linear relationship shown here, and a similar slope calculated over the full 10 days of the nestling period, did not differ when calculated for the total biomass of lerp versus the total biomass arthropod prey delivered. From te Marvelde et al. (2009).

than merely trying to be seen to help without actually providing much benefit.

Bell miner nestlings are sometimes infested by the larvae of the parasitic fly *Passeromyia indecora*, which reduces nestling growth and can be fatal (Poiani 1993). Observational and experimental evidence from our study indicates that helpers and breeding males perform similar levels of nest inspection and nestling preening in order to detect and remove these parasites, with breeding females doing more than any other group member, perhaps due to their constant proximity to the nest (Pacheco et al. 2008). Helper sex and relatedness have no obvious effects on individual levels of this antiparasitic behavior, and there were no audience effects on helper effort, including no responses to the temporary removal of breeding males and females. Thus, as with other forms of helping effort, this unusual form of helping appears similar to parental behavior in being an investment in nestling welfare and fitness by helpers.

As mentioned earlier, experimental playbacks of nestling begging caused similar increases in nest visit rates by breeding males and less-related male helpers (McDonald et al. 2009). This is a clear indication of helping as investment, and mirrors the results found

in other cooperative breeders (Wright 1998) as well as biparental care systems (Wright and Leonard 2002; Royle et al. 2012). In the bell miners, the brood begging experienced during the most recent visit to the nest determines how quickly individuals return to provision the brood next time and the size of the load delivered (Figure 10.3). The scale of these provisioning responses did not differ according to the sex or relatedness of helpers, nor between helpers and parents of either sex (Wright et al. 2010). Such a match in individual responsiveness to the same begging cues by all cooperative group members has been noted previously (Wright 1998), and may be adaptive in integrating group-wide adjustment to changes in brood need in order to ensure stable overall levels of food delivery to the nest. However, this suggestion remains to be confirmed by models assessing both the behavioral and evolutionary dynamics of such cooperative strategies (McNamara et al. 1999; Dobler and Kölliker 2009).

In any case, basing feeding decisions on brood demand experienced during the most recent visit provides the most parsimonious behavioral mechanism for almost all of the patterns of provisioning effort observed in biparental and cooperative helping systems (Wright and Dingemanse 1999). Thus, our initial impression concerning the apparent quietness of bell miner broods appears to have been unjustified, since nestlings in this species signal sufficient variation in nutritional need for their begging to be used by helpers to make fine-tuned adjustments in their provisioning effort in precisely the same way as do parents. In summary, our results indicate that helping in bell miners is based upon individual feeding rules that culminate in provisioning effort that adaptively tracks the nutritional requirements of the brood.

Helper sex and offspring sex ratios show no evidence for group augmentation

The number of bell miner helpers per nest increases gradually with nestling age as brood demand increases (te Marvelde et al. 2009). All individuals resident within a coterie, except the breeding females, therefore appear to join any active nests that require them as helpers

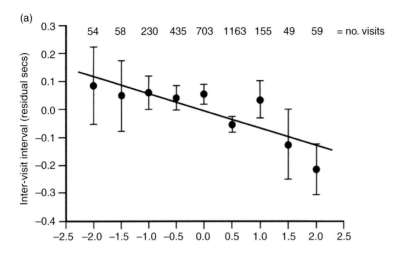

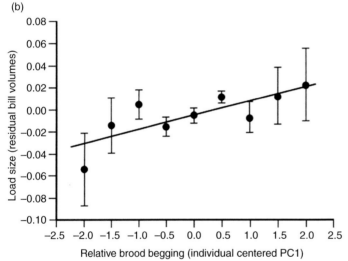

Figure 10.3. The effect of relative brood begging intensity experienced by individuals during their last visit to the nest on mean (± S.E.) within-individual variation in: (a) inter-visit interval (time to return) to the nest with food; and (b) load size. Both results are shown as residuals from a mixed model with individual and nest as random effects. Values are shown for all classes of group member combined, as there were no differences in slope between helpers of different sex and relatedness or between helpers and parents (Wright et al. 2010). The number of nest visits sampled in each level of begging is shown at the top. From Wright et al. (2010).

during the eight-month breeding season. We hypothesize that individuals split their efforts between nests both simultaneously and sequentially according to the different fitness benefits anticipated from investment in provisioning the various broods, and as a trade-off against the personal fitness benefits of investment in

their own foraging needs and the collective defense of the colony.

Helping in bell miners represents a considerable commitment of effort, and in the case of males often extends over many years. Given the lack of any obvious effects of helper age on levels of helping effort (Wright et al. 2010), helping in bell miners does not seem to be based solely on the benefits of skill acquisition (Selander 1964) and any benefits of helping experience must be quite small. It also suggests that helping in this species is unlikely to be unselected (Jamieson and Craig 1987; Jamieson 1989, 1991), notwithstanding its similarity to parental care (Wright 1999b). We therefore now consider a collection of overlapping adaptive hypotheses for any remaining direct fitness benefits that may arise from helping in terms of the production of additional group members (Woolfenden and Fitzpatrick 1978, 1984; Ligon and Ligon 1978, 1983; Connor 1986, 1995; Brown 1987), collectively referred to in more recent publications as "group augmentation" (Kokko et al. 2001; Clutton-Brock 2002; Wright 2007).

Adaptive group augmentation is particularly relevant to an obligate cooperative breeder like the bell miner. Larger coteries lead to improved individual survival and reproduction, and the fission-fusion system of coteries joining together to form larger colonies clearly points to potential advantages of collective defense in larger social groupings (Clarke 1989; Ewen et al. 2003). Bell miners provide a unique opportunity to test the hypothesis of group augmentation. Because female helpers are only resident in the colony for a few months after helping, whereas males remain in their natal colony their entire lives, group augmentation should provide far more benefits for male than female helpers. This suggests that males should be more likely to help and should work harder than females for group augmentation benefits.

Contrary to this prediction, we found no detectable effects of helper age or sex in visit rates, load sizes, prey types, or the probability of helping (Wright et al. 2010). Males are seven times more likely to help than females, but this is a consequence of the sex bias in retention of potential helpers within bell miner colonies, and when they do help then male and female helpers invest more or less equally in provisioning nestlings.

Given that female offspring do not remain in the colony for long, the benefits associated with group augmentation in bell miners should also be heavily biased toward sons and not daughters, or at least targeted more toward male-biased broods. Again, we found no evidence for this prediction with no sex differences in

genetic relatedness to the broods helped, no differences in the sex ratios of broods provisioned by male versus female helpers, and no effect of brood sex ratios on the amount of care provided by male and female helpers (McDonald et al. 2010). As might be expected, male nestlings appear to be slightly more costly to raise (te Marvelde et al. 2009), and bell miners adjust their primary brood sex ratio according to habitat productivity, probably because sons will contribute to building up the size of any colony in need of members, whereas daughters provide dispersers for large mature colonies (Ewen et al. 2003). However, we found no evidence that levels of helping were adjusted to brood sex ratios, and male nestlings were not favored within broods, a result consistent with the apparent lack of any visual or auditory cues as to nestling sex (McDonald et al. 2010). Therefore, for what must be the first time in a study of cooperative breeding (Wright 2007), we were able to test for and reject the hypothesis of group augmentation as an explanation for the evolution of helping.

Kin discrimination using *mew* calls plus population viscosity explains helping

Having failed to find support for the various hypotheses involving direct fitness benefits from helping in bell miners, we are left with the possibility of kin selection for indirect fitness benefits from the provisioning of relatives (Hamilton 1964). For many years this has constituted by far the most widely accepted explanation for adaptive helping behavior (Brown 1987; Stacey and Koenig 1990; Emlen 1997; Cockburn 1998; Koenig and Dickinson 2004), and has been suggested in previous work on bell miners as well (Clarke 1984).

It is important here to distinguish between two potential forms of adaptive kin selection (Hamilton 1964). First, behavioral kin discrimination may create facultative variation in helping effort from recipient to recipient based on pairwise relatedness between members of complex social groups. Alternatively, a more general finding of indiscriminate kin-selected help may result if relatedness within social groups is consistently high enough, as a result of limited dispersal and subsequent population viscosity (Cornwallis et al. 2009). In

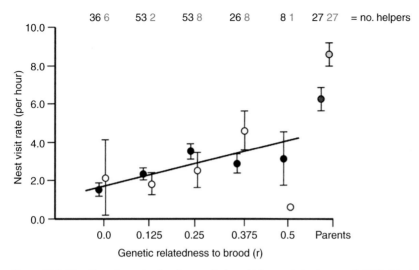

Figure 10.4. The effect of genetic relatedness to the brood (r) on variation in mean ($\pm$ S.E.) visitation rates to the nest by male (closed circles) and female (open circles) helpers. The best-fit line was drawn using parameter estimates from a mixed model for both sexes of helpers combined, and represents largely within-individual variation in helping. For comparison, data are also shown for male (dark gray) and female (light gray) parents. The number of individuals sampled at each level of relatedness is shown at the top (numbers in black are for males and in gray for females). From Wright et al. (2010).

the case of bell miners, we expect to see behavioral kin discrimination because of the large variation in relatedness within coteries. Helping might also be indiscriminate, however, due to the high rates of male philopatry producing large differences in relatedness between both coteries and colonies (Painter et al. 2000).

We found clear evidence for both types of kin selection in bell miners (Wright et al. 2010). Individual helping effort increased linearly with genetic relatedness to the brood and, as predicted by kin selection theory, this occurred to a similar degree in both male and female helpers (Figure 10.4). Interestingly, this result was driven primarily by a within-subjects effect; that is, the same individuals varied their level of help at different broods depending on their genetic relatedness to each brood. This therefore provides one of the best examples to date for behavioral kin discrimination in the form of facultative adjustment in helper effort according to relatedness (Cornwallis et al. 2009). However, unrelated helpers ($r = 0$) of both sexes still provided around half the level of help compared to full sibs ($r = 0.5$), suggesting some degree of indiscriminate kin-selected

helping. Apparently, all individuals provide help to any brood in the coterie up to a certain level, beyond which further increases depend upon their relatedness to the specific brood. In addition, none of these effects can be explained by any confounding effects of helper age (Wright et al. 2010).

The results illustrated in Figure 10.4 hold for both visitation rates and biomass delivered. We can therefore be confident that visitation rates are a reliable proxy of actual helping effort and do not hide significant unmeasured variation in the form of differences in load size or prey type (Wright et al. 2010). This sort of continuous variation in helping effort within individuals has rarely been demonstrated, and kin discrimination on such a fine scale demands an explanation in terms of the behavioral mechanisms involved.

Given the consistent individual variation in bell miner *mew* calls given around the nest, these seem the most likely mechanism for kin discrimination in this system. To compare *mew* call similarities, we used spectrographic cross-correlation (SPCC; Charif et al. 2004). SPCC values (mean $\pm$ S.E.) for our birds varied from a maximum of 0.78 ± 0.01 ($N = 118$) for the same individual recorded on different occasions at the same nest, to a minimum of 0.35 ± 0.01 ($N = 118$) for different individuals recorded at different nests (Figure 10.5a). This pattern of SPCC values clarifies three important issues for our acoustic analysis: (1) the upper limits to repeatability of the same call type within individuals; (2) the additional systematic variation one has to take into account due to the different acoustic environment around each nest; and (3) the lower limits for differences between individuals in *mew* calls that still have to be discernably of the same call type.

We analyzed a total sample of 1985 calls from 125 birds, requiring over 3.9×10^6 correlations to generate the SPCC values showing that male, but not female, *mew* calls encode information concerning genetic relatedness (Figure 10.5b). As might be expected from this result, *mew* call structure appears fixed during the lifetime of an individual, at least during the three years of our study, and is not modified in any obvious way by experience or age. For example, *mew* call structure is unaffected by the *mew* calls of other individuals heard at the nest, either as a nestling or as a young adult (McDonald and Wright 2011). It would therefore be interesting to explore the quantitative genetics of vocal tract morphology in male versus female bell miners, but this was beyond the scope of the current study.

As a result of these findings, we hypothesized that the similarity of a male helper's *mew* call to the breeding male's *mew* call may provide the helper with information concerning its genetic relatedness to the brood (McDonald and Wright 2011). This requires that helpers retain a template of their own *mew* call, which could be genetically inherited or learned through imprinting on the *mew* call of their father or other close male relatives early in life. The cross-fostering experiments necessary to confirm this suggestion have yet to be carried out.

The logic of this hypothesis also suggests that the breeding female's *mew* call should provide helpers with little additional information, since as immigrants female breeders are always unrelated to other colony members except their own offspring and grand-offspring. This could also explain why female *mew* calls do not need to reflect genetic relatedness, since such calls would carry little useful information that would not already

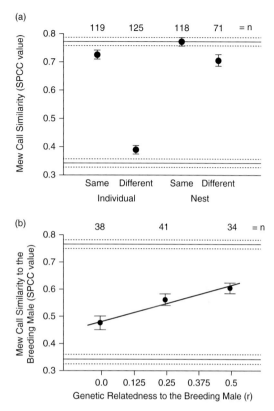

Figure 10.5. Mean (± S.E.) *mew* call similarity (spectrographic cross-correlation [SPCC] coefficients) between exemplars given by: (a) different individuals within nests and the same individual across different nests; and (b) male helpers versus breeding males according to the genetic relatedness between them (with best-fit line). The number of individuals in each comparison is given at the top. Solid and dotted horizontal lines at the top and bottom of each graph represent means (± S.E.) of effective minimum and maximum SPCC values, respectively. From McDonald and Wright (2011).

be known from putative relationships. If *mew* calls are the rule-of-thumb male helpers use to discriminate kin, then *mew* call similarity to the breeding male, but not to the breeding female, should explain more statistical variation in male helping effort than our molecular estimates of genetic relatedness.

Consistent with this prediction, we found that *mew* call similarity to the male breeder had more support as a predictor of variation in male helping effort than

Table 10.1. Linear mixed model selection comparisons explaining within-subject variation in helper effort according to genetic relatedness versus *mew* call similarity (based on SPCC) to the breeding female or breeding male

Model	Model factors	Deviance	K	AICc	ΔAICc
1	Basic	82.9	4	87.0	9.7
2	Basic + genetic relatedness	75.3	5	79.4	2.1
3	Basic + breeding female *mew* call SPCC	84.0	5	88.1	10.8
4	Basic + breeding male *mew* call SPCC	73.2	5	77.3	0

The basic model includes the intercept and helper sex, with individual identity as a random effect. Changes in AICc values are presented relative to model 4, which received the most support. Results were qualitatively similar if all first-order relatives were excluded, since they may have had additional putative information on relatedness to the parents of broods (McDonald and Wright 2011).

did measures of genetic relatedness (Table 10.1). Also as predicted, this was neither the case for call similarity to breeding females nor for the helping effort of female helpers. It is currently unclear exactly how female helpers adjust their levels of care without using *mew* call similarities, but perhaps the relatively short time they spend helping means that they are able use measures of putative relatedness. Our relatively small sample sizes of female helpers limits further investigation in this regard, but female helpers did seem able to adjust their levels of helping according to brood relatedness with a similar accuracy to male helpers (Figure 10.4). The bell miner therefore provides one of the best examples of continuous adaptive within-individual variation in kin-selected helping effort driven by facultative adjustments (Wright et al. 2010), and where a possible mechanism for fine-scale discrimination of kinship has been identified (McDonald and Wright 2011), although more work is now needed to fully confirm this.

Conclusion

Our study of the decision-making process behind helping is one of the few that has been able to address almost all adaptive explanations for the evolution of helping, a feat made possible by the unusual complexity of the bell miner system. It was also facilitated by our goal of collecting unbiased data on all aspects of helping at the nest, since this allowed us to detect crucial details in this kin-directed helping system (Wright et al. 2010).

Bell miners represent one of only a handful of examples of clear kin discrimination among cooperative breeders, and one of the best cases of fine-scale facultative adjustments concerning the level of helping effort, rather than the propensity to help (Cornwallis et al. 2009; Nam et al. 2010). Uniquely, bell miners also exhibit a base-line level of helping by even the least-related individuals in the group, corresponding to the more common finding of indiscriminate helping resulting from relatedness differences between social groups (Cornwallis et al. 2009). These findings therefore provide an example of Hamilton's (1964) two sources of kin selection, namely kin discrimination and population viscosity, and generate critical insight into what this theory predicts with regard to the effects of genetic relatedness on helping behavior (Wright et al. 2010).

Relatedness is calculated as an absolute value in most cooperatively breeding studies, including this one, which can be misleading unless a sufficiently large proportion of the population is sampled in order to obtain an accurate estimate of average relatedness (i.e., $r = 0$) – a value crucial for understanding selection for indirect benefits (Frank 1998). Of equal importance is the fact that absolute measures of relatedness alone fail to capture the specific dimensions of genetic relatedness of interest to the evolution of helping, which include variation in relatedness within social groups needed to favor the evolution of kin discrimination, and the between-group

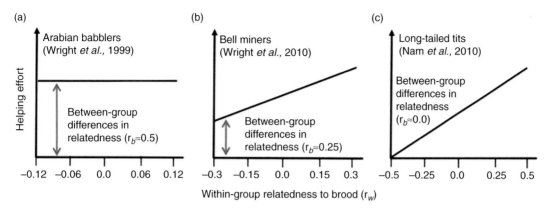

Figure 10.6. Different combinations of the two types of kin-selected helping (kin discrimination and population viscosity) illustrated in terms of simplified linear behavioral reaction norms (BRNs). Hypothetical within-group relatedness (r_w) and between-group relatedness (r_b) values are presented for three examples from the literature. Greater variation in r_w increases the positive slope of the BRN, indicating the degree of adaptive plasticity in kin discrimination. Greater differences in r_b increase the elevation of the BRN at its lowest point indicating the magnitude of any indiscriminate helping (gray arrows and text). Between-group kin selection on its own results in completely indiscriminate helping in (a) Arabian babblers, via high r_b values and little variation in r_w due to very high population viscosity (Wright et al. 1999). Both within- and between-group kin selection are present in (b) bell miners, due to intermediate values of both r_w and r_b producing kin discrimination on top of a base-line level of indiscriminate helping (Wright et al. 2010). Within-group kin selection on its own results in strong kin discrimination in (c) long-tailed tits (*Aegithalos caudatus*) as a result of large variation in r_w values, but helping effort decreases to zero with no indiscriminate helping due to low r_b values resulting from low population viscosity (Nam et al. 2010).

differences in relatedness that select for indiscriminate helping by any and all group members (Cornwallis et al. 2009). Our understanding of kin-selected helping might therefore benefit from a more focused statistical approach that decomposes genetic relatedness into these within-group versus between-group effects. For example, this could be accomplished using mean-centering, as is done routinely in behavioral ecology to test for within- versus between-individual effects (van de Pol and Wright 2009).

This conceptualization of kin-selected helping (Figure 10.6) borrows from recent work on behavioral reaction norms and the associated statistical approach of quantitative genetics to understand sources of phenotypic variation in labile traits such as helping behavior (Dingemanse et al., 2010). The slope of the helping behavioral reaction norm represents behavioral plasticity in terms of the degree of adaptive kin discrimination in helping (Figure 10.4), but here it is more correctly plotted against variation in within-group relatedness.

The intercept of the behavioral reaction norm at its lowest point reflects the level of adaptive indiscriminate helping due to population viscosity and variation in between-group differences in relatedness. It is no coincidence that this decomposition into within- versus between-group kin selection mirrors the approach used in Price's (1970, 1972) equation decomposition that is at the heart of multilevel selection theory (Okasha 2006). Given the mathematical equivalence that is now acknowledged between kin selection and (trait-) group selection (Marshall 2011; but see Okasha 2015), it seems appropriate that tests of kin selection theory should utilize this conceptually attractive feature of multilevel selection theory.

Statistically decomposing kin selection into within- versus between-group relatedness effects provides a simple and powerful empirical tool for distinguishing between the effects of kin discrimination and population viscosity on variation in helping effort expressed within and between individuals (Figure 10.6).

Unfortunately, our observations include too few colonies to properly apply this statistical method to our own data. We therefore suggest that future researchers in cooperative breeding follow this approach using data collected at more appropriate demographic scales, because in this way it should be possible to gain considerably greater understanding of the effects of kin selection on the evolution of adaptive helping behavior.

Acknowledgments

Thanks to Walt and Janis for the opportunity to summarize all of our findings on the bell miners in one place, and for their expert editorial assistance with this chapter. We are grateful to Nick and Joan Hoogenraad and the La Trobe University Wildlife Reserve for kindly allowing us to carry out fieldwork on their land. Luc te Marvelde, Maria Pacheco, Amanda Dare, and James O'Connor assisted with fieldwork, while Joy Tripovich helped extract call exemplars. Anna Lashko, Mike Double, Christine Hayes, and Andrew Cockburn provided facilities for and carried out the molecular analyses at ANU, Canberra. Mike Clarke and Ani Kazem provided input during the early stages of this project. This study was funded by BBSRC grant (5/S19268) to JW while at the University of Wales, Bangor. PGM was also funded by a Macquarie University Fellowship. This research was approved by the La Trobe University Animal Ethics committee (AEC01/19(L)/V2), the Department of Sustainability and Environment (license 10002082) and the Australian Bird and Bat Banding Scheme (A2259), who also provided leg bands.

REFERENCES

Boland, C. R. J., Heinsohn, R., and Cockburn, A. (1997). Deception by helpers in cooperatively breeding white-winged choughs and its experimental manipulation. *Behav. Ecol. Sociobiol.*, 41, 251–256.

Brown, J. L. (1987). *Helping and Communal Breeding in Birds.* Princeton, NJ: Princeton University Press.

Canestrari, D., Marcos J. M., and Baglione V. (2004). False feedings at the nests of carrion crows *Corvus corone corone.* *Behav. Ecol. Sociobiol.*, 55, 477–483.

Charif, R. A., Clark, C. W., and Fristrup, K. M. (2004). *RAVEN 1.2 User's Manual.* Ithaca, NY: Cornell Lab of Ornithology.

Clarke, M. F. (1984). Co-operative breeding by the Australian bell miner *Manorina melanophrys* Latham: a test of kin selection theory. *Behav. Ecol. Sociobiol.*, 14, 137–146.

Clarke, M. F. (1989). The pattern of helping in the bell miner (*Manorina melanophrys*). *Ethology*, 80, 292–306.

Clarke, M. F. and Fitz-Gerald, G. F. (1994). Spatial organisation of the cooperatively breeding bell miner *Manorina melanophrys.* *Emu*, 94, 96–105.

Clutton-Brock, T. H. (2002). Breeding together: kin selection and mutualism in cooperative vertebrates. *Science*, 296, 69–72.

Clutton-Brock, T. H., Russell, A. F., Sharpe, L. L., and Jordan, N. R. (2005). "False feeding" and aggression in meerkat societies. *Anim. Behav.*, 69, 1273–1284.

Cockburn, A. (1998). Evolution of helping behavior in cooperatively breeding birds. *Annu. Rev. Ecol. Syst.*, 29, 141–177.

Connor, R. C. (1986). Pseudo-reciprocity: investing in mutualism. *Anim. Behav.*, 34, 1562–1584.

Connor, R. C. (1995). The benefits of mutualism: a conceptual framework. *Biol. Rev.*, 70, 427–457.

Conrad, K. F., Clarke, M. F., Robertson, R. J., and Boag, P. T. (1998). Paternity and the relatedness of helpers in the cooperatively breeding bell miner (*Manorina melanophrys*). *Condor*, 100, 343–349.

Cornwallis, C. K., West, S. A., and Griffin, A. S. (2009). Routes to indirect fitness in cooperatively breeding vertebrates: kin discrimination and limited dispersal. *J. Evol. Biol.*, 22, 2445–2457.

Dingemanse, N. J., Kazem, A. J. N., Réale, D., and Wright, J. (2010). Behavioural reaction norms: animal personality meets individual plasticity. *Trends Ecol. Evol.*, 25, 81–89.

Dobler, R. and Kölliker, M. (2009). Behavioural attainability of evolutionarily stable strategies in repeated interactions. *Anim. Behav.*, 77, 1437–1434.

Emlen, S. T. (1997). Predicting family dynamics in social vertebrates. In: *Behavioural Ecology: An Evolutionary Approach*, 4th edn, ed. J. R. Krebs and N. B. Davies. Oxford: Blackwell, pp. 228–253.

Ewen, J. G., Crozier, R. H., Cassey, P., Ward-Smith, T., Painter, J. N., Robertson, R. J., Jones, D. A., and Clarke, M. F. (2003). Facultative control of offspring sex in the cooperatively breeding bell miner, *Manorina melanophrys. Behav. Ecol.*, 14, 157–164.

Gaston, A. J. (1978). Ecology of the common babbler *Turdoides caudatus. Ibis*, 120, 415–432.

Hamilton, W. D. (1964). The genetical evolution of social behaviour. II. *J. Theor. Biol.*, 7, 17–52.

Harrison, F., Barta, Z., Cuthill, I. C., and Székely, T. (2009). How is sexual conflict over parental care resolved? A meta-analysis. *J. Evol. Biol.*, 22, 1800–1812.

Haythorpe, K. M. and McDonald, P. G. (2010). Non-lethal foraging by bell miners on a herbivorous insect: potential implications for forest health. *Austral. Ecol.*, 35, 444–450.

Hinde, C. A. (2006). Negotiation over offspring care? – a positive response to partner-provisioning rate in great tits. *Behav. Ecol.*, 17, 6–12.

Jamieson, I. G. (1989). Behavioral heterochrony and the evolution of birds' helping at the nest: an unselected consequence of communal breeding? *Am. Nat.*, 133, 394–406.

Jamieson, I. G. (1991). The unselected hypothesis for the evolution of helping behavior: too much or too little emphasis on natural selection? *Am. Nat.*, 138, 271–282.

Jamieson, I. G. and Craig J. L. (1987). Critique of helping behaviour in birds: a departure from functional explanations. In: *Perspectives in Ethology, vol. 7*, ed. P. Bateson and P. Klopfer. New York: Plenum, pp.79–98.

Johnstone, R. A. and Hinde, C. A. (2006). Negotiation over offspring care – how should parents respond to each other's efforts? *Behav. Ecol.*, 17, 818–827.

Jones, D. A. (1998). Parentage, mate removal experiments and sex allocation in the cooperatively breeding bell miner, *Manorina melanophrys*. M.Sc thesis, Queen's University, Kingston, Canada.

Koenig, W. D. and Dickinson, J. L., eds. (2004). *Ecology and Evolution of Cooperative Breeding in Birds.* Cambridge: Cambridge University Press.

Kokko, H., Johnstone, R. A., and Clutton-Brock, T. H. (2001). The evolution of cooperative breeding through group augmentation. *Proc. R. Soc. London B*, 268, 187–196.

Kokko, H., Johnstone, R. A., and Wright, J. (2002). The evolution of parental and alloparental effort in cooperatively breeding groups: when should helpers pay-to-stay? *Behav. Ecol.*, 13, 291–300.

Ligon, J. D. and Ligon, S. H. (1978). Communal breeding in green woodhoopoes as a case for reciprocity. *Nature*, 276, 496–498.

Ligon, J. D. and Ligon, S. H. (1983). Reciprocity in the green woodhoopoe (*Phoeniculus purpureus*). *Anim. Behav.*, 31, 480–489.

Marshall, J. A. R. (2011). Group selection and kin selection: formally equivalent approaches. *Trends Ecol. Evol.*, 26, 325–332.

McDonald, P. G. (2012). Cooperative bird differentiates between the calls of different individuals, even when vocalizations were from completely unfamiliar individuals. *Biol. Lett.*, 8, 365–368.

McDonald, P. G. and Wright, J. (2008). Provisioning vocalizations in cooperative bell miners: more than a simple stimulus for nestling begging? *Auk*, 125, 670–678.

McDonald, P. G. and Wright, J. (2011). Bell miner provisioning calls are more similar among relatives and are used by helpers at the nest to bias their effort towards kin. *Proc. R. Soc. London B*, 278, 3403–3411.

McDonald, P. G., Heathcote, C. F., Clarke, M. F., Wright, J., and Kazem, A. J. N. (2007a). Provisioning calls of the cooperatively breeding bell miner *Manorina melanophrys* encode sufficient information for individual discrimination. *J. Avian Biol.*, 38, 113–121.

McDonald, P. G., Kazem, A. J. N., and Wright, J. (2007b). A critical analysis of "false-feeding" behavior in a cooperatively breeding bird: disturbance effects, satiated nestlings or deception? *Behav. Ecol. Sociobiol.*, 61, 1623–1635.

McDonald, P. G., te Marvelde, L., Kazem, A. J. N., and Wright, J. (2008a). Helping as a signal and the effect of a potential audience during provisioning visits in a cooperative bird. *Anim. Behav.*, 75, 1319–1330.

McDonald, P. G., Kazem, A. J. N., Clarke, M. F., and Wright, J. (2008b). Helping as a signal: does removal of potential audiences alter helper behavior in the bell miner? *Behav. Ecol.*, 19, 1047–1055.

McDonald, P. G., Kazem, A. J. N., and Wright, J. (2009). Cooperative provisioning dynamics: fathers and unrelated helpers show similar responses to manipulations of begging. *Anim. Behav.*, 77, 369–376.

McDonald, P. G., Ewen, J. G., and Wright, J. (2010). Brood sex ratio does not affect helper effort in a cooperative bird, despite extreme sex-biased dispersal. *Anim. Behav.*, 79, 243–250.

McNamara, J. M., Gasson, C. E., and Houston, A. I. (1999). Incorporating rules for responding into evolutionary games. *Nature*, 401, 368–371.

Mulder, R. A. and Langmore, N. E. (1993). Dominant males punish helpers for temporary defection in Superb Fairy-wrens. *Anim. Behav.*, 45, 830–833.

Nam, K-B., Simeoni, M., Sharp, S. P., and Hatchwell, B. J. (2010). Kinship affects investment by helpers in a cooperatively breeding bird. *Proc. R. Soc. London B*, 277, 3299–3306.

Okasha, S. (2006). *Evolution and the Levels of Selection.* Oxford: Oxford University Press.

Okasha, S. (2015). The relation between kin and multilevel selection: an approach using causal graphs. *Brit. J. Phil. Sci.*, 10.1093/bjps/axu047.

Pacheco, M. L., McDonald, P. G., Wright, J., Kazem, A. J. N., and Clarke, M. F. (2008). Helper contributions to anti-parasite behavior in the cooperatively breeding bell miner. *Behav. Ecol.*, 19, 558–566.

Painter, J. N., Crozier, R. H., Poiani, A., Robertson, R. J., and Clarke, M. F. (2000). Complex social organization reflects genetic structure and relatedness in the cooperatively breeding bell miner, *Manorina melanophrys*. *Mol. Ecol.*, 9, 1339–1347.

Poiani, A. (1993). Social structure and the development of helping behaviour in the bell miner (*Manorina melanophrys*, Meliphagidae). *Ethology*, 93, 62–80.

Price, G.R. (1970). Selection and covariance. *Nature*, 227, 520–521.

Price, G. R. (1972). Extension of covariance selection mathematics. *Ann. Hum. Genet., London*, 35, 485–490.

Reyer, H.-U. (1990). Pied kingfishers: ecological causes and reproductive consequences of cooperative breeding. In: *Cooperative Breeding in Birds: Long Term Studies of Ecology and Behavior*, ed. P. B. Stacey and W. D. Koenig. Cambridge: Cambridge University Press, pp. 527–557.

Royle, N. J., Smiseth, P. T., and Kölliker, M. (2012). *The Evolution of Parental Care*. Oxford: Oxford University Press.

Selander, R. K. (1964). Speciation in wrens of the genus *Camplyorynchus*. *Univ. Calif. Publ. Zool.*, 74, 1–305.

Stacey P. B. and Koenig W. D., eds. (1990). *Cooperative Breeding in Birds: Long-Term Studies of Ecology and Behavior*. Cambridge: Cambridge University Press.

te Marvelde, L., McDonald P. G., Kazem A. J. N., and Wright J. (2009). Do helpers really help? Provisioning biomass and prey type effects on nestling growth in the cooperative bell miner. *Anim. Behav.*, 77, 727–735.

van de Pol, M. and Wright, J. (2009). A simple method for distinguishing within- versus between-subject effects using mixed models. *Anim. Behav.*, 77, 753–758.

Woolfenden, G. E. and Fitzpatrick, J. W. (1978). The inheritance of territory in group-breeding birds. *BioScience*, 28, 104–108.

Woolfenden, G. E. and Fitzpatrick, J. W. (1984). *The Florida Scrub Jay: Demography of a Cooperative-Breeding Bird*. Princeton, NJ: Princeton University Press.

Wright, J. (1997). Helping-at-the-nest in Arabian babblers: signaling social status or sensible investment in chicks? *Anim. Behav.*, 54, 1439–1448.

Wright, J. (1998). Helpers-at-the-nest have the same provisioning rule as parents: experimental evidence from play-backs of chick begging. *Behav. Ecol. Sociobiol.*, 42, 423–429.

Wright, J. (1999a). Altruism as a signal: Zahavi's alternative to kin selection and reciprocity. *J. Avian Biol.*, 30, 108–115.

Wright, J. (1999b). Adaptive versus non-adaptive helping in cooperative breeders. *Behav. Ecol. Sociobiol.*, 46, 437–438.

Wright, J. (2007). Cooperation theory meets cooperative breeding: exposing some ugly truths about social prestige, reciprocity and group augmentation. *Behav. Proc.*, 76, 142–148.

Wright, J. and Dingemanse, N. J. (1999). Parents and helpers compensate for experimental changes in the provisioning effort of others in the Arabian babbler. *Anim. Behav.*, 58, 345–350.

Wright, J. and Leonard, M. L., eds. (2002). *The Evolution of Begging: Competition, Cooperation and Communication*. Dordrecht: Kluwer Academic Press.

Wright, J., Parker, P. G., and Lundy, K. J. (1999). Relatedness and chick-feeding effort in the cooperatively breeding Arabian babbler. *Anim. Behav.*, 58, 779–785.

Wright, J., McDonald P. G., te Marvelde L., Kazem A. J. N., and Bishop C. (2010). Helping effort increases with relatedness in bell miners, but "unrelated" helpers of both sexes still provide substantial care. *Proc. R. Soc. London B*, 277, 437–445.

Zahavi, A. (1977). Reliability in communication systems and the evolution of altruism. In: *Evolutionary Ecology*, ed. B. Stonehouse and C. Perrins, Baltimore, MD: University Park Press, pp. 253–259.

Zahavi, A. (1995). Altruism as a handicap: limitations of kin selection and reciprocity. *J. Avian Biol.*, 26, 1–3.

11

Superb starlings: Cooperation and conflict in an unpredictable environment

Dustin R. Rubenstein

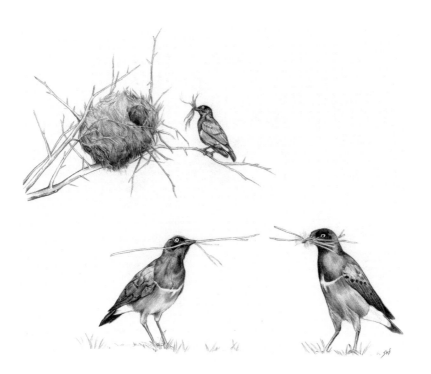

Introduction

The starlings are an Old World family of birds concentrated in the Indo-Malayan and Afrotropical regions (Feare and Craig 1999; Lovette and Rubenstein 2007). Because the European starling (*Sturnus vulgaris*) and common myna (*Acridotheres tristis*) – both of which originated in Eurasia (Lovette et al. 2008) – are among the world's most invasive avian species, starlings are now present on all continents except South America and Antarctica (Feare and Craig 1999).

The African clade of starlings, comprising approximately 45 species, is one of the most socially diverse groups of birds in the world, with nearly 40% of the

Cooperative Breeding in Vertebrates: Studies of Ecology, Evolution, and Behavior, eds W. D. Koenig and J. L. Dickinson.
Published by Cambridge University Press. © Cambridge University Press 2016.

species exhibiting cooperative breeding behavior (Rubenstein and Lovette 2007). Cooperatively breeding starling societies range from simple to complex. Singular breeding species live in simple societies with a single breeding pair and one or a few offspring that delay dispersal and help on the natal territory. In contrast, plural breeding species live in complex societies with multiple breeding pairs and helpers of both sexes (some related to the breeding pair and some not) that can provision multiple nests simultaneously.

In East Africa, the superb starling (*Lamprotornis superbus*) is one of the savanna's most easily recognizable species. It is one of approximately 22 species in the genus *Lamprotornis*, best known for its iridescent blue-green plumage (Lovette and Rubenstein 2007; Maia et al. 2013). Most *Lamprotornis* starlings are gregarious, with many living in cooperatively breeding groups (Feare and Craig 1999). Superb starlings live in large, boisterous kin-based social groups and have one of the most complicated social systems of any bird, making them a particularly good model system for the study of cooperation and conflict.

Study area

Since 2001, I have studied a population of superb starlings in central Kenya at the Mpala Research Centre, Laikipia (0°17′ N, 37°52′ E), between 1,740 and 1,800 m in elevation. This private property, over 200 km² in size, consists of savanna-bushland habitat, a matrix of trees, grass, and bare earth. Mpala lies in the middle of the Laikipia District, a plateau that stretches from the slopes of the Aberdare Mountains and Mt. Kenya in the south and east, to the edge of the Great Rift Valley in the west, to the drier low elevation regions in the north. Annual rainfall at Mpala ranges from nearly 600 mm in the south to less than 350 mm in the north. The study area, consisting of nine marked social groups, is approximately 15 km² in the southern portion of the property where rainfall is highest. Seven social groups have been continuously monitored since April 2001, and two additional groups were added to the study population in January 2002.

Rainfall in this region of central Kenya is highly variable in both time and space (Rubenstein 2011).

From 1999 through 2013, the mean (± standard deviation [S.D.]) amount of annual rainfall at Mpala was 576 ± 184 mm (range = 280 mm in 2000 to 960 mm in 2011) (Figure 11.1a), with most rain falling during the short (October–November; mean = 138 ± 70 mm) and long (March–May; mean = 238 ± 99 mm) rainy seasons (Figure 11.1b). The most variable period of rainfall is the three-month dry season (the pre-breeding period; mean = 59 ± 57 mm, range = 10 mm in 1999 to 215 mm in 2010) between the two rainy seasons (Rubenstein 2011) (Figures 11.1c and 11.1d). Although I have not quantified spatial variation in rainfall within the study area, three of the marked groups occur in a slightly drier region than the other six groups. Thus, territories vary substantially in the amount and timing of annual rainfall, which affects the start and duration of the breeding seasons, and in some years whether groups breed at all during the short rains.

The high variation in rainfall within and across years strongly influences superb starling territory quality through its effects on grass cover, which in turn is highly correlated with insect biomass in this ecosystem (Rubenstein 2007d). Grass cover varies both spatially and temporally, but high quality territories are consistently better relative to low quality territories (Rubenstein 2011). Grass cover is not only influenced by rainfall, but also by topography and soil type, being generally greatest on the tops of ridges and lowest in the valleys where moisture accumulates and bushes and trees predominate.

At Mpala, there are two primary soil types – red sandy loams (Ferric and Chromic Luvisols containing roughly 50% clay and 24% sand; Young et al. 1998) and black cotton soils (Pellic Vertisols containing 15% clay and 74% sand; Augustine 2003). These two soil types support different communities of trees, grasses, and animals (Augustine et al. 2011). Superb starlings are found commonly on both types of soil, and some of the territories with the lowest grass cover occur in the transition zone between the two soil types. Five of the marked social groups in the study population occur on red soils and four on the transition between red and black cotton soils. I have not studied any groups occurring on pure black cotton soils, largely because roads in the black cotton ecosystem become impassable to vehicles during the rainy season when birds are breeding.

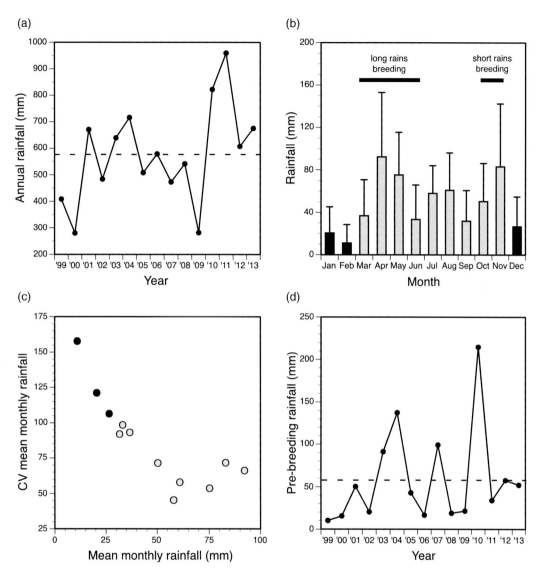

Figure 11.1. Rainfall patterns at the Mpala Research Centre, Kenya from 1998 to 2013. (a) Total annual rainfall from 1999 through 2013. The dashed line indicates the mean annual rainfall during this period (576 mm). (b) Mean (± S.D.) monthly rainfall from June 1998 through December 2013. Black bars indicate the pre-breeding period from December to February. The typical long and short rains breeding seasons are indicated above the bars. (c) Mean monthly rainfall is negatively related to the coefficient of variation (CV) in mean monthly rainfall, indicating that drier months are more variable than wetter months. The three most variable months occur during the pre-breeding period, and are indicated by black circles. (d) Pre-breeding rainfall from 1999 through 2013. The dashed line indicates the mean pre-breeding rainfall during this period (59 mm).

Life history and demography

Distribution and geographical ecology

Superb starlings live primarily in savanna-woodland habitat throughout much of East Africa, but can be found occasionally in arid regions, cultivated areas in wetter regions, and even in towns and suburban gardens. They are omnivorous, feeding on everything from termites, grasshoppers, Lepidoptera larvae, and ants, to berries, small fruits, and seeds (Feare and Craig 1999), and occasionally on mammal carcasses. During the breeding season nestlings are fed insects, primarily caterpillars and grasshoppers. Food resources are apparently not defensible during any season, and individuals do not appear capable of monopolizing food to the exclusion of other group members. Superb starlings are long-lived; in captivity they can live for more than 15 years, and in our study population, some individuals have lived for at least 14 years.

Superb starlings have large territories, often 50 ha or more in size. The landscape at Mpala is saturated with territories and social groups often border multiple other groups. Groups are territorial year-round, but birds spend extensive amounts of time each day off their territories, particularly during the nonbreeding season. When not on their territories, they are usually going to water or searching for food. In the nonbreeding season, groups will often mingle peacefully at the borders of territories to feed on the berries of dry season fruiting trees, and form mixed species flocks with other starling species such as the greater blue-eared glossy starling (*Lamprotornis chalybaeus*) and the Hildebrandt's starling (*L. hildebrandti*). Birds defend their territories in the breeding season, chasing away birds from other groups, particularly individuals that approach nests.

Territories are distributed heterogeneously in bushland habitat with a mix of grassy open areas that birds use for foraging and trees that they use for nesting. At Mpala, superb starling territories invariably encompass at least one grassy glade, a remnant of abandoned pastoralist livestock corals, called bomas, which were used for the overnight containment of livestock (Young et al. 1995). Because large quantities of livestock dung are concentrated in these small areas, both the soil and the vegetation inside glades are nutrient-rich, with insect abundance more than twice that in neighboring bushland sites (Huntzinger 2005). These nutrient-rich hotspots generate a positive feedback loop by attracting ungulate herbivores that continue to urinate and defecate in the glades, thus concentrating nutrients further and enhancing the abundance of insects and wildlife alike (Augustine 2003; Rubenstein 2007d). Nutrient-rich bomas persist as grassland glades on the landscape for decades, thus representing stable high quality areas in an otherwise depauperate landscape. Thus, these hotspots represent predictable patches of resources in otherwise climatically unpredictable environment that allow superb starling social groups to persist as dynasties for generations.

Group and demographic structure

Superb starlings are plural cooperative breeders that live in large territorial groups of up to 40 or more individuals with multiple breeding pairs per group. Mean ($\pm$ S.D.) group size is 25.8 $\pm$ 5.9 (Table 11.1), with 4.3 $\pm$ 2.4 breeders per group during the long rains and 2.6 $\pm$ 1.7 breeders per group during the short rains. The remaining nonbreeding birds are a mix of helpers that provision nestlings and nonbreeder/nonhelpers that neither provision offspring nor breed, but can play an important role in defending nests from predators (Rubenstein 2007b). This category includes birds that would likely have provisioned at a nest had it not been depredated in the egg stage. However, some nonbreeder/nonhelpers do not contribute to breeding in any capacity, even through nest guarding.

The sex ratio of superb starling groups is roughly equal (Table 11.1). Importantly, both sexes of superb starlings help at the nest, although males provision more and make up a higher proportion of the helping individuals than females (Rubenstein 2006). In general, males are the primary philopatric sex and females the primary dispersing sex; from 2002 to 2005, 8 of 11 (73%) birds that immigrated from one marked social group to another were female (Fisher exact test; $P < 0.01$), and

Table 11.1. Patterns of genetic relatedness and demographic structure from nine superb starling social groups monitored from 2002 to 2012

Trait	Mean ± S.D.	Max	Min
Genetic relatedness (r)			
Male	0.12 ± 0.05	0.15	0.02
Female	0.07 ± 0.05	0.21	−0.04
Combined sexes	0.08 ± 0.04	0.14	0.01
Demographic structure			
Number of males	12.8 ± 3.0	19.8	7.8
Number of females	13.3 ± 3.2	23.7	7.8
Group size (males and females)	25.8 ± 5.9	43.6	15.6

Pairwise relatedness values were calculated using Kingroup v2 (Konovalov et al. 2004).

61 of 76 (80%) individuals that immigrated into the study population were females ($P < 0.001$). Dispersal records from the population are limited, but banded birds have been observed in new groups nearly 20 km from where they were born. The majority of dispersal and immigration into new groups occurs during the pre-breeding dry season, although some immigration takes place at other times of the year as well. Females delay dispersal and remain in their natal groups for an average of 2.0 years before they disperse, and 17 of 65 (26%) females remained for ≥ 3 years before dispersing (Rubenstein 2006).

Although some females never disperse from their natal groups, there have only been three apparent cases of a female breeding in the group in which she was born. However, all of these breeding attempts were depredated before parentage could be confirmed with microsatellite markers, so there is no genetic evidence of a female breeding in her natal group. In contrast, male breeders appear to be a mix of natal and immigrant individuals. Determining which birds were actually born into the group is difficult because birds are long-lived and many were alive when the project began in 2001. In any case, 43 of the 112 (39%) males that bred for the first time at least two years after the project began were confirmed to have been born in the group in which they bred. Although this number is almost certainly an underestimate, it suggests that as many as half of the breeding males in groups may be immigrants.

Breeding biology and life history

Although superb starlings have been observed nesting in every month of the year at Mpala, the primary breeding season occurs during the long rains from March to June with a secondary breeding season during the short rains in October to November. The mean (± S.D.) number of nest attempts per group was 5.1 ± 2.8 during the long rains breeding season and 3.4 ± 2.4 during the short rains breeding season. In contrast, the sympatric greater blue-eared glossy starling (a noncooperative breeder) and the Hildebrandt's starling (a facultative cooperative breeder) only breed during the long rains, except during El Niño years, when the rains are particularly prolonged. During these El Niño years, the short and long breeding seasons of the superb starling can blend into one extended breeding season because of high rainfall during the pre-breeding period.

Superb starlings build nests of woven grass in trees, often near the center of the group territory and around the central grassland glade. Breeding pairs always build nests in different trees, which can be both close together or far apart. Although the breeding pair does most of the nest building, helpers occasionally contribute. Nests consist of a closed dome structure, typically with a short tunnel entrance. Pairs will reuse nests in successive breeding seasons, although most get destroyed by weather or other animals within two years. Birds have also been reported to use the abandoned nests of other birds, including those of swallows, swifts, and a variety of species of weavers (Fry et al. 2000; Rubenstein 2006).

Across most of their range, superb starlings nest in thorn trees, primarily in the genus *Acacia* at heights ranging from < 1 m to > 9 m above the ground (mean = 2.8 m). There appears to be no effect of nest height or tree species on the probability of being depredated (Rubenstein 2006). The most abundant tree species in the black cotton soil and transition zone is the whistling thorn acacia (*Acacia drepanolobium*), which is protected from megaherbivores (primarily elephants) by one of four species of symbiotic ant (Goheen and Palmer 2010). Preliminary data suggest that superb starlings may preferentially place their nests in trees defended by the most aggressive ant species, presumably because the ants help protect the nest from predators.

Nest failure is extremely high. From 2001 to 2013, I monitored 862 nest attempts, of which only 172 (27%) fledged any offspring. Of 2,549 eggs laid during this period (mean ± S.D. clutch size = 3.5 ± 0.6), only 333 (13%) fledged, and the mean (± S.D.) proportion of eggs fledging per nest was 0.12 ± 0.29. The high nest failure rate leads to extremely low average lifetime reproductive success for those individuals that attempt to breed: the mean (± S.D.) lifetime reproductive success for females was 2.0 ± 3.0 offspring fledged (range = 0–13; N = 55 females through 2012), and for males was 2.0 ± 3.2 (range = 0–17; N = 41 males through 2012). Nests fail due to abandonment, starvation, and predation, but failure is primarily attributable to the latter, as 92% of complete nest failure is due to predation. Diurnal predators include birds, baboons, snakes, and squirrels and nocturnal predators include genets, mice, and snakes. During the nestling stage, starvation remains an important source of nest failure, particularly during the beginning of the season when some pairs nest before the true onset of the rainy season, and the end of the breeding season when the rains begin to taper off.

Social behavior

Kinship

The male-biased dispersal pattern of superb starlings results in kin structure within a social group that is higher among males (mean r = 0.12) than among females (mean r = 0.07) (Table 11.1). Male kin structure

in particular varies greatly among groups, ranging from r = 0 to 0.26. The group with the lowest average relatedness among males surrounds the Mpala Research Centre where food and water are available year-round. This group is also the largest and has the most transient birds that are banded during the dry season and never seen again, as well as many birds that are only seen in the group for a short period of time.

Although the overall kin structure in most groups is relatively low, this is likely the result of having large groups with multiple unrelated breeding females and a mix of related and unrelated breeding males. Kinship among breeders and helpers has not yet been formally assessed, but the majority of helpers are offspring of the breeding pair or other close relatives. Thus, within the larger, plural breeding group exists smaller subgroups organized around the family unit. So, although the overall mean relatedness among males in the group is relatively low, high pairwise relatedness among many members of the group suggests that kin selection is likely to play an important role in the evolution or maintenance of superb starling societies.

Given the range of kinship values in superb starling groups, individual must have a mechanism to recognize relatives. In at least some cooperatively breeding birds, kinship is assessed through vocalizations (Sharp et al. 2005; McDonald and Wright 2011; Akçay et al. 2013) (see also Chapters 2, 3, and 10). In other species, vocalizations also have been shown to signal group membership (Tyack 2008) or individual identity (Stoddard 1996). Superb starlings make short, stereotyped vocalizations, or flight calls, when approaching conspecifics. Immigrant females are able to learn these flight calls as adults after joining a new social group (Keen et al. 2013). A combination of acoustic recording analyses and playback experiments were used to show that superb starling flight calls are more similar within than among groups, and that individuals respond differently to playbacks from their own group versus those from other groups (Keen et al. 2013). Call similarity was not correlated with genetic relatedness, however, indicating that flight calls are learned and reflect social association and individual identity rather than kinship. Thus, in complex societies with both kin and nonkin group members, signaling individuality and group association, and not just kinship, may be an important mechanism that facilitates cooperation.

Offspring care and nest defense

Superb starlings are apparently obligate cooperative breeders, with >90% of nests having at least one helper feeding nestlings (Rubenstein 2006). Determining whether all nests have helpers – the definition of an obligate cooperative breeder – is a difficult task because nest predation rates are high in this population and the number of attendants at a nest increases with nestling age (Rubenstein 2006). Most of the nests where helpers were not observed were depredated early in the hatchling period, and it is likely that helpers would have been observed feeding nestlings had the nest survived longer. In any case, helping is very important and increases parental fitness; nests where chicks starve have approximately 50% fewer helper visits and provisioning trips per hour than nests where chicks do not starve (Rubenstein 2007c). Only breeding females incubate eggs (and there is no observational or genetic evidence of egg dumping), but once the eggs hatch, social fathers and helpers aide in provisioning offspring. Mothers contribute >50% of the nestling provisioning, while social fathers and helpers split the rest equally. As many as 14 helpers have been observed provisioning at a single nest, but the mean (± S.D.) number of helpers at a nest is 3.3 ± 2.7 ($N = 222$ nests from 2001 to 2014).

Nestling provisioning and helping behavior is extremely complex. Although most nests are attended by helpers that are previous offspring of the breeding pair, helpers can assist at multiple nests simultaneously, and breeders occasionally provision at others' nests after their own nests have failed. Cases of breeders helping at others' nests often involve brother – brother and father – son relationships, but they can also involve less related individuals. In a few cases, one of the breeding individuals that was observed helping at another pair's nest was observed to be paired with one of the other breeders the following breeding season.

Patterns of nestling provisioning vary both in time and space. For example, the proportion of nestling provisioning done by helpers – but not mothers or social fathers – varies among years and is related to the amount of pre-breeding rainfall (Rubenstein 2006). Helpers contribute a greater proportion of the provisioning following dry pre-breeding periods, and a lower proportion following wetter pre-breeding periods. In contrast, the proportion of provisioning done by mothers – but not helpers or social fathers – varies among groups and is related to territory quality. Mothers do a greater proportion of nestling provisioning on lower-quality territories and a lower proportion of provisioning on higher-quality territories (Rubenstein 2006). This result is somewhat surprising and suggests that further study of the temporal and spatial patterns of nestling provisioning is needed.

Superb starlings use a loose sentinel system to protect nests from predators. When parents are actively feeding chicks, at least one group member often perches on the top of a tree within 30 m of the nest. Both helpers and nonbreeder/nonhelpers act as sentinels that will actively alarm call if a potential predator approaches the nest. In experiments involving model predators, mothers were always the first to attack models, but eventually helpers and nonbreeder/nonhelpers attacked models more collectively than either the mother or social father alone (Rubenstein 2006). Thus, although nonbreeder/nonhelpers do not provision nestlings, they appear to play an important role in the group given that nest predation rates are so high. This could at least partially explain why superb starling groups are so large and why birds that neither breed nor provision nestlings are allowed to remain in the group.

Mating system

Superb starlings are socially monogamous with an average of 10% of offspring and 17% of nests resulting from extra-pair fertilizations. Extra-pair paternity is higher in the long rains breeding season (12% of offspring and 19% of nests) than in the short rains breeding season (8% of offspring and 14% of nests). Moreover, extra-pair paternity varies across years, ranging from 0% to 24% of offspring and 0% to 45% of nests. Between 2001 and 2013, molecular analyses also indicated that at least 22% of socially breeding females and 17% of socially breeding males engaged in extra-pair fertilizations at least once.

Although extra-pair paternity is low overall, there is high variation among groups, ranging from 4% to 32% of offspring and 7% to 60% of nests (Rubenstein 2007d). This variation in extra-pair paternity – most of which involves males from outside of the group – is unrelated to group size, genetic relatedness within groups, and pre-breeding rainfall. Instead, rates are correlated with territory quality (as estimated by grasshopper abundance and grass cover) such that extra-pair paternity is highest on low-quality territories with little grass cover and few insects (Rubenstein 2007d). This pattern likely reflects differences in the effectiveness of mate-guarding by males on territories of different quality. Preliminary observations and radio telemetry data suggest that females on lower quality territories forage further from the nest and central glade, indicating that they may have increased opportunity to mate with extra-group males. Thus, territory quality may influence a male's ability to guard his mate, and a female's ability to escape this mate-guarding and seek extra-pair fertilizations from outside the group.

Females exhibit two distinct extra-pair mating strategies: half of females that had extra-pair offspring in their nest (7% of all extra-pair offspring from 2001 to 2005) copulated with extra-pair sires from inside the group, and half (also 7% of all extra-pair offspring) copulated with extra-pair sires from outside the group (Rubenstein 2007a). Females that choose extra-pair mates from inside the group tend to be first-time breeders or those that had few surviving offspring from previous years (Rubenstein 2007a). Because these females have few potential kin helpers, they target unrelated subordinate (i.e., nonsocially paired) males that could potentially help at their nests (Rubenstein 2007a). In nests that survived to hatching, many of these subordinate sires did indeed act as helpers.

In contrast, females that choose extra-pair males from outside the group were able to increase the genetic diversity of their offspring. Offspring produced from extra-group males were more heterozygous – in terms of standardized heterozygosity and internal relatedness – at microsatellite loci than offspring produced by the social mate (Rubenstein 2007a). Females that sought out these extra-group males were those paired to mates that were relatively less heterozygous than themselves. Thus, females can potentially gain both direct benefits, in the form of increased alloparental care, and indirect benefits, in the form of increased offspring genetic diversity, by being promiscuous.

Extra-pair fertilizations are not the only strategy that birds use to make secondary mate choice decisions. Birds can mate-switch, or divorce, if the pair bond is inadequate (Botero and Rubenstein 2012). Mate switching is extremely common in superb starlings, with 45% of breeders of both sexes switching mates at some point during their breeding tenure; between 2001 and 2013, 231 pairs – involving 143 males and 151 females – attempted to breed in the population. Although most of the mate-switching occurs between breeding seasons, 10 cases of divorce within a breeding season have been observed. It is not yet clear why birds divorce within- or among-years, but in nearly all cases both birds remain in the group, and often, both the male and female will re-mate at some point in the future.

Not all pairs are quick to divorce, however, and some remain faithful despite being unsuccessful at breeding. The maximum number of failed breeding attempts in a season by a faithful pair is four, and the maximum breeding tenure for a pair without ever fledging offspring is four years (up to eight breeding attempts). In contrast, the maximum breeding tenure for birds that have bred together successfully is six years. Further work is clearly needed to understand how pairs form and why some end in divorce while others do not.

Synthesizing the social lives of starlings

Social and sexual competition in cooperative breeders

Intense social and sexual competition for breeding opportunities, as is evident in many cooperative breeders (Rubenstein 2012; Young and Bennett 2013), suggests that both males and females may benefit by the use of armaments to compete with same-sex individuals or ornaments to attract mates (Lyon and Montgomerie 2012). Comparative work in the entire group of African starlings has shown that cooperatively breeding species are less sexually dimorphic in plumage and body size than noncooperatively breeding species (Rubenstein and Lovette 2009). This reduced sexual dimorphism occurs in cooperative species because females are more similarly ornamented to the males of their species rather than vice versa. Moreover, females tend to be larger and more ornamented than the females of noncooperatively breeding species. Thus, selection – be it natural, sexual, or social – on traits used in intrasexual competition may be particularly intense in females in cooperatively breeding species, ultimately resulting in trait elaboration in both sexes.

Starling coloration is particularly vivid and appears to be under intense sexual selection. African starlings are the only monophyletic avian group to display all four of the structural color-producing melanosome morphotypes identified in birds (Durrer 1970). The mechanisms of color production have evolved directionally in this group from simple to more complex, resulting in faster color evolution, the occupation of novel regions of color space with new and brighter colors, and accelerated diversification via sexual selection (Maia et al. 2013). Some of the most colorful plumage and complex melanosome morphotypes occur in the *Lamprotornis* group where cooperative breeding behavior is particularly common.

Superb starlings are sexually monomorphic not only in plumage coloration, but also in other socially or sexually selected traits. Adults sing complex and diverse songs with as many as 82 distinct motifs, including all of the motifs used in flight calls (Keen et al. 2013). Although the function of superb starling song is unknown, males and females both sing during the breeding and nonbreeding seasons and there appears to be no differences in the number of motifs that each sex sings, with males producing an average (±S.D.) of 56.1 ± 1.6 motifs (range = 47–64) and females 54.7 ± 1.9 (range = 47–61) (Pilowsky and Rubenstein 2013). Moreover, there were no measurable differences in the structure of male and female songs. Breeder song differs in structure from nonbreeder (both helper and nonbreeder/nonhelper) song, however, with breeders producing songs with a higher proportion of unique motifs per bout than nonbreeders. Additionally, individuals singing in groups produce songs that are more continuous and have longer bouts than those singing

alone. Thus, although the function of superb starling song is still unclear, it may be a signal used by both sexes to establish dominance rank or signal breeding status. Song could also be used to attract mates, but further work on this topic is needed.

As a plural breeding species, superb starlings have relatively low reproductive skew compared to singular breeding species characterized by a single breeding pair because more than one individual of each sex breeds in the group. Since social groups are typically so large, only about 25% of the birds in the group form pairs and breed socially despite the fact that nearly all groups in all years contain nonbreeding immigrant females and (unrelated) philopatric males of breeding age that could presumably pair and breed. Therefore, competition for dominance rank and reproductive conflict over breeding roles and mating opportunities appears to be quite high.

It is not yet clear how dominance status – or for that matter, how mate choice – is achieved in superb starlings, but it is likely that there are separate male and female dominance hierarchies. Observations made at baited feeding platforms have indicated that breeders are dominant to nonbreeder/nonhelpers which are dominant to helpers (Rubenstein 2006). Age likely plays a central role in dominance status, as breeders tend to be older than nonbreeder/nonhelpers, which tend to be older than helpers. Both sexes are aggressive and females often supplant subordinate males at the feeding platforms. Comparisons of glucocorticoid stress hormones in individuals with different breeding roles suggest that aggressive interactions and social suppression of breeding by dominants increases in drier years (Rubenstein 2007b; Rubenstein and Shen 2009). Aggressive interactions – most of which occur in flight – at the end of the pre-breeding period and beginning of the long rains breeding season are also apparently higher in drier years. Thus, environmental factors appear to interact with social factors to influence aggressive interactions, dominance rank, and ultimately breeding roles in superb starling social groups.

The opportunity for multiple pairs to breed in superb starlings social groups – that is, low reproductive skew – sets the stage for strong competition for social rank and high potential reproductive conflict over breeding roles and mating opportunities in both sexes (Rubenstein 2012). This not only influences social structure and creates tension over which birds get to breed and which help, but the similarly high potential for intense reproductive conflict within groups may help explain the monomorphic plumage (Rubenstein and Lovette 2009) and complex but similar vocalizations of males and females (Pilowsky and Rubenstein 2013). Further work is needed to explore signal evolution and maintenance in this and other cooperative breeders, particularly in species or populations where reproductive skew varies among groups.

Environmental uncertainty and the evolution of cooperative breeding

Ecological constraints on dispersal have long been thought to influence the incidence of cooperative breeding behavior in birds. Most barriers to independent breeding, such as a shortage of vacant breeding territories, the costs of dispersal, and difficulties in finding a mate (Hatchwell and Komdeur 2000) are the result of living in a spatially heterogeneous landscape where suitable territories are limiting (Emlen 1982; Koenig et al. 1992). Spatial constraints on dispersal are not the only environmental factor that can influence cooperative breeding behavior, however, as temporal variation in the environment may also be important (Emlen 1982). Comparative analysis in the African starlings (Rubenstein and Lovette 2007), later extended to all terrestrial birds (Jetz and Rubenstein 2011), suggests that cooperative breeders are found more commonly in temporally variable environments where precipitation varies unpredictably from year-to-year. One hypothesis for this relationship is that helpers at the nest may buffer groups against harsh conditions when food becomes limiting (Rubenstein and Lovette 2007).

Contrary to this hypothesis, recent work in hornbills (family Bucerotidae) suggests that cooperative breeders are found in less, not more, variable environments (Gonzalez et al. 2013). Similarly, in acorn woodpeckers (*Melanerpes formicivorus*), having helpers increases fitness only during environmentally favorable years, not in environmentally harsh years (Koenig et al. 2011; Chapter 13). These discrepancies in the role

of environmental variability in favoring cooperation may simply be a taxonomic issue, however, since in Jetz and Rubenstein's (2011) global analysis, cooperative breeding behavior was predicted by rainfall variation in passerines (including starlings), but not in nonpasserines (including hornbills and woodpeckers). Instead, temperature variation, which is indicative of a latitudinal signal, predicted sociality in nonpasserines. Nonetheless, for African starlings, environmental uncertainty in the form of interannual rainfall variation appears to be important in shaping the evolution and maintenance of cooperative breeding behavior.

In superb starlings, nearly all components of their social behavior and breeding life history are related to among-year variation in rainfall. The most climatically variable period of the year occurs during the pre-breeding dry season, when the coefficient of variation in mean monthly rainfall is highest (Figure 11.1c). Pre-breeding rainfall impacts a variety of physiological mediators, including glucocorticoid stress hormones (Rubenstein 2007b) and immune function (Rubenstein et al. 2008). Baseline and stress-induced corticosterone levels are correlated with pre-breeding rainfall in subordinate birds that become helpers but not in the more dominant individuals that become breeders or nonbreeder/nonhelpers during the following breeding season (Rubenstein 2007b). The elevated levels of stress hormones in helpers during the driest years are most consistent with the hypothesis that environmental conditions influence the relative costs of dominance behavior. These rank-related costs in turn affect the degree and intensity of social interactions, and ultimately reproductive decisions and breeding roles (Rubenstein 2007b; Rubenstein and Shen 2009). In contrast to levels of corticosterone, immune function – measured as the capacity for innate immunity in plasma to kill Gram-negative, nonpathogenic bacteria – was lowest in years with dry pre-breeding periods, but did not differ significantly among birds of different breeding roles (Rubenstein et al. 2008).

Annual variation in pre-breeding rainfall has a number of carryover effects to the breeding season. Rainfall variation directly influences maternal body condition, which later impacts offspring sex ratio (Rubenstein 2007c). Mothers in poor body condition during the

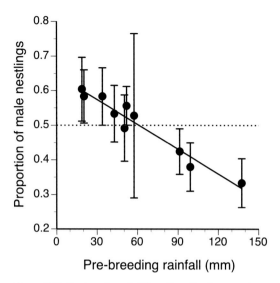

Figure 11.2. Pre-breeding rainfall predicts offspring sex ratio in superb starlings. Females overproduce male offspring in dry years and female offspring in wet years. This figure extends data published in Rubenstein (2007c) through 2013. Only nests where three or four nestlings survived to day 7 after hatching were used in the original analysis and graphed here. Each point is the mean (± S.E.) proportion of male nestlings per nest in a given long rains breeding season. Only years in which three or more nests were sampled were included. The year 2010 was excluded because it was an El Niño year where continuous rainfall meant that there was not a pre-breeding dry season. The total sample size was 80 nests over 11 breeding seasons (range = 3–14 nests per year). The dotted line represents an even 50:50 sex ratio.

years with wetter pre-breeding periods (Figure 11.3), which may be due to greater offspring production, enhanced survival, and/or reduced dispersal. Additionally, the number and proportion of birds that breed for the first time is greater following wetter pre-breeding periods, suggesting that reduced dispersal in high quality years could at least partially influence the group size pattern (Rubenstein 2007b).

Since superb starling physiology, behavior, and life history are affected by among-year variation in rainfall, environmental uncertainty is also likely to influence fitness. Although mean reproductive success for breeding pairs in a group does not appear to be impacted by either temporal (rainfall) or spatial (territorial quality) environmental variation, variance in reproductive success is correlated with among-year variation in rainfall and among-territory variation in grass cover. That is, the standardized variance in reproductive success declines with increasing environmental quality (both rainfall and territory quality), as well as with increasing group size (a proxy for the potential for cooperation and the number of helpers in the group) (Rubenstein 2011). Specifically, in drier years, differences in territory quality are amplified and variance in reproductive success among groups is higher. Thus, environmental uncertainty influences variance in superb starling fitness, but not mean fitness, suggesting that cooperative breeding behavior may itself be a risk-averse strategy that groups use to reduce environmentally induced fecundity variance. Although environmental variation may be the primary force reducing variance in reproductive success in superb starlings, this "bet-hedging hypothesis" applies to any selection pressure that could influence variation in fitness, such as predation and brood parasitism (Rubenstein 2011).

The logic underlying the bet-hedging hypothesis is relatively straightforward. If having helpers in the group reduces the variance in reproductive success across years by limiting complete nest failure in some years, perhaps by preventing nestling starvation in harsh years or by successfully defending a clutch from a nest predator, then selection should favor having helpers in the group even if doing so reduces the mean reproductive output of the group and the mean per capita reproductive success of the breeders. Such declines in mean

pre-breeding period overproduce male offspring when pre-breeding rainfall is low, but overproduce female offspring when rainfall is high (Figure 11.2). Although this pattern appears to contradict the Trivers-Willard hypothesis (Trivers and Willard 1973), it does not because female superb starlings – like most cooperatively breeding birds (Hauber and Lacey 2005) – have a higher variance in reproductive success than males (Rubenstein 2007c). Thus, in accord with the Trivers-Willard hypothesis, mothers should be expected to overproduce female offspring when conditions are best, as is observed in superb starlings.

Pre-breeding rainfall also influences demography and reproductive behavior. Group sizes are larger in

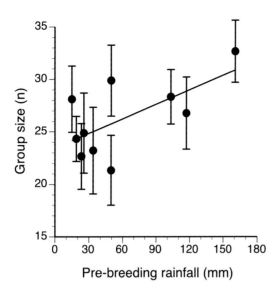

Figure 11.3. Superb starling group size varied with pre-breeding rainfall from 2002 to 2012. Groups were larger in years when more rainfall fell during the pre-breeding period ($F_{1,80} = 14.6$, $P < 0.001$; GLMM includes social group as a random effect to account for repeated measures across years). This pattern may result from increased offspring production, increased survival, and/or decreased dispersal in years with more rainfall during the pre-breeding dry season. The year 2010 was excluded because it was an El Niño year where continuous rainfall meant that there was not a pre-breeding dry season.

per capita reproductive success with increasing group size are common in cooperatively breeding vertebrates. Moreover, similar patterns of declining offspring production with increasing colony size are observed in eusocial insects, where the phenomenon is called Michener's paradox (Michener 1964). Of course, reducing years of complete nest failure will inevitably lead to a slight increase in the mean in addition to a reduction in the variance. This may explain why in superb starlings there is no relationship between group size and mean reproductive success (Rubenstein 2011), rather than a negative relationship.

If having helpers is a form of insurance that breeders use to minimize fecundity variance, then we expect the bet-hedging hypothesis to be most relevant to species living in large social groups. Of course, as group

size increases with the retention of more subordinate individuals, reproductive conflict over breeding opportunities is likely to increase (Shen et al. 2014). One way for breeders to reduce this potential conflict may be to allow others in the group to breed, and thus, plural breeding could evolve. This scenario predicts that plural breeding is more likely to be found in systems where among-year variation in fecundity is high. Although this prediction has not been explored in detail, most plural breeding birds are found in semi-arid environments similar to those of the superb starling (Brown 1987).

Clearly more data from superb starlings and other cooperatively breeding species are needed to test the bet-hedging hypothesis. In general, the bet-hedging hypothesis should be tested in plural cooperatively breeding species where some but not all females in a social group reproduce. For species with variation in social structure among groups or populations, groups with helpers would be predicted to have a higher geometric mean fitness but not arithmetic mean fitness than groups without helpers. Moreover, for closely related species with different social systems living in similar environments, cooperative and noncooperative breeders should show different relationships in mean and variance in fitness with environmental and demographic parameters. Ultimately, researchers must consider how selection on variance in fitness, rather than on mean fitness alone, might influence cooperation and conflict in cooperatively breeding species.

At broad geographic and taxonomic scales, the degree of among-year variation in precipitation influences the incidence of cooperative breeding behavior in African starlings (Rubenstein and Lovette 2007) and more generally in all terrestrial birds, at least in the passerine lineage (Jetz and Rubenstein 2011). This temporal variability hypothesis suggests that living in kin-structured family groups and having helpers-at-the-nest allows birds to buffer environmental conditions when they are harsh and take greater advantage of conditions when they are good (Rubenstein and Lovette 2007). This appears to be the case for the plural breeding superb starling, where pre-breeding rainfall influences stress hormones, immune function, maternal body condition, and sex allocation, as well as the adoption of different breeding roles, levels of parental care, the intensity of reproductive conflict within groups, and demographic structure. Although mean reproductive success in groups is not directly influenced by rainfall variation, variance in reproductive success is related to pre-breeding rainfall. Cooperative breeding in superb starlings, specifically having large, plural breeding groups with many potential helpers, may therefore be an adaptation to reduce complete nest failure by buffering groups against environmental uncertainty and protecting nests against predators.

In summary, superb starlings appear to be able to reduce environmentally induced fecundity variance in both time and space by living in complex, plural breeding groups. Having a stable pool of subordinate individuals available to act as helpers to feed nestlings appears essential in this obligate cooperative breeder because poor quality years occur frequently and unpredictably. Indeed, when females lack access to potential helpers, they are willing to recruit helpers through extra-pair fertilizations with subordinate males within the group (Rubenstein 2007a). Moreover, subordinate individuals also play an important role in nest defense. When the mean lifetime reproductive success for both males and females is only two offspring fledged, preventing even a single nest predation event could more than double an individual's reproductive output. Thus, nearly all aspects of the superb starling's social life, including the evolution and maintenance of its complex plural cooperatively breeding social system, are influenced by the climatically variable savanna ecosystem in which they live. Superb starlings, however, are a cosmopolitan and wide-ranging East African species that can also be found occasionally in more mesic and more xeric environments. It will be interesting to compare the behavior, life history, and physiology of superb starlings living in deserts and forests to those in the savanna.

Conclusion

Superb starlings are endemic to the savannas of East Africa and have one of the most complicated lifestyles of any cooperatively breeding bird. They are an obligately cooperative species, with nearly all nests having helpers that provision nestlings. Group sizes are among the largest of any cooperatively breeding bird studied, and each group has multiple breeding pairs that can be assisted in caring for offspring by more than a dozen helpers. Superb starlings have a female-biased dispersal pattern, which results in higher genetic relatedness among males than among females. These sex-biased patterns of dispersal and philopatry result in a patriarchal society, and although both sexes help, males do more of the nest provisioning than females.

Although nearly all breeding females immigrate into the group, surprisingly, nearly half of the breeding males also appear to be immigrants. This likely explains the relatively low overall relatedness among males and among females. Both sexes of superb starlings also compete intensively for breeding opportunities, which may have implications for the evolution of sexually or socially selected traits like plumage coloration and song in this species. Breeding positions are constantly in flux, and divorce is frequent in this population. However, pairs are generally faithful and extra-pair paternity is on average quite low (10% of offspring and 17% of nests), even though promiscuous females can gain a variety of direct fitness benefits, such as helper recruitment, and indirect fitness benefits, such as increased offspring genetic diversity. Despite low overall promiscuity, extra-pair paternity varies greatly among groups and is influenced by territory quality, with higher rates on lower quality territories with reduced grass cover and lower insect abundance. This pattern is likely the result of females escaping mate-guarding on the lower quality territories where all individuals need to forage further from the nest and the central glade.

Superb starlings live in a variable environment where the amount of rainfall and duration of the rainy season varies unpredictably from year-to-year. Annual variation in precipitation during the most variable period of the annual cycle, the pre-breeding dry season, influences all aspects of life for superb starlings, including breeding roles, stress physiology, immune function, helping behavior, reproductive conflict, and demographic structure. Moreover, cooperative breeding itself may be an adaptation to this uncertain climate, as allowing subordinate helpers to remain in the group may be a risk-averse strategy used by dominant breeders to minimize environmentally induced fecundity variance. Ultimately, the complicated lifestyle of the superb starling, and the degree of cooperation and conflict within their complex societies, is tied directly to the spatially and temporally variable savanna environments in which this plural breeder lives.

Acknowledgments

I thank Kathleen Apakupakul, Sarah Guindre-Parker, and Lea Pollack for providing constructive comments on this chapter and collecting some of the data. Much of the field data were collected by Tyler Davis, James Ekiru, Rebecca Harris, Godffrey Manyass, Brynn McCleery, Gabriel Rana, and Julius Rongore. This project would not exist without the continued support and insights from Wilson Nderitu who began working on the project at its inception in 2001. Elizabeth Adkins-Regan, Stephen Emlen, Irby Lovette, Daniel Rubenstein, and Martin Wikelski provided guidance in the project's early stages. I acknowledge the Kenyan National Commission for Science, Technology and Innovation, the Kenyan National Environmental Management Authority, the National Museums of Kenya Ornithology Department, the Kenya Wildlife Service, the Columbia Global Centers | Africa, and the Mpala Research Centre for enabling this work. The study was funded by fellowships from the Howard Hughes Medical Institute, the Smithsonian Institution, the Cornell University College of Agriculture and Life Sciences, and the Miller Foundation for Basic Research at the University of California, Berkeley. Additionally, support came from grants from the National Science Foundation (IBN-407713, IOS-1257530), the American Museum of Natural History Chapman Fund, the American Ornithologists' Union, the Wilson Ornithological Society, the Society for Integrative and Comparative Biology, the Animal Behavior Society, the Andrew W. Mellon Foundation, the Harvard Travellers Club, the Society of Sigma Xi, the Cornell University Graduate School, the Cornell University Mario Einaudi Center for International Studies, the Cornell University Department of Neurobiology and Behavior, the Cornell Laboratory of Ornithology Benning Fund, Cornell Sigma Xi, the Museum of Vertebrate Zoology at the University of California, Berkeley, and the Columbia University Earth Institute.

REFERENCES

Akçay, C., Swift, R. J., Reed, V. A., and Dickinson, J. L. (2013). Vocal kin recognition in kin neighborhoods of western bluebirds. *Behav. Ecol.*, 24, 898–905.

Augustine, D. J. (2003). Long-term, livestock-mediated redistribution of nitrogen and phosphorus in an East African savanna. *J. Appl. Ecol.*, 40, 137–149.

Augustine, D. J., Veblen, K. E., Goheen, J. R., Riginos, C., and Young, T. P. (2011). Pathways for positive cattle-wildlife interactions in semiarid rangelands. In: *Conserving Wildlife in African Landscapes: Kenya's Ewaso Ecosystem*, ed. N. J. Georgiadis. Washington, D.C.: Smithsonian Institution Scholarly Press, pp. 55–71.

Botero, C. A. and Rubenstein, D. R. (2012). Fluctuating environments, sexual selection and the evolution of flexible mate choice in birds. *PLoS One*, 7, e32311.

Brown, J. L. (1987). *Helping and Communal Breeding in Birds: Ecology and Evolution*. Princeton, NJ: Princeton University Press.

Durrer, H. (1970). Schillerfarben der stare (Sturnidae) [Iridescent colors of the starlings (Sturnidae)]. *J. Ornithol.*, 111, 133–153.

Emlen, S. T. (1982). The evolution of helping. 1. An ecological constraints model. *Am. Nat.*, 119, 29–39.

Feare, C. and Craig, A. (1999). *Starlings and Mynas*. Princeton, NJ: Princeton University Press.

Fry, C.H., Keith, S., and Urban, E.K. (2000). *The Birds of Africa*. San Diego, CA: Academic Press.

Goheen, J. R. and Palmer, T. M. (2010). Defensive plant-ants stabilize megaherbivore-driven landscape change in an African savanna. *Curr. Biol.*, 20, 1768–1772.

Hatchwell, B. J. and Komdeur, J. (2000). Ecological constraints, life history traits and the evolution of cooperative breeding. *Anim. Behav.*, 59, 1079–1086.

Hauber, M. E. and Lacey, E. A. (2005). Bateman's principle in cooperatively breeding vertebrates: the effects of nonbreeding alloparents on variability in female and male reproductive success. *Integr. Comp. Biol.*, 45, 903–914.

Huntzinger, M. (2005). How do distantly related herbivores that share food resources interact? Ph.D. thesis, University of California, Davis, USA.

Jetz, W. and Rubenstein, D. R. (2011). Environmental uncertainty and the global biogeography of cooperative breeding in birds. *Curr. Biol.*, 21, 72–78.

Keen, S. C., Meliza, C. D., and Rubenstein, D. R. (2013). Flight calls signal group and individual identity but not kinship in a cooperatively breeding bird. *Behav. Ecol.*, 24, 1279–1285.

Koenig, W. D., Pitelka, F. A., Carmen, W. J., Mumme, R. L., and Stanback, M. T. (1992). The evolution of delayed dispersal in cooperative breeders. *Q. Rev. Biol.*, 67, 111–150.

Koenig, W. D., Walters, E. L., and Haydock, J. (2011). Variable helper effects, ecological conditions, and the evolution of cooperative breeding in the acorn woodpecker. *Am. Nat.*, 178, 145–158.

Konovalov, D. A., Manning, C., and Henshaw, M. T. (2004). KINGROUP: a program for pedigree relationship reconstruction and kin group assignments using genetic markers. *Mol. Ecol. Res.*, 4, 779–782.

Lovette, I. J. and Rubenstein, D. R. (2007). A comprehensive molecular phylogeny of the starlings (Aves: Sturnidae) and mockingbirds (Aves: Mimidae): congruent mtDNA and nuclear trees for a cosmopolitan avian radiation. *Mol. Phylogen. Evol.*, 44, 1031–1056.

Lovette, I. J., McCleery, B. V., Talaba, A. L., and Rubenstein, D. R. (2008). A complete species-level molecular phylogeny for the "Eurasian" starlings (Sturnidae: *Sturnus, Acridotheres*, and allies): recent diversification in a highly social and dispersive avian group. *Mol. Phylogen. Evol.*, 47, 251–260.

Lyon, B. E. and Montgomerie, R. (2012). Sexual selection is a form of social selection. *Phil. Trans. R. Soc. London B*, 367, 2266–2273.

Maia, R., Rubenstein, D. R., and Shawkey, M. D. (2013). Key ornamental innovations facilitate diversification in an avian radiation. *Proc. Natl. Acad. Sci. (USA)*, 110, 10687–10692.

McDonald, P. G. and Wright, J. (2011). Bell miner provisioning calls are more similar among relatives and are used by helpers at the nest to bias their effort towards kin. *Proc. R. Soc. London B*, 278, 3403–3411.

Michener, C. D. (1964). Reproductive efficiency in relation to colony size in hymenopterous societies. *Insectes Sociaux*, 11, 317–341.

Pilowsky, J. A. and Rubenstein, D. R. (2013). Social context and the lack of sexual dimorphism in song in an avian cooperative breeder. *Anim. Behav.*, 85, 709–714.

Rubenstein, D. R. (2006). The evolution of the social and mating systems of the plural cooperatively breeding superb starling, *Lamprotornis superbus*. Ph.D. thesis, Cornell University, Ithaca, NY, USA.

Rubenstein, D. R. (2007a). Female extrapair mate choice in a cooperative breeder: trading sex for help and increasing offspring heterozygosity. *Proc. R. Soc. London Ser. B*, 274, 1895–1903.

Rubenstein, D. R. (2007b). Stress hormones and sociality: integrating social and environmental stressors. *Proc. R. Soc. London Ser. B*, 274, 967–975.

Rubenstein, D. R. (2007c). Temporal but not spatial environmental variation drives adaptive offspring sex allocation in a plural cooperative breeder. *Am. Nat.*, 170, 155–165.

Rubenstein, D. R. (2007d). Territory quality drives intraspecific patterns of extrapair paternity. *Behav. Ecol.*, 18, 1058–1064.

Rubenstein, D. R. (2011). Spatiotemporal environmental variation, risk aversion and the evolution of cooperative breeding in birds. *Proc. Natl. Acad. Sci. (USA)*, 108, 10816–10822.

Rubenstein, D. R. (2012). Family feuds: social competition and sexual conflict in complex societies. *Phil. Trans. R. Soc. London B*, 367, 2304–2313.

Rubenstein, D. R. and Lovette, I. J. (2007). Temporal environmental variability drives the evolution of cooperative breeding in birds. *Curr. Biol.*, 17, 1414–1419.

Rubenstein, D. R. and Lovette, I. J. (2009). Reproductive skew and selection on female ornamentation in social species. *Nature*, 462, 786–789.

Rubenstein, D. R. and Shen, S.-F. (2009). Reproductive conflict and the costs of social status in cooperatively breeding vertebrates. *Am. Nat.*, 173, 650–661.

Rubenstein, D. R., Parlow, A. F., Hutch, C. R., and Martin, L. B., II (2008). Environmental and hormonal correlates of immune activity in a cooperatively breeding tropical bird. *Gen. Comp. Endocrin.*, 159, 10–15.

Sharp, S. P., McGowan, A., Wood, M. J., and Hatchwell, B. J. (2005). Learned kin recognition cues in a social bird. *Nature*, 434, 1127–1130.

Shen, S.-F., Akçay, E., and Rubenstein, D. R. (2014). Group size and social conflict in complex societies. *Am. Nat.*, 183, 301–310.

Stoddard, P. K. (1996). Vocal recognition of neighborhoods by territorial passerines. In: *Ecology and Evolution of Acoustic Communication in Birds*, ed. D. E. Kroodsma, and E. H. Miller. Ithaca, NY: Cornell University Press, pp. 356–374.

Trivers, R. L. and Willard, D. E. (1973). Natural selection of parental ability to vary the sex ratio of offspring. *Science*, 179, 90–92.

Tyack, P. L. (2008). Convergence of calls as animals form social bonds, active compensation for noisy communication channels, and the evolution of vocal learning in mammals. *J. Comp. Physiol.*, 122, 319–331.

Young, A. J. and Bennett, N. C. (2013). Intra-sexual selection in cooperative mammals and birds: why are females not bigger or better armed? *Phil. Trans. R. Soc. London B*, 368 20130075.

Young, T. P., Patridge, N., and Maccrae, A. (1995). Long-term glades in acacia bushland and their edge effects in Laikipia, Kenya. *Ecol. Appl.*, 5, 97–108.

Young, T. P., Okello, B. D., Kinyua, D., and Palmer, T. M. (1998). KLEE: A long-term multi-species herbivore exclusion experiment in Laikipia, Kenya. *African J. Range Forage Sci.*, 14, 92–104.

12

Seychelles warblers: Complexities of the helping paradox

Jan Komdeur, Terry Burke, Hannah Dugdale, and David S. Richardson

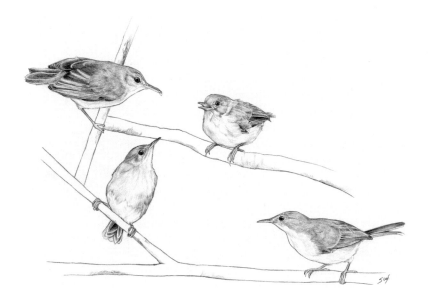

Introduction

The Seychelles warbler (*Acrocephalus sechellensis*), a passerine endemic to the Seychelles archipelago, is a facultatively cooperative breeder that lives either in pairs or small groups. Breeding groups normally consist of a dominant pair and one to three subordinates, although up to nine have been observed. Subordinates can be of either sex, and are often offspring that have delayed dispersal and remained in their natal territory (Komdeur

1992; Richardson et al. 2002; Eikenaar et al. 2008, 2010). By the 1960s the last remnant population of this then critically endangered species was confined to Cousin Island (Figure 12.1). Subsequent conservation actions, including the restoration of forest habitat and the establishment of new populations through translocations, have provided unique opportunities to study the evolutionary ecology of cooperative breeding in this species.

We have followed the entire world population of the Seychelles warbler since our study started in 1981. In

Cooperative Breeding in Vertebrates: Studies of Ecology, Evolution, and Behavior, eds W. D. Koenig and J. L. Dickinson.
Published by Cambridge University Press. © Cambridge University Press 2016.

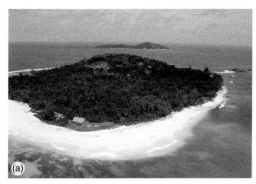
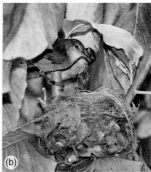

Figure 12.1. (a) Cousin Island, with Cousine Island in the distance. Photograph by David Richardson. (b) Seychelles warblers feeding a nestling. Photograph by Danny Ellinger. See plate section for color figure.

1997, however, we increased the intensity of work on Cousin and since then nearly all individuals, including fledglings, have been captured, ringed, blood sampled, sexed, and monitored for breeding and status. Molecular tools have been used to assign the sex and genetic parentage of young birds and to determine levels of relatedness between individuals. In addition, a comprehensive set of behavioral, life history, and annual fitness parameters have been recorded for nearly all individuals, providing important opportunities for assessing changes in social behavior. The lack of interisland dispersal (Komdeur et al. 2004a), combined with sampling of the entire population, provides a rare opportunity to monitor the survival, reproduction, and lifetime fitness of all individuals within the population.

Our long-term research program into cooperative breeding, hand-in-hand with conservation actions, has created an experimental system in which we can attempt to unravel the factors that alter the cost-benefit trade-offs of cooperative breeding. Over time, this system has become proof of the power of the experimental methods and of the corrective value of long-term studies, where iterative examination with longer-term data sheds new insights on short-term findings. Here we detail various findings that have allowed us to uncover how changing social and ecological factors influence the form and function of reproductive competition and cooperation in the Seychelles warbler. We also outline how molecular genetic tools have given us a better understanding of the species' cooperative breeding

system and the selective factors that favor switching between different forms of cooperative and independent breeding.

Distribution and conservation

The Seychelles warbler is a small (13–19 g) passerine endemic to the Seychelles archipelago in the Indian Ocean (Safford and Hawkins 2013; Figure 12.2). In the 1870s this species was recorded on the islands of Mahé, Marianne, Félicité, and Cousine (Oustalet 1878; Figure 12.2). It probably also occurred historically on most of the Seychelles islands, which made up a single large island during the last ice age (Collar and Stuart 1985). This assumption is supported by the large effective population sizes estimated for the pre-bottleneck Seychelles warbler population using museum samples from the 1800s (Spurgin et al. 2014).

The destruction of natural habitat for the planting of coconut trees (*Cocos nucifera*), along with the introduction of mammalian predators in the early 1900s, resulted in the warbler's extirpation from nearly all the islands where they previously occurred. Only on Cousin Island, which remained free of predators (Collar and Stuart 1985), did the warblers survive, with only 26–50 individuals remaining between 1940 and 1967 (Crook 1960; Loustau-Lalanne 1968; Spurgin et al. 2014). Cousin Island was purchased by a consortium led by BirdLife International (then the International

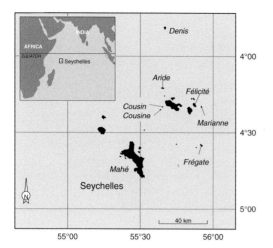

Figure 12.2. The location of the Seychelles in the Indian Ocean (inset) and the inner granitic islands in detail, including Cousin (0.29 km²), Cousine (0.25 km²), Aride (0.68 km²), Denis (1.42 km²), Félicité (2.68 km²), Frégate (2.19 km²), Marianne (0.96 km²), and Mahé (154 km²).

Council for Bird Preservation) in 1968 and designated as a nature reserve to save the Seychelles warbler from extinction. Habitat restoration was successful and, by 1982, much of Cousin was again covered with native forest (Bathe and Bathe 1982). As a consequence, the warbler population recovered and since 1982 has been at a carrying capacity of about 320 adults inhabiting around 110 territories that cover all but the bare rock areas of Cousin (Figure 12.3). This ratio of birds to territories also means there has been a considerable surplus of (unpaired) adult birds on the island since the point of saturation (Komdeur 1992; Brouwer et al. 2009, 2012).

The flight apparatus of the Seychelles warbler does not differ from that of other long-distance migratory *Acrocephalus* warblers (Komdeur et al. 2004a). Nonetheless, interisland dispersal is virtually nonexistent. During the 28 years of this study only six individuals were recorded to have crossed the sea between islands. Given the low probability of any new warbler populations establishing by themselves, and the vulnerability of a single small population, four new populations were established by translocation of birds from Cousin to the islands of Aride and Cousine in 1988 and

1990, respectively (29 individuals each time; Komdeur 1994a), Denis in 2004 (58 individuals; Richardson et al. 2006), and Frégate in 2011 (59 individuals; Wright et al. 2014; Figure 12.2). In contrast to the food limitation observed on Cousin, where a shorter breeding season was the norm, warblers on the new islands experienced higher food availability and initially bred year-round (Komdeur et al. 1995). This resulted in an initial increase in annual productivity of up to ten-fold compared to the population on Cousin (Komdeur 1996a). As each population increased, productivity declined, presumably because of the increased density of the population (Brouwer et al. 2009). Most recent population sizes are estimated at 210 warblers on Cousine in 2007 (van de Crommenacker and Richardson 2007), 1850 on Aride in 2003 (Orchard 2004), 300 on Denis in 2013 (J. van de Woude, unpubl. data), and 80 on Frégate in 2013 (Teunissen 2013) (Figure 12.4). The world population of Seychelles warblers is now estimated at 2750 adult birds across five islands and the conservation status of the Seychelles warbler has been reduced from endangered to vulnerable (IUCN 2013).

Natural history: Seychelles warblers

Territoriality and breeding biology

The Seychelles warbler is socially monogamous, and paired dominant birds often remain with the same partner on the same breeding territory for life (Komdeur 1992; Richardson et al. 2007). The pair bond can last up to 14 years (S. A. Kingma, unpubl. data). Seychelles warblers are largely insectivorous, mainly gleaning invertebrate prey from the undersides of leaves. As such, resource abundance, a major aspect of territory quality, can be evaluated by estimating the number of invertebrates on the undersides of leaves and extrapolating from this to estimate prey abundance according to the amount of foliage in each territory (Komdeur 1992; Brouwer et al. 2006). On Cousin, prey abundance has been measured monthly on each territory during the main breeding periods (June to September) for most years since 1987; the same technique has been used to measure prey abundance in

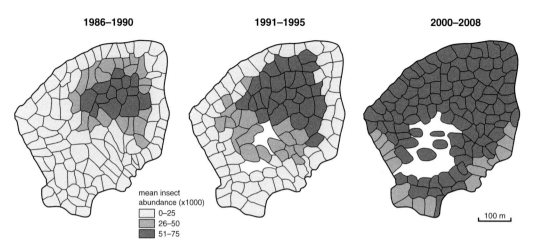

Figure 12.3. Cousin Island outline with Seychelles warbler territories drawn in and mean insect abundance present in each territory during the periods 1986–1990 (from Komdeur 1992), 1991–1995, and 2000–2008 (J. Komdeur, unpubl. data).

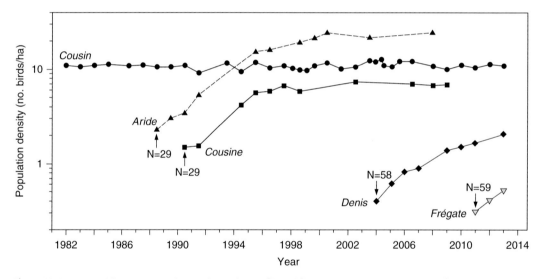

Figure 12.4. Temporal fluctuations in the population density (*In* scale) of Seychelles warblers on Cousin (saturated), Aride (census focused on the accessible plateau area of 5.2 ha; saturated), Cousine (saturated), Denis (increasing phase), and Frégate (increasing phase) islands. Arrows with sample sizes (*N* birds) indicate the introduction of birds to each island. Initial densities differ both because of the different numbers of birds introduced and large differences in the sizes of the islands (Cousin: 0.29 km², Aride: 0.68 km², Cousine: 0.25 km², Denis: 1.42 km², Frégate: 2.19 km²). Figure updated from Brouwer et al. (2009).

various years on the other islands since their populations were founded. Our results show that insect food supply is highly seasonal and that warblers time their breeding such that the production of nestlings is synchronized with the periods of highest prey abundance (Komdeur 1996a) with peaks of nest building between May and August and again, to a lesser extent, between December and February.

Most breeding pairs and groups produce one clutch per year (Komdeur 1996a), with clutches normally consisting of just one egg, although ~13% of nests contain two or three eggs (Richardson et al. 2001). Incubation, which is by the female, lasts 17–19 days, and nestlings are fed by both sexes for 18–20 days prior to fledging, and then for up to four months before reaching independence. This is an extremely long period of dependence; no other known passerine has a six-month period of dependence. Indeed, the mean fledging period for other passerines is only about one tenth as long (Bennett and Owens 2002). Nonetheless, first-year survival is relatively low: 61% of fledglings survive the first year compared to an annual survival of 84% in adults (Brouwer et al. 2006). Like many other tropical bird species, the Seychelles warbler is long-lived, with an average life expectancy of around five years once they reach adulthood and a maximum recorded lifespan of 17 years (Barrett et al. 2013).

The breeding system

Seychelles warbler territories are normally occupied by a single dominant pair-bonded male and female. However, about 30% of territories contain subordinate males and/or females that are sexually mature birds lacking a suitable independent breeding opportunity (Komdeur 1992; Richardson et al. 2002, 2007). This is demonstrated by the fact that birds transplanted to previously uninhabited islands immediately breed independently rather than becoming helpers or subordinate cobreeders. Furthermore, vacancies created in the source population by the translocation of breeders are filled immediately by subordinates from other territories (see "Indirect fitness benefits to subordinates").

Female subordinates normally remain on their natal territory, while ~25% of male subordinates move to a new territory to take up a subordinate position (Richardson et al. 2002). In any given breeding attempt, approximately 44% of subordinate females lay eggs within the dominant pair's nest, while only 15% of subordinate males sire offspring within the group (Richardson et al. 2001); we define such birds as "subordinate cobreeders." The remaining subordinates that have not successfully reproduced (either by siring

young or laying eggs) may help to raise the chicks, either by aiding in nest building (mainly females), incubation (females), guarding the clutch (mainly males), or provisioning (males and females) (Komdeur 1994b; Richardson et al. 2003a, 2003b); we define these birds as "helpers" in that breeding attempt. Subordinates that neither help nor breed successfully are defined as "nonhelping subordinates."

There is no evidence of egg dumping; females (subordinate or otherwise) do not lay eggs in extra-group nests. Similarly, male subordinates never gain paternity outside the group (Richardson et al. 2002). However, extra-group paternity is common, with about 44% of offspring fathered by dominant males from other territories (Richardson et al. 2001; Hadfield et al. 2006). Populations also include a variable, and difficult to define, number of floaters of both sexes that have failed to find a breeding or subordinate position and wander over the island without residing in a territory (Komdeur and Edelaar 2001; Eikenaar et al. 2008).

The costs and benefits of cooperative breeding

In most species the inferred fitness benefits from helping are substantially lower than those from breeding independently. Consequently, cooperative behavior is generally considered to be a suboptimal fitness strategy (Emlen 1982; Lessells 1991; Dickinson et al. 1996; Dickinson and Hatchwell 2004). Therefore, in order to understand its evolution it is important to know what determines when and where cooperative breeding behavior occurs. With this in mind, the route to cooperative breeding may best be viewed as a two-step process: first, the decision by an individual to forgo independent breeding and become a subordinate in a group, and second, the decision by a subordinate to help the dominants to raise offspring (Emlen 1982). The first step is usually attributed to the existence of ecological constraints on independent breeding, such as a shortage of breeding territories or mates (the "ecological constraints" hypothesis; Emlen 1982, 1991), combined with the benefits of remaining in the natal group (the "benefits of philopatry" hypothesis; Brown 1978;

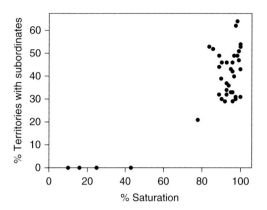

Figure 12.5. The percentage of territories with subordinates in relation to habitat saturation in a given year for the Seychelles warblers on Cousin Island between 1959 and 2013. Habitat saturation was measured as the number of territories present in that year divided by the maximum number of territories recorded in a year ($N = 121$). Figure amended from Komdeur et al. (2008).

Stacey and Ligon 1987, 1991; Ekman et al. 2004; Covas and Griesser 2007). The second step is attributable to a variety of potential fitness benefits, both indirect and direct (Stacey and Koenig 1990; Dickinson and Hatchwell 2004).

In the Seychelles warbler, cooperative breeding was first observed in 1973, when the population of adult birds started to be greater than the number of breeding positions available on territories. At this point, most, but not all, suitable breeding habitat on Cousin was occupied (Komdeur 1992). Interestingly, however, cooperative breeding occurred well before the island was completely saturated (Figure 12.5), indicating that factors other than habitat saturation per se also influence cooperative breeding.

Group living

Early on in our study, young independent males dispersed more often and earlier from their natal territories than young independent females (Komdeur 1996b). This was thought to be because females are usually born on higher-quality territories than males (Komdeur et al. 1997, see "Sex allocation"), and as there

is a positive correlation between the length of time for which independent offspring delay dispersal and the natal territory quality, females ended up delaying dispersal longer than males. This sex-bias in dispersal behavior disappeared later in the study, however, apparently as a result of females starting to disperse earlier, rather than males delaying dispersal longer (Eikenaar et al. 2007, 2010).

We suspect that temporal changes in demography, most likely higher reproductive output per territory due to improved and less variable habitat quality, rather than differences in local density or social conditions, caused the observed changes. In particular, the change in male dispersal behavior coincided with a change in spatial food resource availability. Early on, mean insect numbers were highest in the center of the island and decreased gradually toward the coast (Figure 12.3), but with the restoration of the coastal vegetation insect numbers there increased significantly (Komdeur and Pels 2005). Consequently, the proportion of high-quality territories on the island increased (van de Crommenacker et al. 2011), even though the total number of territories, and Seychelles warblers, has remained similar (Brouwer et al. 2009). Given this change in food abundance across a more or less stable population and the concomitant increase in the quality and reproductive output of territories over the years (Komdeur and Pels 2005), we suspect that food-related fitness consequences drive the dispersal behavior of males, although further work is needed to confirm this.

Helping behavior

Helping is not an inevitable consequence of group living. Both within and among cooperatively breeding species, considerable variation exists in whether, and to what extent, individuals help. Furthermore, helping in many species is biased with respect to the subordinate sex. In most cooperatively breeding birds, male-biased delayed dispersal and helping is the norm (Cockburn 1998; Berg et al. 2009; Cornwallis et al. 2009). Seychelles warblers were originally thought to be an exception in that females were more likely to delay dispersal and become subordinate helpers/cobreeders than males, with 88% of subordinates being female helpers/cobreeders in 1986–1990 (Komdeur 1996b). As mentioned above, this bias toward helpers being females decreased over time to 68% in later years (Richardson et al. 2002) and subsequently disappeared altogether (Eikenaar et al. 2010).

Additionally, a small proportion of birds (14% of females and 3% of males) became subordinates, usually for the second time, after being deposed as dominant breeders. Many of these (68% of the females) were observed to actively help kin and are therefore termed "grandparent helpers" (Richardson et al. 2007). These observations suggest that helping is not a stable trait, but rather a plastic response to local conditions. The key, then, is to assess and understand how different costs and benefits, to both the helpers and the helped, interact to determine this variation.

Indirect fitness benefits to subordinates

For helpers to gain indirect benefits their activities must result in a net benefit to those they help (Hamilton 1964). In the Seychelles warbler, the presence of helpers on high quality territories with high prey abundance increases the number of young produced on a territory: the removal of helpers, from groups with one helper on high-quality territories, resulted in lower reproductive success for the breeding pair compared with control pairs (Komdeur 1994b). A later study demonstrated that the total amount of provisioning to nestlings significantly affects fledging success and first-year survival. Importantly, this improvement was correlated with the number of birds actually helping, not with the total number of birds in the territory including nonhelping subordinates (Brouwer et al. 2012). Furthermore, cross-fostering of nestlings between territories confirmed that it is the number of helpers in the territory where they are reared that determines the survival of offspring, thus ruling out the possibility that offspring quality is confounding the helper effect. Overall, the number of fledglings produced on a territory per breeding attempt increases by 18% for each helper present, even after excluding direct subordinate parentage (Richardson et al. 2002).

Since Seychelles warblers can breed independently in their first year, why do some individuals become subordinates? Individuals that remain as subordinates in high-quality territories and later breed there have higher lifetime fitness than those that disperse from high-quality territories at one year of age and breed in lower-quality territories. Breeding pairs without helpers on high-quality territories produce on average 0.85 fledglings each year compared to only 0.19 fledglings on low-quality territories. Furthermore, a helper on a high-quality territory can increase the dominant pair's reproductive success by 0.77 fledglings from 0.85 to 1.62 fledglings per year, about four times the output from the low-quality territories. This increase, and the fact that subordinates are normally helping their parents, means that subordinates increase their own indirect benefits by remaining as helpers (Komdeur 1992).

At the time these results were published we assumed that all female helpers were nonbreeding helpers. Later work indicated that these "helpers" included both true nonbreeding helpers and subordinate cobreeders (Richardson et al. 2001). To the extent that these birds were actually cobreeders, they would have gained even greater fitness benefits by remaining with their parents.

We were able to experimentally verify the importance of territory quality to cooperative breeding by creating new breeding opportunities when removing breeding adults for translocation to new islands. Initially, in the source population, the breeding vacancies created were filled by subordinates from territories of equivalent or poorer quality, never by subordinates from superior territories, for which helping remained a better option than breeding (Komdeur 1992). On the new islands, initially all translocated individuals bred as independent pairs. However, after a few years, when all the high-quality areas were occupied, individuals again chose to help on high-quality territories rather than to breed independently on low-quality territories. These results support both the benefits of philopatry (Stacey and Ligon 1987, 1991) and the ecological constraints hypotheses (Emlen 1982, 1991), which differ only in the emphasis they place on the costs of leaving versus the benefits of staying (Komdeur 2003).

Cooperatively breeding species are often long-lived, have stable and strong natal philopatry, and a relatively long period of extended parental care during which they associate with family members (Stacey and Koenig 1990; Emlen 1991; Arnold and Owens 1998; Hatchwell and Komdeur 2000; Cornwallis et al. 2009). Most subordinates become helpers after delaying dispersal from their natal territory. In such situations, conditions exist that may assist subordinates to gain indirect fitness benefits through helping: first, since parents are long-lived, helpers on their natal territories will be caring for subsequent related offspring, and second, the extended care period may allow subordinates ("ego") to develop a simple rule: help any individual ("b") that fed ego when ego was a nestling to raise b's subsequent broods, as b is likely to be ego's parents. However, in groups where individuals differ in how related they are to each other and to the brood because of high turnover of breeders or infidelity, direct kin discrimination will be required if potential helpers are to maximize their indirect benefits.

In the Seychelles warbler, males more often become subordinates on nonnatal territories than females and so subordinate males are no more related to the groups' nestlings than one would expect by chance (Richardson et al. 2002). Female subordinates are, therefore, more related to the nestlings than male subordinates. Thus, the kin-selected benefits of helping are more important for female subordinates. Even within the sexes, however, levels of relatedness and the amount of helping vary substantially within and among subordinates. Female subordinates that gain parentage in the nest appear to assess this fact accurately and always provision (Richardson et al. 2003a, 2003b). For nonparent female subordinates, provisioning is positively correlated with their genetic relatedness to the nestlings and thus their potential indirect fitness gain (Figure 12.6).

In contrast, male subordinates rarely obtain paternity in the brood that they help (Richardson et al. 2001) and are usually less related to the nestlings. These males provision considerably less than subordinate females and their contribution is not influenced by their relatedness to the nestling (Richardson et al. 2003a, 2003b).

Relatedness between subordinates that remain in their natal territory and nestlings is lower than one would theoretically expect for first-order relatives (mean $r = 0.13$). This occurs for two reasons: first, males

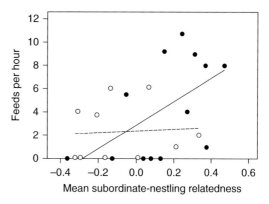

Figure 12.6. Provisioning rates by subordinate female (filled circles) and male (empty circles) nonparents in relation to relatedness between the subordinate and the nestling. There is a positive relationship between provisioning and subordinate–nestling relatedness for female subordinates (solid line; $F_{1,11} = 4.82$, $P = 0.05$, $R^2 = 0.31$) but not for male subordinates (broken line; $F_{1,8} = 0.04$, $P = 0.86$, $R^2 = 0.00$). From Richardson et al. (2003a).

from outside the group are responsible for siring about 40% of offspring (Richardson et al. 2001; Hadfield et al. 2006). This extra-group paternity dramatically reduces the degree of relatedness between subordinates and the offspring they may help, as only 36% share the same father, even if the same male remains dominant in the territory across their birth years. Second, subordinate females commonly lay an egg within the dominant's nest (44% successfully produce offspring in a breeding season; Richardson et al. 2002). Thus, the offspring, including those now acting as subordinates, in a territory with multiple females may have different mothers, both within and between breeding seasons. The consequently reduced relatedness between subordinates and the helped nestlings (mean $r = 0.16$; Richardson et al. 2003b) means that the indirect benefits of helping are relatively small, and substantially less than was expected before we were able to assess relatedness directly using molecular techniques.

Surprisingly, despite these complications, subordinate females appear to possess a mechanism for inferring their kinship to nestlings and direct help toward those to which they are related. With its long period of parental care, kin discrimination is based

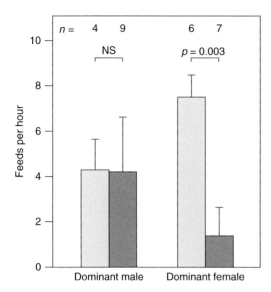

Figure 12.7. Mean provisioning (± S.E.) by subordinate female nonparents in relation to the presence (light gray bars) or absence (dark gray bars) of their putative parents (dominant males $t_{11} = 0.02$; females $t_{11} = 3.71$). n denotes sample size. From Richardson et al. (2003a).

on association and is achieved through learning the identity of parents. The subordinate female's provisioning of the nestlings is best predicted by the continued presence of the dominant female – her putative mother – that raised her. Because the putative mother's continued presence reliably indicates a subordinate's relatedness to the nestling (Richardson et al. 2003a, 2003b), the use of this cue is effective in maximizing the indirect benefit that subordinates gain from their efforts (Figure 12.7).

In contrast, the continued presence of the dominant male that raised the subordinate is not used to determine when to help. From an evolutionary perspective this makes sense because the high frequency of female infidelity means that the continued presence of the same dominant male does not predict reliably that subordinates are related to the nestling.

Cross-fostering experiments focusing on breeding pairs without female helpers have confirmed that the subordinate's decision to help is based on the identity of the female parent, rather than a direct assessment of her relatedness to the nestling. For nestlings that later became subordinates, their decision to help was associated only with the continued presence of the dominant female (their putative mother) irrespective of whether the subordinate was cross-fostered, and therefore regardless of their actual genetic relatedness to that female (Figure 12.8).

It is clear, however, that the cue just outlined will only work for subordinates that were raised in a territory without female helpers present. It remains to be investigated whether and how subordinates that were raised in groups of multiple females discriminate kin. For example, if mothers provide more food than helpers, then the subordinates might base their decision to help on the continued presence of the female that fed them the most. Alternatively, since both the breeding and helping females within a group are often related (Richardson et al. 2002), the subordinate may help to feed the nestling if either potential mother remains present, as this will still indicate subordinate–nestling relatedness, although to a lesser degree.

Even after taking into account subordinate–nestling relatedness, considerable variation in the extent of helping behavior remains unexplained (Richardson et al. 2002). To gain a full and accurate picture of the role of indirect benefits in helping, the costs of helping, and not just the benefits, need to be considered. In the Seychelles warbler, helping appears to be costly and condition dependent. Female subordinates that help have lower body mass at the end of the season than female subordinates that do not help (van de Crommenacker et al. 2011). Consequently, body condition has a positive effect on an individual's decision to help: only those individuals that are in good condition prior to the breeding season will help. Results such as these in the Seychelles warbler and in other species such as meerkats (*Suricata suricatta*; Russell et al. 2003; Chapter 17), suggest that helpers may be only using energy that is surplus to their requirements. If this is true, are there any actual costs of helping? Unless the proximate costs lead to a reduction in future survival and fitness, there may not be any ultimate cost of helping. So, by refining their helping decisions based on their condition, helpers may be able to obtain an indirect benefit at little or no long-term cost.

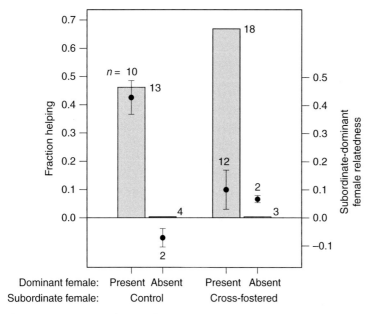

Figure 12.8. The fraction (gray bars) of control and cross-fostered female subordinates that helped to feed nestlings during their second year of life in relation to the continued presence of the dominant females and dominant foster females ($\chi^2 = 1.3$, d.f. = 1, $P = 0.25$), and in relation to the new dominant females that replace the dominant (foster) females that raised the subordinates (absent). Only those subordinates that could have been helpers, that is, where nests with young were present in their natal territory, were included ($N = 38$ individuals). Circles indicate mean relatedness of subordinates ($\pm$ S.E.) to the dominant females and dominant foster females that raised the subordinates and were still present on the territory (present; $t_{20} = 3.48$, $P = 0.002$) or to new dominant females that replaced the dominant (foster) females that raised the subordinates (absent). n denotes the number of subordinates. From Komdeur et al. (2004b).

Direct fitness benefits of helping

It has been suggested that only 10% of the variation in helping behavior can be explained by indirect benefits (Griffin and West 2002). Thus indirect fitness benefits alone are unlikely to fully explain this phenomenon. An alternative explanation is that helpers may increase their own survival and future reproduction by cooperating with others. Here we do not consider all the various possible ways that subordinate individuals might improve their direct fitness, but instead focus on those that appear to be important in the Seychelles warbler system.

Acquisition of parentage

As discussed earlier, female subordinate Seychelles warblers often gain parentage within their own group

by laying an egg in the dominant bird's nest (Richardson et al. 2001). In contrast, male subordinates rarely gain parentage. As a result, the direct fitness benefits gained through parentage by female subordinates are over three times higher than those gained by male subordinates (Figure 12.9). Importantly, in both sexes the direct benefits of helping are up to six times higher than the indirect benefits when direct breeding benefits were included. This suggests that direct benefits are more important in the maintenance of cooperative breeding in the Seychelles warbler than are indirect benefits.

Accumulation of breeding experience

By helping to raise the dominant birds' offspring, subordinates may gain breeding experience, allowing them

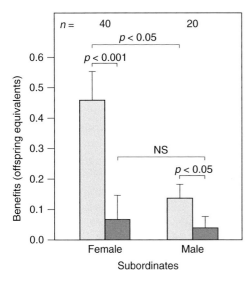

Figure 12.9. Fitness benefits (± S.E.) of cooperative breeding gained by female and male subordinates (1997–1999). Both female and male subordinates gain significantly higher direct (pale columns) compared to indirect (dark columns) breeding benefits (female: $z = 4.22$, males: $z = 2.39$). Direct breeding benefits were significantly higher in females than in males ($z = 2.29$), but there was no significant difference between the sexes in indirect benefits ($z = 0.21$). n denotes sample size. From Richardson et al. (2002).

to be more productive when they achieve a breeding territory of their own in the future (Komdeur 1996c; Hatchwell et al. 1999). In the Seychelles warbler, this idea was tested by translocating similar-aged females and males with different breeding and helping experience. On the new islands, newly formed pairs, where one partner only had helping experience and the other had breeding experience, produced their first fledgling as fast as pairs in which both partners were experienced breeders, and significantly faster than pairs consisting of an inexperienced breeder with no helping experience and an experienced breeder (Komdeur 1996c). Inexperienced females took more than a year to produce a first fledgling, but only four months when they had helping experience. Females with either helping or breeding experience built stronger nests that were less prone to be blown away by wind, and spent more time incubating, resulting in higher hatching success than

for inexperienced females. Once the previously inexperienced birds fledged young themselves, they were then able to produce a second fledgling in the same time as experienced birds, suggesting that they had by then learned all the necessary skills.

In this study, we presumed that all the female helpers were nonbreeders and that all dominant females had bred. However, our later work indicated that 44% of helper females in territories with genotyped offspring were assigned maternity, so it is likely that some of the female helpers included were subordinate cobreeders. Either way, this study shows that the females that gain breeding experience as subordinates do better when subsequently breeding as a dominant for the first time than females without breeding experience. Given that some "helping" females may have been cobreeders, however, it does not unequivocally demonstrate that "helping" females do better as a breeder as a result of the experience or skills gained from their behavior.

Territorial inheritance

Helping may lead to higher status within the group and, hence, greater success when competing for a territory after the death of its owner of the same sex as the helper (Zack 1990; Koenig et al. 1992; Balshine-Earn et al. 1998; Leadbeater et al. 2011). Alternatively, helping can result in higher productivity and thus a larger group size, which may make the group more competitive compared to neighboring groups. If the group then increases the size of its territory by outcompeting neighboring groups, the helper may eventually be able to take over a portion of the territory as its own breeding territory (Emlen 1991).

In the Seychelles warbler, territory inheritance is rare and not linked to helping: of the 219 monitored subordinates, only 3.7% (five males and three females) inherited their natal territory (Eikenaar et al. 2008). However, of the males that remained on their natal territory as subordinates, 78% budded off a small portion of the territory for themselves without having ever been a helper (Komdeur and Edelaar 2001). Those males that did help never budded off part of the territory and never inherited a breeding territory after the death or experimental removal of the dominant male (Eikenaar et al. 2008).

Territory inheritance is therefore almost exclusively linked to budding, and not helping, and even then only accounts for about 4% of cases of territory acquisition.

That it is only male subordinates that are able to bud off a new territory may be because male subordinates gain fewer fitness benefits from helping than female subordinates (Figure 12.9). Plus, if helping is costly in terms of condition, males may do better by refraining from helping and instead harboring their resources to mount a challenge to bud off part of a territory and expel intruders.

Pay-to-stay

This hypothesis proposes that individuals that do not help are punished and may be evicted from the territory (Gaston 1978; Balshine-Earn et al. 1998). Importantly, the "resources" that the helpers are paying to get access to are not necessarily food. For example, where subordinates join and help in a group other than their natal group, the goal of helping may be to form social or breeding relationships with nonkin (Croft et al. 2004). This could well be one of the reasons why, in the Seychelles warbler, males – the sex that gains lower fitness benefits from helping on the natal territory than female subordinates – often disperse to become subordinates on nonnatal territories, while females normally remain on their natal territory as subordinates (Richardson et al. 2002). If this is true, the fitness benefits to subordinate males on nonnatal territories should be higher than those to males on natal territories; this remains to be tested.

Group augmentation

Helping may result in the production of more individuals, causing the group to grow larger. This may increase the survival chances of all individuals in the group, because larger groups are better at competing with other groups or deterring predators (Kokko et al. 2001; Clutton-Brock 2002, 2009). Under this scenario, helpers not only gain benefits for themselves, but also benefit other individuals in the breeding group.

In the Seychelles warbler, helpers have both a short- and long-term effect on offspring fitness: the number of helpers in a territory is positively associated with both the offspring's chances of reaching adulthood and its late-life survival as an adult (Figure 12.10). Importantly, larger group size per se does not appear to be beneficial to adults, as individuals living in larger groups had lower survival probabilities than those living in small groups (Figure 12.11). Predation of warbler eggs and nestlings occurs, but adult warblers suffer virtually no predation pressure on Cousin Island; therefore competition for food is the most probable cause of this reduction in adult survival with increasing group size.

Overall, however, the negative effect of increasing group size on individual survival may be counterbalanced by a gain in the reproductive success of subordinates (Richardson et al. 2002). For example, in larger groups, female subordinates may have a higher chance of becoming cobreeders, although this remains to be investigated. Finally, lower survival benefits in larger groups may form an additional selection pressure on subordinates to help rear related offspring in order to gain a compensatory benefit (at least for female subordinates) or to disperse and join a smaller group to offset the negative effects of increasing group size as an adult.

Sex allocation

In the Seychelles warbler, the advantage of having helpers depends on territory quality. Helpers are beneficial for dominant birds on high-quality territories because they improve the reproductive success of breeding pairs. Unassisted dominant females on high-quality territories maximize their fitness by biasing the sex ratio of eggs to females (Figure 12.12) thus producing a greater proportion of female offspring that are likely to become helping subordinates in subsequent years (Komdeur 1996b, Komdeur et al. 1997). When the group includes helping female subordinates, the dominant birds not only gain an increase in their own productivity, but also gain the indirect benefits associated with subordinate females breeding (Richardson et al. 2002). In contrast, unassisted dominant females on medium-quality territories produced sex ratios around parity, and on low-quality territories, where the presence of subordinates is costly for breeding pairs because of competition for food, unassisted dominant females maximize

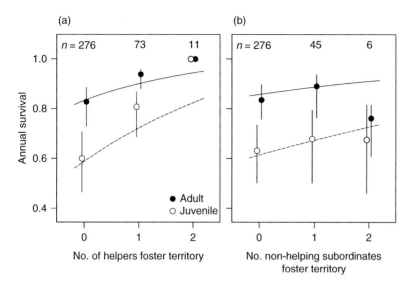

Figure 12.10. Annual adult and juvenile survival probabilities (± S.E.) in relation to (a) the number of helpers in the rearing territory, and (b) the number of nonhelpers in the rearing territory. n denotes the number of individuals that were monitored for survival in their first year of life and subsequently for annual adult survival. From Brouwer et al. (2012).

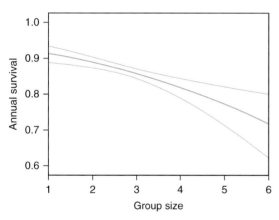

Figure 12.11. Adult survival (± 95% confidence interval) probabilities for an average year (thick lines) in relation to average group size inhabited as an adult. From Brouwer et al. (2006).

their fitness by biasing the egg sex-ratio toward males (Figure 12.12), thus producing a greater proportion of male offspring that will disperse from the natal territory and avoid competing for food with the breeding pair.

This ability to bias the sex ratio, and its link to territory quality, was confirmed during the establishment

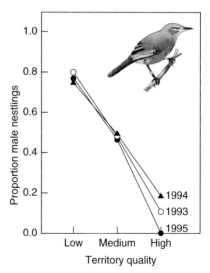

Figure 12.12. Sex ratio of nestlings produced by pairs in relation to quality of breeding territory (low-, medium- and high-quality territories; 1993–1995). Young were hatched from one-egg clutches only. No additional young were present on the territory. From Komdeur et al. (1997).

of a new population on Aride Island. Breeding pairs that were transferred from low- to high-quality territories switched from producing 90% sons to producing 85% daughters. Breeding pairs that were switched between high-quality territories showed no change in sex ratio, producing 80% daughters before and after the switch (Komdeur et al. 1997). Sex-specific embryonic mortality between egg laying and hatching can be ruled out, because the sexes of dead embryos were not biased toward the less adaptive sex (Komdeur et al. 1997, 2002).

We have been able to experimentally confirm the differing fitness consequences of unassisted breeding pairs producing daughters or sons on high- and low-quality territories, respectively. Young nestlings were cross-fostered between unassisted breeding pairs on high- and low-quality territories that were feeding a nestling of the putatively adaptive sex. Pairs breeding on high-quality territories that were allocated foster daughters gained significantly higher inclusive fitness benefits than those raising foster sons, whereas the reverse was true for pairs breeding on low-quality territories (Figure 12.13). These findings provide strong evidence that sex allocation in the Seychelles warbler is adaptive to the breeding pair.

An alternative route to cooperative breeding

In cooperative breeding species helpers are often younger, pre-reproductive individuals that have not yet acquired an independent breeding position (Brown 1987; Cockburn 1998; Koenig and Dickinson 2004; West et al. 2007). In a few long-lived mammalian species, however, older post-reproductive individuals have been documented to provide kin-directed cooperative behavior (Packer et al. 1998; Pavelka et al. 2002). In the Seychelles warbler, we found that some dominant breeders, mainly females, were deposed from their breeding position (Richardson et al. 2007). Importantly, the new dominant females that replaced them were more closely related to the deposed females than one would expect by chance (mean $r = 0.29$); indeed, they are often their daughters. Some of these

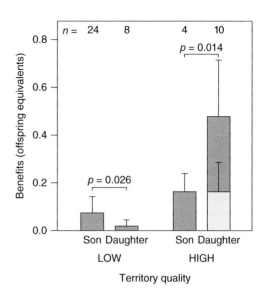

Figure 12.13. Inclusive fitness benefits accrued to focal breeding pairs by producing sons or daughters (1985–1986) on low- and high-quality territories. Fitness benefits (± S.D.; indirect = dark columns, direct = pale columns) were expressed in terms of additional number of yearlings produced by the focal breeding pair through help of their first-generation offspring. The dispersal tactics and reproduction of all first-generation offspring were recorded throughout their lives. *P* values for differences between sons and daughters were determined by two-tailed Mann–Whitney *U* test. *n* denotes number of breeding pairs. Analyses from Komdeur (1998).

deposed females left the territory to become floaters, but 68% remained as subordinate females if, apparently, the quality of the territory was sufficiently high to support another subordinate. Of the demoted subordinates, 64% became helpers for the new dominant female. As of yet, no clear direct benefits have been identified as being gained by these deposed females. It is clear, however, that by helping these new, related dominant females to reproduce, they can gain indirect benefits (Richardson et al. 2007).

In the few other species (including humans) where post-reproductive helping occurs, the cessation of reproduction by older females appears to be a strategy linked to senescence (Packer et al. 1998; Pavelka et al. 2002). This does not appear to be the case in Seychelles warblers. Dominant breeders do not become subordinates as part of a strategy linked to a senescent reduction in their own reproductive output. Indeed many demoted individuals are substantially younger (average age 5.2 years; Richardson et al. 2007) than the age at which reproductive senescence occurs (from age 8 years onward, Hammers et al. 2012).

The observation that adults that have lost a dominant breeding position help their younger relatives is important because this represents an alternative route to cooperative breeding. Becoming a helper is not necessarily an effective strategy for all adult females challenged by a rival, however. The effectiveness of the strategy depends on the degree of relatedness between the demoted female and the new dominant female.

A recent study suggests that an alternative response might be available. If a female dominant allows a subordinate related female helper to cobreed in the same nest she will gain indirect fitness benefits comparable to a demoted nonreproducing female that becomes a helper (Hammers et al. 2012), but in addition the dominant female gains the direct fitness benefits from laying her own egg. For a dominant female it would then be better to allow another subordinate female to become a joint-nester than to be demoted and instead help a new unrelated or less-related dominant female. It remains to be investigated why this does not always happen and why some females become demoted helpers and not cobreed while others adopt the joint-nesting strategy.

Conclusions and prospects

Our study shows that the occurrence of group living and helping behavior in Seychelles warblers can be explained by several ecological and social variables. We discussed the fitness implications resulting from these behaviors, not only for the subordinates but also for the dominants with which they share the territory. Moreover, we also demonstrated that the expression of dispersal behavior and cooperative breeding change over time, and differently for males and females. Despite the long-term nature of our study, however, we are still left with many unresolved questions.

Understanding variation in natal dispersal between and within the sexes

Our study has demonstrated large spatial and temporal variation in the natal dispersal behavior of young Seychelles warblers. At the beginning of our study, young males dispersed from their natal territories more often than females, but later in the study both males and females showed similar natal dispersal. The observed change was the result of females starting to disperse earlier and not the result of a change in the quality of the territories on which males and females were born. We can think of several possible explanations for this change, but the most likely appears to be changes in fitness gained by females dispersing at younger ages. In the beginning of the study period (1982–1990) none of the dispersing female subordinates were observed as floaters and all settled as dominant breeders (Komdeur 1992), whereas later in the study (1995–2005) 16% of dispersing female subordinates became floaters (Eikenaar et al. 2007). These floater females do not gain parentage (there is no egg dumping), and are therefore excluded from reproducing. This increase in the number of female floaters over time suggests that females have more difficulty recruiting into the breeding population and that the fitness gains from leaving the natal territory may have declined over time. If this is true, then the fitness gains from remaining on the natal territory as a subordinate must also have declined, since otherwise it is hard to explain the increased dispersal of females.

To understand the evolution of delayed dispersal, it is important to relate variation in timing of natal dispersal to inclusive fitness benefits gained over the lifetime. This would involve a comparison of fitness costs and benefits before dispersal (remaining on the natal territory as a subordinate) versus the costs and benefits after natal dispersal until death. Furthermore, experiments are needed to show a causal relationship between the timing of natal dispersal and the resultant fitness payoffs. For example, natal dispersal could be delayed by decreasing the group size in which the subordinate lives by removing individuals, or natal dispersal could be advanced by removing a parent (Eikenaar et al. 2007).

In cases where a parent was replaced by a stepparent either naturally or because of the removal of the parent for translocation, young dispersed from the natal territory earlier but were less likely to occupy a breeding vacancy in the next year (Eikenaar et al. 2007). This may indicate that under such circumstances, subordinates cannot postpone dispersal until the best moment, but may be forced out at suboptimal times. The decision to delay natal dispersal may therefore be an adaptive strategy employed by the subordinate to wait until the chances of gaining a breeding position are high.

Furthermore, when a parent was replaced by a stepparent, the likelihood of dispersal was higher for male than female subordinates (Eikenaar et al. 2007). The logic behind this could be that the stepparent could gain fitness benefits if a female subordinate engages in joint nesting (Richardson et al. 2002). Stepparents may evict unrelated subordinates, given the costs of group living (Brouwer et al. 2006), but this counteracts the observation that a dominant pair sometimes tolerates immigrant male subordinates. To investigate parental tolerance, detailed observations on agonistic interactions between subordinates and (step)parents are required.

Understanding the evolution of variation in helping behavior between and within the sexes

Future studies should also focus on the evolutionary causes of sex-biased helping. Our study has demonstrated that female Seychelles warblers gain more direct benefits through cooperation than do males. This may explain the female bias in helping behavior observed early in the study. What, however, are the factors that drive males to disperse earlier and help less? In order to answer this question we need to know what fitness gains are made by early-dispersing males and females relative to the alternative of staying.

We can suggest several ultimate explanations for the observed sex differences:

(1) *Territory ownership is more important for males than for females.* For males, this is a near prerequisite for reproduction, whereas females can reproduce by joint nesting (Richardson et al. 2001, 2002). In other words, males should obtain a territory at the earliest age possible, because every year that a male remains a subordinate is a year with no or very limited reproduction. Given the importance of territory ownership, competition over breeder vacancies may be more intense for males than for females. This is supported by the fact that experimentally created male vacancies were occupied faster than female vacancies (Eikenaar et al. 2009).

(2) *Reduced costs of dispersing by males.* There may be fewer costs of dispersal for males than females, because males may be more readily accepted into new groups. However, it is unknown how or why group members may benefit from the presence of an immigrant male subordinate.

(3) *Higher fitness benefits to males of joining other groups as subordinates.* The higher competition for male vacancies, and the limited fitness benefits accrued from males remaining on the natal territory, might explain why a considerable fraction of males disperse and become subordinates in other groups. Males might disperse and join groups smaller than their natal group to improve their survival prospects, or they might join a group with an old dominant male to improve their chances of reproducing with the dominant female while the dominant male is still alive, or in order to inherit the territory after his death. Males may move to other groups to avoid inbreeding in their natal territory, and choose to become subordinates in groups where they are less related to the females to avoid inbreeding when the males at a later stage become dominants in these group. However, there is as yet no evidence of inbreeding avoidance (Richardson et al. 2004; Eikenaar et al. 2008). Indeed, breeding between first-order relatives is relatively frequent, resulting in >5% of all offspring, despite negative fitness effects in poor-quality seasons (Richardson et al. 2004). Clearly, we lack an understanding of what drives temporal variation in natal dispersal by males and females.

In the Seychelles warbler there is also variation among individuals in whether or not they provide help if there is an opportunity to do so, at least in females. Preliminary analyses suggest that subordinate females that help produce more fledglings over their lifetime than subordinate females that do not help. This was not due to these helping female subordinates having higher annual survival, but instead because they have higher lifetime reproductive success than nonhelping female subordinates (H. Dugdale et al. unpubl. data). Why, then, do not all subordinate females become helpers when an opportunity arises? This may be linked to their relatedness to the dominant female, as discussed earlier, but there may also be other reasons. For example, it might be that only subordinates in sufficiently high condition can afford to help. In the Seychelles warbler there is evidence that declines in condition are associated with helping, and that the expression of helping behavior is determined by body condition (van de Crommenacker et al. 2011, 2012). Up to now, condition-dependence in dispersal has rarely been incorporated into models of helping strategies (Heinsohn and Legge 1999; Russell et al. 2003; Covas and Griesser 2007; Lawson Handley and Perrin 2007).

Finally, in our studies of the Seychelles warbler we were able to estimate the direct lifetime fitness benefits – the total number of fledglings produced – as a result of helping. It is extremely difficult, however, to assess all the inclusive fitness benefits that are gained. We have a good long-term database on individual-level dispersal behavior and helping strategies, social and environmental parameters, and a genetic pedigree. But it is still a very challenging and complex task to compare an individual's potential inclusive fitness benefit from dispersal versus that gained from remaining in the group and subsequently helping, or not. This is because of hidden effects. For example, helping can also have long-term fitness effects for the offspring that have received helped (i.e., greater later-life survival; Brouwer et al. 2012), and living in groups itself can have costs irrespective of helping. Nonetheless, the unique features of the Seychelles warbler study offer the opportunity to answer this, and other, important questions.

Acknowledgments

We are grateful to Nature Seychelles for allowing us to work on Cousin Island, providing accommodation and facilities and for collaborating with us on various aspects of the warbler conservation and research. The Department of Environment and the Seychelles Bureau of Standards gave permission for fieldwork and blood sampling. We thank numerous students and colleagues for help in the field and for sharing their ideas, including Iain Barr, Emma Barrett, Dorte Bekkevold, Karen Blaakmeer, Lyanne Brouwer, Tom Clarke, Corine Eising, Janske van de Crommenacker, Arjan Dekker, Damian Dowling, Jan Drachmann, Hannah Edwards, Cas Eikenaar, Danni Gilroy, Frank Groenewoud, Martijn Hammers, Ian Hartley, Kim Hutchins, Sjouke Kingma, Kees van Oers, Lewis Spurgin, Thor Veen, Jildou van der Woude, David Wright, and many more. The genetic analyses undertaken at the University of Sheffield were undertaken by Francine Jury and Patricia Salguiero, with the support of Deborah Dawson and Andy Krupa, and at Groningen University were undertaken by Marco van der Velde. We also thank Sjouke Kingma, David Wright, and Lewis Spurgin for their helpful comments on this chapter. We are extremely grateful for the financial support provided by the Netherlands Organization for Scientific Research, the U.K. Natural Environmental Research Council, the Australian Research Council, the EU Marie Curie Fellowship Programme, the Schure-Beijerinck-Popping Foundation, the Dobberke Foundation for Comparative Psychology, the Lucie Burgers Foundation for Comparative Behaviour Research, and the Universities of East Anglia, Groningen, and Sheffield.

REFERENCES

Arnold, K. E. and Owens I. P. F. (1998). Cooperative breeding in birds: a comparative test of the life history hypothesis. *Proc. R. Soc. London B*, 265, 739–745.

Balshine-Earn, S., Neat, F. C., Reid, H., and Taborsky, M. (1998). Paying to stay or paying to breed? Field evidence for direct benefits of helping behavior in a cooperatively breeding fish. *Behav. Ecol.*, 9, 432–458.

Barrett, E. L. B., Burke, T., Hammers, M., Komdeur, J., and Richardson, D. S. (2013). Telomere length and dynamics predict mortality in a wild longitudinal study. *Mol. Ecol.*, 47, 41–53.

Bathe, G. M. and Bathe, H. V. (1982). *Territory size and habitat requirements of the Seychelles Brush warbler* Acrocephalus (Bebrornis) sechellensis. Cambridge: International Council for Bird Preservation, Internal Report.

Bennett, P. M. and Owens, I. P. F. (2002). *Evolutionary Ecology of Birds–Life Histories, Mating Systems, and Extinction*. Oxford: Oxford University Press.

Berg, E. C., Eadie, J. M., Langen, T. A., and Russell, A. F. (2009). Reverse sex-biased philopatry in a cooperative bird: genetic consequences and a social cause. *Mol. Ecol.*, 18, 3486–3499.

Brouwer, L., Richardson, D. S., Eikenaar, C., and Komdeur, J. (2006). The role of group size and environmental factors on survival in a cooperatively breeding tropical passerine. *J. Anim. Ecol.*, 75, 1321–1329.

Brouwer, L., Tinbergen, J. M., Both, C., Bristol, R., Richardson, D. S., et al. (2009). Experimental evidence for density-dependent reproduction in a cooperatively breeding passerine. *Ecology*, 90, 729–741.

Brouwer, L., Richardson, D. S., and Komdeur J. (2012). Helpers at the nest improve late-life offspring performance: evidence from a long-term study and a cross-foster experiment. *PLoS One*, 7, e33167.

Brown, J. L. (1978). Avian communal breeding systems. *Annu. Rev. Ecol. Syst.*, 9, 123–155.

Brown, J. L. (1987). *Helping and Communal Breeding in Birds: Ecology and Evolution.* Princeton, NJ: Princeton University Press.

Clutton-Brock, T. H. (2002). Breeding together: kin selection and mutualism in cooperative vertebrates. *Science*, 296, 69–72.

Clutton-Brock, T. (2009) Cooperation between non-kin in animal societies. *Nature*, 462, 51–57.

Cockburn, A. (1998). Evolution of helping behavior in cooperatively breeding birds. *Annu. Rev. Ecol. Syst.*, 29, 141–177.

Collar, N. J. and Stuart, S. N. (1985). *Threatened Birds of Africa and Related Islands.* Cambridge: ICBP/IUCN Red Data Book Part 1. International Council for Bird Preservation.

Cornwallis, C. K., West, S. A., and Griffin, A. S. (2009). Routes to indirect fitness in cooperatively breeding vertebrates: kin discrimination and limited dispersal. *J. Evol. Biol.*, 22, 2445–2457.

Covas, R. and Griesser, M. (2007). Life history and the evolution of family living in birds. *Proc. R. Soc. London B*, 274, 1349–1357.

Croft, D. P., Krause, J. and James, R. (2004). Social networks in the guppy (*Poecilia reticulata*). *Biol. Lett.*, 271, 516–519.

Crook, J. (1960). *The Present Status of Certain Rare Land-birds of the Seychelles Islands.* Unnumbered Seychelles Government Bulletin, Department of the Environment, Victoria.

Dickinson, J. L. and Hatchwell, B. J. (2004). The fitness consequences of helping. In: *Ecology and Evolution of Cooperative Breeding in Birds*, ed. W. D. Koenig and J. L. Dickinson. Cambridge: Cambridge University Press, pp. 48–66.

Dickinson, J. L., Koenig, W. D., and Pitelka, F. A. (1996). Fitness consequences of helping behavior in the western bluebird. *Behav. Ecol.*, 7, 168–177.

Eikenaar, C., Richardson, D. S., Brouwer, L., and Komdeur, J. (2007). Parent presence, delayed dispersal, and territory acquisition in the Seychelles warbler. *Behav. Ecol.*, 18, 874–879.

Eikenaar, C., Komdeur, J., and Richardson, D. S. (2008). Natal dispersal patterns are not associated with inbreeding avoidance in the Seychelles warbler. *J. Evol. Biol.*, 21, 1106–1116.

Eikenaar, C., Richardson, D. S., Brouwer, L., Bristol, R., and Komdeur, J. (2009). Experimental evaluation of sex differences in territory acquisition in a cooperatively breeding bird. *Behav. Ecol.*, 20, 207–214.

Eikenaar, C., Brouwer, L., Komdeur, J., and Richardson, D. S. (2010). Sex biased natal dispersal is not a fixed trait in a stable population of Seychelles warblers. *Behaviour*, 147, 1577–1590.

Ekman, J, Dickinson, J. L., Hatchwell, B. J., and Griesser, M. (2004). Delayed dispersal. In: *Ecology and Evolution of Cooperative Breeding in Birds*, ed. W. D. Koenig and J. L. Dickinson. Cambridge: Cambridge University Press, pp. 35–47.

Emlen, S. T. (1982). The evolution of helping. I. An ecological constraints model. *Am. Nat.*, 119, 29–39.

Emlen, S. T. (1991). The evolution of cooperative breeding in birds and mammals. In: *Behavioural Ecology: an Evolutionary Approach*, 3rd edn, ed. J. R. Krebs and N. B. Davies. Oxford: Blackwell, pp. 301–337.

Gaston, A. J. (1978). The evolution of group territorial behavior and cooperative breeding. *Am. Nat.*, 112, 1091–1100.

Griffin, A. S. and West, S. A. (2002). Kin selection: fact and fiction. *Trends. Ecol. Evol.*, 17, 15–21.

Hadfield, J. D., Richardson, D. S., and Burke, T. (2006). Towards unbiased parentage assignment: combining genetic, behavioural and spatial data in a Bayesian framework. *Mol. Ecol.*, 15, 3715–3730.

Hammers, M., Richardson, D. S., Burke, T., and Komdeur, J. (2012). Age-dependent terminal declines in reproductive output in a wild bird. *PLoS One*, 7, e40413.

Hamilton, W. D. (1964). The genetical evolution of social behaviour I and II. *J. Theor. Biol.*, 7, 1–52.

Hatchwell, B. J. and Komdeur, J. (2000). Ecological constraints, life history traits and the evolution of cooperative breeding. *Anim. Behav.*, 59, 1079–1086.

Hatchwell, B. J., Russell, A. F., Fowlie, M. K., and Ross, D. J. (1999). Reproductive success and nest-site selection in a cooperative breeder: effect of experience and a direct benefit of helping. *Auk*, 116, 355–363.

Heinsohn, R. G. and Legge, S. (1999). The cost of helping. *Trends Ecol. Evol.*, 14, 53–57.

IUCN (2013). *IUCN Red List of Threatened Species.* Version 2013.2. www.iucnredlist.org.

Koenig, W. D. and Dickinson, J. L., eds. (2004). *Ecology and Evolution of Cooperative Breeding in Birds.* Cambridge: Cambridge University Press.

Koenig, W. D., Pitelka, F. A., Carmen, W. J., Mumme, R. L., and Stanback, M. T. (1992). The evolution of delayed dispersal in cooperative breeders. *Q. Rev. Biol.*, 67, 111–150.

Kokko, H., Johnstone, R. A., and Clutton-Brock, T. H. (2001). The evolution of cooperative breeding through group augmentation. *Proc. R. Soc. London B*, 268, 187–196.

Komdeur, J. (1992). Importance of habitat saturation and territory quality for evolution of cooperative breeding in the Seychelles warbler. *Nature*, 358, 493–495.

Komdeur, J. (1994a). Conserving the Seychelles warbler *Acrocephalus sechellensis* by translocation from Cousin Island to the islands of Aride and Cousine. *Biol. Conserv.*, 76, 143–152.

Komdeur, J. (1994b). Experimental evidence for helping and hindering by previous offspring in the cooperative-breeding Seychelles warbler *Acrocephalus sechellensis*. *Behav. Ecol. Sociobiol.*, 34, 175–186.

Komdeur, J. (1996a). Seasonal timing of reproduction in a tropical bird, the Seychelles warbler: a field experiment using translocation. *J. Biol. Rhythms*, 11, 333–346.

Komdeur, J. (1996b). Facultative sex ratio bias in the offspring of Seychelles warblers. *Proc. R. Soc. London B*, 263, 661–666.

Komdeur, J. (1996c). Influence of helping and breeding experience on reproductive performance in the Seychelles warbler: a translocation experiment. *Behav. Ecol.*, 7, 326–333.

Komdeur, J. (1998). Long-term fitness benefits of egg sex modification by the Seychelles warbler. *Ecol. Lett.*, 1, 56–62.

Komdeur, J. (2003). Daughters on request: about helpers and egg sexes in the Seychelles warbler. *Proc. R. Soc. London B*, 270, 3–11.

Komdeur, J. and Edelaar, P. (2001). Male Seychelles warblers use territory budding to maximize lifetime fitness in a saturated environment. *Behav. Ecol.*, 12, 706–715.

Komdeur, J. and Pels, M. D. (2005). Rescue of the Seychelles warbler on Cousin Island, Seychelles: the role of habitat restoration. *Biol. Conserv.*, 124, 305–313.

Komdeur, J., Huffstadt, A., Prast, W., Castle, G., Mileto, R., et al. (1995). Transfer experiments of Seychelles warblers to new islands: changes in dispersal and helping behaviour. *Anim. Behav.*, 49, 695–708.

Komdeur, J., Daan, S., Tinbergen, J., and Mateman, C. (1997). Extreme adaptive modification in sex ratio of the Seychelles warbler's eggs. *Nature*, 385, 522–525.

Komdeur, J., Piersma, T., Kraaijeveld, K., Kraaijeveld-Smit, F., and Richardson, D. S. (2004a). Why Seychelles warblers fail to recolonize nearby islands: unwilling or unable to fly there? *Ibis*, 146, 298–302.

Komdeur, J., Burke, T., and Richardson, D. S. (2004b). Experimental evidence that kin discrimination in the Seychelles warbler is based on association and not on genetic relatedness. *Proc. R. Soc. London B*, 271, 963–969.

Komdeur, J., Eikenaar, C., Brouwer, L., and Richardson, D. S. (2008). The evolution and ecology of cooperative breeding in vertebrates. In: *Encyclopedia of Life Sciences*. Chichester: John Wiley and Sons, Ltd, pp. 1–8.

Lawson Handley, L. J. and Perrin, N. (2007). Advances in our understanding of mammalian sex-biased dispersal. *Mol. Ecol.*, 16, 1559–1578.

Leadbeater, E., Carruthers, J. M., Green, J. P., Rosser, N. S., and Field, J. (2011). Nest inheritance is the missing source of direct fitness in a primitively eusocial insect. *Science*, 333, 874–876.

Lessells, C. M. (1991). The evolution of life histories. In: *Behavioural Ecology: An Evolutionary Approach*, 3rd edn, ed. J. R. Krebs and N. B. Davies. Oxford: Blackwell, pp. 32–68.

Loustau-Lalanne, P. (1968). *The Seychelles, Cousin Island Nature Reserve*. Cambridge: International Council for Bird Preservation, Internal report.

Orchard, D. (2004). Aride Seychelles warbler Census. In: *Annual Report 2003. Aride Island Nature Reserve, Seychelles*, ed. M. Betts. Royal Society of Wildlife Trusts, unpublished report.

Oustalet, M. E. (1878). Etude sur la faune ornithologique des isles Seychelles. *Bull. Soc. Philomath. Paris*, 7, 161–206.

Packer, C., Tatar, M., and Collins, A. (1998). Reproductive cessation in female mammals. *Nature*, 392, 807–811.

Pavelka, M. S. M., Fedigan, L. M., and Zohar, S. (2002). Availability and adaptive value of reproductive and postreproductive Japanese macaque mothers and grandmothers. *Anim. Behav.*, 64, 407–414.

Richardson, D. S., Jury, F. L., Blaakmeer, K., Komdeur, J., and Burke, T. (2001). Parentage assignment and extra-group paternity in a cooperative breeder: the Seychelles warbler (*Acrocephalus sechellensis*). *Mol. Ecol.*, 10, 2263–2273.

Richardson, D. S, Burke, T., and Komdeur, J. (2002). Direct benefits explain the evolution of female biased cooperative breeding in the Seychelles warblers. *Evolution*, 56, 2313–2321.

Richardson, D. S., Komdeur, J., and Burke, T. (2003a). Altruism and infidelity among warblers. *Nature*, 422, 580.

Richardson, D. S., Burke, T., and Komdeur, J. (2003b). Sex-specific associative learning cues and inclusive fitness benefits in the Seychelles warbler. *J. Evol. Biol.*, 16, 854–861.

Richardson, D. S., Komdeur, J., and Burke, T. (2004). Inbreeding in the Seychelles warbler: environment-dependent maternal effects. *Evolution*, 58, 2037–2048.

Richardson, D. S., Bristol, R., and Shah, N. J. (2006). Translocation of the Seychelles warbler *Acrocephalus sechellensis* to establish a new population on Denis Island, Seychelles. *Conserv. Evidence*, 3, 54–57.

Richardson, D. S., Burke, T., and Komdeur, J. (2007). Grandparent helpers: the adaptive significance of older, postdominant helpers in the Seychelles warbler. *Evolution*, 31, 2790–2800.

Russell, A. F., Sharpe, L. L., Brotherton, P. N. M., and Clutton-Brock, T. H. (2003). Cost minimization by helpers in cooperative vertebrates. *Proc. Natl. Acad. Sci. (USA)*, 100, 3333–3338.

Safford, R. and Hawkins, F. (2013). The Seychelles warbler. In: *The Birds of Africa: Volume VIII: The Malagasy Region: Madagascar, Seychelles, Comoros, Mascarenes*. London: Christopher Helm, pp. 758–760.

Spurgin, L., Wright, D. J., van der Velde, M., Collar, N. J., Komdeur, J., et al. (2014). Museum DNA reveals the demographic history of the endangered Seychelles warbler. *Evol. Applic.*, 7, 1134–1143.

Stacey, P. B. and Koenig, W. D., eds. (1990). *Cooperative Breeding in Birds: Long-term Studies of Ecology and Behavior*. Cambridge: Cambridge University Press.

Stacey, P. B. and Ligon, J. D. (1987). Territory quality and dispersal options in the acorn woodpecker, and a challenge to the habitat-saturation model of cooperative breeding. *Am. Nat.*, 130, 654–676.

Stacey, P. B. and Ligon, J. D. (1991). The benefits-of-philopatry hypothesis for the evolution of cooperative breeding: variation in territory quality and group-size effects. *Am. Nat*, 137, 831–846.

Teunissen, N. (2013). A newly translocated population of the Seychelles warbler: is there evidence for interspecific competition with Seychelles white-eyes? M.Sc. thesis, Groningen University, The Netherlands.

van de Crommenacker, J. and Richardson, D. S. (2007) Monitoring and Studying the Seychelles warbler: fieldwork on Cousine Island. Report from the University of East Anglia, U.K./ University of Groningen, Netherlands.

van de Crommenacker, J., Komdeur, J., and Richardson, D. S. (2011). Assessing the cost of helping: the roles of body condition and oxidative balance in the Seychelles warbler (*Acrocephalus sechellensis*). PLoS One, 6, e26423.

van de Crommenacker, J., Richardson, D. S., Koltz, A. M., Hutchings, K., and Komdeur, J. (2012). Parasitic infection and oxidative stress are associated and vary with breeding activity in the Seychelles warbler. *Proc. R. Soc. London B*, 279, 1466–1476.

West, S. A., Griffin A. S., and Gardner, A. (2007). Evolutionary explanations for cooperation. *Curr. Biol.*, 17, 661–672.

Wright, D. J., Shah, N. J., and Richardson, D. S. (2014). Translocation of the Seychelles warbler *Acrocephalus sechellensis* to establish a new population on Frégate Island. *Conserv. Evidence*, 11, 20–24.

Zack, S. (1990). Coupling delayed breeding with short-distance dispersal in cooperatively breeding birds. *Ethology*, 86, 265–286.

13

Acorn woodpeckers: Helping at the nest, polygynandry, and dependence on a variable acorn crop

Walter D. Koenig, Eric L. Walters, and Joseph Haydock

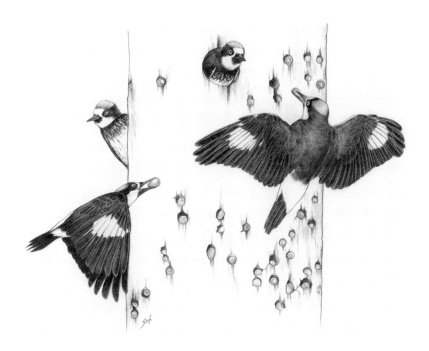

Introduction

The acorn woodpecker (*Melanerpes formicivorus*) plays an important role in the history of cooperative breeding. It was one of the earliest species for which cooperative breeding was noted with more than two individuals feeding at a single nest as well as apparent mate-sharing (Myers 1915; Leach 1925; Michael

1927). Subsequently, in his classic *Animal Dispersion in Relation to Social Behaviour*, V. C. Wynne-Edwards singled out the acorn-storing habits of this species as a means by which birds assessed the food supply and adjusted their breeding so as to avoid overexploitation of resources. Indeed, Wynne-Edwards suggested that acorn storing was "the perfect example of an epideictic rite, combining as it does a sampling of the

Cooperative Breeding in Vertebrates: Studies of Ecology, Evolution, and Behavior, eds W. D. Koenig and J. L. Dickinson.
Published by Cambridge University Press. © Cambridge University Press 2016.

food-supply, a territorial symbol (the tree), and social competition" (Wynne-Edwards 1962: 325). Four years later, cooperative breeding in this species was predicted to be based (this time accurately) on kinship in G. C. Williams's *Adaptation and Natural Selection*, written to counter the group-selectionist bent of Wynne-Edwards (Williams 1966).

It was but a few years after Williams' prediction, itself an outgrowth of W. D. Hamilton's (1964) papers introducing inclusive fitness theory, that Michael and Barbara MacRoberts began a study of acorn woodpeckers at Hastings Reservation in central coastal California, a field station run by the Museum of Vertebrate Zoology at the University of California, Berkeley. During the years of their work from 1968 to 1974 they banded 139 birds and described many aspects of their ecology and social behavior (MacRoberts and MacRoberts 1976). It is their study that the senior author took up in July 1974 and has worked on continuously ever since along with a series of students and collaborators, most recently the two coauthors of this manuscript. The work summarized here is thus a product of over 40 years of study during which time we have banded over 5,500 individuals and followed over 1,600 nests. We also refer when appropriate to earlier parallel studies conducted by Peter Stacey at Water Canyon, New Mexico and The Research Ranch in southeastern Arizona (Stacey and Bock 1978; Stacey 1979a, 1979b), updating results summarized in Koenig and Stacey (1990).

Acorn woodpeckers are a New World species found in oak woodlands along the Pacific Coast of North America between southern Washington State and Baja California, the American Southwest, and the mountains of western Mexico, Central America, and northern Colombia. On the Pacific Coast of California, where our study was conducted, adults (but not fledglings up until their prebasic [or postjuvenal] molt several months after fledging) are sexually dichromatic and slightly, but significantly, sexually dimorphic in size (mean ± standard deviation [S.D.] mass of adult males is 80.1 ± 4.7 g [$N = 345$] compared to 76.5 ± 4.7 g [$N = 432$] for females). Acorn woodpeckers eat a diverse array of insects, which they primarily flycatch and glean from bark, as well as on sap and fruit, including most prominently

acorns harvested from oaks (mostly trees of the genus *Quercus*) and store in individually-drilled holes in storage trees, or granaries. Vertebrates, including small lizards, bats, and nestling swallows, are also eaten occasionally (Fajer et al. 1987). Exceptions to their extensive use of stored acorns include populations that have been observed in central Mexico (Koenig and Williams 1979) and Colombia (Kattan 1988), which do not necessarily store acorns, and a few populations in the southwestern United States that are known to be migratory (Stacey and Bock 1978).

No population of acorn woodpeckers has yet been described that does not facultatively breed cooperatively, although group size varies considerably, from a mean of 4.5 birds (range 2–15) during the spring breeding season at Hastings Reservation to a mean of 2.2 birds (range 2–3) in the largely migratory (and mostly noncooperatively breeding) population studied by Stacey at the Research Ranch in Arizona. Groups in a third population studied by Stacey in Water Canyon, New Mexico, were intermediate in size (Koenig and Stacey 1990). Of the small proportion of groups at the Research Ranch that contained more than a pair, most were trios that included a nonbreeding helper. Thus, cooperative polygamy was absent in the Research Ranch population, and even helpers were uncommon and only found among groups that managed to gather and store enough food to remain resident through the winter (Stacey and Bock 1978).

In contrast, at Hastings Reservation, 39% of groups consist of breeding pairs, 31% of groups consist of at least two cobreeder males (maximum = 8) and one breeder female; 9% consist of at least two joint-nesting females (maximum = 4) and one breeder male, and 14% are polygynandrous groups consisting of two or more cobreeder males and at least two joint-nesting females (data from 1,481 group-years studied during the breeding season between 1972 and 2012). The presence of nonbreeding helpers in a group is similarly variable: of the 1,481 group-years, 42% had no helpers and 58% had between one and 10 helpers (mean ± S.D. = 1.55 ± 1.85), which are of both sexes but slightly male-biased (of 2253 helpers, 1294 [57.4%] were male). Thus, there is considerable variability in group composition both within and between populations.

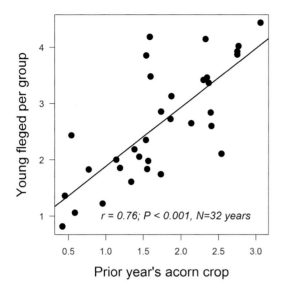

Figure 13.1. Mean young fledged per group versus the prior autumn's acorn crop.

Along the Pacific Coast of the United States, where acorn woodpeckers are resident and dependent on stored acorns, populations are largely restricted to areas with at least two species of oaks, most likely because the higher diversity reduces the probability of an acorn crop failure, and populations vary less in numbers from year to year in areas where the diversity of oak species is greater (Bock and Bock 1974; Koenig and Haydock 1999). The strong effect of the acorn crop on the demography of acorn woodpeckers within a population is vividly demonstrated by the catastrophic effects of acorn crop failures on group composition and population size (Hannon et al. 1987) and, conversely, a strong correlation between the size of the acorn crop and subsequent reproductive success of the population (Figure 13.1) including autumnal nesting – a relatively rare event among temperate-zone birds – in years of particularly prolific acorn crops (Koenig and Stahl 2007). The relationship between reproductive success and the prior autumn's acorn crop is considerably stronger than the relationship between reproductive success and other environmental factors, including rainfall or temperature during either the winter or the breeding season (Koenig et al. in press).

Oaks are in general mast-fruiting species among which the acorn crop is a "pulsed" resource whose availability varies greatly not only seasonally but from year to year (Koenig et al. 1994). For the acorn woodpeckers, seasonal access to acorns is supplemented with alternative food resources and acorn storage, while variability in acorn availability from year to year is reduced as a result of oak species diversity. At Hastings Reservation, for example, birds have access to between three and five species of oaks, depending on the location of their territory. Nonetheless, populations are subject to considerable variability in conditions from year to year, which has effects not only on reproductive success but on survivorship, population size, group composition, and the behavior of individuals within groups (Koenig et al. in press).

Except for years of acorn crop failures and a few populations (such as that studied by Stacey in Arizona), groups are resident and territorial throughout the year, defending their territory intraspecifically against intruders from other groups and interspecifically from a wide range of other birds and mammals that try to steal acorns from their granaries (MacRoberts and MacRoberts 1976). Birds do, however, regularly foray outside their usual home ranges, foraging for acorns when the crop is poor (Koenig et al. 2008) and (as non-breeding helpers) searching for reproductive vacancies (Koenig et al. 1996). Breeder dispersal also occurs, and is surprisingly common, with 10%, or if we include birds that left the study area and returned, 25% of birds leaving the first territory on which they hold breeding status. Breeding dispersal occurs primarily to avoid incest or to move to a territory of higher quality (Haydock et al. unpubl. data).

Cooperation and competition

Social and genetic mating system

Acorn woodpecker groups are family-based and, as indicated above, consist of two categories of birds: breeders and helpers. Breeder males consist of a coalition of brothers or of fathers and their sons, all of which compete for matings with the breeder female(s).

Similarly, breeder females are a coalition of sisters or a mother and her daughter, all of which generally lay their eggs in a single nest cavity. Because of communal nesting, a group has only a single nest at a time regardless of its composition; only one exception to this rule has been found during the study thus far. Helpers are offspring from the communal nests that delay dispersal and remain in their natal group but do not participate in breeding. Helpers remain in their natal territory for a variable length of time during which they contribute to group activities including acorn storage, feeding of nestlings, and territorial defense, while engaging in forays off the territory in search of reproductive vacancies elsewhere (Koenig et al. 1996).

Birds within groups are consequently all genetically closely related to each other (siblings or parent/offspring), the exception being that the breeder males are generally unrelated to the breeder females. Nonetheless, birds within groups exhibit an impressive array of competitive, as well as cooperative, behaviors. Among breeder males, competition for matings is expressed by mate guarding, but strong mate-guarding behavior only occurs when there are two or more cobreeder males within a group and not when there is only a single breeder male and one or more helper males – the latter constrained from attempting to breed because of incest avoidance. These attributes indicate that mate guarding is an expression of within-group competition rather than related to guarding against copulations by extra-group males (Mumme et al. 1983a). Meanwhile, competition between cobreeder females is expressed most dramatically by egg destruction whereby a breeder female laying an egg will have it removed from the nest by another breeder female in the group up until the latter is about to lay her first egg (Mumme et al. 1983b; Koenig et al. 1995). Eggs removed from a nest are taken to a horizontal limb where a crevice provides a suitable spot to hold it and then eaten by all group members, including the female that laid it.

Egg destruction by joint-nesting females is particularly detrimental in terms of delaying breeding, since it can take a week or more for two females to synchronize their egg-laying so as to produce a communal clutch, and even longer when there are three joint-nesting females. Moreover, a high proportion of eggs are potentially lost; in one case in which three females attempted to breed together, 15 of 23 eggs (65%) were destroyed and only eight were eventually incubated (Koenig et al. 1995). Such competition reduces the relative benefit of female joint nesting compared to male cobreeding, presumably contributing to the greater incidence of the latter: 47% of 1,481 group-years involved two or more cobreeder males compared to 23% that involved two or more joint-nesting females. Overall, the mean (± standard error [S.E.]) number of cobreeding males per group is 1.73 ± 0.03 whereas the mean number of joint-nesting females per group is 1.22 ± 0.02; similarly, the proportion of males cobreeding with at least one other male is 71% compared to 41% of females that nest jointly with one (rarely more) other females.

Beyond influencing the relative costs and benefits of cobreeding, the outcome of these interactions is very different for the two sexes. Because of egg destruction, joint-nesting females share maternity more equally than expected by chance (Haydock and Koenig 2002, 2003). Breeder males, however, exhibit high reproductive skew, with one male monopolizing paternity of a brood approximately two-thirds of the time. Tests of reproductive skew versus estimates of ecological constraints on independent reproduction and on relatedness failed to find consistent support for transactional models of reproductive skew, whether assuming complete control on the part of a single dominant individual ("concessions" models) or assuming that dominants have limited or incomplete control ("restraint" models) (Haydock and Koenig 2003). This suggests that factors not necessarily considered in these models such as competitive interactions among potential breeders and mate choice are important determinants of parentage.

Between broods sired by the same set of males, however, there is frequent switching of paternity, raising the possibility that males share paternity equally on a brood by brood, rather than a nestling by nestling, basis. In other words, paternity of a brood may be a fair "winner take all" game in which the probability of winning is equal, rather than paternity of each chick being determined independently. If so, it explains the observation that male paternal care among cobreeders

Table 13.1. Behavior of cobreeder males vis-à-vis their realized paternity at nests

	Sex	Bird with more parentage did more	Bird with less parentage did more	P-value
Behavior at nests				
Provisioning	Males	31	19	0.12
	Females	12	12	1.0
Nest sanitation	Males	12	22	0.12
	Females	7	6	1.0
Brooding and incubation	Males	15	15	1.0
	Females	5	8	0.58
Nocturnal roosting in the nest (males only)		Male with some paternity	Male with no paternity	
Roosted	Males	9	7	1.0
Did not roost	Males	9	6	
		Male with majority of paternity	Male with minority of paternity	
Roosted	Males	4	11	0.14
Did not roost	Males	9	6	

None of the behaviors appear to correlate with paternity, consistent with the hypothesis that cobreeder males do not know whether they have paternity or not in a particular nest.

is uncorrelated with realized paternity. That is, the male who sires all or most of the young in any particular nest is often not the male that contributes the most paternal care at the nest or even one of the birds that spends the night in the nest incubating eggs or brooding young (Table 13.1). Apparently males do not have information on whether they have successfully sired young in a particular nest, but behave as if they may have done so regardless of the actual outcome.

One caveat to this conclusion may be when a large number of males – four or more – share breeding status in a group. In such cases, which typically result from helper males inheriting breeding status following the death and replacement of their mothers by one or more unrelated females, younger, subordinate males may have such a low probability of successfully siring young that for all practical purposes they are nonbreeding helpers. Such cases are not common, however; only 6.4% of groups contained four or more (maximum of eight) cobreeder males. A similar situation resulting in the exclusion of one or more individuals from

reproduction may apply to the rare cases when four females share breeder status, which has occurred in only <1% ($n = 10$) of group-years.

Characterizing the social mating system is thus problematic to the extent that a significant proportion of males considered to be "breeders" may not successfully sire offspring in any particular nest or within a given year. Furthermore, copulations are rarely observed, and thus there is little behavioral evidence to support assertions regarding which males are or are not "attempting" to breed. Because the breeding success of such birds is constrained by reproductive competition rather than incest avoidance, however, we consider them cobreeders rather than helpers, as explained in Chapter 20.

We tested this approach with experiments in which we removed eggs in nests with cobreeder males (i.e., males unrelated to the breeder female) shortly after laying in order to force groups to renest, and then compared paternity in the eggs artificially incubated from the first (experimental) nest with paternity

Table 13.2. Switching of majority paternity (the male siring the most young) across nests produced by the same coalition of cobreeder males within the same breeding season

Comparison		Switched	Did not switch	% switching
N cobreeder males	2	21	28	43
	2+	10	11	48
Relationship of male	Father/son	7	9	44
cobreeders	Siblings	24	30	44
N joint-nesting females	1	18	33	35
	2	13	6	68

There is no significant difference in the tendency for switching in relation to male coalition size or relationship of cobreeders (Fisher exact tests; $P > 0.05$). Switching is, however, significantly higher in groups containing two joint-nesting females compared to those with only a female ($P < 0.02$).

in the renesting attempt. Switching of paternity is common, regardless of male coalition size, whether cobreeders were brothers or a father and his son, or even the number of breeder females in the group, although switching is more common in groups with two joint-nesting females than those with only a single breeder female (Table 13.2). These results support the assumption that males unrelated to the breeder females in a group are all at least "hopeful breeders," even if they fail to sire young during any particular nesting attempt.

One way in which the mating system of acorn woodpeckers is straightforward is in the absence of extra-group parentage. No offspring whose parentage has been determined thus far has been unambiguously identified as having been the result of intraspecific nest parasitism, quasiparasitism, or an extra-group mating on the part of a female. This is consistent with the conclusion reached from mate-guarding indicating that mate-guarding is a behavior directed toward cobreeder males within the group rather than against the unlikely possibility that females will attempt to mate outside their social unit (Mumme et al. 1983a; Dickinson et al. 1995).

In summary, the mating system of the acorn woodpecker is opportunistically polygynandrous, with groups consisting of between one and eight related, cobreeding males competing for matings with a lesser number (usually one or two but rarely as many as four) joint-nesting females, plus their offspring (up to 10 of either sex) from prior years that participate in all group activities with the exception of mating. Joint-nesting females generally share maternity equally within nests; cobreeder males exhibit significant reproductive skew on a nest by nest basis, but switching is common and paternity is egalitarian across nests, except possibly for subordinate males and females in unusually large coalitions. Mating is always within the group; extra-group paternity or egg-dumping is at most rare.

Reproductive vacancies and incest avoidance

The close genetic relatedness combined with the opportunity for multiple individuals of both sexes to breed makes acorn woodpeckers ideal for investigating the importance of incest avoidance. Particularly key is the question of how groups persist through time, specifically when they are faced with a reproductive vacancy following the death or disappearance of all breeders of one sex. (The death of cobreeders does not result in a reproductive vacancy as long as at least one breeder of that sex is still present.)

Reproductive vacancies are of interest for several reasons. First, they are not generally filled by birds from within the group, but rather by coalitions of sibling helpers from elsewhere. Second, vacancies are often not filled quietly, but rather following contests called "power struggles" involving helpers (often fighting in coalitions of same-sex siblings) from many territories away competing for the right to fill the vacancy (Koenig 1981; Hannon et al. 1985). Exactly how birds recognize vacancies is not known for sure; there is some evidence that surviving birds within groups advertise vacancies by means of increased rates of vocalization (Hannon et al. 1985), but vacancies are sometimes detected in less than an hour, even among groups still containing adult helpers of the missing sex, and it seems possible, albeit untested, that foraying birds are sufficiently familiar with the individuals in some groups that they are able to detect when a reproductive vacancy exists through some other means and act accordingly.

Power struggles end when one coalition of birds successfully drives off competing coalitions to the periphery of the territory, from where the losing birds eventually return home and resume their status as nonbreeding helpers. In general, the largest participating coalition wins power struggles, and after a victory, members of the coalition may all remain and become cobreeders in the new territory. This is not always the case, however, particularly among females, for which competition to fill vacancies is particularly intense, and sometimes large winning coalitions subsequently break up, leaving a smaller, more tractable number of females to breed in the new territory while the remaining coalition members fill a vacancy elsewhere or return home.

Reproductive vacancies are often filled very quickly, but exceptions occur when there are nonbreeding helpers of the missing sex present within the group. The presence of such helpers can significantly delay the filling of a vacancy, and if several are present, they can result not only in failure to fill the vacancy but also in failure of the group to subsequently breed. Because such groups contain adult, reproductively competent birds of both sexes that are all close genetic relatives, this loss of reproduction is directly attributable to incest avoidance, and is estimated to cost the population 9.2–12.1% in overall reproductive potential and decrease the population rate of increase by as much as 2.3% year^{-1} (Koenig et al. 1999). Eventually, the helpers of the missing sex either find a vacancy elsewhere and disperse, after which the unfilled vacancy is quickly filled, or the group breeds incestuously. The latter occurs approximately 4% of the time, a rate comparable to that observed in other cooperatively breeding species (Rowley et al. 1993; Haydock et al. 2001). Thus, incest occurs, but is avoided under most circumstances.

The most notable aspect of power struggles, however, is as an indication of the intense competition for breeding opportunities. Power struggles can last for days and involve dozens of birds; helpers are clearly willing to fight extensively for the possibility of gaining a reproductive position in the population, even one that they then must share with siblings. The duration of power struggles and the number of intruders competing are both positively correlated with the size of the territory's granary (Hannon et al. 1985); thus, territory quality plays a role in determining the amount of competition to fill vacancies. Nonetheless, the fact that birds fight to such an extent for the chance to fill a vacancy is unambiguous evidence that breeding and cobreeding are preferred options compared to being a nonbreeding helper. It is unknown, however, why power struggles only take place when vacancies exist since it seems likely that large coalitions of siblings could displace smaller coalitions and enhance their breeding opportunities without waiting for an actual vacancy to arise.

Sexual conflict and sexual selection

Sexual conflict and sexual selection have yet to be studied in detail in acorn woodpeckers, but there is reason to believe that one or both may play an important role in their social behavior. Group reproductive success increases with all categories of birds, but breeders of both sexes gain by having as many breeders of the opposite sex help feed their young as they can and lose (on a per breeder basis) by sharing breeding status with cobreeders (Figure 13.2). Thus, as in the dunnock *Prunella modularis* (Davies 1992), this results in potential conflicts of interest between the sexes that may help explain the variability observed in the mating system.

Sexual conflict may also help explain why the act of mating is so secretive, with copulations almost never being observed during a female's fertile period. Our current best guess is that copulation takes place within nest cavities in such a way that obscures potential

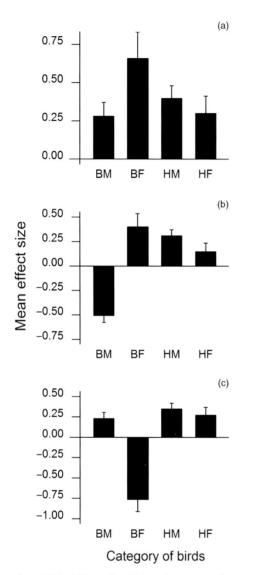

Figure 13.2. (a) Mean (± 2 S.E.) number of young fledged per group as a function of group composition (BM = breeder males; BF = breeder females; HM = helper males; HF = helper females). The effect size of each of the four categories is significant ($P < 0.001$). (b) Mean (± 2 S.E.) number of young fledged per breeder male as a function of group composition; all effects are $P < 0.001$ except that of helper females ($P = 0.004$). (c) Mean (± 2 S.E.) number of young fledged per breeder female as a function of group composition; all effects are $P < 0.001$. Analyses by linear mixed-effects models with "year" as a random effect. N group-years = 1,366; N years = 41.

paternity. Since males then have little or no information as to their success relative to their cobreeders, this sets the stage for male sharing of paternal duties that is uncorrelated with actual paternity (Table 13.1). Why acorn woodpeckers have evolved such a system rather than copulating frequently out in the open, as do, for example, red-cockaded woodpeckers *Picoides borealis* (Chapter 4), southern pied babblers *Turdoides bicolor* (Chapter 7), and lions *Panthero leo* (Schaller 1972) is unknown. In any case, it is important that all male cobreeders have had at least an opportunity to mate, since males denied mating access may subsequently destroy the nest and force renesting (Koenig 1990).

The role of sexual selection is even less well understood. Thus far we have detected no morphological, age-related, or behavioral correlates of paternity success, and thus whether any mate choice is taking place based on such characters seems unlikely. Given the significant reproductive skew among males at individual nests, female choice and sperm competition is possible, although the high frequency of paternity switching from one nest to the next would reduce variance in success among males, thus rendering it unlikely that significant sexual selection could result. Such findings, combined with the absence of extra-group mating, suggest that the greatest opportunity for sexual selection is likely to occur during power struggles and competition over the filling of reproductive vacancies.

Sex ratio evolution

The population sex ratio is slightly, but significantly, male biased. Over the 33 years from 1980 to 2012, the mean sex ratio (expressed as percent males) of breeders in the population during the breeding season was 58.1% (range 51.1 to 63.4%), while the mean sex ratio of helpers was an almost identical 57.7% (range 41.2 to 75.0%). The biased sex ratio of breeders can thus be explained in part by the sex-bias among helpers, but is in addition driven by the more destructive competitive interactions among joint-nesting females compared to cobreeder males, as discussed earlier. Also contributing to the bias is a higher mortality rate among breeder females, whose mean annual survivorship is 75.3% (range 61.0 to 95.2%) compared to 79.5% (range 70.0 to

93.5%) for breeder males (mean annual survivorship from 1 September to 31 August of all birds with complete data from 1979–1980 to 2011–2012). The higher mortality rate of females appears to occur mainly during the spring and summer, and thus is most likely related to the higher cost of reproduction incurred by breeder females, including costs of egg formation and nest care, the latter of which (except for nocturnal brooding, which, as in other woodpecker species, is primarily done by males) is performed disproportionately by breeder females (Koenig and Mumme 1987).

The biased sex ratio of helpers is also due to a combination of factors. First, the sex ratio of young birds surviving to independence (defined as the time of the postjuvenal molt about three months postfledging) is 54%, a significant male bias due to faster nestling growth and lower postfledging mortality of males, since the sex ratio of eggs appears to be either even or slightly female-biased (Koenig et al. 2001). Subsequently, there is a small bias toward male fledglings becoming helpers (59% of male fledglings become helpers compared to 53% of females), and males tend to remain slightly longer as helpers than females (the mean number of years males remain as a helper is 1.57 vs. 1.48 for females).

The ultimate cause of the male sex ratio bias among helpers is more difficult to determine. The major hypotheses for sex ratio variability all predict either a female bias or a male bias smaller than that observed (Koenig et al. 2001), including local resource competition, sexual size dimorphism, and the repayment model (Emlen et al. 1986; Koenig and Walters 1999), the last of which proposes that helpers repay part of the cost of their production by assisting their parents in subsequent breeding attempts. We have also yet to detect any evidence of facultative sex ratio manipulation within broods (Koenig et al. 2001), although producing broods of predominantly one sex or the other would seem to be potentially beneficial by increasing the size and competitiveness of sibling coalitions.

Helpers and provisioning behavior

Nonbreeding helpers make up a third of the population (33.8%) during the breeding season. Furthermore,

as mentioned previously, there are only minor differences in the proportion of fledglings of the two sexes that remain as helpers. There are, however, substantial differences in the proportion that attain breeding status in their natal territory (inherit), which is considerably more common for males than females (23.7% of males [$N = 577$] vs. 4.6% of females [$N = 482$]), and, conversely, in the proportion that disappear or leave the study area (57.8% of males vs. 76.1% of females). The former is a direct result of the greater incidence of female reproductive vacancies, which in turn is due to the greater size of male cobreeding coalitions and the lower survivorship of breeder females. The latter parallels the increased competition females experience for breeding vacancies and greater dispersal distance of females, whose root-mean-square dispersal distance is estimated at 0.53–9.57 km compared to 0.22–2.90 km for males (Koenig et al. 2000). As a result of these differences, acorn woodpecker groups are generally patrilineal; the mean (± S.E.) length of male lineages in groups present for at least six years between 1979 and 2012 was 4.95 ± 0.38 years (range 1–31), significantly greater than lineage length for females, which was 3.63 ± 0.38 years (range 0–20).

Helpers contribute to all aspects of group behavior, including acorn storage, granary defense, incubation, and feeding of young, although typically at lower levels than that of breeders (Mumme et al. 1990). The patterns of provisioning behavior are affected by a variety of variables, including not only sex and status (breeder or nonbreeding helper) but also nestling age, brood size, temperature, date, group size, and time of day (Koenig and Walters 2012a). Breeder females brood and feed nestlings more than do breeder males, and breeders brood and provision at higher rates than helpers. Helper males are more likely than helper females to feed nestlings overall, but in paired comparisons of male and female helpers at the same nest, helper females feed significantly more than helper males, contrary to the expectation that helper males should invest more in provisioning young because of the patrilineal nature of acorn woodpecker groups. There are no differences between helper males and helper females in their tendency to reduce provisioning rates with increasing group size (compensatory care), or to adjust their provisioning rates to experimental changes in brood size (Koenig and Walters 2012b). Helpers do not adjust their feeding rates to changes in brood size to the same extent as breeders, however, a surprising result given that helpers might be expected to devote the extra time and energy afforded by reduced brood sizes to alternative activities such as foraying in search of reproductive vacancies.

Helpers exhibit a strong dominance hierarchy related to body size, which in turn is correlated with hatching order within broods (Stanback 1994). Overwinter survival of larger, dominant fledglings is greater than that of smaller subordinates, but among birds surviving their first winter, there are no differences related to dominance in the proportion that act as helpers or ultimately inherit their natal territory (Koenig et al. 2011a). Interestingly, in analyses of broods in which only one of two male broodmates became a helper instead of dispersing, the bird becoming a helper is more likely to have been the smaller, subordinate rather than the larger, dominant male, a result opposite that found in Siberian jays (*Perisoreus infaustus*; Chapter 1) and red-cockaded woodpeckers (Chapter 4).

Helpers help to raise birds that are related to them by an estimated mean $r = 0.45$ (Koenig and Mumme 1987), and thus, perhaps unsurprisingly, kinship is a particularly important aspect of helping behavior in this species. Of 1,366 helpers whose social parentage was known, 1,204 (88.1%) were helping birds that were breeding in the group when they were born, while 148 (10.8%) were helping stepparents of one sex or the other and were thus raising half-siblings, and only 14 (1.0%) were apparently provisioning unrelated offspring. Thus, virtually all helpers are offspring of the breeders they assist.

The effects of helpers on reproductive success of the group and survival of breeders vary depending on several factors. Overall, each helper at a nest contributes an average of 11% of the brooding time (10.6% for males; 10.9% for females) and about 15% of feeding visits (13.6% for males; 15.9% for females) (Figure 13.3), less than an average breeder but still a significant amount of effort (Koenig and Walters 2012a). The fitness effects of helping behavior vary significantly between the sexes and with the prior year's acorn crop (Koenig et al. 2011b).

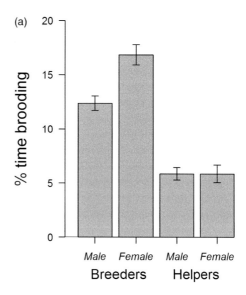

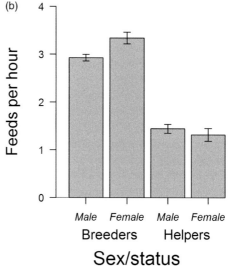

Figure 13.3. (a) Mean (± S.E.) brooding time and (b) mean (± S.E.) provisioning rates by sex and status. Brooding includes only watches conducted during the first 11 days of the nestling period. From Koenig and Walters (2012a).

The effect of helper females on reproductive success is positive but not statistically significant and is unrelated to the acorn crop (Figure 13.4b). In contrast, the effect of helper males is strongly dependent on the prior year's acorn crop: the better the acorn crop, the more beneficial

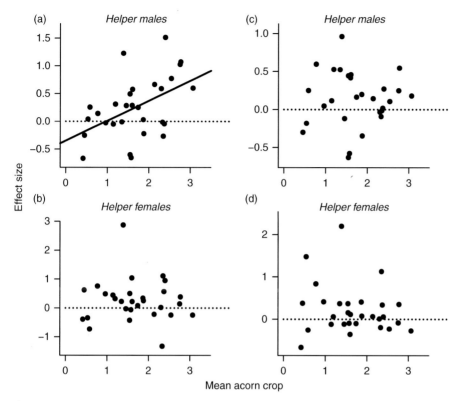

Figure 13.4. Effect size of (a) helper males and (b) helper females on mean annual reproductive success of groups as a function of the mean acorn crop based on linear regressions for individual years controlling for group composition and prior breeder experience; (c) and (d) are identical analyses using only data from first spring nests; thus, the positive effects of helper males in good acorn years are due entirely to additional nesting attempts rather than increased brood size. Correlations: (a) $r = 0.49$, $P < 0.01$; (b) $r = -0.03$, $P = 0.86$; (c) $r = 0.03$, $P = 0.88$; (d) $r = -0.17$, $P = 0.37$. $N = 29$ years.

a helper male is to group reproduction, whereas following a poor acorn year, each helper male correlates with a small reduction in group success (Figure 13.4a). This effect appears to be due almost entirely to an enhanced frequency of second nests in good years rather than increased brood size (Figures 13.4c, 13.4d).

Breeder male survivorship is increased when helpers of either sex are present, but again only when conditions are favorable, either in terms of a large acorn crop, on a high-quality territory, or among experienced breeders. Our data do not provide any evidence for "concealed" helper effects (Russell et al. 2007) such as, for example, females laying smaller eggs when assisted by helpers (Koenig et al. 2009).

In summary, helpers have a positive effect on the fitness of breeders – through increased survivorship and (at least for male helpers) increased fledging success – that is greater when ecological conditions are favorable. This pattern has not been described previously, and contrasts markedly from findings for other cooperative breeders that have been examined in which the effect of helpers is greater when conditions are poor (Magrath 2001; Covas et al. 2008). This latter, more common result is predicted by the hypothesis that cooperative breeding is an evolutionary response to ecological conditions that are so poor that cooperation among more than two individuals is required for success (the "hard life" hypothesis). Helpers in acorn woodpeckers are clearly not necessary for successful reproduction. Instead, helpers, particularly males, provide significant benefits but only when conditions are favorable to begin with.

The overall fitness effects of helping are consequently not simple to estimate, since they vary depending on conditions, and particularly on the acorn crop, which itself varies greatly from year to year (Koenig et al. 1994). We approached this problem by performing a simulation estimating the lifetime fitness effects of a helper on breeders depending on the acorn crop and quality of the territory (Koenig et al. 2011b). Results suggest that on average, a bird delaying dispersal and helping for one year will increase the fitness of a breeder by 8–18% over the number of offspring the breeder would otherwise expect to produce over its lifetime (Table 13.3). Of these values, between 35 and 48% of the fitness benefits conferred by helpers are due to future indirect fitness; that is, increased fitness via enhanced survivorship of breeders (Mumme et al. 1989). The fitness benefits of helping are thus nontrivial, but are still much less than those gained by breeding.

There are at least two important caveats to this conclusion. First, helpers may gain direct fitness benefits from provisioning and other cooperative behaviors (Clutton-Brock 2002). These potentially include: maintaining access to resources on the territory ("pay-to-stay;" Mulder and Langmore 1993); gaining skills that allow them to be more successful when they become breeders later in life (the "skills" hypothesis; Selander 1964); enhancing their social status in a way that increases their future access to resources or mates (Zahavi 1995); or having their help reciprocated, either from the nestlings they help feed (Ligon and Ligon 1978) or by "group augmentation" – increasing the overall success of the group (Brown 1987; Kokko et al. 2001; Kingma et al. 2014).

Although we have not tested all these hypotheses in acorn woodpeckers, we have found no evidence to support those that we have examined (Koenig and Walters 2011). Helpers increase their provisioning rates with age, but in paired comparisons, helper males that fed young at higher rates had no greater reproductive success later in life than less helpful helper males, contrary to the key prediction of the skills hypothesis that such experience should enhance future fitness. And although males that fed more as second-year helpers remained as helpers significantly longer and were more likely to inherit their natal territory than male helpers that fed less, this result is most likely a consequence of differences in dispersal behavior – specifically, that helpers devoting more time to searching for reproductive vacancies rather than provisioning offspring are more likely to find and fill a reproductive position in the population – rather than the birds' prior feeding history, contrary to the key prediction of the pay-to-stay hypothesis. Thus, indirect, kin-selected benefits appear to provide the primary, if not the only, benefits gained by helpers through their provisioning behavior.

The second caveat to the conclusion that helpers gain primarily indirect fitness benefits is that we have no evidence that the positive effects they confer are causally related to their provisioning rather than some other cooperative behavior, a question that arises both because of the highly variable behavior of helpers and the lack of any obvious correlation between the overall fitness effects of helpers and their provisioning behavior (W. Koenig and E. Walters, unpubl. data). This problem, which arises in almost all cooperative breeders, is an important one: many helpers do not, in fact, provision at nests, and if their fitness effects are the same as those that do, it leaves wide open the question of "why helpers help?" We hope to address this problem in the future using new tracking technologies that will allow us to monitor the location of helpers as well as their behavior.

Endocrinology of helping

Neither sex nor breeding status (helper or breeder) affect pre-breeding season levels of luteinizing hormone, indicating that helpers are as capable of achieving breeding condition as are breeders (M. Stanback and J. Wingfield, unpubl. data). Breeding status, but not body weight or age, correlate with pre-breeding testosterone (T) levels in males, but although T levels are elevated and testes are larger

Table 13.3. Estimated lifetime number of young fledged (S = mean fitness) by a breeder living as a pair and as a consequence of the presence of a single male or female helper and whether the bird resides on a low- or a high-quality territory

	Helper male effect on				Helper female effect on			
	Breeder male		Breeder female		Breeder male		Breeder female	
	Low-quality territory	High-quality territory	Low-quality territory	High-quality territory	Low-quality territory	High-quality territory	Low-quality territory	High-quality territory
S_{nh} (mean fitness, no helper)	5.59	8.65	5.14	9.63	5.58	8.65	5.14	9.63
S_{1h} (mean fitness, 1 helper)	6.57	9.99	5.75	10.57	6.51	9.94	5.63	10.40
$S_{1h,R}$ (1 helper, effects on current reproduction only)	6.10	9.27	5.63	10.31	5.95	9.08	5.48	10.10
$S_{1h,S}$ (1 helper, effects on future survivorship only)	6.03	9.32	5.28	9.87	6.12	9.47	5.30	9.91
Combined benefit (% of S_{nh})	0.99 ± 0.27 (18%)	1.34 ± 0.31 (16%)	0.61 ± 0.25 (12%)	0.94 ± 0.28 (10%)	0.92 ± 0.07 (16%)	1.29 ± 0.08 (15%)	0.49 ± 0.02 (10%)	0.78 ± 0.03 (8%)
Current indirect fitness (% of combined benefit)	0.51 ± 0.23 (52%)	0.62 ± 0.25 (46%)	0.47 ± 0.23 (77%)	0.68 ± 0.26 (72%)	0.36 ± 0.01 (39%)	0.43 ± 0.01 (33%)	0.33 ± 0.01 (68%)	0.48 ± 0.01 (61%)
Future indirect fitness (% of combined benefit)	0.44 ± 0.05 (45%)	0.68 ± 0.06 (51%)	0.13 ± 0.01 (21%)	0.25 ± 0.02 (26%)	0.54 ± 0.06 (58%)	0.82 ± 0.07 (64%)	0.15 ± 0.02 (31%)	0.29 ± 0.02 (37%)

The mean effect of the helper (± S.D.) is divided into the fraction enhancing breeder reproduction (current indirect fitness) and the fraction increasing breeder survivorship (future indirect fitness).

Source: From Koenig et al. (2011b).

in breeders than helpers, helpers also have elevated T levels and larger testes during the breeding season compared to the nonbreeding season, indicating some degree of reproductive competence. Among males, body weight but not breeding status influence pre-breeding levels of corticosterone, indicating that their incomplete reproductive state is not due to glucocoricoid-mediated stress imposed by dominant breeders. Similarly, there are no direct effects of dominance status on corticosterone levels, pre-breeding T levels, or testis size.

These findings support the hypothesis that the absence of reproductive activity on the part of helpers is voluntary and not due to reproductive suppression by older, dominant individuals. This is consistent with the results indicating that reproductive roles are determined primarily by incest avoidance rather than reproductive competition, although the latter is still important in terms of the relative success of individual birds in cobreeding coalitions.

Evolution of cooperative breeding

Acorn woodpeckers at Hastings Reservation live under conditions of what has traditionally been referred to as habitat saturation. The clearest support for this statement is that birds fight to fill reproductive vacancies, unambiguously demonstrating that helpers value the opportunity to become a breeder in the population over helping. Indeed, competition is so fierce that birds often form coalitions in order to successfully win power struggles, implying that even a shared breeding position is a superior fitness option compared to serving as a helper.

Until recently, we believed that granaries were the resource most likely to be limiting territorial establishment and thus driving delayed dispersal in the Hastings population. We have now tested this hypothesis by means of an experiment in which we compared sets of four potentially useable sites not previously inhabited by acorn woodpeckers, experimentally adding artificial granaries with 1,500 storage holes to site 1, two artificial nest cavities to site 2, both artificial granaries and two nest cavities to site 3, and nothing to control site

4. After three years, the number of groups in the population increased by 17%, with artificial nesting cavities attracting more new groups than artificial storage facilities (E. Walters and W. Koenig, unpubl. data). As such, acorn woodpeckers are similar to red-cockaded woodpeckers in which nesting and roosting cavities are key ecological constraints driving delayed dispersal (J. Walters et al. 1992).

On the one hand, this is surprising in that acorn woodpecker cavities are not modified in any discernable way and are typically used communally for roosting, with up to 14 roosting in the same cavity, whereas red-cockaded woodpecker cavities are not only specially modified by the birds with a resin barrier to deter predators (Kappes and Sieving 2011) but also only used for roosting by one bird at a time. On the other hand, over 50% of acorn woodpecker nests are in previously excavated cavities (Wiebe et al. 2006), and we have observed groups apparently unable to nest when their nest cavity was taken over by European starlings (*Sturnus vulgaris*). In any case, these observations suggest that the excavation of new nesting holes is difficult and support the conclusion that cavities are an important resource to some extent driving cooperative breeding in this species.

In summary, the main proximate factors driving group living in acorn woodpeckers, both through delayed dispersal of offspring and coalition formation and mate-sharing among breeders, are the ecological constraints imposed by limited nesting cavities and the need for access to granary facilities in which to store acorns. Two predictions of this hypothesis are first, the number of groups should vary little from year to year relatively compared to the number of birds in the population, and second, there should be at best a modest relationship between the number of groups and key resources that vary from year to year – primarily the acorn crop. A factor confounding these tests is that the population size has not been constant throughout the course of the study: both the number of birds and number of groups within the core study area have increased, with the latter rising from 19 in 1980 to 54 in 2012 (Figure 13.5), at least in part because of an increase in canopy cover on the study area (McMahon et al. 2015). In contrast, group size has remained constant

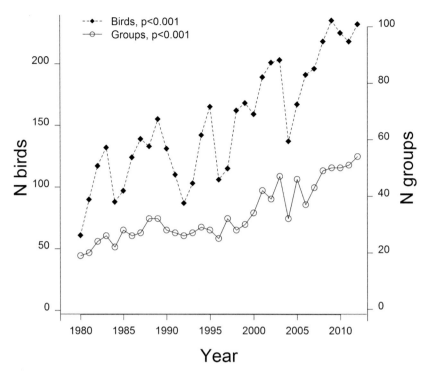

Figure 13.5. Population size through time at the Hastings Reservation study site. Correlations: $r = 0.86$ (N birds vs. year); $r = 0.92$ (N groups vs. year). $N = 33$ years (1980 to 2012).

(correlation between birds per group and year: $r = 0.12$, $P = 0.5$). In order to control for long-term changes in habitat we calculated the residuals from regressions of the number of groups and birds on year and used these values to estimate variability and the effects of the acorn crop.

Results support the first prediction: the variance in number of groups within the core study area between 1980 and 2012 was 20.4, significantly less than the variance in the number of birds in the population (580.7; variance test, $P < 0.001$) and variances of any of the four categories of birds (variance in breeder males = 119.8; breeder females = 86.2; helper males = 125.8; helper females = 90.4; paired variance tests, all $P < 0.002$).

Less clear are results regarding the second prediction: all components of population size, including the number of groups and group size, varied significantly and positively with either the acorn crop the prior year or (in the case of helpers and group size) with the acorn

crop two years earlier (Table 13.4). Thus, following large acorn crops, both the number of groups and the number of birds increase in the population, the latter primarily due to increased number of groups rather than changes in group size. With access to lots of acorns, groups are reproductively very successful, resulting in more helpers and larger groups the following year.

We can compare relative variation in the relevant parameters by log-transforming the number of birds and groups, thereby rendering their variances independent of scale (Lewontin 1966) and comparable to variance in the *ln*-transformed acorn crop. The results confirm that variability in the (*ln*-transformed) acorn crop (variance = 0.545) is several times greater than variance in the (*ln*-transformed) number of groups (0.083) which in turn is less than variance in (*ln*-transformed) overall population size (0.113).

The significant relationship between population size and resources raises a question regarding the

Table 13.4. Correlations between the residuals of regressions of group composition on year vs. the acorn crop in year x-1 (the prior autumn) and year x-2 (the year before that)

Category	Acorn crop year x-1	Acorn crop year x-2
N groups	0.46**	-0.26
N birds	0.35*	0.30
N birds per group	0.02	0.59***
N breeder males	0.36*	-0.16
N breeder females	0.56***	-0.32
N helper males	-0.01	0.60***
N helper females	-0.08	0.55**

*$P < 0.05$; **$P < 0.01$; ***$P < 0.001$.

habitat saturation hypothesis, which is predicated on the underlying fundamental processes restricting independent reproduction being relatively stable from year to year (Koenig and Pitelka 1981; Emlen 1982). Clearly this is not the case to the extent that both the number of birds and number of groups covary with the acorn crop. Specifically, conditions become more or less favorable depending on the acorn crop and in a good year a modest proportion of territories that would otherwise not be inhabited become suitable for colonization. Given this situation, it is possible that averaging across all years underestimates the importance of helping, particularly in years when the acorn crop is poor, and thus that helpers are not making the best of a bad job but rather choosing a situation that is either the best alternative when resources are unfavorable (Magrath 2001) or exercising a "bet-hedging" strategy designed to minimize variance in fitness under conditions of high spatiotemporal variation (Rubenstein 2011).

The first of these possibilities conforms to the "hard life" hypothesis discussed earlier, and is not supported by the finding that the fitness benefits of male helpers is greatest when the acorn crop is good rather than poor (Figure 13.4; Koenig et al. 2011). The second, bet-hedging hypothesis predicts that variance in fecundity decreases with increasing sociality. There are several approaches to addressing this question, but in general our analyses indicate that although relative fecundity variance (measured by the coefficient of

variation in the number of young fledged) is reduced in more social groups, the decrease is not enough to compensate for the decrease in mean fecundity as measured by the per capita number of young fledged (Table 13.5). Thus, in general, bet-hedging does not appear to play an important role in acorn woodpecker populations, although it is still possible that reduced fecundity variance may provide a significant benefit to some aspects of group living in years of poor acorn crops (Koenig and Walters 2015).

Because groups consist of close relatives, nonbreeding helpers gain indirect (kin) fitness benefits from helping, especially when the acorn crop is good. As discussed above, we have yet to demonstrate any significant direct fitness benefits of helping. One benefit that has frequently been proposed for helpers, however, is the potential for inheriting a high-quality territory (Stacey and Ligon 1991; Kokko et al. 2001; Clutton-Brock 2002; Covas and Griesser 2007). This is a potentially important phenomenon in acorn woodpeckers, particularly for males given their high rate of inheritance. Countering this hypothesis, however, is that a significant number of birds inheriting their natal territory (22% of males and 12% of females) did so after dispersing and assuming a breeding position elsewhere in the population (Haydock et al. unpubl. data). Thus, in our population, at least, inheritance of the natal territory is not dependent on delayed dispersal. Similar to species with redirected helpers (Chapters 1 and 2), birds apparently monitor their natal territory even *after* they have dispersed elsewhere and potentially return to breed there should a (nonincestuous) breeding opportunity arise. Such cases devalue the importance of delayed dispersal to helping and territorial inheritance, and increase the relative value of kin-selected benefits to the frequency of delayed dispersal and helping behavior.

Conclusion

Acorn woodpeckers do not live in a particularly stable environment, being dependent on a highly variable acorn crop. Thus, there is an argument for cooperative breeding in this system being an adaptation to cope

Table 13.5. Comparison of fecundity variance (CV) and mean estimated fitness for groups divided by an index of sociality measured by total group size, number of cobreeder males, number of cobreeder females, and the presence/absence of helpers

Index of sociality	Relatively nonsocial	Relatively social	Wilcoxon V	P-value
Fecundity variance (CV)				
Total group size[a]	77.7 ± 7.2	72.6 ± 4.6	205	0.04
Cobreeder males[b]	86.4 ± 7.5	71.2 ± 5.2	410	0.02
Cobreeder females[b]	78.9 ± 5.8	75.0 ± 5.9	332	0.37
Presence of helpers[c]	77.7 ± 8.7	58.8 ± 5.6	210	0.03
Estimated fitness[d]				
Total group size[a]	0.67 ± 0.10	0.60 ± 0.05	285	0.48
Cobreeder males[b]	1.14 ± 0.18	0.86 ± 0.08	289	0.13
Cobreeder females[b]	1.24 ± 0.18	1.03 ± 0.12	132	0.04
Presence of helpers[c]	0.71± 0.10	0.64 ± 0.06	252	0.47

Values are means ± SE. Analyses by Wilcoxon paired signed-rank test. N = 33 years (except for presence of helpers, where N = 23 years for CV and N = 29 for fitness).

[a] Pairs vs. groups, except for 10 years in which there were not enough pairs (or variance was undefined) where comparison is for pairs plus trios vs. groups of 4+ birds.

[b] Groups with one breeder vs. two or more cobreeders; all groups had one breeder of the other sex and no helpers.

[c] Pairs without vs. pairs with one or more helpers of either sex.

[d] Estimated using the method described by Frank and Slatkin (1990); for details, see Koenig and Walters (2015).

Source: From Koenig and Walters (2015).

with highly variable and unpredictable conditions, as was proposed originally by Emlen (1982) and more recently expanded by Rubenstein and his colleagues (Chapter 11), and supported by the apparent reduction in fecundity variance exhibited by larger, more social groups (Koenig and Walters 2015). Nonetheless, the population generally lives under conditions of habitat saturation, with access to the key resources of nesting cavities and storage facilities acting as ecological constraints driving delayed dispersal on the part of offspring and coalition formation and subsequent polygynandry on the part of breeders.

Thus, competition for territories sets the stage for delayed dispersal on the part of offspring and coalition formation on the part of helpers attempting to improve their chances of gaining a reproductive opportunity. But why help? For cobreeders, provisioning behavior appears to be driven by the direct fitness benefit of parentage, or at least the opportunity of parentage,

combined with the indirect fitness benefits of kinship with cobreeders. Both females and males share parentage relatively equitably, within individual nests (for females) and across nests (for males). We suspect that individuals that have copulatory access or have laid eggs in the nest have little information regarding their own parentage, but as we have shown, parentage is equally likely for all but the most subordinate of breeders. Given these circumstances, all breeders contribute to raising offspring, because they have a relatively equal chance of being a successful parent and, if not, gain the indirect benefits of assisting relatives.

The fitness benefits of provisioning offspring for non-breeding helpers appear to be primarily, if not exclusively, indirect through kinship. Not all possible routes to achieving direct fitness benefits have been tested, but thus far, our data do not support either the skills or the pay-to-stay hypotheses. Helper males gain significant indirect fitness benefits, particularly in good acorn years; in contrast, male helpers do not appear to gain benefits in poor acorn years, and female helpers do not incur significant indirect fitness benefits from helping except by enhancing breeder survivorship. Several key questions remain, however: why do breeders allow helpers to remain in poor acorn years?; why do female helpers provision when they appear to confer little or no fitness benefit?; what, exactly, are male and female helpers doing differently that leads to these differences?; and are the observed benefits due to provisioning behavior per se or some other behavior on the part of helpers?

Also remaining is a thorough explanation for the differences among populations. Three populations have been studied in detail thus far, and each differs significantly from the others, resulting in strikingly different conclusions regarding the factors driving cooperative breeding (Koenig and Stacey 1990). With populations stretching through Mexico, Central America, and into Colombia, there is significant potential to further explore the existence and significance of variability in social behavior of this species, potentially yielding important new insights into the evolution and maintenance of complex social systems.

Acknowledgments

We are particularly grateful to Michael and Barbara MacRoberts, Ron Mumme, Sue Hannon, Mark Stanback, Philip Hooge, and Janis Dickinson for their many contributions to the study over the years, along with the help of the 139 field assistants that have assisted with the project since 1980. The study would not have been possible without the long-term support of the Museum of Vertebrate Zoology, UC Berkeley, Hastings Natural History Reservation, and the National Science Foundation. The manuscript was improved by the comments of Janis Dickinson and Bruce Lyon.

REFERENCES

Bock, C. E. and Bock, J. H. (1974). Geographical ecology of the acorn woodpecker: diversity versus abundance of resources. *Am. Nat.*, 108, 694–698.

Brown, J. L. (1987). *Helping and Communal Breeding in Birds: Ecology and Evolution.* Princeton, NJ: Princeton University Press.

Clutton-Brock, T. (2002). Breeding together: kin selection and mutualism in cooperative vertebrates. *Science*, 296, 69–72.

Covas, R. and Griesser, M. (2007). Life history and the evolution of family living in birds. *Proc. R. Soc. London B*, 274, 1349–1357.

Covas, R., Du Plessis, M. A., and Doutrelant, C. (2008). Helpers in colonial cooperatively breeding sociable weavers *Philetairus socius* contribute to buffer the effects of adverse breeding conditions. *Behav. Ecol. Sociobiol.*, 63, 103–112.

Davies, N. B. (1992). *Dunnock Behaviour and Social Evolution.* Oxford: Oxford University Press.

Dickinson, J. L., Haydock, J., Koenig, W. D., Stanback, M. T., and Pitelka, F. A. (1995). Genetic monogamy in single-male groups of acorn woodpeckers, *Melanerpes formicivorus. Mol. Ecol.*, 4, 765–770.

Emlen, S. T. (1982). The evolution of helping. I. An ecological constraints model. *Am. Nat.*, 119, 29–39.

Emlen, S. T., Emlen, J. M., and Levin, S. A. (1986). Sex-ratio selection in species with helpers-at-the-nest. *Am. Nat.*, 127, 1–8.

Fajer, E. D., Schmidt, K. J., and Eschler, J. G. (1987). Acorn woodpecker predation on cliff swallow nests. *Condor*, 89, 177–178.

Frank, S. A. and Slatkin, M. (1990). Evolution in a variable environment. *Am. Nat.*, 136, 244–260.

Hamilton, W. D. (1964). The genetical evolution of social behaviour. I, II. *J. Theor. Biol.*, 7, 1–52.

Hannon, S. J., Mumme, R. L., Koenig, W. D., and Pitelka, F. A. (1985). Replacement of breeders and within-group conflict in the cooperatively breeding acorn woodpecker. *Behav. Ecol. Sociobiol.*, 17, 303–312.

Hannon, S. J., Mumme, R. L., Koenig, W. D., Spon, S., and Pitelka, F. A. (1987). Poor acorn crop, dominance, and decline in numbers of acorn woodpeckers. *J. Anim. Ecol.*, 56, 197–207.

Haydock, J. and Koenig, W. D. (2002). Reproductive skew in the polygynandrous acorn woodpecker. *Proc. Natl. Acad. Sci. (USA)*, 99, 7178–7183.

Haydock, J. and Koenig, W. D. (2003). Patterns of reproductive skew in the polygynandrous acorn woodpecker. *Am. Nat.*, 162, 277–289.

Haydock, J., Koenig, W. D., and Stanback, M. T. (2001). Shared parentage and incest avoidance in the cooperatively breeding acorn woodpecker. *Mol. Ecol.*, 10, 1515–1525.

Kappes, Jr., J. J. and Sieving, K. E. (2011). Resin-barrier maintenance as a mechanism of differential predation among occupants of red-cockaded woodpecker cavities. *Condor*, 113, 362–371.

Kattan, G. (1988). Food habits and social organization of acorn woodpeckers in Colombia. *Condor*, 90, 100–106.

Kingma, S. A., Santema, P., Taborsky, M., and Komdeur, J. (2014). Group augmentation and the evolution of cooperation. *Trends Ecol. Evol.*, 29, 476–484.

Koenig, W. D. (1981). Space competition in the acorn woodpecker: power struggles in a cooperative breeder. *Anim. Behav.*, 29, 396–409.

Koenig, W. D. (1990). Opportunity of parentage and nest destruction in polygynandrous acorn woodpeckers, *Melanerpes formicivorus. Behav. Ecol.*, 1, 55–61.

Koenig, W. D. and Haydock, J. (1999). Oaks, acorns, and the geographical ecology of the acorn woodpecker. *J. Biogeogr.*, 26, 159–165.

Koenig, W. D. and Mumme, R. L. (1987). *Population Ecology of the Cooperatively Breeding Acorn Woodpecker*. Princeton, NJ: Princeton University Press.

Koenig, W. D. and Pitelka, F. A. (1981). Ecological factors and kin selection in the evolution of cooperative breeding in birds. In: *Natural Selection and Social Behavior: Recent Research and New Theory*, ed. R. D. Alexander and D. W. Tinkle. New York: Chiron Press, pp. 261–280.

Koenig, W. D. and Stacey, P. B. (1990). Acorn Woodpeckers: group-living and food storage under contrasting ecological conditions. In: *Cooperative Breeding in Birds: Long-term Studies of Ecology and Behavior*, ed. P. B. Stacey and W. D. Koenig. Cambridge: Cambridge University Press, pp. 413–453.

Koenig, W. D. and Stahl, J. T. (2007). Late summer and fall nesting in the acorn woodpecker and other North American terrestrial birds. *Condor*, 109, 334–350.

Koenig, W. D. and Walters, E. L. (2011). Age-related provisioning behaviour in the cooperatively breeding acorn woodpecker: testing the skills and the pay-to-stay hypotheses. *Anim. Behav.*, 82, 437–444.

Koenig, W. D. and Walters, E. L. (2012a). Brooding, provisioning, and compensatory care in the cooperatively breeding acorn woodpecker. *Behav. Ecol.*, 23, 181–190.

Koenig, W. D. and Walters, E. L. (2012b). An experimental study of chick provisioning in the cooperatively breeding acorn woodpecker. *Ethology*, 118, 566–574.

Koenig, W. D. and Walters, E. L. (2015). Temporal variability and cooperative breeding: testing the bet-hedging hypothesis in the acorn woodpecker. *Proc. R. Soc. London B*, 282, 20151742.

Koenig, W. D. and Walters, J. R. (1999). Sex-ratio selection in species with helpers at the nest: the repayment model revisited. *Am. Nat.*, 153, 124–130.

Koenig, W. D. and Williams, P. L. (1979). Notes on the status of acorn woodpeckers in central Mexico. *Condor*, 81, 317–318.

Koenig, W. D., Mumme, R. L., Carmen, W. J., and Stanback, M. T. (1994). Acorn production by oaks in central coastal California: variation in and among years. *Ecology*, 75, 99–109.

Koenig, W. D., Mumme, R. L., Stanback, M. T., and Pitelka, F. A. (1995). Patterns and consequences of egg destruction among joint-nesting acorn woodpeckers. *Anim. Behav.*, 50, 607–621.

Koenig, W. D., Van Vuren, D., and Hooge, P. N. (1996). Detectability, philopatry, and the distribution of dispersal distances in vertebrates. *Trends Ecol. Evol.*, 11, 514–517.

Koenig, W. D., Stanback, M. T., and Haydock, J. (1999). Demographic consequences of incest avoidance in the cooperatively breeding acorn woodpecker. *Anim. Behav.*, 57, 1287–1293.

Koenig, W. D., Hooge, P. N., Stanback, M. T., and Haydock, J. (2000). Natal dispersal in the cooperatively breeding acorn woodpecker. *Condor*, 102, 492–502.

Koenig, W. D., Stanback, M. T., Haydock, J., and Kraaijeveld-Smit, F. (2001). Nestling sex ratio variation in the cooperatively breeding acorn woodpecker (*Melanerpes formicivorus*). *Behav. Ecol. Sociobiol.*, 49, 357–365.

Koenig, W. D., McEntee, J. P., and Walters, E. L. (2008). Acorn harvesting by acorn woodpeckers: annual variation and comparison with genetic estimates. *Evol. Ecol. Res.*, 10, 811–822.

Koenig, W. D., Walters, E. L., and Haydock, J. (2009). Helpers and egg investment in the cooperatively breeding acorn woodpecker: testing the concealed helper effects hypothesis. *Behav. Ecol. Sociobiol.*, 63, 1659–1665.

Koenig, W. D., Walters, E. L., and Haydock, J. (2011a). Fitness consequences of within-brood dominance in the cooperatively breeding acorn woodpecker. *Behav. Ecol. Sociobiol.*, 65, 2229–2238.

Koenig, W. D., Walters, E. L., and Haydock, J. (2011b). Variable helpers effects, ecological conditions, and the evolution of cooperative breeding in the acorn woodpecker. *Am. Nat.*, 178, 145–158.

Koenig, W. D., Walters, E. L., Knops, J. M. H., and Carmen, W. J. (In press). Acorns and acorn woodpeckers: ups and downs in a long-term relationship. In: *Proceedings of the 7th California Oak Symposium: Managing Oak Woodlands in a Dynamic World*. Pacific SW Forest & Range Exp. Station Gen. Tech. Rep.

Kokko, H., Johnstone, R. A., and Clutton-Brock, T. H. (2001). The evolution of cooperative breeding through group augmentation. *Proc. R. Soc. London B*, 268, 187–196.

Leach, F. A. (1925). Communism in the California woodpecker. *Condor*, 27, 12–19.

Lewontin, R. C. (1966). On the measurement of relative variability. *Syst. Zool.*, 15, 141–142.

Ligon, J. D. and Ligon, S. H. (1978). Communal breeding in green woodhoopoes as a case for reciprocity. *Nature*, 276, 496–498.

MacRoberts, M. H. and MacRoberts, B. R. (1976). Social organization and behavior of the acorn woodpecker in central coastal California. *Ornith. Monogr.*, 21, 1–115.

Magrath, R. D. (2001). Group breeding dramatically increases reproductive success of yearling but not older female scrub-wrens: a model for cooperatively breeding birds? *J. Anim. Ecol.*, 70, 370–385.

McMahon, D. E., Pearse, I. S., Koenig, W. D., and Walters, E. L. (2015). Tree community shifts and acorn woodpecker population increases over three decades in a California oak woodland. *Can. J. For. Res.*, 45, 1113–1120.

Michael, E. (1927). Plurality of mates. *Yosemite Nature Notes*, 6, 78.

Mulder, R. A. and Langmore, N. E. (1993). Dominant males punish helpers for temporary defection in superb fairy-wrens. *Anim. Behav.*, 45, 830–833.

Mumme, R. L., Koenig, W. D., and Pitelka, F. A. (1983a). Mate guarding in the acorn woodpecker: within-group reproductive competition in a cooperative breeder. *Anim. Behav.*, 31, 1094–1106.

Mumme, R. L., Koenig, W. D., and Pitelka, F. A. (1983b). Reproductive competition in the communal acorn woodpecker: sisters destroy each other's eggs. *Nature*, 306, 583–584.

Mumme, R. L., Koenig, W. D., and Ratnieks, F. L. W. (1989). Helping behaviour, reproductive value, and the future component of indirect fitness. *Anim. Behav.*, 38, 331–343.

Mumme, R. L., Koenig, W. D., and Pitelka, F. A. (1990). Individual contributions to cooperative nest care in the acorn woodpecker. *Condor*, 92, 360–368.

Myers, H. W. (1915). A late nesting record for the California woodpecker. *Condor*, 17, 183–185.

Rowley, I., Russell, E. M., and Brooker, M. G. (1993). Inbreeding in birds. In: *The Natural History of Inbreeding and Outbreeding*, ed. N. W. Thornhill. Chicago: University of Chicago Press, pp. 304–328.

Rubenstein, D. R. (2011). Spatiotemporal environmental variation, risk aversion, and the evolution of cooperative breeding as a bet-hedging strategy. *Proc. Natl. Acad. Sci. (USA)*, 108, 10816–10822.

Russell, A. F., Langmore, N. E., Cockburn, A., Astheimer, L. B., and Kilner, R. M. (2007). Reduced egg investment can conceal helper effects in cooperatively breeding birds. *Science*, 317, 941–944.

Schaller, G. B. (1972). *The Serengeti Lion: A Study of Predator-prey Relations*, Chicago: University of Chicago Press.

Selander, R. K. (1964). Speciation in wrens of the genus *Campylorynchus. Univ. Calif. Publ. Zool.*, 74, 1–305.

Stacey, P. B. (1979a). Habitat saturation and communal breeding in the acorn woodpecker. *Anim. Behav.*, 27, 1153–1166.

Stacey, P. B. (1979b). Kinship, promiscuity, and communal breeding in the acorn woodpecker. *Behav. Ecol. Sociobiol.*, 6, 53–66.

Stacey, P. B. and Bock, C. E. (1978). Social plasticity in the acorn woodpecker. *Science*, 202, 1298–1300.

Stacey, P. B. and Ligon, J. D. (1991). The benefits of philopatry hypothesis for the evolution of cooperative breeding: variance in territory quality and group size effects. *Am. Nat.*, 137, 831–846.

Stanback, M. T. (1994). Dominance within broods of the cooperatively breeding acorn woodpecker. *Anim. Behav.*, 47, 1121–1126.

Walters, J. R., Copeyon, C. K., and Carter, III, J. H. (1992). Test of the ecological basis of cooperative breeding in red-cockaded woodpeckers. *Auk*, 109, 90–97.

Wiebe, K. L., Koenig, W. D., and Martin, K. (2006). Evolution of clutch size in cavity-excavating birds: the nest site limitation hypothesis revisited. *Am. Nat.*, 167, 343–353.

Williams, G. C. (1966). *Adaptation and Natural Selection*, Princeton, NJ: Princeton University Press.

Wynne-Edwards, V. C. (1962). *Animal Dispersion in Relation to Social Behaviour*, Edinburgh: Oliver and Boyd.

Zahavi, A. (1995). Altruism as a handicap – the limitations of kin selection and reciprocity. *J. Avian Biol.*, 26, 1–3.

14

Taiwan yuhinas: Unrelated joint-nesters cooperate in unfavorable environments

Sheng-Feng Shen, Hsiao-Wei Yuan, and Mark Liu

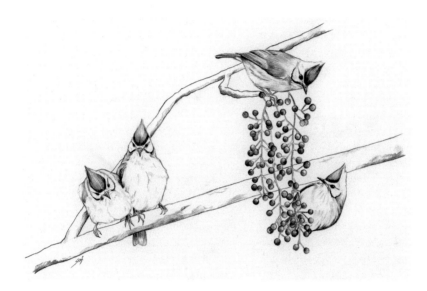

Introduction

The cooperative breeding behavior of Taiwan yuhinas (*Yuhina brunneiceps*) – an endemic to Taiwan – was first described by Yamashina (1938) more than 70 years ago. He observed 4–8 birds attending the same nest and, based on the different color patterns of the eggs, inferred that there were 2–3 females laying eggs communally. However, there is no subsequent detailed study on Taiwan yuhinas until we started our pilot work in 1995.

Taiwan yuhinas are elevational migrants and are widely distributed at elevations ranging from 800–2,800 m during breeding season and at somewhat lower elevations in the winter. They primarily inhabit natural forests but also breed in fragmented and disturbed habitats. Yuhinas are open-cup nests and they build their nests in concealed places as diverse as small ferns near the ground, fruit trees, dense epiphytes, underneath concrete roofs, and various trees. It is the most abundant breeding bird species in the mountainous areas of Taiwan (Koh and Lee 2005).

Cooperative Breeding in Vertebrates: Studies of Ecology, Evolution, and Behavior, eds W. D. Koenig and J. L. Dickinson.
Published by Cambridge University Press. © Cambridge University Press 2016.

Taiwan yuhinas are joint-nesting plural breeders (Brown 1978; Vehrencamp and Quinn 2004) in which several monogamous pairs defend a group territory and females lay eggs in joint nests. They are very different from cooperative breeders that form groups with kin, usually through offspring staying in the natal groups, but in some cases also cobreeding with relatives (Vehrencamp and Quinn 2004). In such kin-based cooperative breeders helpers and cobreeders are typically making the "best of a bad job" and are remaining in their natal group in order to gain a small indirect fitness benefit that is essentially better than nothing at all. By examining the fitness of joint nesting and the ecological drivers of cooperation in Taiwan yuhinas, we sought to explore direct fitness benefits of cooperation and the selective pressures favoring cooperation in a system where indirect fitness benefits and natal philopatry were not part of the equation. This led to investigation of insider-outsider conflict, a framework we believe is necessary for understanding group membership in cooperative breeders, but that can also be extended to explore determinants of group size and group composition in a broader spectrum of cooperative breeding systems (Giraldeau and Caraco 1993; Higashi and Yamamura 1993). The yuhina study is thus an example of how studying an unusual species allows us to test existing hypotheses while also expanding the theoretical approaches and understandings.

Description of study population and methods

We conducted our study in a seminatural environment at Meifeng Highland Experimental Farm of National Taiwan University in central Taiwan (24°05′N, 121°10′E, elevation 2,150 m). Our study focused on a 50 ha area with a system of small roads that allowed us to monitor the activity of the breeding groups. The study site was mixed with greenhouses, orchards of temperate fruits, meadows, Japanese cryptomeria (*Cryptomeria japonica*) plantations, and various ornamental trees surrounded by natural forests consisting mainly of Fagaceae and Lauraceae.

Although we started our pilot study in 1995, the difficulty of reaching yuhina nests – mostly built at the edge of the thin branches with average height of 7 m – severely limited our data collection. The problem was solved in 2004 when we started using a cherry picker to reach their nests across the rugged terrain, allowing us to reach 75% of nests instead of the 30% of nests we could get to by climbing ladders or trees. Prolonged rainfall in the spring and typhoons were additional factors limiting of our data collection. Since 2004, however, we have employed transponder and digital video recording systems, which can operate 24/7 regardless of weather conditions. This ability to collect behavior data under all weather conditions has enabled us to investigate the crucial ecological determinant of yuhinas' social behaviors. The work we summarize here is based on studies involving many students and undergraduate volunteers between 1995 and 2012.

Social and genetic mating system

During 1997–1998, 2001, and 2004–2007, we sampled 103 groups of yuhinas for 161 group-years and found 318 nests. Group members defend a common territory throughout the breeding season and take care of the same nest during nest building, incubation, nestling provisioning, and fledgling. Breeding group sizes of yuhinas range from two to eight individuals. Most commonly, yuhina groups are comprised of four individuals, which comprised 41.3% of groups (Figure 14.1a) and 45% of nests (Figure 14.1b). Only 22 groups (13.7%) consisted of two birds, and such groups were often unstable. Thus, over 86% of the yuhina breeding groups we observed were engaged in cooperative breeding.

Within groups, Yuhinas form socially monogamous pairs. Pair relationships can be easily identified during egg-laying, when the male and female move together, and are often separated from other group members. Genetic parentage data, determined by microsatellite markers, confirmed that 72.5% of offspring ($N = 294$) are sired by social pairs. Among the 81 offspring sired outside of social pairs, 47 (58.0%) were sired by males within the same group and 34 (42.0%) were sired by males of other groups. Subordinate (β) females are

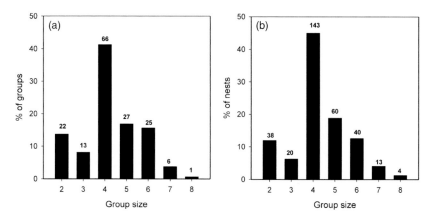

Figure 14.1. Group size distributions in terms of (a) group-years and (b) nesting attempts. Numbers above each bar indicate sample sizes.

more likely to produce offspring sired by extra-pair fathers than the dominant females (α) in low rainfall condition, whereas, the rank of the males does not influence their probability of siring extra-pair offspring. A minority of groups (28.6%) include an unpaired individual. Unpaired group members were both male ($N = 20$) and female ($N = 12$) and originated via three routes: delayed dispersal by offspring, immigration from another group, and groups' members that had lost their mates. The unmated helpers from the first two routes were mostly genetically related individuals; 12 of 13 cases of male helpers and 5 of 7 cases of female helpers were related ($r > 0.25$) to at least one existing group member.

We monitored the membership of each group and determined the position of each bird within the group hierarchy based on displacement and chasing behavior. For both males and females, particular individuals consistently initiated chases with and displaced same-sex members of their group. We determined dominance hierarchies for each sex based on these consistent patterns of chasing and displacement with the most α individuals being those that consistently chased and displaced all other same-sex group-mates. In larger groups, γ individuals were chased by both α and β individuals. We also found that γ males never sang territorial songs when α or β males were present unless groups were involved in intergroup conflicts

at the territory boundaries. When both α and β males were present at the same time and at least one was singing *to-mi-ju*, the α male sang significantly more (14.1 ± 9.3 min⁻¹) than the β male (5.0 ± 7.6 min⁻¹). In 50% of the song observations ($N = 50$) the β male did not sing at all when the α male was present (Yuan et al. 2004).

Most yuhina offspring disperse from their natal territories soon after they fledge. Only 4.2% of fledglings ($N = 167$), including six males and one female, remained in their natal territory into the next breeding season. Genetic data also indicate that most groups consist of nonrelatives: the average genetic relatedness between same-sex group members was low (0.079 for male dyads and -0.003 for female dyads), and only 20.2% of 317 within-group dyads ($N = 317$) were comprised of kin. There was also a low proportion of closely-related kin ($r > 0.25$) in groups (26.4% and 14% for male and female dyads, respectively). The relatedness of male dyads within breeding groups was, however, significantly higher than female dyads (Mann-Whitney U test; $P = 0.01$). In addition, the proportion of closely-related male dyads was significantly higher than the proportion of closely-related female dyads ($\chi^2 = 6.81$, df = 1, $P = 0.009$).

To understand the mechanisms of nonkin group formation, we examined breeding vacancy replacements of both sexes and birds of different ranks. We found that social queuing for breeding vacancies

Table 14.1. Resolutions of reproductive vacancies in Taiwan yuhinas

Breeding vacancies	Mate remained in the group	Alpha	Beta	Gamma	Unpaired	Insider total	Insider available?			Outsider total	N[b]	Total
							M[a]	N	Y			
Alpha females	No	0	5	0	3	8	0	0	7	7	1	16
	Yes	0	9	0	0	9	0	1	14	15	2	26
Beta Females	No	1	0	0	1	2	3	8	6	17	1	20
	Yes	2	0	4	2	8	3	6	2	11	4	23
Total		3	14	4	6	27	6	15	29	50	8	85
Alpha males	No	0	9	4	2	15	0	0	1	1	1	17
	Yes	0	5	1	1	7	0	2	5	7	1	15
Beta males	No	1	1	1	4	7	1	6	5	12	1	20
	Yes	1	0	3	1	5	1	10	4	15	1	21
Total		2	15	9	8	34	2	18	15	35	4	74

[a] Whether insiders were available is unknown.

[b] Instances of breeding vacancies were not resolved.

and dominant status are common in males but not females. Specifically, 73% of α male vacancies were filled by lower-ranked within-group males (insiders), while only 44% of α females, 26% of β females, and 31% of β male vacancies were filled by insiders (Table 14.1).

Group benefits

Group size effects

We tested two types of grouping benefits: "resource access" (RA) benefits derived from access to critical resources controlled by the group, and "socially produced" (SP) benefits resulting from social cooperation among group members. If groups form for RA benefits, we predict that per capita productivity will decrease as group size increases, as seen in many cooperatively breeding birds. Alternatively, if yuhinas form groups because of SP benefits, the per capita productivity is expected to increase with group size until it achieves the most productive size.

A breakdown of the components of reproductive success as a function of group size reveals some of the costs and advantages of group living. Nest failure is high – 77% – as a result of abandonment, predation, and severe weather. Nevertheless, we found a hump-shaped relationship between nesting success and group size, with the peak at the median group size of 4 and 5 ($z = 2.76$, $P < 0.01$, $N = 443$ nests; Figure 14.2a). Although total clutch size increases with group size (Figure 14.2b), the per-pair clutch size decreases (Figure 14.2c). A similar decrease is evident for the number of fledglings produced in successful nests. Finally, groups of median size had more nesting attempts within a season than did groups at the tail ends of the group size distribution. Summing these fitness components, we found that the relationship between breeding success and group size is largely influenced by nesting success rate and thus is again hump-shaped with a peak at the median group size (Figure 14.2d).

How does group size influence survival and lifetime fitness? Individuals in larger groups had significantly higher survival probabilities than individuals in smaller group sizes with the exception of α males (Tarone-Ware log-rank test, $\lambda^2 = 5.41$, $P = 0.02$, $N = 55$; Figure 14.3a). Combining the survival probability of individuals and annual breeding success, the estimated lifetime reproductive success of individuals in median group sizes is greater than that of individuals in larger groups, and individuals in groups smaller than the median have the lowest lifetime reproductive success (Figure 14.3b).

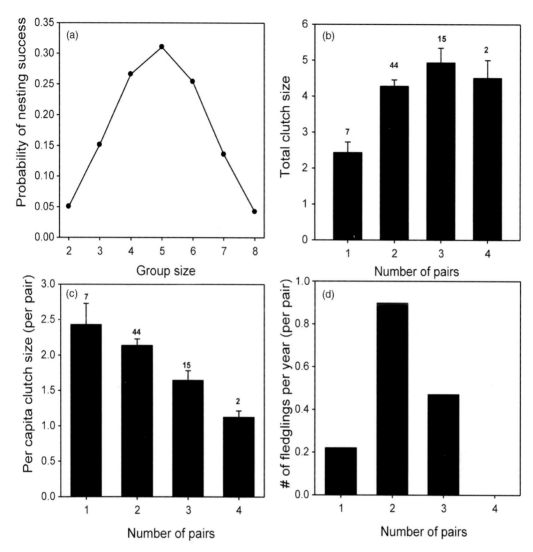

Figure 14.2. The relationships between group size and (a) probability of nesting success, (b) total clutch size of a group, (c) average per capita clutch size of a pair, and (d) average total number of fledglings per pair in a season, calculated by multiplying average number of nesting attempts in a season, probability of nesting success, and per capita fledglings per pair in successful nesting attempts. Error bars represent standard errors.

Nest concealment, parental activity, and nest predation

Our results suggest stabilizing selection on group size around a mean of about four individuals per group. These results beg the question of how yuhinas gain from living in groups rather than breeding independently. Given that selection acts primarily through total nest failure and adult survivorship, we hypothesized that the threat of predation plays an important role in selection for breeding in groups.

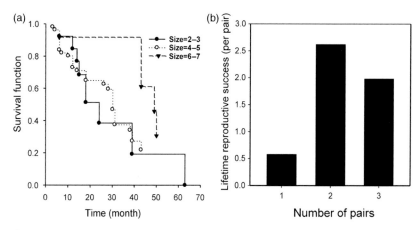

Figure 14.3. (a) The Kaplan-Meier survival function of individuals ($N = 82$) in different group sizes, and (b) the lifetime reproductive success of yuhinas vs. group size, obtained by multiplying the average number of fledglings per pair in a season by the survival probability of individuals in different group sizes.

Yuhinas seldom mob predators; consequently, we focused on the effects of nest site and parental activity on nest predation. These specific behavioral and ecological factors are likely to interact with each other as determinants of nesting success. Our observational data indicate that nest predation during the nestling stage is not higher than during incubation, despite higher visitation rates. To understand the possible cause of this puzzling result, we conducted both observational and experimental studies to disentangle the effects of nest site and parental activity on nest predation. Among the 10 nest site characteristics we measured, foliage cover above the nest was the most important factor influencing nest predation risk. We also found that the average foliage cover was lowest in nests that were depredated during incubation, higher in nests that were depredated during nestling period, and highest in successful nests, suggesting that there is a graded effect of the amount of foliage cover on nest success (Figure 14.4a).

Concealment of individual nests can be conflated with overall vegetation density near the nest. To test the role of local nest concealment on predation risk compared to the role of overall vegetation density (Chalfoun and Martin 2009), we experimentally increased nest concealment by adding a small artificial cloth above nests. Rates of predation on treated nests with added cover decreased 67% compared to controls ($P = 0.03$). Thus local nest concealment appears to play a crucial role influencing nest predation rate regardless of surrounding vegetation density.

Next we investigated the effect of parental activity on nest predation. In natural nests, nest survival rates did not differ between the nestling and incubation periods. However, after controlling for the nest concealment effect, nest survival was 97% higher during incubation than during the nestling period (Cox survival analysis, stage: $P = 0.015$; cover: $P = 0.004$), suggesting that nests surviving to the nestling stage were concealed more effectively than nests that were depredated. We then investigated the influence of parental activity on nest predation by placing eggs in nests constructed by yuhinas in previous nesting attempts, thus mimicking the scenario of no parental activity (Cresswell 1997; Martin et al. 2000). Survival of artificial clutches in which parental activities were absent was higher than for naturally laid clutches at the nestling stage, but not during the incubation stage (parental activity: $P = 0.02$; incubation: $P = 0.91$). These results indicate that parental activities have a negative impact on nest survival.

To test for a potential interaction between nest concealment and parental activity, we experimentally

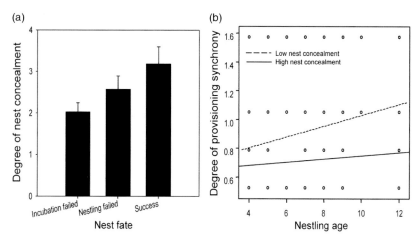

Figure 14.4. (a) Nest concealment in three groups of nests divided by whether nests were depredated during incubation, depredated during the nestling stage, or successful. Higher degree of nest concealment indicates denser vegetation cover above a nest. (b) The relationship among provisioning synchrony, nest concealment, and nestling age in two-pair groups. Provisioning synchrony is represented by arcsine transformation of the number of provisioning individuals in the same trip divided by group size.

placed eggs in inactive nests to examine nest predation compared to that experienced for the same nest during the prior "real" nesting attempt. Rates of predation on these "inactive" nests with eggs, surprisingly, did not differ among nests that previously failed during the incubation stage, failed during the nestling stage, or successfully fledged young (GLMM: $\chi^2 = 2.64$, df = 2, $P = 0.27$). Also, in contrast to natural nests, there was no effect of foliage cover on nest survival in the artificial clutches where parental activity was absent ($P = 0.19$). Similarly, foliage cover did not differ between nests with artificial clutches that were depredated versus successful (Mann-Whitney U test, $P = 0.19$), while foliage cover was significantly higher in natural nests that were successful than the unsuccessful ones (Mann-Whitney U test, $P = 0.02$). These results indicate that the concealment effect of the nest site only influences nest predation in conjunction with parental activity, possibly through a "track-covering" effect whereby better nest concealment lowers the probability of predators detecting nests through observing parents making feeding trips to the nest. We conclude that the degree of nest concealment has an important influence on the group provisioning strategy of yuhinas, as we will see in the following section.

Influence of group size on nesting success

Given that nest concealment and parental activity are the key determinants of nest success, we investigated how group size influences nest concealment and parental activity. Our results indicate that larger groups did not choose better nest sites than did smaller groups (cover: $P = 0.76$). Group size also had little effect on overall feeding rates due to an interaction between group size and the number of group members provisioning nests at the same time.

Adult yuhinas generally feed nestlings in groups instead of alone, potentially reducing the probability of being found by predators, as found in several other avian species (Raihani et al. 2010). Only 10.5% of the 1,393 feeding trips were solo visits, while in 67% of visits more than half the group members provision at the same time. The number of feeding trips per hour increases with nestling age ($P = 0.002$), but is not influenced by group size ($P = 0.58$) or brood size ($P = 0.20$); instead, significantly more individuals arrive at the nest together to feed during each feeding trip in larger groups ($P < 0.001$). Thus, although the total hourly feeding rate increases with nestling age ($P < 0.001$) and brood size ($P = 0.017$), it is not influenced by group size, even though larger groups generally have larger broods. This suggests that there is no nutritional benefit for nestlings of being in a large group.

In addition, we found that group members are more likely to synchronize their provisioning in more exposed nest sites and when nestlings are older and need more food (Figure 14.4b, interaction between nest cover and nestling age: $P = 0.02$). These results suggest that yuhinas synchronize their provisioning to reduce the number of feeding trips, which may reduce the probability of nests being detected by predators in large groups. Group size also influences other aspects of breeding including individuals' workloads, which are lower during both incubation and feeding in larger groups. Larger groups also renest faster after nest failure and build larger nests with more nesting material, which hold up better when conditions are poor.

These results suggest that our finding that individuals in groups of median sizes (four and five) achieve the highest lifetime reproductive success can be attributed to trade-offs that differ among group sizes. Birds have lower per capita share of reproduction in larger groups, but they minimize the cost of exposure to nest predators by synchronizing their feeding in large groups while enjoying the benefits of load-lightening, faster renesting, and more effective buffering of nests against predation and severe weather (Shen 2002; Yuan et al. 2005). In smaller groups the clustered interfeeding interval will be shorter, the load lightening less, and the nests more likely to be found by predators.

Group size and composition

The insider-outsider conflict framework

Due to the complex interactions between group size and benefits for individuals living in or joining groups, we introduce the concept of insider-outsider conflict (IOC) – the tension between potential joiners ("outsiders") and current group members ("insiders") – and use it to organize the disparate properties of social animals, including grouping benefits, group size, kinship composition, and group stability. The concept of insider-outsider conflict was first described by Sibly

(1983), who questioned the stability of the most productive group size, measured in terms of per capita productivity. The reason for this is that although it is often in an insider's interest to maintain the most productive group size, when joining the group yields higher fitness than being solitary, outsider(s) will still gain by joining it, thereby driving group size to become larger than the insider's optimum.

The concept of insider-outsider conflict was later developed more formally to incorporate the effects of inclusive fitness and the distinction between insider and outsider control of group membership (Higashi and Yamamura 1993; Giraldeau and Caraco 1993, 2000). Accordingly, the grouping benefit, measured by the relationship between per capita productivity and group size, is a key factor influencing the resolution of insider-outsider conflict and resulting group size. Kinship is another important determinant of group size, especially when group size is larger than the most productive group size.

We focus on per capita productivity – instead of individual's share of reproduction, or reproductive skew – because the minimum requirement for group formation is that per capita productivity must be greater than the average solitary payoffs, regardless of the relatedness among group members and personal share of reproduction. For example, if the total group productivity is G, β individual gets p share of group productivity and α gets the remaining $(1-p)$ share. For β individual to prefer forming a group with α, her fitness in the group, Gp, must be great than if she breeds on her own (S). Thus, the inequality $Gp > S$ must hold. Similarly, $G(1-p) > L$ must be true for α, where L is the solitary breeding payoff of α. Summing the above two inequalities together, we can obtain $G > S + L$ and thus $G/2 > (S+L)/2$, which proves that, for the formation of a social group, per capita productivity must be greater than the average solitary payoffs (Keller and Reeve 1994). This approach allows us to simplify the analysis for understanding the insider-outsider conflict as well as making the empirical studies on group formation more feasible.

The power of the IOC framework is that it simultaneously considers the interests of both current group members (insiders) and potential joining members (outsiders) – both offspring and unrelated immigrants – and their relationship with group benefit. If current group members such as parents have control over group membership, IOC models predict that more-closely related kin will be more likely to be accepted into the group when the group size is larger than the most productive size, which, in turn, results in even larger observed group size than optimal. In contrast, if outsiders – offspring or unrelated immigrants – have more control over group membership, observed group size is predicted to be smaller when potential joiners are kin than nonkin. This is because a more-closely related potential joiner, such as the offspring of current group members, is better off avoiding kin competition.

We focus on the insiders-control version of IOC models because it is biologically more realistic for cooperative breeders, predicting that:

(1) Group size will converge to slightly larger than the most productive group size in terms of per capita productivity.
(2) Groups will be most stable when their sizes are close to the most productive size.
(3) The mean genetic relatedness will increase with group size assuming insider control of group membership.

We tested these predictions using our long-term data on group benefit, group size, and group composition.

Dynamics of group size and group membership

To investigate the dynamics of group size in light of insider-outsider processes, we quantified the directions of changes in group size and factors influencing the group stability of a group. We found that among groups that changed size in successive nesting attempts within the breeding season, large groups of six to eight tended to decrease in size. Specifically, 76.5% of large groups became smaller ($N = 13$); mid-size groups of four to five both decreased (33.3%) and increased (66.7%) in size ($N = 21$); and small groups of two or three either left their territories and disappeared ($N = 10$) or increased in size ($N = 11$). In only one case did a small group decrease further to a single pair. These results indicate that yuhinas converge on groups of four and five, the most productive groups, as predicted by the IOC model.

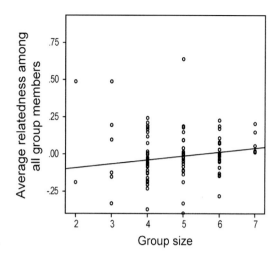

Figure 14.5. The relationship between average pairwise relatedness among group members and group size.

Our results also demonstrate that the stability of groups of four and five, defined as the probability of remaining the same size between consecutive nesting attempts within the same breeding season, was 86.5%, significantly higher than the stability of groups of two and three (69.2%) and groups of six to eight (69.1%). This result, again, suggests that the grouping benefit is the crucial factor influencing the size of social groups.

To test the IOC predictions of group formation and to understand the role of kinship in the formation of yuhina groups, kinship structures were compared for small and large groups. Overall, 57 of 147 groups-years (38.8%) contained at least one related dyad. As predicted by the IOC model, average relatedness among group members increased with group size ($P < 0.01$, Figure 14.5). Therefore, as predicted by the IOC model, individuals were more likely to live with kin in large groups than in small groups, because relatives are more likely to be accepted by insiders when group size is larger than the optimal size.

Social queuing and resolution of breeding vacancies

Several factors affected the resolution of breeding vacancies. Since two-pair groups were the most common, there were significantly more insiders available to fill α vacancies (95.7%, $N = 69$) than β vacancies (56.5%, $N = 69$; $\chi^2 = 18.3$, $P < 0.001$; 14.1). Whether an insider is queuing for the breeding vacancy has a significant effect on the resolution of β vacancies, which are more likely to be filled by insiders (56.4%, $N = 39$), if insiders are available compared to if they are not (28.6%, $N = 77$; Fisher exact test, $P = 0.005$). Thus, nonkin emigrants were more likely to join groups as subordinates when group sizes were smaller than the most productive size. In contrast, while most α and β vacancies were filled (92.4%, $N = 158$), vacancies created due to disappearance of lower-ranking individuals were significantly less likely to be replaced (8.6%, $N = 70$; Fisher exact test, $P < 0.001$), as predicted by the IOC model, because group sizes were larger than the most productive size.

In addition, α females had a key influence on the resolution of α-male vacancies: unrelated outsider-males were more likely to fill α-male vacancies when the α female remained in the group (50%, $N = 14$) than when the α female also disappeared (6.3%, $N = 16$; Fisher exact test, $P = 0.01$). Whether opposite-sex breeders remained in the group did not affect the resolution of breeding vacancies for other breeding roles (Table 14.1). This demonstrates that the mating interest of the insiders – here, accepting unrelated mates by α females – is an important mechanism for the formation of nonkin groups.

Balance of cooperation and competition

Given that most groups are composed of nonkin, potential conflict among group members is expected to be high and stability of groups low. Here we describe both the sharing conflict, including conflict over offspring quantity and quality, and the conflict over investing in the common good – joint nests – including collective incubation and provisioning young. We then examine how social and environmental factors influence the resolution of these conflicts.

Competitive strategies over offspring quantity and quality

We investigated two interference-type competitive strategies that involve overt aggression – tussling during egg laying and egg tossing, and two exploitative-type competitive strategies that are indirect ways of competing for group resources – laying more eggs and early onset of incubation (Shen et al. 2012). During egg laying, we discovered that female group members often aggressively compete for access to the nest with tussling behaviors; a first-come female occupies the nest while other laying female(s) stands on her back and tries to push her out of the nest to lay her egg. All tussling and egg laying attempts occurred early in the morning, usually within 5 min of the first male songs. Tussling behavior occurred at almost all nests (97%, $N = 36$) in which more than one female laid eggs on the same day.

Several lines of evidence suggest that tussling is an important competitive strategy influencing the number of eggs that females can lay in the communal clutch. In 39% ($N = 61$) of tussling events, one female prevented the other female from laying. Nevertheless, longer tussling duration was associated with more females successfully laying eggs and resulted in a more egalitarian share of reproduction between dominants and subordinates. In addition, tussling events were more likely to occur before nocturnal incubation started, when the benefit of laying eggs was higher (86%, [$N = 57$] of cases, compared to 43% [$N = 28$] of cases on the days after nocturnal incubation started; Fisher exact test, $P < 0.01$). This benefit arises because eggs laid before the onset of nocturnal incubation usually hatch earlier (Shen et al. 2012).

Egg tossing is another interference-type competitive strategy, but occurred in only 7.0% ($N = 43$) of nests that we were able to observe prior to egg laying. In all three cases, eggs were removed immediately after tussling behaviors ended. To further test the role of egg tossing, we conducted model egg addition experiments in nine nests at various stages during egg laying. No egg tossing occurred in any of the cases where a model egg was added. Model eggs were incubated for more than ten days and mostly removed by parents at the end of the incubation period. Thus, egg tossing does not appear to be an important competitive strategy for yuhinas.

For communal breeders, the number of offspring produced can also be an important exploitative competitive strategy, because group members share limited resources. In yuhinas, offspring body weight

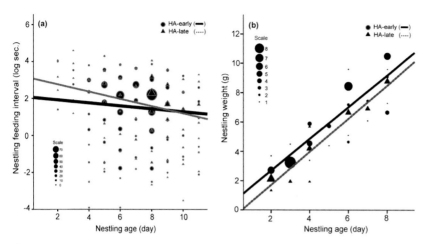

Figure 14.6. The relationship between hatch order (early hatching or late hatching) in asynchronously hatching nests and (a) the nestling feeding interval (interval between two feeding events for a nestling) and (b) nestling weight, at different ages.

decreased, and both the absolute number and proportion of offspring that died increased, as joint brood size increased. Thus, laying more eggs increases an individual's personal share of group resources but potentially drives the joint clutch size larger than the most productive size in terms of total young fledged. Early onset of nocturnal incubation is another exploitative competitive strategy because eggs laid after incubation onset hatch later and thus chicks from late eggs are at a competitive disadvantage. The number of eggs hatching on the first day significantly increases with the number of eggs incubated on the first day of nocturnal incubation. Thus, asynchronous hatching and an early chick advantage are associated with early onset of nocturnal incubation.

These results suggest that tussling, laying more eggs, and onset of nocturnal incubation are interconnected strategies. Females that successfully compete and lay more eggs in the first two days of the egg-laying period are also more likely to start nocturnal incubation, which then favors their own offspring at the expense of their cobreeders. In 94.7% ($N = 19$) cases with two or three breeding females, females that initiated nocturnal incubation were first-day egg layers, but only 40.9% ($N = 22$) of females that did not initiate nocturnal incubation were first-day layers (Fisher exact test, $P < 0.001$). Lay order is also associated with dominance;

the initiator of incubation was the α female in 11 cases, β female in six cases, and γ female in one case. Early onset of nocturnal incubation thus ensures that the female that successfully competed to lay more eggs also has earlier-hatching eggs, which have a competitive growth advantage because they are heavier than late-hatching nestlings (Figure 14.6a) and they obtain food at shorter time intervals in the asynchronously hatching nests (Figure 14.6b).

Ecology and social conflict

In our high-altitude and subtropical montane cloud forest study site, rainfall is an unfavorable ecological condition for the birds. Overcast, foggy, and rainy weather often prevail for many hours, forcing birds to perform most of their activities in the rain. Among other things, rainfall reduces nestling provisioning rates (GLMM, $F_{1,288} = 23.4$, $P < 0.001$) and results in fewer nests being initiated. The percentage of nests initiated on days preceded by a three-day average daily rainfall > 5 mm was smaller (45.2%, $N = 330$) than the percentage (53.3%, $N = 362$) when the preceding three-day average rainfall was < 5 mm ($\chi^2 = 4.6$, $df = 1$, $P = 0.03$). Although more rainfall could potentially increase biomass production and thus have a positive effect on subsequent provisioning rates, this was apparently not the

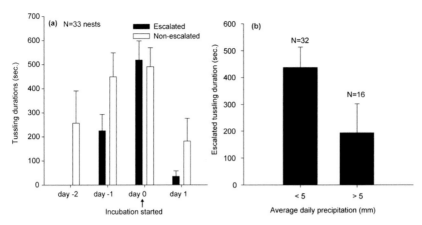

Figure 14.7. Tussling duration in relation to (a) onset of nocturnal incubation and (b) average daily rainfall before the onset of nocturnal incubation; sample size represents number of tussling events. Day 0 represents the day nocturnal incubation starts, on which females lay eggs in the early morning and the nocturnal incubator starts incubating eggs that evening. Day -1 indicates one day before the day nocturnal incubation starts.

case: nestlings from nests initiated during high rainfall periods on average received similar numbers of provisioned items (GLMM, $F_{1,91} = 0.7$, $P = 0.39$) of similar size (GLMM, $F_{1,26} = 0.7$, $P = 0.42$) than nestlings from nests initiated during low rainfall periods. Thus, more rainfall during the egg laying period did not result in better or worse conditions for provisioning young (Shen et al. 2012).

We developed a game-theoretical model to investigate the relationship between ecological conditions and social conflict in the context of communal breeding (Shen et al. 2012). We assumed that when conditions are poor, the cost of producing offspring is higher and an individual young's fitness declines with increasing brood size. We also assumed that an offspring's share of group resources is determined by parents' competitive effort, while the cost of this competitive effort also increases when environmental conditions are harsh. The key predictions of the model are that social conflict and the number of offspring produced will, unsurprisingly, decrease when conditions are poor. Counterintuitively, however, individual offspring fitness and total group productivity can increase as ecological conditions decline. This is because poor ecological conditions increase the cost of competition and thus prevent the "tragedy of the commons."

We used average rainfall in the three days before nocturnal incubation to represent ecological conditions because this is the period in which all three competitive strategies (tussling, egg laying, and onset of nocturnal incubation) take place. As predicted, we found that cobreeding females were involved in less intense tussling events during period of high rainfall when ecological conditions were poor and before the start of nocturnal incubation, but that the length of tussling was not affected by group size (Figures 14.7a and 14.7b).

Rainfall had a significant effect on the number of eggs produced and offspring quality. As predicted, more eggs were produced when ecological conditions were favorable (low rainfall). The number of total surviving offspring, however, was lower in nests initiated during favorable ecological conditions than those initiated during poor conditions (Figure 14.8a), because when there was less rain, eggs were more likely to be added to a clutch after incubation had started compared to nests initiated when there was more rain (Fisher exact test, $P < 0.01$; Figure 14.8b). As a consequence, hatching was significantly more likely to be asynchronous when there was less rain (67%, $N = 21$ nests) than when there was more rain (18%, $N = 11$ nests; Fisher exact test, $P = 0.02$). Also as predicted, nestlings grew significantly faster and heavier and thus nestling condition was better in

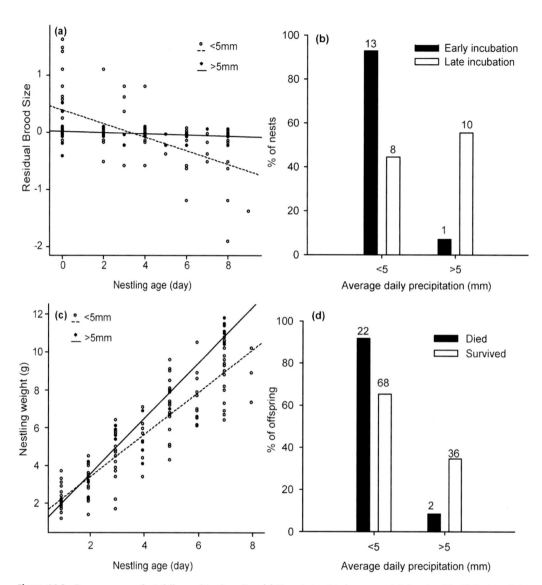

Figure 14.8. Consequences of rainfall on yuhina breeding. (a) The relationship between rainfall and residual joint-brood size. Day 0 represents number of eggs. (b) The relationship between rainfall and the occurrence of different onsets of nocturnal incubation. (c) The relationship between rainfall and nestling weight. (d) The fates of offspring in relation to average daily rainfall before the onset of nocturnal incubation. "Survived" nestlings successfully fledged.

nests with eggs laid during poor ecological conditions (Figure 14.8c). As a consequence, late-hatching nestlings were more likely to die in nests with eggs laid during favorable conditions (Fisher exact test, $P = 0.01$; Figs. 14.8c and 14.8d). The "tragedy of the commons" scenario, whereby individuals compete for a higher share of group resources at the cost of group productivity, was thus avoided during unfavorable conditions.

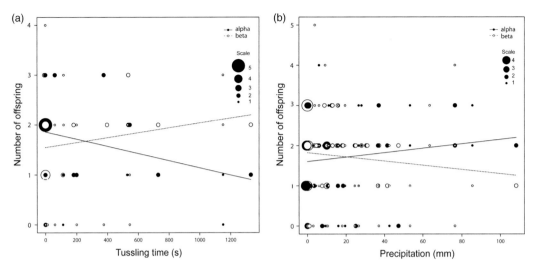

Figure 14.9. Number of offspring sired by α and β individuals in relation to (a) tussling duration and (b) precipitation. Tussling duration was negatively influenced by precipitation.

Reproductive share and ecology

As we have shown above, higher rainfall reduces tussling duration, number of eggs laid, and, indirectly, asynchrony, and thus poor environmental conditions counterintuitively increase group productivity by reducing social conflict. Here we summarize how ecology and different competitive strategies affect the share of group resources among group members in terms of both offspring quantity and quality.

We found that the duration of tussling events, measured as the sum of tussling time during and one day before the day that nocturnal incubation starts, differentially influences the number of offspring that dominants and subordinates sired for both sexes (GLMM, interaction between hierarchy and tussling time, $P = 0.02$, $N = 85$). Specifically, the number of subordinates' offspring increased with increasing tussling duration, but decreased for the dominants. Since the duration of tussling is mainly mediated by rainfall, we also found that subordinates had more offspring than dominants when ecological conditions were good, whereas dominants had more offspring when conditions were poor (GLMM, interaction between hierarchy and precipitation, $P < 0.05$, $N = 203$, Figure 14.9).

Individuals not only compete for parentage, they also compete for offspring quality. Overall, dominants had significantly heavier offspring than subordinates, but this pattern was especially pronounced under favorable environmental conditions when tussling was more intense. These results suggest that ecological conditions have a critical influence on the strategies and outcome of the within-group conflict. The interference-type competitive strategy – tussling during egg laying – is more important in determining reproductive sharing and offspring quality when environmental conditions are favorable, presumably because the costs of competition are lower. In contrast, the exploitative-type competitive strategy – simply having the ability to lay more and earlier eggs in poor ecological conditions – is the key determinant of the differential reproductive patterns between dominants and subordinates.

Cooperation and conflict during collective parental care

Individuals do not discriminate their own eggs or nestlings, as demonstrated by our model-egg addition and nestling swapping experiments. Thus, collective incubation and provisioning young is a collective action problem – group members invest jointly in a common good and each can free ride on each other's effort. Here, we investigate the effects of the two potential types of collective good – offspring quality and quantity – on cooperative parental care during incubation.

Our results show that offspring quality, represented by nestling body weight, but not quantity, is the key determinant of an individual's incubation effort. Furthermore, we found that the benefits of heavier, more competitive, offspring can only be obtained by investing in early onset of nocturnal incubation. The underlying reason for this is that parents initiating nocturnal incubation were usually the first-day layers. By incubating earlier and also investing more both in diurnal and nocturnal incubation, they had heavier (and presumably earlier hatching) nestlings.

With respect to cooperation, there is an important difference in the way that quality and quantity of offspring are determined in yuhinas. The number of offspring produced is determined during the egg-laying stage, *before* parental investment in incubation and provisioning begins. Chick quantity therefore has less ability to inhibit free-riding (Eadie and Lyon 2011). The quality of offspring, represented by offspring body weights, is determined by both priority of egg laying and onset of nocturnal incubation. These late hatched, low-quality offspring were also more likely to die because of their inability to compete for food (Figure 14.8c).

Early onset of nocturnal incubation simultaneously involves both cooperation and competition because it entails both a contribution to group benefit – group members share the workload during incubation – and provides a competitive advantage to heavier chicks. Our study thus demonstrates the importance of timing and highlights a novel source of asymmetric benefit – investing in parental care to enhance the competitive ability of offspring – for understanding the mechanisms of stabilizing cooperation.

Alternative feeding tactics and nestling competition

Whether differently ranked individuals employ alternative reproductive tactics has received relatively little attention in social systems with clear dominance hierarchies such as yuhinas. We hypothesize that subordinates – usually with late hatching and, thus, lighter nestlings – should use alternative tactics when provisioning young to increase the chance of channeling food to their offspring.

In general, heavier nestlings are more likely to obtain food, and lighter nestlings need to spend more effort by raising their heads higher and getting closer to parents in order to obtain food. Thus heavier nestlings are competitively superior. However, at the level of group performance, we found that food distribution among nestlings was more evenly distributed, and fewer nestlings begged during large-party feeding bouts compared with small-party feeding bouts. This is because large-party provisioning caused multiple feeding events to occur in a bout, with short time intervals averaging 49 s, whereas feeding trips were, on average, 7 min apart (Figure 14.10a, Shen et al. 2010). The shorter feeding event intervals resulted in fewer nestlings begging for food and more even food distribution among nestlings (Figure 14.10b).

In addition, we found that subordinates adjusted their sequences of feeding nestlings during a provisioning trip as a strategy to achieve shorter feeding intervals: subordinates were more likely to feed the nestlings in the later sequences as their provisioning frequency increased (GLMM, $N = 415$, $P = 0.035$), whereas the feeding sequences of the dominants were not influenced by their provisioning effort. As a consequence, dominants were more likely to feed the heavier nestlings and the subordinates were more likely to feed the lighter ones (GLMM, $N = 529$, $P = 0.002$, Figure 14.11). These results reveal that even though lighter nestlings are generally in inferior competitive condition, their subordinate parents adopt feeding tactics that shorten the feeding event interval and, in turn, increase the probability of their lighter nestlings obtaining food.

The evolution of cooperative breeding: resource access and socially produced benefits

Taiwan yuhinas do not form their social groups through delayed dispersal of offspring. Instead, most

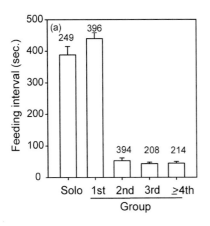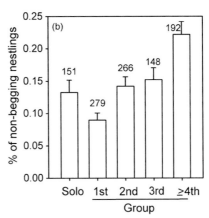

Figure 14.10. (a) Feeding event intervals for different provisioning trip types and for feeding events within sequences. (b) The percentage of nonbegging nestlings for different provisioning trip types and feeding events within sequences. "Solo" refers to feeding trips by a single individual and "group" refers to trips by more than one individual. "1st" represents the first adult to feed a nestling during a feeding trip and so on. The feeding interval for a solo provisioning event is the interval since the last time any nestling at that nest was fed.

offspring disperse from their natal territories and groups are mainly composed of nonkin, although the rare unmated helpers are mostly comprised of kin. Traditionally, groups formed by nonkin individuals and formed through offspring delayed dispersal are viewed as two distinct routes in the evolution of cooperative breeding (similar to the subsocial and parasocial routes in social insects). Most studies have employed the classic "why stay?" and "why help?" framework to address the later scenario from the perspective of offspring fitness. For example, the ecological constraints hypothesis states that grown young delay dispersal and remain in their natal social groups when ecological constraints severely lower the expected fitness payoff of the alternative options, of either dispersing to breed independently or floating.

One drawback of the ecological constraints hypothesis is the lack of the predictive power above the species level, since numerous species seemingly face equally strong ecological constraints but do not exhibit delayed dispersal of offspring. As several authors have pointed out, the overgenerous definition of constraints – including everything from lack of breeding vacancies in stable environment to inability of rear young independently

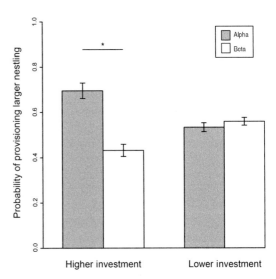

Figure 14.11. The probability of α and β individuals feeding heavier nestlings was differentially influenced by the provisioning effort. "Higher investment" and "lower investment" represent cases in which individuals fed nestlings more or less than the average of all group members in a given hour, respectively.

in fluctuating environments – can make it too easy to identify constraints post hoc.

In addition, a recent large-scale comparative study, including all avian species, showed that cooperative breeding is more common in environments with high degrees of between-year variation in climate, particularly rainfall (Jetz and Rubenstein 2011). This study poses a special difficulty for the ecological constraints hypothesis based on habitat saturation because habitat saturation should be less likely to occur in highly variable environments (Cockburn and Russell 2011). Moreover, a recent review has also shown that groups include nonrelatives more frequently than often thought in cooperative breeders (Riehl 2013). Thus, solely focusing on delayed dispersal by offspring is too narrow for understanding the evolution of cooperative breeding in general.

To overcome these difficulties, we first identify two major categories of group benefits – RA benefits, which derive from access to critical resources controlled by the group, and SP benefits, which results from social cooperation among group members (Alexander 1974; Emlen 1982; Koenig et al. 1992; Rankin et al. 2007; Chapter 20). The RA benefits concept assumes that group-controlled resources are important for survival and reproduction. This is most likely to be true when population density is high (leading to habitat saturation) and critical resources are spatially and temporally distributed so as to be defensible by groups. If RA benefits are the key for the group formation, per capita productivity will decrease as group size increases because the fixed amount of group resource must be shared among more individuals when group size is larger. In contrast, SP benefits are generated by active social coordination between group members and leads to greater efficiency in social activities, such as group foraging, cooperative caring young, and cooperative defense against predators. As a consequence, per capita productivity in SP benefits in cooperatively breeding groups will *increase* as group size increases until each reaches its maximal level, then decrease as group size increases further.

Toward a predictive framework of cooperative breeding

Two evolutionary routes to cooperative breeding societies

One crucial difference between the two categories of benefits is that the optimal group size is solitary pair in resource-access type of groups and is larger than a pair in groups driven by SP benefits. Thus, in the RA type of groups, insiders will be more likely to accept kin than nonkin to join the group to increase their inclusive fitness through increasing their relative's future fitness, such as inheriting the good quality territory or simply increase their survival. Family groups thus are inherently unstable as predicted by the original ecological constraints hypothesis. In contrast, for the SP type of groups, if group size is smaller than the most productive size, insiders may allow both kin and nonkin to join the group to increase their direct fitness, although relatives will be preferred because of their common genetic interests. Social groups of this type can be stable for years because staying at natal territory is no longer a suboptimal option (i.e., dispersal is not delayed), as described in the group augmentation scenario (Kokko et al. 2001).

Not every case that offspring stay in the natal group should be viewed as "delayed" dispersal. We propose to define delayed dispersal as "offspring joining the natal group with size larger than its optimal size." Thus, delayed dispersal is only important for the formation of RA type of social groups. On the contrary, in SP groups, delayed dispersal could occur when group sizes are larger than the most productive size and thus influences stable group size and genetic composition but not the initial formation of the group. Of course, offspring can stay and join their natal groups in the socially produced type of group when group size is smaller than the most productive size. But, in this case, groups will be stable and exhibit higher variation of genetic relatedness among group members than in the RA type of group.

The distinction between RA and SP benefits might help explain why early interspecific comparative studies in birds had difficulty finding any consistent relationship between the incidence of cooperative breeding and ecological or environmental factors. This is because both the original benefits of philopatry hypothesis (Stacey and Ligon 1987, 1991) and Emlen's (1982) broadened ecological constraints hypothesis included both RA benefits and the need for SP benefits. Instead, because both kin and nonkin can form SP groups, we argue that the two routes – RA and SP benefits – to the evolution of cooperatively breeding is a more complete framework than artificially classifying cooperative breeding species into group formation through offspring delayed dispersal and by nonkin individuals.

The problem of "delayed dispersal" occurs in both stable and fluctuating environments and thus lack of predictive power can also be resolved. RA benefits play the more important role in explaining the link between life history traits (Arnold and Owens 1998; Russell 1989; Hatchwell and Komdeur 2000), habitat saturation, and natal philopatry in a stable environment. In contrast, SP benefits – mainly due to the advantages of having more individuals provision and defend offspring when conditions for breeding are unfavorable – will be more important in cases of harsh, variable, and unpredictable environments.

Ecological consequences of sociality

Although sociality is often thought to have played a critical role in allowing modern humans to expand rapidly across the earth to exploit a more diverse range of environments than the African savannas in which our ancestors evolved (Laland et al. 2001), the equivalent question of the relationship between sociality and the ecological consequences of a species has received little attention in nonhuman animals (Sun et al. 2014). We propose that if SP benefits are the key benefit for the evolution of cooperative breeding, groups should allow social species to live in a broad range of conditions and cope with a variety of environmental challenges such as predation risk, fluctuating climates, or interspecific competition (Jetz and Rubenstein 2011; Gonzalez et al. 2013; Shen et al. 2014). In contrast, when a species form groups for RA benefits, sociality is a consequence of high population density – which suggests that solitary individuals of the species are already well adapted to

the environment. Therefore, sociality is an adaptation to intraspecific challenges such as competition with conspecific groups or with members of their own group over a lack of breeding vacancies or critical resources (Emlen 1982; Reeve and Hölldobler 2007; Gonzalez et al. 2013). As a consequence, forming social groups should enable individuals to specialize in a single stable environment. We believe that cooperatively breeding birds are especially suitable for testing this novel "social conquest" hypothesis, given that their phylogeny, social systems, geographic distributions, and abundances are relatively well known.

Conclusion

By identifying two types of benefits, we synthesize the ecological constraints hypothesis with insider-outsider conflict (IOC) theory that simultaneously considers the interests of current group members (insiders) and the potential joiners (outsiders) to provide a predictive framework for the evolution of cooperative breeding. The distinction between the two categories of group benefit identifies the key ecological bases for the evolution of cooperative breeding and the IOC concept helps us understand how social factors such as group size and genetic relatedness influence the stability and composition of social groups. Thus, this framework allows us to resolve previous confusion and the lack of predictive power of existing theories. It also generates novel predictions for variation of kinship structure and identifies novel research directions for studies of cooperative breeding.

The IOC concept also provides a general framework to simultaneously consider the interests of current group members (insiders) and potential joiners' (outsiders) for studying the evolution of cooperative breeding. Applying the IOC model, how a grouping benefit varies with group size – represented by per capita productivity – plays a crucial role in influencing group formation, size, and composition. In yuhinas, median group sizes are the most productive due to the balancing forces between the social benefits – reducing work load to coping with harsh environment – and the costs – higher within-group conflict over offspring number and quality – associated with larger group size. Thus, we predict and confirm that, in yuhinas, nonkin are more likely to be accepted by insiders in groups that are smaller than the most productive size than larger groups, because there is less potential conflict between a joining outsider and current group members. These questions – such as group formation or variation in size and kinship composition of social groups – remain poorly explored both theoretically and empirically and more attention is clearly needed to achieve a complete understanding of the evolution of cooperative breeding.

Acknowledgments

We thank the editors, Walt Koenig and Janis Dickinson, for inviting us to write this chapter and for providing helpful comments. We also thank Stephen Emlen, Sandra Vehrencamp, Kern Reeve, Dustin Rubenstein, and Rufus Johnstone for their advice and support for this long-term study. SFS greatly appreciates the support of Director Wen-Hsiung Li at Academia Sinica. We also thank P.-F. Lee, I.-H. Chang, Sylvester Karimi, C.-C. Lin, S.-Y. Chang, T.-Y. Hsieh, Q.-D. Zhong, S.-W. Fu, F.-Y. Huang, C.-J. Chang, Y.-H. Chang, I.-F. Liao, K.-C. Cheng, H.-C. Chen, T.-N. Yuan, S.-F. Chan, S.-C. Pan, K.-Y. Lin, S.-Y. Tsai, and more than 30 volunteers from the NTU Nature Conservation Students' Club, Department of Life Science and School of Forestry and Resource Conservation, and the staffs in Mei-Feng highland experimental farm for their help in the field and lab. This research was funded by Ministry of Science and Technology of Taiwan (100-2621-B-001-004 and 103-2918-I-001-006 to SFS and HWY), Career Development Award, Academia Sinica, and Cornell University through the Lab of Ornithology, Department of Neurobiology and Behavior, and a Hu Shih Memorial Award (to SFS).

REFERENCES

Alexander, R. D. (1974). The evolution of social behavior. *Annu. Rev. Ecol. Syst.*, 5, 325–383.

Arnold, K. E. and Owens, I. P. F. (1998). Cooperative breeding in birds: a comparative test of the life history hypothesis. *Proc. R. Soc. London B*, 265, 739–745.

Brown, J. L. (1978). Avian communal breeding systems. *Annu. Rev. Ecol. Syst.*, 9, 123–155.

Chalfoun, A. D. and Martin, T. E. (2008). Habitat structure mediates predation risk for sedentary prey: experimental tests of alternative hypotheses. *J. Anim. Ecol.*, 78, 497–503.

Cresswell, W. (1997). Nest predation: the relative effects of nest characteristics, clutch size and parental behaviour. *Anim. Behav.*, 53, 93–103.

Cockburn, A. and Russell, A. F. (2011). Cooperative breeding: a question of climate? *Curr. Biol.*, 21, R195–R197.

Eadie, J. McA. and Lyon, B. E. (2011). The relative role of relatives in conspecific brood parasitism. *Mol. Ecol.*, 20, 5114–5118.

Emlen, S. T. (1982). The evolution of helping I. An ecological constraints model. *Am. Nat.*, 119, 29–39.

Giraldeau, L. A. and Caraco, T. (1993). Genetic relatedness and group size in an aggregation economy. *Evol. Ecol.*, 7, 429–438.

Giraldeau, L. A. and Caraco, T. (2000). *Social Foraging Theory*. Princeton, NJ: Princeton University Press.

Gonzalez, J.-C. T., Sheldon, B. C., and Tobias, J. A. (2013). Environmental stability and the evolution of cooperative breeding in hornbills. *Proc. R. Soc. London B*, 280, 20131297.

Hatchwell, B. J. and Komdeur. J. (2000). Ecological constraints, life history traits and the evolution of cooperative breeding. *Anim. Behav.*, 59, 1079–1086.

Higashi, M. and Yamamura, N. (1993). What determines animal group size? Insider-outsider conflict and its resolution. *Am. Nat.*, 142, 553–563.

Jetz, W. and Rubenstein, D. R. (2011). Environmental uncertainty and the global biogeography of cooperative breeding in birds. *Curr. Biol.*, 21, 72–78.

Keller, L. and Reeve, H. K. (1994). Partitioning of reproduction in animal societies. *Trends Ecol. Evol.*, 9, 98–102.

Koenig, W. D., Pitelka, F. A., Carmen, W. J., Mumme, R. L., and Stanback, M. T. (1992). The evolution of delayed dispersal in cooperative breeders. *Q. Rev. Biol.*, 67, 111–150.

Koh, C.-N. and Lee, P.-F. (2005). Spatial structure of Taiwan yuhinas (Yuhina brunneiceps) population density and its correlations to environmental variables. *Taiwan J. Sci.*, 20, 283–292.

Kokko, H., Johnstone, R. A., and Clutton-Brock. T. H. (2001). The evolution of cooperative breeding through group augmentation. *Proc. R. Soc. London B*, 268, 187–196.

Laland, K. N., Odling-Smee, J., and Feldman, M. W. (2001). Cultural niche construction and human evolution. *J. Evol. Biol.*, 14, 22–33.

Martin, T. E., Scott, J., and Menge, C. (2000). Nest predation increases with parental activity: separating nest site and parental activity effects. *Proc. R. Soc. London B*, 267, 2287–2293.

Raihani, N. J., Nelson-Flower, M. J., Moyes, K., Browning, L. E., and Ridley, A. R. (2010). Synchronous provisioning increases brood survival in cooperatively breeding pied babblers. *J. Anim. Ecol.*, 79, 44–52.

Rankin, D. J., Bargum, K., and Kokko, H. (2007). The tragedy of the commons in evolutionary biology. *Trends Ecol. Evol.*, 22, 643–651.

Reeve, H. K. and Hölldobler, B. (2007). The emergence of a superorganism through intergroup competition. *Proc. Natl. Acad. Sci. (USA)*, 104, 9736–9740.

Riehl, C. (2013). Evolutionary routes to non-kin cooperative breeding in birds. *Proc. R. Soc. London B*, 280, 2013–2245.

Russell, E. M. (1989). Cooperative breeding: a Gondwanan perspective. *Emu*, 89, 61–62.

Shen, S.-F. (2002). Ecology of cooperatively breeding Taiwan yuhinas (*Yuhina brunneiceps*) in Meifeng areas. M.Sc. thesis, National Taiwan University, Taipei, Taiwan.

Shen, S.-F., Chen, H.-C., Vehrencamp, S. L., and Yuan, H.-W. (2010). Group provisioning limits sharing conflict among nestlings in joint-nesting Taiwan yuhinas. *Biol. Lett.*, 6, 318–321.

Shen, S.-F., Vehrencamp, S. L., Johnstone, R. A., Chen, H.-C., Chan, S.-F., et al. (2012). Unfavourable environment limits social conflict in *Yuhina brunneiceps*. *Nature Comm.*, 3, 885.

Shen, S.-F., Akçay, E., and Rubenstein, D. R. (2014). Group size and social conflict in complex societies. *Am. Nat.*, 183, 301–310.

Sibly, R. M. (1983). Optimal group size is unstable. *Anim. Behav.*, 31, 947–948.

Stacey, P. B. and Ligon, J. D. (1987). Territory quality and dispersal options in the acorn woodpecker, and a challenge to the habitat-saturation model of cooperative breeding. *Am. Nat.*, 130, 654–676.

Stacey, P. B. and Ligon, J. D. (1991). The benefits-of-philopatry hypothesis for the evolution of cooperative breeding: variation in territory quality and group size effects. *Am. Nat.*, 137, 831–846.

Sun, S.-J., Rubenstein, D. R., Chen, B.-F., Chan, S.-F., Liu, J.-N., et al. (2014). Climate-mediated cooperation promotes niche expansion in burying beetles. *eLife* 3, e02440.

Vehrencamp, S. L. and Quinn, J. S. (2004). Joint laying systems. In: *Ecology and Evolution of Cooperative Breeding in Birds*, ed. W. D. Koenig and J. L. Dickinson. Cambridge: Cambridge University Press, pp. 177–196.

Yamashina, M. Y. (1938). Die Lebensweise einiger wenig bekannter Sylviiden aus Ostasien. *J. Ornithol.*, 86, 497–515.

Yuan, H.-W., Liu, M., and Shen, S.-F. (2004). Joint nesting in Taiwan yuhinas: a rare passerine case. *Condor*, 106, 862–872.

Yuan, H.-W., Shen, S.-F., Lin, K.-Y., and Lee, P.-F. (2005). Group-size effects and parental investment strategies during incubation in joint-nesting Taiwan yuhinas (*Yuhina brunneiceps*). *Wilson Bull.*, 117, 306–312.

15

Guira cuckoos: Cooperation, infanticide, and female reproductive investment in a joint-nesting species

Regina H. Macedo

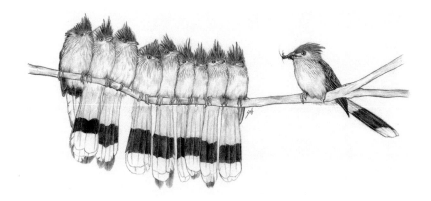

Introduction

Cooperatively breeding birds are species where "more than two individuals rear the chicks at one nest" (Emlen and Vehrencamp 1985), and were first described over a century ago by Australian naturalists (Ashby 1912; Boland and Cockburn 2002). Studies show that the social structure and mating patterns of such species vary widely, and may depend on numerous factors, such as phylogeny, number of individuals of each sex, levels of relatedness among individuals, habitat and climatic characteristics, among other possibilities. A relatively rare form of cooperative breeding is plural breeding with communal nesting (or joint-nesting), characterized by the occurrence of two or more breeding individuals of the same sex that care for the young.

In such species, sharing of reproductive opportunities among individuals may occur among both males and females, and the degree of sharing generates reproductive skew that may vary from 0 (egalitarianism) to 1 (monopolization of reproduction by one individual) (Magrath et al. 2004).

Here I describe the biology of the guira cuckoo (*Guira guira*), a species that combines some of the customary cooperative breeding traits with the added complexities of plural breeding in communal nests. The questions I have subjected to in-depth investigation over the course of this study include: (1) what are the possible selective pressures favoring the evolution of communal nesting? (2) can kin selection explain cooperation? (3) what are the costs and benefits of group living? (4) how does the group resolve conflicts? (5) is

Cooperative Breeding in Vertebrates: Studies of Ecology, Evolution, and Behavior, eds W. D. Koenig and J. L. Dickinson.
Published by Cambridge University Press. © Cambridge University Press 2016.

breeding relatively egalitarian or do some group members monopolize reproduction? and (6) can transactional models of reproductive cooperation and conflict improve our understanding of this system?

The guira cuckoo

Guira cuckoos (see cover photo) belong to the subfamily Crotophaginae, one of six subfamilies in the family Cuculidae. This clade is characterized by social nesting habits instead of the parasitic behaviors for which many of the other cuckoos are known. The Crotophaginae include four species that share the unique form of cooperative breeding described above: plural breeding with a joint-nesting system (Davis 1940, 1941, 1942). In these species, social groups consist of several females that lay their eggs in a single nest, resulting in a shared clutch of offspring. Worldwide, only a handful of species exhibit such characteristics, which inevitably raises questions about the convergence of taxonomic, evolutionary, and ecological factors that promote this breeding system.

The Crotophaginae consist of the monotypic guira cuckoo (*G. guira*) and three species of *Crotophaga*: the greater ani (*C. major*), the groove-billed ani (*C. sulcirostris*), and the smooth-billed ani (*C. ani*). All four species are Neotropical, with overlapping ranges extending from the Rio Negro in Argentina northward through South and Central America and into Texas and Florida in the United States (Davis 1942; Sick 2001). They also share somewhat similar morphology and general behaviors, exhibiting medium-sized bodies (30–46 cm; about 100 g), long tails, terrestrial foraging habits, lethargic gliding flight, and the habit of sunning themselves with outspread wings (Skutch 1959). Earlier accounts of the natural history of crotophagines were followed by more conceptually based studies describing the theoretical foundations of the social and breeding systems of the four species: groove-billed ani in Costa Rica (Vehrencamp 1977, 1978; Vehrencamp et al. 1986; Koford et al. 1990); smooth-billed ani in Florida and Puerto Rico (Loflin 1983; Quinn and Startek-Foote 2000; Schmaltz et al. 2008a, 2008b); greater ani in Panama (Riehl and Jara 2009; Riehl 2010a, 2010b); and guira cuckoo in Brazil.

Guira cuckoos occupy open and semi-open habitats from the Amazon region in northern Brazil southward through most of Brazil, Bolivia, Argentina, Paraguay and Uruguay. Throughout their range they are associated with savanna, scrubby, and altered habitats, including urbanized areas such as parks and gardens, and are not found in forested regions. The guira cuckoo differs markedly in appearance from its crotophagine cousins. Instead of being black, as are the anis, the guira cuckoo has whitish-buff underparts and face, dark grey dorsum and a long tail, a spiky orangish crest that is erected when the bird is agitated, orange bill and iris, and grayish-green legs. Males and females are indistinguishable. Guira cuckoos are highly social and usually found in flocks of 4 to 15 birds foraging on the ground. One of the earliest accounts describes a pet bird kept in an Argentinean household, the eggs of which were pronounced as "beautiful beyond compare" and of an "exquisite turquoise blue" (Farley 1924). Also noted in Farley's account was the bird's capacity to lay numerous eggs: "The bird was prodigal with her eggs; seemed, in short, to have an egg-laying gift." These first descriptive reports mentioned that guira cuckoo eggs were frequently found on the ground, attributing this to accidental or erratic egg-laying behavior.

A long period elapsed before the "egg-laying gift" was further scrutinized from a scientific perspective. The social nesting habits of the guira cuckoo were first described in detail by Davis (1940), who observed that nests were attended by more than a pair of birds and that groups often had more than one simultaneously active nest in their territories. He described communal clutches of 14 and 18 eggs, thus confirming joint-nesting. The rudiments of ecological hypotheses to explain cooperative breeding can be discerned in his account, as when he explains: "Thus it is likely that in many cases the habitat encourages the birds to build a communal nest."

Moving beyond the initial suggestion that poor nest-building skills, predators, or clumsiness accounted for the frequency of eggs found on the ground, Davis (1940) suggested, although not explicitly, the possibility of egg ejection for the smooth-billed ani: "... a colony of fifteen birds dropped six eggs, some as far as twelve feet away from the nest." Ultimately, Vehrencamp (1977) directly observed female groove-billed anis rolling eggs out of the nest, providing the solution to the mystery. My work confirmed that guira cuckoos exhibit similar behavior.

Study area and methods

I studied guira cuckoos for 10 breeding seasons (typically August to March), spanning the years from 1987 to 2001, near the capital city of Brasilia, Brazil. Here I summarize my analyses of this system thus far; unfortunately, urban development around Brasilia no longer allows me to continue this long-term study. My field site in the central Cerrado biome of Brazil (15°47′S, 47°56′W; altitude 1,158 m) covered an area of approximately 20 km², composed mostly of a mosaic of tropical savanna and semi-cultivated fields and gardens. The Cerrado biome is highly seasonal, with a rainy period between October and March, wherein most of the year's precipitation occurs (0.8–2.0 m), and mean annual temperatures of 22–27°C. The endemic, undisturbed savanna in the study site was composed of herbaceous vegetation with shrubs and small trees (3–4 m) that include numerous species of Leguminosae, Vochysiaceae, Myrtaceae, Melastomataceae, and Rubiaceae. Within this matrix of natural savanna, the study site also encompassed many landowners' private properties, including pastures, lawns, and gardens.

Breeding of guira cuckoos in central Brazil coincides with the rainy season, and groups retain the same territories for several years, although these usually remain vacant during the driest part of the year. General field methods included capturing adults using a lure trap with live cuckoos as lures and mist nets, banding them for individual identification, taking blood samples to determine genetic parentage, and conducting behavioral observations to determine territorial occupation, group size and composition, intergroup and interindividual interactions, and provisioning of young.

Natural history and demography

Only rarely (8 of 182 [4.4%] nesting attempts) did we observe a single bird or a pair defending a territory and

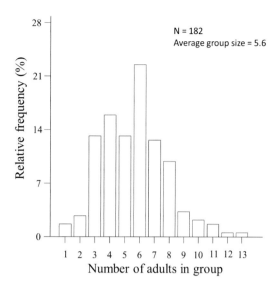

Figure 15.1. Distribution of guira cuckoo group sizes. $N = 182$ groups over 10 years between 1987 and 2001.

attempting to build a nest. Group size averaged 5.6 and ranged from solitary, unpaired birds occupying a territory (3 cases) to a group of 13 birds (Figure 15.1). The most common group size was six (23% of groups), with groups of more than nine birds representing only 8% of all cases.

Guira cuckoos are highly territorial, and groups remain in residence for as long as nine months each year, usually foraging and remaining within 300 m of their nests. At the peak of the dry season many groups abandon their territories and merge with other groups. Although we were unable to track these birds during these periods to find out exactly where they go, we occasionally saw very large assemblages of more than 20 birds foraging together in irrigated areas or near streams. When the rains start the previous territory holders usually once again occupy the territories.

Groups are not composed exclusively of family members and their offspring, although group members are in some cases genetically related (see "The role of direct and indirect fitness benefits"). I rarely observed groups engaging in aggressive behavior along territorial borders, possibly because territories are large and the habitat is not fully saturated. Groups actively defend their territories against intruders, however. Average territory size for five groups in urban areas of Brasilia (mapped in 2002–2003 using 95% adaptive kernel) was 57.0 ± 10.8 ha (range: 68.9–134.5 ha), and groups overlapped very little. I found no correlation between the sizes of these groups and their territories, although this may have been a consequence of the small sample and relative homogeneity among the sizes of the groups.

One of the most curious features of the urbanized landscape occupied by guira cuckoos in central Brazil is the Paraná pine (*Araucaria angustifolia*), introduced as an ornamental species and planted extensively in gardens and along pasture edges. This tree, a conifer native to southern Brazil, has thick, triangular and razor-sharp leaves that cover most of the tree and is the guira cuckoo's preferred nesting site in disturbed landscapes. In its absence, birds typically nest in tall trees with thorny branches or use dense bamboo thickets – vegetation that provides protection from terrestrial predators. Groups occasionally used more than one Paraná pine simultaneously within their territories, and renesting attempts of the same group within the same season usually took place in different Paraná pines.

Guira cuckoos generally forage in groups both within and outside their territories. They are terrestrial foragers that consume large arthropods and small vertebrates such as lizards, snakes, amphibians, and mice, among other potential prey. In addition to foraging on the ground, guira cuckoos occasionally prey on other birds' nestlings, and one individual was even seen capturing a blue-black grassquit (*Volatinia jacarina*) as it executed its courtship leap. Adults appear to search for their quarry using loosely organized herding behavior, with individuals a few meters apart slowly walking over the ground in the same general direction, within visual contact of one another. Quite frequently when one bird catches a large prey, a nearby individual rapidly runs or flies over and attempts to steal it.

Nestlings consume prey that is first killed by the adult before being offered, head first, to the nestlings. In three nests where food items were quantified and their size estimated through focal observations of adult feeding behavior, we found that food items can sometimes be larger than the nestling itself, although the majority (90%) of prey fed to chicks were smaller invertebrates

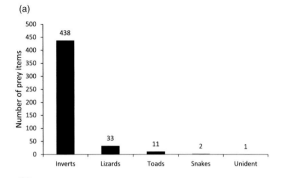

(a)

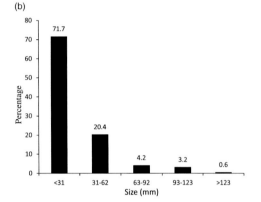

(b)

Figure 15.2. Feeding contributions (*N* = 485 items) brought by adults to nestlings in three communal guira cuckoo nests in central Brazil relative to (a) type of prey; and (b) size of prey.

(Figure 15.2). Sometimes nestlings need several hours to swallow and digest the largest food items such as amphibians and snakes. Nest provisioning behavior by the adults in each group appears to be highly variable, and frequency of feeding differed significantly among adults in five of seven nests (*N* = 2,396 feeding trips) monitored between 1987 and 1990. Although it appears that all group members visit the nest frequently, the number of food items delivered may vary widely since visits do not always indicate prey delivery. In one group composed of six adults, for example, two adults, both of which visited the nest several times, brought only a single food item out of 438 total feedings observed. The genetic data linking these adults to the chicks, however, remain to be analyzed to answer the question of whether relatedness to chicks may influence provisioning rates.

The habitat saturation hypothesis (Selander 1964), postulating that key elements in the habitat are scarce leading a population to occupy all suitable habitat in a region, is potentially applicable to the guira cuckoo system for a number of reasons. Offspring remain within their natal territories for at least one breeding season, and occasionally longer. The extended breeding season often allows a group to produce more than one brood of young, generating overlap between nestlings and juveniles. Finally, groups often contain nonbreeding adults of both sexes (Macedo et al. 2004a; Lima et al. 2011). Presumably, if suitable habitat were available, sexually mature offspring could disperse and adults in larger groups that are excluded from breeding would be able to find alternative breeding sites.

We used a two-pronged approach to test whether dispersal options of cooperative groups are constrained by a saturated habitat. First, we used data from the 1994–1995 breeding season to compare habitat attributes of territories occupied by guira cuckoo groups with those of unoccupied sites. Second, using a broader database from four breeding seasons, we asked whether elements of the vegetation affected breeding parameters of groups and examined the occupancy patterns of territories in the study site (Macedo and Bianchi 1997).

We assumed that the presence of the Paraná pine was one of the important features of a desirable territory. Additionally, the suitability of a territory for a guira cuckoo group could be even more dependent on prey abundance in the substrate and other features, so we assessed a broad array of habitat variables in 14 sites occupied by groups and in nine adjacent and ecologically similar sites that remained vacant during the breeding season. All sites contained at least one but as many as 31 Paraná pines that could be used as nesting sites. We measured 13 variables in each site, including substrate coverage and height, canopy coverage, number and height of shrubs and trees, several measures relative to the number and importance of the Paraná pines and also invertebrate prey abundance and biomass, expecting that some of these would be good predictors of occupancy by guira cuckoo groups. Contrary to our expectation, multivariate discriminant analysis failed to distinguish between occupied and

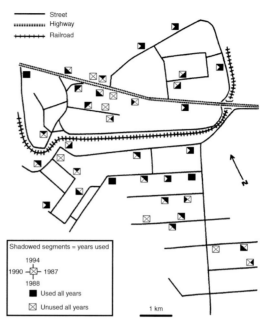

Figure 15.3. Study site map showing the spatial distribution of guira cuckoo nesting sites (squares) during four breeding seasons in central Brazil. Redrawn from Macedo and Bianchi (1997).

empty sites. Additionally, none of the variables differed significantly between empty and occupied sites, with the exception of prey abundance, which was higher in empty sites, mostly due to a single outlier site with high prey abundance.

We also evaluated the possible link between habitat variables and group attributes, using 13 groups that bred 17 times in four different breeding seasons (1987, 1988, 1990, 1994). There was no linear relationship between group size and number of Paraná pines when considering either the largest group size over the years or mean group size. When considering all habitat variables, only the proportion of grass cover was significantly associated with group size.

Finally, the occupancy pattern recorded over four breeding seasons does not suggest a saturated habitat (Figure 15.3). Although there were a few sites that were considered suitable but that were always left unoccupied (empty squares), there were several sites that were occupied in some years and not in others (some segments of square shaded). In fact, in a few cases a group

Table 15.1. Characteristics of breeding groups of guira cuckoos in central Brazil, from 1988 to 2001

Variable	Mean ± S.D. (N)	Range
Group size	5.6 ± 2.2 (182)	1–13
Number of females	2.8 ±1.8 (36)	1–7
Communal clutch size	7.7 ± 4.5 (199)	1–24
Eggs ejected	3.5 ± 3.7 (183)	0–24
Eggs hatched	3.6 ± 3.1 (109)	0–11
Chicks died	2.8 ± 2.6 (78)	0–11
Chicks fledged	2.3 ± 2.0 (101)	0–9

of guira cuckoos that occupied a site in one year had an empty neighboring site within a kilometer that had been occupied in prior years, and thus presumably suitable for breeding. These results suggest that dispersal of individuals to nearby or more distant sites with suitable habitats and optimal nesting spots in the form of Paraná pines was apparently not constrained by a saturated habitat.

Social organization and mating system

Groups often leave their territories during June to August, the driest part of the year in central Brazil, but return at the beginning of the rainy season. When groups remain in their territories throughout the dry season, they wander widely and far beyond their borders. The largest group we monitored had 13 members, and up to seven females may share a communal clutch (Table 15.1). Group composition remains relatively stable through each breeding season and even across a few seasons, but changes are not rare. Groups sometimes renest as many as five times within a breeding season if nests fail. The offspring remain in their natal groups for 2–3 months and then usually disperse, although in a few cases adult offspring remained in their natal units for more than one breeding season. We were unable to band the nestlings consistently, since by the time they can be banded they are also capable of leaving the nest. Thus, offspring retention within the group for more than one season may occur more frequently than we were able to document.

Genealogies of breeding groups were studied for a sample of 51 breeding attempts, sampling adults, eggs, and chicks to estimate relatedness among adult group members as well as parentage (Lima et al. 2011). There was a high degree of variability in relatedness between group members, ranging from low (mean pairwise $r = -0.22$) to high (mean $r = 0.51$). In 30% of groups ($N = 20$), intragroup males were more closely related to each other than to males outside their groups. For females this analysis was only possible for one group, in which females were not more related to each other than expected by chance. Our results indicate low levels of incest, with 2 of 11 (18%) male-female dyads more related to each other than expected by chance and 2 of 225 (1%) offspring from two different nests being the apparent result of an incestuous mating. Taken together, our results are consistent with female-biased dispersal in which sons are more likely to be retained or to form breeding coalitions than are daughters, but they also suggest that kinship is not the primary basis of cooperative breeding in this species.

Shared breeding appears to occur in all groups. That is, all nests contain multiple individuals of both sexes that produce offspring, although not all group members reproduce in each nesting event (Quinn et al. 1994; Macedo et al. 2004a; Lima et al. 2011). We used yolk protein electrophoresis for identifying egg maternity for 195 eggs from 34 nesting bouts produced by 22 groups over two years. Communal clutches in these joint nests ranged from 1 to 19 eggs, but many were reduced through egg ejection. Results indicated that multiple females contributed eggs to nests, and in one rare case, seven females laid a total of 16 eggs. We found that there were no groups where all of the females reproduced in all consecutive nesting bouts, implying that some females are excluded from breeding or unable to breed in particular nesting events (Cariello et al. 2002). On the other hand, we also found that in some groups a subset of females participated in all nesting bouts, suggesting that some females dominate the breeding scenario for at least part of a group's history. In general, female laying order changes across nesting bouts so that no single female monopolizes breeding opportunities for long periods. Breeding patterns of males appear to be similar to those of females in that group membership does not automatically result in siring offspring in any particular nesting event (Lima et al. 2011). Such temporal variation in parentage reduces the level of reproductive skew within groups, at least over the long term (Macedo et al. 2004a), similarly to what has been found for acorn woodpeckers (Chapter 13).

Despite retaining group membership and residing in one territory over different seasons, individuals of both sexes sometimes wander far from their territories and visit groups that may be over 6 km away. I also detected one case where a female produced chicks in nests of two different groups 6 km apart during the same season, albeit in nonoverlapping breeding events. Either this case was one of brood parasitism, unlikely because of the distance between territories, or the female changed groups midseason. In either case, it demonstrates that group members sometimes travel long distances to explore different groups and territories.

Historically, social monogamy has been reported for all three *Crotophaga* species, with observations of conspicuous formation of pair bonds. Polyandry and polygyny have also been suspected, even when observations of paired individuals prevailed (Davis 1942). In groove-billed anis, groups are composed of socially monogamous pairs, but the genetic mating system has yet to be studied (Vehrencamp and Quinn 2004). In smooth-billed anis, there is evidence that genetic monogamy is not always the rule, and analyses suggest the existence of polygamy, intraspecific brood parasitism, and extra-pair fertilization (Startek 1997). In the greater ani, 75–81% of nestlings are produced by socially monogamous pairs, but extra-pair matings are common, and both males and females mate with multiple partners both within and outside the group (Riehl 2012).

Guira cuckoos depart from this pattern of conspicuous social monogamy, since no behavioral pair bonding is evident. Our genetic analyses indicate that mating patterns vary widely among groups, but polygamous mating prevails (72% of nests), with polygynandry being most frequent (28% of nests). Monogamy was estimated to occur in 5–28% of nesting attempts (Lima et al. 2011). We considered genetic monogamy as prevalent in a group when no offspring resulted from extra-pair fertilizations. For example, in a group

monitored in 2001 composed of four males and four females, five offspring were generated by the four male-female pairs, with no evidence that any of the birds parented offspring outside of their pair bond. An example of a polyandrous mating, monitored in 2001, was in a group that consisted of three females and four males that produced six offspring. In this case, one female produced two offspring with one of the males and a third chick with another male. The three additional chicks were produced by two genetically monogamous pairs (one and two chicks, respectively).

Polygynandrous matings, which occurred frequently, were cases where some males and females within groups produced chicks with more than one partner. One example, from 1998, was a group composed of three males and two females that produced five chicks. The two females each mated with two males. One of the males sired offspring with both females while the other two males mated monogamously.

From nest building to infanticide

Guira cuckoo groups in central Brazil build conspicuous, bulky, open-cup structures with large twigs and lined with fresh leaves that are constantly renovated by the adults during egg-laying and incubation. The earliest clutch we found was initiated in July, typically the driest month of the year, while the latest clutch in the season was laid in May with 90% of all nesting attempts concentrated within a four-month period from August to November. These peak breeding months correspond to the early rainy season when insects are relatively abundant (Pinheiro et al. 2002; Silva et al. 2011).

Guira cuckoo eggs are round to elliptical and exhibit large variation in size, ranging from 15.8 to 32.3 g (mean = 24.6 ± 2.9 g; $N = 509$ eggs). They are turquoise blue and their outer surface is covered with a lacelike white pattern of splotches and lines composed of vaterite (Figure 15.4), a polymorph of calcium carbonate that has been found in the eggshells of the smooth-billed ani and a few other birds including some species of Pelecaniformes. The patterns of its deposition in guira cuckoo eggs are astonishingly beautiful, and merit

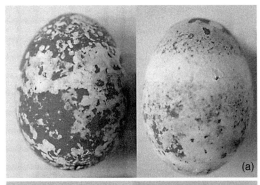

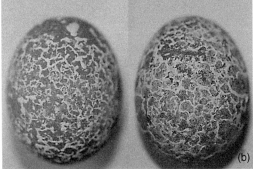

Figure 15.4. (a) Two eggs laid by the same female in one nesting event, showing the large degree of variation for eggs laid by the same female. (b) Two eggs laid by different females in consecutive nesting bouts of the same group, showing the possible similarity of eggs produced by different females. From Cariello et al. (2004).

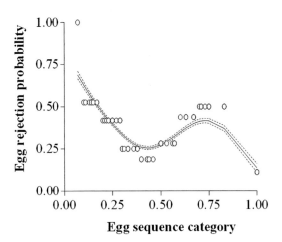

Figure 15.5. The relationship between egg ejection probability and egg sequence index; curve fitted by a cubic spline. The open circles represent the probability of egg ejection according to its position in the communal clutch. Redrawn from Macedo et al. (2004b).

Board and Perrott's (1979) suggestion that they are similar to Wedgewood pottery.

Communal clutches vary in size from 1 to 24 eggs produced by up to seven females. Not all eggs laid are incubated, however, as these joint clutches are usually reduced through egg-ejection carried out by group members: of 239 completed clutches, egg ejection carried out by members of the social group took place in 89%. Egg ejection is correlated with the number of females in the group, but not with group size, which suggests that female competition drives this behavior.

Egg ejection as first described in detail for groove-billed anis was explained as being perpetrated by females that had not yet laid any eggs, thus implying that females could not recognize their own

eggs (Vehrencamp 1977). In support of this conjecture, the highest probability of egg ejection for guira cuckoo clutches occurs early during the egg-laying sequence – what I call the "egg laying-ejection phase" when eggs typically are ejected as soon as they are laid (Figure 15.5). It is fairly common for eggs to be ejected on the same day they are laid, but eggs are also ejected after incubation has started, however. This raises the possibility that group females can discriminate among eggs, perhaps by differentiating freshly laid from older eggs, which could allow them to discriminate and eject eggs laid after they have laid their own eggs. This possibility has been verified experimentally for the greater ani, where group members use this recognition rule to eject eggs laid out of synchrony by extra-group parasites (Riehl 2010a).

The 24 eggs laid in one nesting attempt mentioned earlier were entirely destroyed by sequential ejection of eggs as they were laid. In cases such as this, the group is apparently trapped in the egg laying-ejection phase. Given such cases, it is perhaps not surprising that we find no correlation between group size and the communal clutch size of incubated eggs, almost certainly because group size does not correspond to the number of breeding females in the group or participating in a

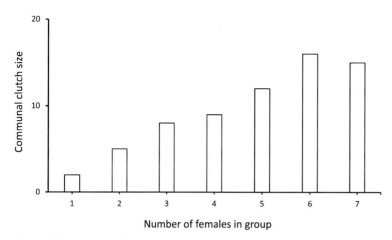

Figure 15.6. Communal clutch size (number of eggs incubated) relative to the number of females based on data from 36 groups where female identities were verified genetically.

particular nesting bout. Using only breeding bouts from groups for which we had genetically identified females ($N = 36$ groups), we verified that the number of females laying eggs is closely associated not only with the communal clutch size ($r = 0.88$, $P < 0.001$; Figure 15.6), but also with the number of eggs ejected ($r = 0.36$, $P = 0.04$; $N = 34$). This suggests that as the number of females sharing reproduction increases, so does the extent of conflict involving egg investment and ownership of the incubated clutch.

Incubation lasts 10 days and eggs within a nest usually hatch within 24 h (75% of 28 clutches monitored during hatching), although hatching periods of up to four days were observed. Nestlings grow very rapidly, and if the nest is approached on the fifth or sixth day after hatching, nestlings can potentially leave the nest and scramble around the branches, and may fall or leap to the ground. Chicks can fledge as early as 12 days after hatching, but more typically around day 15.

Although predation, inferred from whole clutch or brood disappearance along with visible damage to the nest, was rare and involved only 5–6% of eggs and chicks, the developmental period from egg to fledging is fraught with hazards. Many eggs do not last long after being laid, and after hatching few chicks survive to fledge. The most typical cause of mortality for both eggs and chicks was ejection from the nest, carried out

by adult group members. Of 1,530 eggs monitored, only 900 (58.8%) became part of the incubated clutch due to the ejection by group members (Figure 15.7). Of these, only 389 survived to hatching (43.2% of eggs incubated, 25.4% of eggs laid). Brood reduction after hatching is also common, with 227 of 389 hatchlings (58%) surviving to fledge on day 15.

Infanticide was first suspected when I noticed the almost daily disappearance of chicks from their nests, usually during the first few days after hatching. Occasionally, dead or wounded chicks were found on the ground under the nest. Eventually, I observed adults killing chicks and pieced together a predictable pattern. First, most victimized nestlings are less than six days old. A young chick is either tossed directly over the rim of the nest by one of the group's adults or carried 30–40 m from the nest and dropped to the ground. The chick is then attacked not only by the infanticidal adult, but by other members of the group. In none of the observed attacks did any adult attempt to defend the chick after it was on the ground. Paradoxically, one adult observed killing a chick had previously cared for chicks in the communal nest. None of the killed chicks was ever seen to be cannibalized by adults.

There are several hypotheses for why birds might benefit by eliminating chicks from a brood. One, dating back to Lack (1947, 1954), proposes that birds

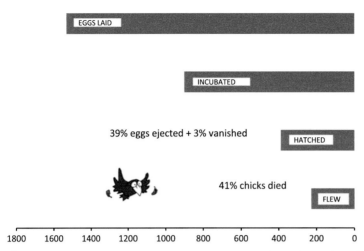

Figure 15.7. Number of eggs laid, incubated, and hatched over 10 years. Losses shown between each category are approximately: 40% between laying and incubation; 55% between incubation and hatching; and 41% between hatching and fledging.

deliberately lay more eggs than they normally can rear. If breeding conditions are favorable, then extra eggs represent a bonus for the parents if they survive to fledge. If conditions are marginal, one or more chicks can be sacrificed to help ensure the survival of other offspring. This explanation does not appear to be applicable to the brood reduction in guira cuckoos given that several entire broods were eliminated through infanticide.

Alternatively, infanticide may be performed by individuals to enhance their own reproductive opportunities within the group (Hrdy 1979). For example, if one or more adults were initially denied an opportunity to breed because of the lack of a partner or early ejection of all its eggs, those individuals could improve their future chances of breeding by disrupting the current nesting bout through egg ejection and infanticide (Koenig 1990). In support of this hypothesis, groups that lose all of their eggs and chicks renest within a shorter time interval (mean = 34.9 days) than groups with surviving chicks (mean = 65.7 days; Macedo 1994). Additional work will be necessary to conclusively test whether sexually selected infanticide in guira cuckoos provides a robust explanation for the frequent brood reduction and total nest failure observed in this species.

Female reproductive manipulation: how much is an egg worth?

Oscar Wilde once remarked that "An egg is always an adventure; the next one may be different," and biologically, egg variability has important consequences, since in many species larger eggs result in larger chicks with higher chances of survival (Williams 1994). There are several other egg traits that are in some cases associated with offspring fitness, including yolk androgen concentrations, relative amounts of yolk and albumin, and various specific nutrients (Schwabl et al. 1997; Badyaev et al. 2005). Ideally, females should invest maximally in each, but there are trade-offs, since nutrient allocation to eggs is energetically costly, and current investment in an egg or clutch potentially reduces female condition and thus investments in future reproduction. The adaptive modification of clutch or egg characteristics in response to social or mating circumstances remains one of the more elusive yet exciting facets of bird breeding biology (Sheldon 2000; Drummond et al. 2008; Paquet et al. 2013).

Adaptive adjustment of maternal allocation to eggs may be particularly valuable for guira cuckoo females, since eggs face the possibility of eviction and, upon hatching, chicks are confronted with possible infanticide. Given the competitive context that involves obtaining a breeding slot and space in the communal nest for their eggs, females have several options. Since the habitat is not saturated and potential mates are not limiting, they could presumably go off with a male and attempt to breed on their own. As this is rarely observed, we assume that the advantages of group living outweigh the costs. Are there maternal effects that increase those benefits or minimize their costs?

Egg loss for guira cuckoos represents a significant energetic cost, given that their eggs are relatively large, averaging 25 g in mass, about 16% of female body mass (Macedo 1992). Do females adjust their egg investment according to the probability of ejection? We examined this issue by asking the following questions (Macedo et al. 2004b): (1) is there a relationship between the position of an egg in the laying sequence of the communal clutch, probability of ejection, and number of breeding females? (2) does the nutrient content of eggs reflect social circumstances? (3) does the position of the female in the egg-laying queue influence her investment in the clutch? and (4) do female egg manipulation decisions translate into differences in chick size and survival?

Patterns of egg ejection vary greatly from nest to nest, although the most common pattern is the sequential ejection of freshly-laid eggs at the beginning of egg-laying by the group. A direct comparison between ejected eggs and eggs retained for incubation showed that the latter had significantly larger yolks and thinner shells. Additionally, we found that in groups with more females (and therefore larger communal clutches), eggs are larger in mass and albumin content, although not in yolk content. Also, for communal clutches of all sizes, females that enter the laying sequence first not only suffer a high rate of egg ejection and lay eggs with lower nutrient content but lay more eggs than females that lay last. Last-laying females derive benefits because larger eggs produce heavier chicks that are less likely to suffer infanticide than small chicks. Thus, the production of larger eggs and a smaller clutch by late-laying females may reflect a trade-off between the costs of egg production and the probability of their loss through ejection.

We also analyzed whether maternal androgen investment in eggs was associated with possible female laying tactics that reflect the competitive environment of groups, again finding that the social context of communal breeding influences individual reproductive tactics (Cariello et al. 2006). When females laid up to three eggs in communal clutches, their first egg had lower androgen concentrations than the second and third eggs, and these first-laid eggs had a higher chance of being ejected. One hypothesis for this finding, which has also been observed in smooth-billed anis (Schmaltz et al. 2008b), is that differential androgen allocation favoring later eggs – which are more likely to survive the ejection period – may result in chicks that are more active and aggressive, which could in turn lead to dominance and increased survival within the communal brood. We also found that androstenedione, but not testosterone, yolk concentrations were higher in larger communal clutches, again lending support to the idea that chicks in more competitive social environments may benefit from higher androgen concentrations. The link between yolk androgens and chick phenotype remains to be explored in the context of survival within communal broods, however.

The role of direct and indirect fitness benefits

The costs of group living in all four crotophagines are particularly evident, including egg burial and ejection (Vehrencamp et al. 1986, Macedo et al. 2004a, 2004b; Schmaltz et al. 2008a; Riehl and Jara 2009), as well as known or suspected infanticide (Macedo and Melo 1999; Macedo et al. 2001; Riehl and Jara 2009; Quinn et al. 2010). Female laying tactics, as described above, can attenuate some of these drawbacks. What, however, are the advantages to group living?

One benefit of sociality in many cooperative breeders is the opportunity to gain indirect fitness by helping relatives. Such indirect fitness benefits do not appear to play a significant role in either smooth-billed or greater anis, both of which have been shown to have low levels of relatedness among group members (Blanchard 2000; Riehl 2011). The situation in guira cuckoos appears to be more complex, with relatedness among adult group members varying considerably among groups.

In about a third of the population, adult males within groups are more closely related than expected by chance (Lima et al. 2011). This suggests that at least in some cases male philopatry, or joint dispersal by male kin, results in kin associations. In several groups, non-breeding males were genetically related to the group's progeny, indicating that these male helpers may be reaping indirect fitness benefits. Retention of male offspring in natal territories, joint dispersal by male kin, or both may explain male group composition in guira cuckoos. Indirect fitness benefits are unlikely to be gained by females, however, given that they disperse much greater distances from their natal territories than do males.

Thus far there has been little focus on the potential direct benefits of social life in this taxon. Larger groups with three or more pairs in greater anis have lower rates of nest predation, even when controlling for nest-site quality (Riehl 2011). Thus, at least in this species, the main factor selecting for group living and breeding appears to be the direct benefits associated with more efficient nest defense against predators in larger groups and their ability to defend better nesting sites. For smooth-billed anis, lowered predation probably plays an important role selecting for group living as well, since groups exhibit a sentinel system where a single bird gives alarm calls from an elevated site (Loflin 1983). There is also some evidence that groups provide protection against nest predators (Quinn and Startek-Foote 2000). In the case of guira cuckoos, birds exhibit "nest-attendance" behavior (Macedo 1994) whereby adults take turns perching near the nest after feeding chicks, a behavior which may provide protection for the nest from both predators and infanticidal group members. Thus, both direct and indirect fitness benefits may play a role in group living and breeding in this species.

Conclusions

The guira cuckoo, along with its ani relatives, is strikingly different from the other cooperative breeders discussed in this book. In most of these other species, dependent offspring are retained in their natal territories and help their parents rear younger siblings. Most are constrained from breeding by incest avoidance, many are limited in their dispersal options because of habitat saturation, and nearly all typically live in family groups where indirect fitness benefits are crucial. In guira cuckoos the genetic structure of groups exhibits great variability, and while some groups may include genetically related birds, others are unrelated. Furthermore, groups usually contain several breeders of both sexes, generating a considerable amount of complexity in terms of competitive and cooperative interactions. Thus, the guira cuckoo is a species in which social living and cooperative breeding are not necessarily associated with indirect fitness benefits (Figure 15.8). Furthermore, group living persists despite the availability of alternative breeding sites. Even more notable is that individuals continue to live in groups despite intense reproductive competition in the form of egg ejection and infanticide.

When groups are nonkin-based, they are expected to exhibit similarities with the anis in terms of increased importance of behaviors and patterns that promote direct fitness benefits, such as increased vigilance for predators and higher incidences of group foraging. Because of the low kinship among group members, however, they might also be expected to exhibit higher levels of reproductive competition in the form of egg ejection and infanticide. In guira cuckoo groups that are kin-based, the conflicts of interest generated by the shared breeding might potentially be attenuated due to the higher levels of kinship, resulting in lower reproductive competition and in indirect fitness benefits (Figure 15.8). Kinship in itself does not necessarily safeguard against intense reproductive competition, however, as illustrated by the egg destruction behavior exhibited by female acorn woodpeckers (Chapter 13). In general, benefits to individuals should depend on the specific profile of the group, and may vary along a gradient reflecting the genetic composition of the group and the degree of conflict resulting from reproductive competition.

In conclusion, the subfamily Crotophaginae is ideally suited to examine how kinship mediates the trade-offs between direct benefits and reproductive competition. Comparative analyses of all four species should contribute toward a better understanding of the numerous

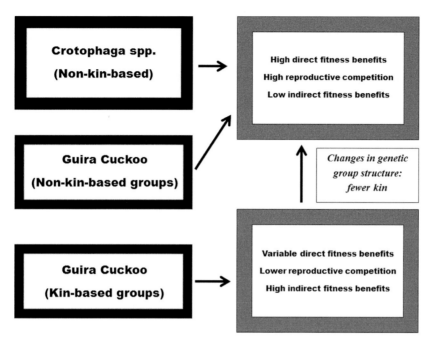

Figure 15.8. Diagram showing the consequences, in terms of benefits and costs, for kin and nonkin-based group living crotophagine species.

selective pressures and evolutionary routes that can lead to group living and, more specifically, to shared reproduction and joint nesting.

Acknowledgments

I am grateful to Walt Koenig and Janis Dickinson for inviting me to contribute this chapter, and to their thorough and insightful comments. I am indebted to numerous students over the years, including Carlos A. Bianchi, Mariana Cariello, Marcos R. Lima, Celine Melo, Laura Muniz, and Angela Pacheco. I would also like to single out Jeff Graves and Hubert Schwabl, who participated in my quest for answers. James Quinn shared my initial interest for the guira cuckoos and provided many helpful insights. I am most grateful to Hugh Drummond and Christina Riehl for their valuable comments on previous versions of this manuscript. The Universidade de Brasília provided logistic support that kept my research afloat in difficult periods, and long-term financial support was generously provided by the National Geographic Society and CNPq (Brazil research funding council). I am forever indebted to my parents, who contributed not only financially, but with support and enthusiasm. My husband, Carlyle, helped to carry ladders and scaffolds and has always been available to discuss ideas. I also thank my daughters, Natasha and Chantal, for enduring my frequent absences, my single-minded focus on "bird topics," and numerous intrusions of field-related issues into our family life.

REFERENCES

Ashby, E. (1912). The *Malurus. Emu*, 11, 254.

Badyaev, A. V., Schwabl, H. G., Young, R. L., Duckworth, R. A., Navara, K. J., et al. (2005). Adaptive sex differences in growth of pre-ovulation oocytes in a passerine bird. *Proc. R. Soc. London B*, 272, 2165–2172.

Blanchard, L. (2000). An investigation of the communal breeding system of the smooth-billed ani (*Crotophaga ani*). M.Sc. thesis, McMaster University, Hamilton, Ontario, Canada.

Board, R. G. and Perrott, H. R. (1979). Vaterite, a constituent of the eggshells of the nonparasitic cuckoos, *Guira guira* and *Crogophaga ani. Calcif. Tissue Int.*, 29, 63–69.

Boland, C. R. J. and Cockburn, A. (2002). Short sketches from the long history of cooperative breeding in Australian birds. *Emu*, 102, 9–17.

Cariello, M. O., Schwabl, H. G., Lee, R. W., and Macedo, R. H. (2002). Individual female clutch identification through yolk protein electrophoresis in the communally-breeding guira cuckoo (*Guira guira*). *Mol. Ecol.*, 11, 2417–2424.

Cariello, M. O., Lima, M. R., Schwabl, H. G., and Macedo, R. H. (2004). Egg characteristics are unreliable in determining maternity in communal clutches of guira cuckoos *Guira guira. J. Avian Biol.*, 35, 117–124.

Cariello, M. O., Macedo, R. H., and Schwabl, H. G. (2006). Maternal androgens in eggs of communally breeding guira cuckoos (*Guira guira*). *Horm. Behav.*, 49, 654–662.

Davis, D. E. (1940). Social nesting habits of the smooth-billed ani. *Auk*, 57, 179–218.

Davis, D. E. (1941). Social nesting habits of *Crotophaga major. Auk*, 58, 179–183.

Davis, D. E. (1942). The phylogeny of social nesting habits in the Crotophaginae. *Q. Rev. Biol.*, 17, 115–134.

Drummond, H., Rodríguez, C., and Schwabl, H. G. (2008). Do mothers regulate facultative and obligate siblicide by differentially provisioning eggs with hormones? *J. Avian Biol.*, 39, 139–143.

Emlen, S. T. and Vehrencamp, S. (1985). Cooperative breeding strategies among birds. In: *Experimental Behavioral Ecology*, ed. B. Hölldobler and M. Lindauer. Stuttgart: Gustav Fischer, pp. 359–374.

Farley, J. A. (1924). Argentine birds. *Auk*, 41, 169–170.

Hrdy, S. B. (1979). Infanticide among animals: a review, classification, and examination of the implications for the reproductive strategies of females. *Ethol. Sociobiol.*, 1, 13–40.

Koenig, W. D. (1990). Opportunity of parentage and nest destruction in polygynandrous acorn woodpeckers, *Melanerpes formicivorus. Behav. Ecol.*, 1, 55–61.

Koford, R. R., Bowen, B. S., and Vehrencamp, S. L. (1990). Groove-billed anis: joint-nesting in a tropical cuckoo. In: *Cooperative Breeding in Birds: Long-term Studies of Ecology and Behavior*, ed. P. B. Stacey and W. D. Koenig. Cambridge: Cambridge University Press, pp. 335–355.

Lack, D. (1947). The significance of clutch size. *Ibis*, 89, 302–352.

Lack, D. (1954). *The Natural Regulation of Animal Numbers*. London: Oxford University Press.

Lima, M. R., Macedo, R. H., Muniz, L., Pacheco, A., and Graves, J. (2011). Group composition, mating system and relatedness in the communally breeding guira cuckoo in central Brazil. *Auk*, 128, 475–486.

Loflin, R. K. (1983). Communal behaviors of the smooth-billed ani (*Crotophaga ani*). Ph.D. thesis, University of Miami, Coral Gables, Florida.

Macedo, R. H. (1992). Reproductive patterns and social organization of the communal guira cuckoo (*Guira guira*) in central Brazil. *Auk*, 109, 786–799.

Macedo, R. H. (1994). Inequities in parental effort and costs of communal breeding in the guira cuckoo. *Neotr. Ornithol.*, 5, 79–90.

Macedo, R. H. and Bianchi, C. (1997). Communal breeding in tropical guira cuckoos *Guira guira*: sociality in the absence of a saturated habitat. *J. Avian Biol.*, 28, 207–215.

Macedo, R. H. and Melo, C. (1999). Confirmation of infanticide in the communally breeding guira cuckoo. *Auk*, 116, 847–851.

Macedo, R. H., Cariello, M. O., and Muniz, L. (2001). Context and frequency of infanticide in communally breeding guira cuckoos. *Condor*, 103, 170–175.

Macedo, R. H., Cariello, M. O., Graves, J., and Schwabl, H. (2004a). Reproductive partitioning in communally breeding guira cuckoos, *Guira guira. Behav. Ecol. Sociobiol.*, 55, 213–222.

Macedo, R. H., Cariello, M. O., Pacheco, A., and Schwabl, H. (2004b). Significance of social parameters on differential nutrient investment in guira cuckoo (*Guira guira*) eggs. *Anim. Behav.*, 68, 485–494.

Magrath, R. D., Johnstone, R. A., and Heinsohn, R. G. (2004). Reproductive skew. In: *Ecology and Evolution of Cooperative Breeding in Birds*, ed. W. D. Koenig and J. L. Dickinson. Cambridge: Cambridge University Press, pp. 157–176.

Paquet, M., Covas, R., Chastel, O., Parenteau, C., and Doutrelant, C. (2013). Maternal effects in relation to helper presence in the cooperatively breeding sociable weaver. *PLoS One*, 8, e59336.

Pinheiro, F., Diniz, I. R., Coelho, D., and Bandeira, M. P. S. (2002). Seasonal pattern of insect abundance in the Brazilian cerrado. *Austral Ecol.*, 27, 132–136.

Quinn, J. S. and Startek-Foote, J. M. (2000). Smooth-billed ani (*Crotophaga ani*). In *The Birds of North America*, ed. A. Poole. Ithaca: Cornell Lab of Ornithology; retrieved from the Birds of North America Online: http://bna.birds.cornell.edu/bna/species/539

Quinn, J. S., Macedo, R. H., and White, B. N. (1994). Genetic relatedness of communally breeding guira cuckoos. *Anim. Behav.*, 47, 515–529.

Quinn, J. S., Samuelsen, A., Barclay, M., Schmaltz, G., and Kahn, H. (2010). Circumstantial evidence for infanticide of chicks of the communal smooth-billed ani (*Crotophaga ani*). *Wilson J. Ornithol.*, 122, 369–374.

Riehl, C. (2010a). A simple rule reduces costs of extragroup parasitism in a communally breeding bird. *Curr. Biol.*, 20, 1830–1833.

Riehl, C. (2010b). Egg ejection risk and hatching asynchrony predict egg mass in a communally breeding cuckoo, the greater ani (*Crotophaga major*). *Behav. Ecol.*, 21, 676–683.

Riehl, C. (2011). Living with strangers: direct benefits favour non-kin cooperation in a communally nesting bird. *Proc. R. Soc. London B*, 278, 1728–1735.

Riehl, C. (2012). Mating system and reproductive skew in a communally breeding cuckoo: hard-working males do not sire more young. *Anim. Behav.*, 84, 707–714.

Riehl, C. and Jara, L. (2009). Natural history and reproductive biology of the communally breeding greater ani (*Crotophaga major*) at Gatún Lake, Panama. *Wilson J. Ornithol.*, 121, 679–687.

Schmaltz, G., Quinn, J. S., and Lenz, C. (2008a). Competition and waste in the communally breeding smooth-billed ani: effects of group size on egg-laying behaviour. *Anim. Behav.*, 76, 153–162.

Schmaltz, G., Quinn, J. S., and Schoech, S. J. (2008b). Do group size and laying order influence maternal deposition of testosterone in smooth-billed ani eggs? *Horm. Behav.*, 53, 82–89.

Schwabl H., Mock, D. W., and Gieg, J. A. (1997). A hormonal mechanism for parental favouritism. *Nature*, 386, 231.

Selander, R. K. (1964). Speciation in wrens of the genus *Campylorhynchus*. *Univ. Calif. Publ. Zool.*, 74, 1–305.

Sheldon, B. C. (2000). Differential allocation: tests, mechanisms and implications. *Trends Ecol. Evol.*, 15, 397–402.

Sick, H. (2001). *Ornitologia Brasileira*, 3rd edn. Rio de Janeiro, Brazil: Editora Nova Fronteira.

Silva, N. A. P., Frizzas, M. R., and Oliveira, C. M. (2011). Seasonality in insect abundance in the "Cerrado" of Goiás State, Brazil. *Rev. Bras. Entomol.*, 55, 79–87.

Skutch, A. F. (1959). Life history of the groove-billed ani. *Auk*, 76, 281–317.

Startek, J. M. (1997). Microsatellite DNA analysis of the communal breeding system of the smooth-billed ani (*Crotophaga ani*) in southwest Puerto Rico. M.Sc. thesis, McMaster University, Hamilton, Ontario, Canada.

Vehrencamp, S. L. (1977). Relative fecundity and parental effort in communally nesting anis, *Crotophaga sulcirostris*. *Science*, 197, 403–405.

Vehrencamp, S. L. (1978). The adaptive significance of communal nesting in groove-billed anis (*Crotophaga sulcirostris*). *Behav. Ecol. Sociobiol.*, 4, 1–33.

Vehrencamp, S. L., Bowen, B. S., and Koford, R. R. (1986). Breeding roles and pairing patterns within communal groups of groove-billed anis. *Anim. Behav.*, 34, 347–366.

Vehrencamp, S. L. and Quinn, J. S. (2004). Joint laying systems. In: *Ecology and Evolution of Cooperative Breeding in Birds*, ed. W. D. Koenig and J. L. Dickinson. Cambridge: Cambridge University Press, pp. 177–196.

Williams, T. D. (1994). Intraspecific variation in egg size and egg composition in birds: effects on offspring fitness. *Biol. Rev.*, 68, 35–59.

16

Cichlid fishes: A model for the integrative study of social behavior

Michael Taborsky

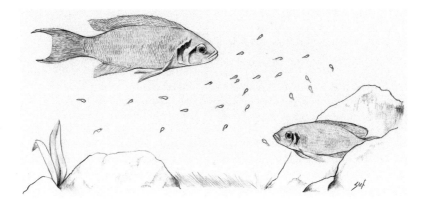

Introduction

Cooperative breeding – characterized by the joint care of young produced primarily by dominant group members – is widespread in animals, including invertebrates, birds, and mammals (Brown 1987; Stacey and Koenig 1990; Solomon and French 1997; Bourke 2011). Unequal partitioning of reproduction or "reproductive skew" is paramount for this type of social system (Hager and Jones 2009). Usually, groups form by the extended philopatry of offspring, which causes high degrees of relatedness within groups (Koenig et al. 1992; Bourke 2011). Therefore, kin selection has been considered to be the major explanatory framework for the cooperative behavior of group members having no or a lower share of the group's reproduction (Hamilton 1964; Griffin and West 2003; Bourke 2011).

The story is quite different in fish, where cooperative breeding has been described in roughly 25 species of cichlids and a few other species (Taborsky 1994). In the cooperatively breeding fish species investigated thus far, relatedness among adult group members on average seems to be low. This makes fish extremely well suited to study the importance of evolutionary mechanisms other than kin selection that can generate advanced sociality.

At first glance, it is puzzling why cooperative breeding is so rare (< 0.1% of 32,700 known fish species). Most importantly, the majority of fish species show little or no brood care. Their specialty is rather to produce large offspring numbers – quantity instead of quality – and leave them without any postfertilization care. In fish taxa showing brood care, typically only one parent takes responsibility, often caring for several

Cooperative Breeding in Vertebrates: Studies of Ecology, Evolution, and Behavior, eds W. D. Koenig and J. L. Dickinson.
Published by Cambridge University Press. © Cambridge University Press 2016.

clutches at a time (Breder and Rosen 1966; Blumer 1979, 1982). Such efficiency is possible because young fish are usually not fed by their parents and offspring protection is a sharable benefit. Therefore, the effort required to care for them hardly rises with increasing offspring numbers (Blumer 1979; Sargent and Gross 1986). Consequently, only a relatively small number of fish species have biparental care (Sargent and Gross 1986), an apparent precondition for the evolution of cooperative breeding (Komdeur and Ekman 2010). If the number of biparental species is taken as baseline, the percentage of cooperatively breeding fish species is more comparable to that of mammals and birds (ca. 3.5%, based on estimated number of fish species with biparental care; Blumer 1982; Gross and Sargent 1985). In addition, relatively few social and breeding systems of fishes have been studied, and thus there may be quite a few cooperatively breeding fishes that have not yet been detected.

The greatest number of cooperatively breeding fish species occurs among the cichlids (family Cichlidae) of the East African Rift Valley's Lake Tanganyika. In this deep and ancient lake, some 70 species of cichlids do not raise their young in the mouth like the majority of African lacustrine cichlids, but instead attach eggs to substrate and care for the brood by biparental guarding (Brichard 1978; Kuwamura 1997; Konings 1998). Often this involves keeping predators at bay by aggressive behavior, providing shelters, for instance by digging out holes under stones or collecting empty gastropod shells, cleaning eggs and larvae, and supplying eggs with oxygen by fanning. About one-third of these biparental "substrate brooders" of Lake Tanganyika breed cooperatively (Taborsky 1994; Heg and Bachar 2006).

The reproductive and social systems of these cooperative cichlids vary substantially. Groups may include different numbers of immatures, for instance, whereas the number of mature subordinate helpers varies within narrower limits (with means usually varying between one and three males and/or females; Heg et al. 2005a; Taborsky 2009). Relatedness among group members varies both between species (very low in *Julidochromis ornatus*, Awata et al. 2005; rather high in *Neolamprologus multifasciatus*, Kohler 1997; Taborsky

2009) and within species (Dierkes et al. 2005), which may have strong and unexpected effects on cooperation among group members (Stiver et al. 2005; Zöttl et al. 2013a). Reproduction may be highly skewed among group members (as described here for *Neolamprologus pulcher*) or rather balanced (*J. ornatus*, Awata et al. 2005). Different forms of cooperative breeding and other manifestations of cooperative reproduction in fish, including non-cichlids, have been discussed elsewhere (Taborsky 1994, 2009).

Neolamprologus pulcher as a model

As yet, most information on cooperative breeding in fishes has been collected from one of the Lake Tanganyika substrate brooders, the lamprologine cichlid *Neolamprologus pulcher* (Wong and Balshine 2011). *N. pulcher* occurs in rocky habitats around the sublittoral zone of the lake. Originally the fish of northern populations were described as *Lamprologus brichardi*, whereas the southern populations were described as *L. (savoryi) pulcher* (Poll 1974). A lake-wide genetic comparison of different populations revealed no clear-cut separation between these two morphs, but rather a gradual clinal variation in which differences increased with the distance between sampled populations. Thus, both morphs are now referred to as *N. pulcher* (Duftner et al. 2007). Incidentally, *pulcher* is Latin for "beautiful," which many view as appropriate name.

Social system

Breeding units or "groups" of *N. pulcher* usually consist of a dominant pair of breeders and a variable number of subordinate individuals ranging widely in size. In the north of the lake, a few breeder pairs have been found without helpers (~5%), whereas breeding units lacking helpers are extremely rare in southern populations (< 1%; Taborsky and Limberger 1981; Heg et al. 2005b). Hence it seems justified to categorize *N. pulcher* as an obligatory cooperative breeder. On average, groups include a pair of dominant breeders and between five and six subordinate helpers ≥ 15 mm standard length (SL) (Taborsky and Limberger 1981; Balshine et al.

2001; Heg et al. 2005b), with helper numbers ranging between 1 and 30 per group.

Virtually all subordinate group members help defend, maintain, and improve the territory as well as care for the brood, which is why subordinates are generally referred to as "helpers." Groups defend a territory consisting of a breeding shelter and a variable number of additional shelters, which may be monopolized by individual group members but are typically shared by several of them (Taborsky 1984; Balshine et al. 2001; Werner et al. 2003). A small space around these shelters is also part of the defended area (≤ 0.33 m^2; Taborsky and Limberger 1981).

In addition to group members, the population contains two types of nonreproductive individuals of both sexes that do not belong to breeding groups. In the north of the lake, sexually mature nongroup members are part of stable aggregations surrounding group territories (ca. 20% of the population, with a significant male bias; Taborsky 1982, 1984). Such individuals do not have access to individual shelters, but they grow much faster than group members and are candidates for potential territory takeovers if an opportunity arises. In southern populations, individuals that do not belong to breeding groups defend individual shelters outside of group territories, which they may share with one or two conspecifics called "group independents." Such individuals make up about 5% of the population (Stiver et al. 2004; Heg et al. 2005a).

The social system of *N. pulcher* is particularly well suited to increasing our understanding of the evolution of sociality, because several features diverge significantly from those of most other cooperative breeders. These include:

(1) Due to indeterminate growth, group members vary greatly in body size, and the efficiency of most cooperative tasks depends on size. This is effectively a size-specific specialization in the division of labor (size-dependent polyethism; Bruintjes and Taborsky 2011).

(2) Reproductive skew within groups differs between males and females and is contingent on group composition (Heg et al. 2008a).

(3) Groups consist of a mixture of related and unrelated individuals. Relatedness among breeders and helpers declines with increasing age of the latter. That is, the largest and most efficient helpers are usually unrelated to their beneficiaries (Dierkes et al. 2005).

(4) Transactions between breeders and helpers over the amount of cooperative effort that subordinates deliver provide opportunities to understand why subordinates pay to stay in the territory of dominants by helping to raise and protect the latters' broods (Bergmüller and Taborsky 2005). In this situation, relatedness can even reduce cooperative effort (Zöttl et al. 2013a). Thus, cooperative breeding reflects reciprocal trading of commodities.

(5) One particular ecological factor – predation pressure – is the dominating ecoevolutionary trigger of this social system (Taborsky 1984; Heg et al. 2004a). It explains colonial breeding, extended philopatry, altruistic effort of helpers that pay to stay in a safe territory, strategic growth of helpers, and the degree of reproductive skew within groups.

In addition to these features, *N. pulcher* is exceptionally well suited for observational and experimental studies both under natural and standardized laboratory conditions. One or several territories of natural size can be easily hosted in a moderately sized aquarium; all behaviors can be easily observed and individuals can be tracked around the clock; the behavior in seminatural laboratory settings does not differ in most aspects from behavior shown in the field; the complex behavioral repertoire including roughly 30 agonistic, affiliative, and submissive behaviors exerted among group members can be directly observed, video recorded, and experimentally manipulated; groups can be artificially composed of individuals with different sizes, sexes, behavioral types ("personalities"), and degrees of relatedness and familiarity; individuals respond well to experimental alterations of their ecology, social environment, and behavior; and important ecological parameters, such as predation, habitat structure, food, and shelter can be easily manipulated. Furthermore, the physiological and genetic mechanisms controlling behavior can be experimentally studied, as will be outlined below; the recent assembly of the genome sequence of *N. brichardi/pulcher* further facilitates this endeavor (Brawand et al. 2014).

This combination of unique features is the reason why, arguably, *N. pulcher* is among the best understood cooperative breeders regarding the ultimate and proximate mechanisms responsible for its sociality.

In contrast to most other systems, this largely rests on experimental scrutiny, applied both in the laboratory and field.

Ecology

N. pulcher settles in diverse habitats ranging from pure rock with few holes and crevices to finely structured habitats consisting mainly of empty gastropod shells and small stone rubble (Taborsky and Limberger 1981). Often, extensive colonies dwell on sand substrate that is interspersed with rocks, where group members dig out the required shelters from underneath stones by removing sand with their mouths (Bruintjes and Taborsky 2011). Territories consist usually of a semi-sphere of about 25–50 cm radius around one or several shelters and their main function is to provide protection from predators (Taborsky 1984; Balshine et al. 2001).

Territories contain only little food, and sexually mature group members (≥ 35 mm SL) feed primarily on zooplankton in the water column (Taborsky 1982, Gashagaza 1988; Bruintjes et al. 2010). Only small offspring, from fry stage to about 3 cm SL, feed from the bottom and plankton exclusively inside the defended area. The food consists mainly of crustaceans. The fact that food is acquired predominantly outside the territory means that resources within territories are not highly depreciable. Even though there is some competition for shelter space among subordinate group members (Balshine et al. 2001; Werner et al. 2003), group size is not strongly limited by resource competition among group members. Nonetheless, food abundance significantly affects the behavior of group members, including interactions among each other and the work load they take on (Bruintjes et al. 2010).

Demography

For their size, *N. pulcher* are very long-lived. Individuals can live > 4 years in the field, and in the aquarium some fish have exceeded 10 years of age, corresponding to a slow growth rate and a rather low reproductive output (especially without brood care helpers; Taborsky 1982; Skubic et al. 2004). Like most fish taxa, *N. pulcher* exhibits indeterminate growth, that is, individuals do not stop growing when reproductively mature. Size is of paramount importance for dominance rank within groups and for the success of aggressive interactions with members of other groups (Taborsky 1985; Hamilton et al. 2005; Reddon et al. 2011a). Growth depends on social rank, group composition, and probably also on cooperative effort, which is very energy demanding (Taborsky 1984; Grantner and Taborsky 1998; Riebli et al. 2011, 2012).

Group structure

Breeder males often defend more than one group – a harem – each consisting of a dominant female breeder and subordinate helpers (Limberger 1983; Desjardins et al. 2008a; Wong et al. 2012). Such polygynous males regularly visit the group territories, which may be up to 7 m apart (Figure 16.1). Females and helpers do not switch between groups in such harems, so "groups" consist of the breeding female, a varying number of helpers and young, and a male breeder that may also be associated with other such groups. Groups are usually aggregated in colonies ranging in size from a few groups up to several hundred (Heg et al. 2008b).

Within groups there is a strict dominance hierarchy, with rank determined by body size, even if such differences are small. A number of aggressive displays, overt attacks including physical contact, and affiliative and submissive behaviors are involved in the establishment and maintenance of dominance relationships among group members (Taborsky 1982, 1984; Hamilton et al. 2005). There are sex-specific differences in aggression of dominant breeders toward subordinate helpers (Mitchell 2009a), but rank among helpers is not sex-specific (Dey et al. 2013), even though sex can affect dominance acquisition among same-size subordinates (Riebli et al. 2012), and growth patterns (Hamilton and Heg 2008).

Reproduction

Reproduction is highly skewed within groups, with dominant breeders producing the majority of offspring. Nevertheless, both male and female helpers participate in reproduction to a variable extent (Taborsky 2009).

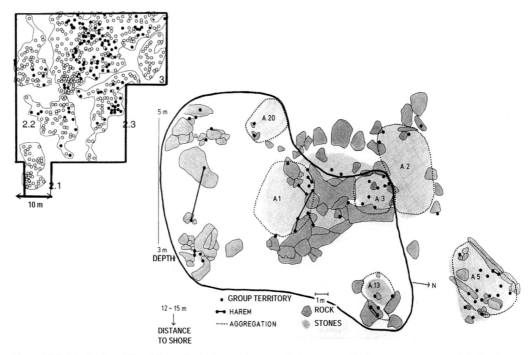

Figure 16.1. Distribution of *N. pulcher* territories in a northern population at 3–5 m depth near Magara, Burundi (Taborsky and Limberger 1981). Insert on top left: Distribution of *N. pulcher* (open circles) and *N. savoryi* (closed circles) territories at 10–11.5 m depth in a southern location at Kasakalawe Point, Zambia (Heg et al. 2008b). *N. savoryi* is a similar sized cooperative breeder with territories and space requirements resembling those of *N. pulcher* (Heg et al. 2005a, 2008b). In this southern population, the habitat consists of a sand layer with half submerged rocks (ca. 5–20 cm in diameter) under which group members dig out shelters. Apparently, this allows a much higher density of breeding groups than the rocky habitat in the depicted northern population. Harems are not marked in this southern location. Note the different scales of the two pictures. Bold black lines mark the borders of the respective study areas.

Mature male helpers try to fertilize eggs by surreptitious sneaking when the dominant territory owners spawn. Mature female helpers can produce independent clutches in a different shelter within the group territory or rarely add eggs to the clutch of a dominant female (< 1% of clutches; Heg et al. 2008a).

While some helpers of both sexes produce their own offspring in the groups where they help, most are nonbreeding helpers. Five experimental laboratory studies and one observational field study have provided parentage data for 403 broods containing 17,535 young (Table 16.1). In all of these studies, one to four mature helpers were present in addition to the dominant breeders, which corresponds to the natural situation. Although results varied among studies, comparison of pooled data indicates no significant sex difference in the proportion of broods involving some reproduction by helpers (19.1% for males vs. 13.8% for females; $N = 403$ broods, Fisher exact test, $P = 0.15$), but female helpers produced a significantly higher proportion of young than did male helpers (14.5% for females vs. 4.5% for males of larvae or free-swimming fry; $N = 17,535$ young, $\chi^2 = 220$, df = 1, $P < 0.0001$). Two studies in which male and female helpers were present in equal numbers corroborate these results (Heg et al. 2006, 2008a). In these studies, the proportion of broods in which male helpers produced young was significantly higher than the proportion of broods produced by female helpers (18.4% vs. 7.9% of 114 broods; Fisher exact test; $P = 0.03$), whereas again the number of offspring

Table 16.1. Numbers and proportions of broods completely or partially produced by helpers, and numbers and proportions of offspring (i.e., hatched larvae or free-swimming fry) produced by male and female helpers

	Male helpers			Female helpers			Reference
	Number assigned to helper	Total number	Percent assigned to helper	Number assigned to helper	Total number	Percent assigned to helper	
Broods	6	44	13.6	1	44	2.3	Heg et al.
Young	57	1,185	4.8	30	1,185	2.5	2006
Broods	15	70	21.4	8	70	11.4	Heg et al.
Young	37	1,365[a]	2.7	108	1,352[a]	8.0	2008a
Broods	3	19	15.8				Dierkes et al.
Young	30	294	10.2				1999
Broods[b]	5	10[a]	50.0	0	12[a]	0	Bruintjes et al.
Young	14	191[a]	7.3	0	217[a]	0	2011
Broods				27	102	26.5	Heg and Hamilton
Young				2066	11,051	18.7	2008
Broods				25	153	16.3	Zöttl et al.
Young				264	3,392	7.8	2013a

Bruintjes et al. (2011) studied natural broods in the field, whereas all other studies involved experimentally controlled groups in the laboratory containing one or two reproductively mature male and/or female helpers.

[a] The number of broods or offspring produced with male helpers present differed slightly from the number of broods or offspring produced with female helpers present.

[b] Only broods of groups with potentially mature helpers are considered (inferred from size and state of genital papilla; $N = 7$ broods with one, 1 with two and 2 with three mature male helpers present; $N = 7$ broods with one, 3 with two and 2 with four mature female helpers).

produced by female helpers exceeded the number of offspring produced by male helpers (5.4% vs. 3.7% of 2,550 young; $\chi^2 = 8.6$, df = 1, $P = 0.003$).

Due to sperm competition with the male territory owner, male helpers can apparently sire only a small number of young in their territory (mean = 4.8 young/brood), whereas female helpers produce on average 40.5 young/brood *if* they lay a clutch. If more than one mature male helper is present in a territory, the most dominant male helper sires more young than if he is the only male helper (Heg et al. 2008a; Mitchell et al. 2009a). In addition, male helpers can sire offspring parasitically in neighboring territories as well (Heg et al. 2006). The reproductive success of male helpers apparently depends on the composition of their own group and on reproductive opportunities in their neighborhood.

Cooperation

Immature and mature helpers of both sexes help in all duties of brood care, territory defense, and maintenance. Tasks are shared unequally, dependent on size, sex, and status of group members, and on current demands (Taborsky and Limberger 1981; Taborsky 1984; Desjardins et al. 2008b, 2008c). If several demands appear concurrently, helpers specialize in territory maintenance, whereas female breeders focus on direct brood care and both breeders engage in defense (Taborsky et al. 1986). Among helpers, large individuals may defend more frequently than smaller ones (Taborsky and Limberger 1981), or they may specialize in digging while smaller helpers defend the breeding shelter against egg predators (Bruintjes and Taborsky 2011).

Costs of cooperation

The effort helpers and breeders show in brood care, territory maintenance, and defense is costly with respect to energy, time, and risk. Energy consumption is increased particularly by digging (six-fold increase of routine metabolic rate; Grantner and Taborsky 1998) which is mainly performed by helpers and female breeders. Dominant male breeders, in contrast, usually invest little in territory maintenance, but instead engage in aggressive behaviors, which are energetically less demanding. Regarding direct brood care, energetically demanding fanning behavior is mainly shown by breeder females, whereas cheaper egg cleaning behavior is shared between breeder females and helpers (Taborsky and Grantner 1998; Zöttl et al. 2013c).

The energy budgets of group members are mainly determined by standard metabolism. Social behaviors such as aggression and submission among group members make up the bulk of the behavioral time budgets of both breeders and helpers, with aggression dominating the time and energy budgets of breeders, and submissive behavior those of helpers (Taborsky and Grantner 1998). Among cooperative behaviors, territory maintenance, which besides digging includes also removal of stones, shells, and particles ("carrying") as well as substrate cleaning (cleaning walls and ceiling of the breeding shelter), fills a considerable proportion of the behavioral time budget of helpers and female breeders (Taborsky 1982). This brings about high energetic costs, as these behaviors, especially digging and carrying, use much energy. During breeding, digging was found to be responsible for nearly 20% and 25% of behavioral metabolic costs in helpers and female breeders, respectively, with expenses varying among different stages of the breeding cycle (Taborsky and Grantner 1998). Helpers of both sexes dig similarly often, but large helpers take a greater share than small ones when challenged by experimental addition of sand (Bruintjes and Taborsky 2008, 2011).

Depending on demand, helpers take over a substantial amount of territory defense against conspecifics and predators (Bruintjes and Taborsky 2008; Heg and Taborsky 2010; Zöttl et al. 2013b). Large, piscivorous predators are attacked most often by male breeders, followed by female breeders and large helpers. Defense against dangerous predators is often shared, and strategic risk sharing among group members is suggested by significant positive correlations between group size and the per capita attack frequencies of breeders and large helpers against experimentally deployed large predators (Heg and Taborsky 2010). Such behavior apparently reduces mortality risk, since members of large groups survived experimental exposure to predation better despite their higher defense effort (Heg et al. 2004a).

Helpers grow more slowly than individuals living outside of reproductive groups (Taborsky 1984). This can be due both to their submissive status in the group and to their cooperative investment in energetically demanding activities. Experimental evidence shows, however, that the speed of growth depends also on strategy: helpers stay small to remain tolerated in a territory while accumulating reserves for boosting growth after they leave the territory in preparation of independent breeding (Taborsky 1984; Heg et al. 2004b).

Benefits of cooperation

The offspring produced in the territory are the primary beneficiaries of cooperative care, as the helpers present in the group substantially raise their survival chances (Brouwer et al. 2005). However, benefits to breeders arise also through enhanced reproduction in the presence of helpers made possible by the reduced energy expenditure of breeders in the presence of helpers (Taborsky 1984). With increasing helper number, for example, female breeders reduce egg size (Taborsky et al. 2007). Apparently, females with many helpers can afford this economy measure of producing smaller young because of the greater protective effect of a larger group, which increases offspring survival.

Helpers benefit from increased survival through the protection they get in the territory, which results from access to safe shelters and the defensive effort of large group members against dangerous predators (Taborsky 1984). This protective function of large group members (including breeders and large helpers) is so important that at least in the best studied population in the south of Lake Tanganyika, there are hardly any individuals living on their own (Stiver et al. 2004). Furthermore, helper-sized fish given the choice prefer larger groups (Reddon et al. 2011b), which persist longer (Heg et al. 2005b). Experimental manipulation of predation risk revealed that members of large groups benefit from higher survival (Heg et al. 2004a).

Benefits to helpers also accrue from the possibility of sharing reproduction in a safe territory (Table 16.1). As there are numerous duties when attempting to monopolize a safe place to live, the sharing of these duties can increase efficiency, allowing individuals to save effort without losing the benefits. Furthermore, in *N. pulcher* joint offspring production can affect cooperation. When male helpers in the field sired part of the offspring produced in a territory, they increased their defensive effort against egg predators (Bruintjes et al. 2011).

Division of labor

The efficiency of cooperation is strongly determined by the specialization of individuals in different tasks. In *N. pulcher*, indeterminate growth causes group members to differ in size, and consequently dominance status, which correlates with age and is affected by social and environmental conditions (Taborsky 1984; Skubic et al. 2004; Hamilton and Heg 2008). This variation in size provides the basis for temporal behavioral specialization of group members in divergent cooperative tasks (temporal polyethism). Field and laboratory experiments showed that the tasks breeders and helpers of different sizes perform depend on the intrusion of competitors and the type of predators, and on the need for direct brood care and sand removal (Taborsky et al. 1986; Bruintjes and Taborsky 2011; Zöttl et al. 2013b). Female breeders generally seem to prioritize defense of the territory regardless of the type of intruder, whereas helpers and male breeders distinguish more strongly between different types of threat (Desjardins et al. 2008c).

When large or medium-sized *L. elongatus* predators were introduced into large cages containing parts of *N. pulcher* colonies in their natural environment, 30% of aggressive displays and attacks were performed by large helpers, whereas female breeders contributed 26% and male breeders nearly 44% of aggressive acts. In contrast, the share of medium sized helpers was only 0.3%, while small helpers did not attack these predators at all (Heg and Taborsky 2010).

Load lightening and compensation

When different group members cooperate in the performance of duties, loads may be lightened for each participant. However, selection should favor individuals that hold back investment if others will compensate (Houston et al. 2005; Johnstone et al. 2014). This problem is particularly relevant if several individuals share the effort, as in cooperatively breeding groups (Johnstone 2011).

In *N. pulcher*, the cooperative effort of helpers in brood care and territory maintenance reduces the load to female breeders, which can in turn increase their reproductive rate (Taborsky 1984; Heg 2008). Females with helpers are apparently less stressed than those without helpers, as indicated by reduced egg cortisol levels (Mileva et al. 2011). In addition, females lay smaller eggs when receiving more help, as mentioned earlier. Experiments reveal that load-lightening effects and negotiation over brood care determine the investment decisions of both breeders and helpers. When helpers were experimentally prevented from sharing in direct brood care, the female breeder compensated for the lack of help by increasing her egg cleaning effort and the removal of sand from the breeding shelter (Zöttl et al. 2013c). Nevertheless, the total amount of brood care and breeding shelter maintenance was lower when the female breeder was not supported by her helper. This shows that the idleness of brood care helpers is only partially compensated by the dominant, as predicted by theoretical models (McNamara et al. 2003). After the experimental prevention of help, *N. pulcher* helpers increased their effort in these duties, thereby compensating for withheld cooperative investment in the preceding time period.

In another experiment, the effect of the helpers' compensation of withheld cooperation on their subsequent investment in brood care was tested by either allowing the dominant breeders to interact with the behaviorally manipulated helper or not (Schreier

2013). Compensatory help after a period of withheld cooperation was only found when direct interactions between dominant breeders and subordinate helpers were allowed, highlighting the importance of negotiations for the latters' propensity to fulfill costly altruistic tasks. Compensatory responses of helpers to prevented help, but without manipulation of the dominants' behavior, were also revealed by other laboratory and field experiments (Bergmüller and Taborsky 2005; Fischer et al. 2014).

Evolutionary mechanisms underlying cooperative breeding

Cooperative breeding has two critical components: the delayed (or withheld) dispersal of subordinate group members, and their cooperative care of young that are not their own (Komdeur 2006). These two components of sociality, reflecting decisions of group membership and cooperation, are subject to different ecological and social conditions although they likely evolve in concert (Aktipis 2004; Hamilton and Taborsky 2005a; Hochberg et al. 2008).

Why delay dispersal?

Several hypotheses attempt to explain delayed dispersal of subordinates focusing either on the costs of dispersing or the benefits of staying (Emlen 1982; Koenig et al. 1992; Stacey and Ligon 1991). In *N. pulcher*, there are clear benefits of philopatry. Individuals in the size range of helpers gain a substantial survival benefit from the defensive efforts of large group members, particularly the dominant breeders (Taborsky 1984). Helpers experimentally separated from their home territory are not accepted in other groups (Taborsky and Limberger 1981), and even if helpers can switch into a different group, this occurs only rarely (~3.5% of helpers in a sample of 205 genotyped individuals from 31 groups; Dierkes et al. 2005). In southern populations of *N. pulcher*, almost all individuals are members of a group that includes a breeding pair (Heg et al. 2005a, 2005b). In contrast, in the north of Lake Tanganyika the majority of sexually mature fish live in permanent,

nonreproductive aggregations that provide protection and serve as a reservoir of breeders ready to fill vacancies (Taborsky and Limberger 1981).

In addition to affecting survival, prolonged residence in the natal territory determines the opportunity to reproduce, even if reproductive skew is high (Table 16.1). Staying home means a safer but lower reproductive output than leaving and breeding independently; it also provides a chance to inherit breeding status if the same-sex breeder disappears (Balshine-Earn et al. 1998; Stiver et al. 2006). Such territory inheritance is sex-specific, with female helpers inheriting the territory from their mother or sister in 19% of cases (this was more likely in large than in small groups), whereas male helpers inherited their parental territory only in 3% of the surveyed groups (these are minimum estimates; Dierkes et al. 2005).

Males are less likely to inherit and more likely to disperse. In a northern population, nonbreeding aggregations consisted of twice as many males than females, whereas within breeding groups the sex ratio of similar sized individuals was exactly opposite (Taborsky 1984, 1985). Accordingly, in a southern population dispersal distances of males were greater than those of females (Stiver et al. 2007).

When one or both breeders were experimentally removed from groups containing large, sexually mature helpers, northern population helpers failed to take over the vacant dominant position, whereas in a southern population the largest helper took over in 7 of 18 replicates (Taborsky and Limberger 1981; Balshine-Earn et al. 1998). Parallel experiments in this latter population showed that larger female helpers were more likely to take over a vacant dominant breeder position than were larger male helpers (Stiver et al. 2006), corroborating the higher territory inheritance probability of female than male helpers.

The striking difference in territory inheritance patterns between the north and south of Lake Tanganyika is probably due to different population structure. As outlined earlier, in the north most sexually mature individuals live in stable aggregations located next to breeding territories. In contrast, in the south there are no aggregations of nonreproductives, and only about 5% of individuals do not belong to a breeding group.

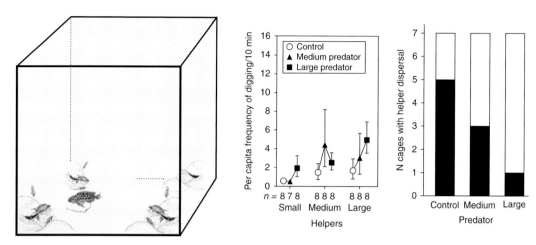

Figure 16.2. Results from a field experiment in which the predation risk was experimentally varied by adding either no (control), a medium, or a large predator (*Lepidiolamprologus elongatus*) to an 8 m³ cage containing part of a natural *N. pulcher* colony (left panel; 21 cages (replicates) were used in total). Middle panel: Digging effort of small, medium and large helpers in the three experimental situations. In the large predator treatment, large helpers in particular engaged a lot in digging out a shelter that was experimentally covered with sand. Depicted are means ± standard error (S.E.) and sample sizes (*N* groups). Right panel: Number of experimental cages in which helpers dispersed (black) of 7 cages each per treatment. After Heg et al. (2004a), Heg and Taborsky (2010).

Hence, takeovers there often involve large helpers or breeders of neighboring groups (Stiver et al. 2006). The resulting mean relatedness between social mates does not differ from a pattern generated by random pair formation, which suggests neither avoidance nor preference of pairing with relatives. Disregard of existing relatedness was suggested also by gonadal investment of subordinates living in social groups, as this was not correlated with their relatedness to the opposite-sex dominant breeder in the group (Stiver et al. 2008).

Dispersal decisions of helpers depend primarily on the risk of predation, but they are also influenced by the availability of vacant breeding positions and the quality of the home territory. In a field study of a population dwelling on a mixed rock/sand habitat, experimental provisioning of territories at the edge of a colony did not cause subordinate group members to disperse and breed independently, but territories provided at similar distances *within* the colony were readily inspected and taken over both by *N. pulcher* and the closely related, syntopic cooperative breeder *N. savoryi* (Heg et al. 2008b). When in contrast the quality of the home territory was diminished by experimentally reducing the

number of shelters, helper numbers in such territories declined (Balshine et al. 2001). Laboratory experiments revealed that breeding habitat availability significantly affects dispersal decisions (Bergmüller et al. 2005a), but habitat saturation is not a prerequisite of delayed dispersal: depending on body size, subordinate individuals often prefer to stay with dominants, even if they are unrelated and alternative options to breed independently are available (Taborsky 1985, Heg et al. 2011). When joining an unfamiliar group, helpers prefer to join large over small groups and groups containing large, more dominant individuals, in spite of incurring greater aggression and a reduced chance of inheriting the territory (Jordan et al. 2010; Reddon et al. 2011b). This again suggests that the primary function of group membership is protection against predation.

Experimental manipulation of predation risk in the field (Figure 16.2) showed that helpers adjust their behavior, spacing pattern, and dispersal propensity to the level of predation risk (Heg et al. 2004a; Heg and Taborsky 2010). Even when dispersal vacancies were available to helpers, they dispersed principally only when large predators were excluded from the area (Figure 16.2). This seems to reflect an adaptive response to current predation risk, as in the presence of large predators, membership in large groups significantly increased survival. Hence, the decision to delay dispersal is apparently triggered by an ecological constraint – predation risk – that contrasts with constraints observed in many other cooperative breeders, where dispersal is limited primarily by the availability of territories or breeding habitat (Emlen 1982; Koenig et al. 1992). Similarly, in Siberian jays (*Perisoreus infaustus*), predation seems to select for philopatry due to effective antipredator behavior of parents, but in the jays, where subordinates do not help, protection is typically withheld from unrelated group members (Griesser et al. 2006; Chapter 1).

Reproductively mature helpers survey their environment not only for local predation risk, but also for suitable breeding habitat and for groups they may join. When helpers were experimentally provided with dispersal opportunities that either did or did not contain breeding substrate, they only dispersed when breeding opportunities were supplied (Bergmüller et al. 2005a). This coincided with a significant reduction of submissive and helping behaviors while still in their home group and with a significant increase in body mass. Thus, helpers strategically reduce effort at home to accumulate reserves for their own reproduction once they have decided to leave and breed independently. These experimental results were corroborated by field data showing that helpers reduced cooperative antipredator defense in their home territories shortly before they dispersed, while helpers inheriting their natal territories did not do so (Zöttl et al. 2013d).

In the field, helpers spend about 5% of their time visiting other groups that can serve as a refuge if conditions turn unfavorable in their home territories (Bergmüller et al. 2005b). Experimentally increasing the perceived risk in the home territory with a fish predator dummy resulted in helpers taking shelter in one of the previously visited territories and even in some cases dispersing to that territory. Such visits to other groups occur more often when helpers are part of a long queue in their home territory, suggesting that helpers may use these visits not only as an insurance strategy, but also

to explore future reproductive opportunities in neighboring groups.

Why help?

Four evolutionary mechanisms may select for the apparently altruistic behavior of helpers (Lehmann and Keller 2006): (1) reciprocity (e.g., commodity trading among group members), (2) direct selfish benefits, (3) kin selection, and (4) genetic correlation between altruism and identifier genes ("greenbeard genes"). In *N. pulcher*, the first three of these mechanisms are apparently present, but it seems that reciprocity is most important for the cooperative behavior of large, sexually mature helpers. There is no evidence for greenbeard genes in this species, hence this mechanism will not be considered.

Reciprocity

Subordinate group members can entail costs to dominants because of resource competition. This may be compensated by cooperative behavior of subordinates, implying that "helping-at-the-nest" serves as "payment of rent" (Gaston 1978; Kokko et al. 2002). In *N. pulcher*, helpers have been shown to pay for being allowed to stay (Taborsky 1985), which provides them with resource access (safe shelters; Heg et al. 2008b), protection due to group antipredator defense (Taborsky 1984), and opportunities to reproduce (Table 16.1). The costs helpers can incur to dominants include competition for shelters, behavioral expenditure diminishing growth and reproductive competition (Dierkes et al. 1999; Balshine et al. 2001; Heg and Hamilton 2008; Heg et al. 2008a; Mitchell et al. 2009a, b). The latter is indicated also by a positive correlation of the testis mass of male breeders with the number of male helpers (Fitzpatrick et al. 2006).

If accepting subordinates is costly to dominants, the latter will be selected to demand compensation (Kokko et al. 2002; Hamilton and Taborsky 2005b). The ensuing pay-to-stay mechanism involves four components: (1) a latent threat to idle subordinates (Cant 2011), (2) an increase in cooperation by subordinates in response to threats or sanctions (Raihani et al. 2012), (3) a demand-driven propensity for dominants to exert pressure on subordinates to make themselves useful (Taborsky 1985), and (4) a scaling of the response of subordinates to the demands of dominants based on the subordinates' outside options (Bergmüller et al. 2005a).

These components have been experimentally identified in the interactions among group members. Dominants regularly exert aggression toward subordinate group members and may evict subordinates from their territory, thereby posing a latent threat (Taborsky 1985; Dierkes et al. 1999). In particular, dominants may punish subordinates for being idle when help is needed, as revealed by manipulation of subordinates' behavior in the field (Fischer et al. 2014). Subordinates increase help after being experimentally prevented from helping, which may appease dominants preemptively (Bergmüller and Taborsky 2005) or constitute a response to increased aggression of dominants (Fischer et al. 2014).

Dominants expel subordinates from their territories in the absence of predators and competitors, that is, when they are not needed, and readily reaccept them when threat of competition or predation is experimentally increased (Taborsky 1985). Increased demand by territory intrusion pressure may lead to the acceptance of unrelated and unfamiliar helpers (Zöttl et al. 2013b).

Subordinates adjust their effort when their outside options are manipulated. If they are provided with an opportunity to disperse and breed independently, in a safe environment, they reduce the help they provide to dominant breeders (Bergmüller et al. 2005a). In contrast, if the benefits of group membership are experimentally increased by raising predation risk, helpers increase their effort with each aggressive act received from dominants (Heg and Taborsky 2010). Although helpers reduce their effort prior to dispersing to a breeding position elsewhere, they maintain high investment when staying to take over their natal territory (Zöttl et al. 2013d).

Why do we consider this somewhat enforced trading of commodities an example of "reciprocity" rather than "coercion?" Both parties have alternative options, so when the costs of cooperation reach an unacceptable level for one of them, they can end the relationship; dominants by expelling the subordinate, and helpers by leaving the group. Cooperation cannot be completely enforced by dominants; it can only be demanded up to a point where benefits to be gained by outside options of the subordinate partner exceed the benefits it can obtain in the group (Cant and Johnstone 2009). By attacking helpers that do not fulfill the demand, dominants can modify the cooperative propensity of subordinates through imposing costs of idleness, but they cannot make subordinates help if they do not provide benefits in return. Hence, the concept of "reciprocal trading" adequately describes pay-to-stay scenarios such as observed in *N. pulcher*. It will be a worthwhile challenge for future studies to unravel evolutionarily stable negotiation rules of reciprocating group members.

Direct selfish benefits

Behaviors that benefit others may also provide selfish benefits to the actor. For instance, if a helper removes sand from the breeding shelter, this benefits the offspring of dominants growing up in the same cavern, but the helper may also derive benefits from hiding in the enlarged shelter when threatened by a predator. Hence, the benefits provided by helpers to dominant breeders may be a side effect of selfish behavior. Mutual benefits to group members also accrue to helpers by positive effects on group size, given that large group size enhances survival and is thus beneficial, an effect that has been referred to as "group augmentation benefits" (Kokko et al. 2001; Kingma et al. 2014). If group augmentation benefits select for helping behavior, two conditions must be fulfilled: fitness benefits of helpers must increase with group size, and helping must drive larger group size.

Both conditions are met in *N. pulcher*. In nature, helpers survive better in large than in small groups (Heg et al. 2004a, 2005a). Benefits of producing additional group members may also result when helpers take over their natal territory, if these group members will then help to raise the offspring of the former helper (long-term group augmentation benefits, or "delayed reciprocity;" Ligon and Ligon 1978; Wiley and Rabenold 1984; Kingma et al. 2014). In *N. pulcher*, female helpers frequently (~20%) inherit territories (Dierkes 2005), creating opportunities for delayed reciprocity. Delayed

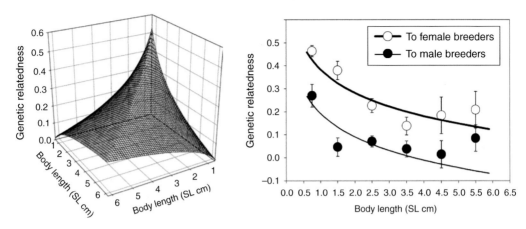

Figure 16.3. (a) Genetic relatedness between helpers of different size (i.e., age) within *N. pulcher* groups measured in the field (*N* = 3,288 helpers). The slopes of the relatedness landscape reveal that average relatedness declines with increasing age, and that helpers within age cohorts are much more closely related than those between cohorts. (b) Within-group relatedness of helpers to male and female breeders. The average degree of relatedness to breeders declines with size (i.e., age) of the helpers due to the natural turnover rate of breeders, and the decline in relatedness to male breeders is much greater than that to female breeders due the higher turnover rate of male territory owners. From Dierkes et al. (2005).

benefits of group augmentation may also accrue if helpers disperse jointly with the recruits they have helped to produce, but we have no evidence for joint dispersal of helpers and recruits in *N. pulcher*.

Subordinates increase the production of dominants' offspring, and hence increase group size by helping, in two ways: they lighten the workload of female breeders who thereby produce larger clutches, and they increase the survival of young (Taborsky 1984; Brouwer et al. 2005). Hence, both conditions for selection based on group augmentation benefits are fulfilled, suggesting that this mechanism plays a role in driving helping decisions.

Kin selection

Above-average relatedness within groups is a standard condition in cooperative breeders because group formation is typically based on delayed dispersal (Koenig et al. 1992). Kin selection will take effect if subordinates and dominants are related, and if subordinates raise the production of dominants' offspring. The latter condition applies to *N. pulcher* as outlined earlier, whereas the first condition is only partly met.

N. pulcher groups consist of a mixture of related and unrelated individuals. On the one hand, above average relatedness is caused by the delayed dispersal of young, which is responsible for significant age-assortative genetic relatedness among subordinates within groups (age cohorts, Dierkes et al. 2005; Figure 16.3a). On the other hand, relatedness between subordinates and dominants is diminished by the fact that helpers stay in the territory after one or both dominant breeders are replaced by unrelated immigrants (Taborsky and Limberger 1981; Balshine-Earn et al. 1998). This happens regularly, and as a result the relatedness between sexually mature helpers and dominant male breeders is not greater than the population mean. Mean relatedness between female breeders and their sexually mature helpers is also low, but significantly higher than the average relatedness level in the population (Dierkes et al. 2005; Figure 16.3b). This sex difference in relatedness of helpers is mainly caused by sex-specific replacement rates, with male rates exceeding those of females, combined with a greater propensity of males to disperse, resulting in about 20% of groups involving matrilines compared to virtually no groups involving patrilines. The greater dispersal distances of males in comparison to females (Stiver et al. 2007) may also affect this sex-specific relatedness pattern.

In addition, relatedness between breeders of both sexes and helpers is reduced by the production of extra-pair young. Although the numbers of extra-pair young produced by helpers of both sexes is generally low (Table 16.1), unrelated neighboring males also fertilize some of the eggs produced in a territory (Stiver et al. 2009; Bruintjes et al. 2011), further reducing relatedness within groups.

There is nonetheless scope for kin selection being important via relatedness to the female breeder (Figure 16.3b). In addition, *N. pulcher* of helper size have been shown to recognize kin, apparently by phenotype matching (Le Vin et al. 2010). These conditions may select for altruistic helping especially in small, young helpers (Bruintjes and Taborsky 2011), as relatedness declines with helper size. The asymmetrical relatedness between helpers and male vs. female breeders predicts that helping effort should differ depending on the sexes involved. This has been corroborated by field data showing that helpers related to female breeders invest more in cooperative defense than helpers unrelated to female breeders, whereas helpers unrelated to the male breeder showed higher defense effort than related ones (Stiver et al. 2005). The first result supports an effect of kin selection, whereas the latter result suggests the importance of paying rent for being allowed to stay in the territory.

The relative importance of kin selection and reciprocity can be determined by experimental manipulation of relatedness between helpers and beneficiaries. *N. pulcher* is one of the few systems were this can be done because of the natural dynamics of group formation. As a result, groups can be experimentally assembled of related or unrelated members, and we can expect that members of such groups will respond to the variation of relatedness in a meaningful way if relatedness is important for the selection of helping behavior. This approach has been used by two experimental laboratory studies. In the first, helping levels were compared between groups made up of helpers related to both breeders and groups with helpers unrelated to both breeders. The work effort of helpers

in the unrelated treatment exceeded that of helpers in the related treatment by roughly ten-fold (Stiver et al. 2005).

In the second study, female helpers were either daughters or sisters, or unrelated to the female breeder, while they were always unrelated to the male breeder. This study focused on direct brood care (egg cleaning and fanning), because these behaviors clearly have costs (Taborsky and Grantner 1998) but do not entail direct fitness benefits and thus are unambiguously altruistic. Again, unrelated helpers showed more care for dominant females' broods than did related helpers (Figure 16.4). In addition, they also invested more effort in digging out the breeding shelter, which is energetically demanding (Grantner and Taborsky 1998). When egg cannibalism of helpers was experimentally simulated, unrelated helpers responded with increased alloparental care, whereas related ones did not (Zöttl et al. 2013a). Hence, both studies confirm that helping behavior is better explained by reciprocity (pay-to-stay) than by indirect, kin-selected fitness benefits. Furthermore, experiments showed that individuals given the choice to settle with related or unrelated individuals avoid the former (Heg et al. 2011), which indicates that subordinates may even prefer reciprocal to kin-based relationships in their group.

Helping personality

Consistent behavioral variation among individuals of a group or population, known as "animal personalities" (Reale et al. 2010), is particularly interesting in species with long-term, close social relationships such as cooperative breeders because they may facilitate social coexistence and enhance potential synergies of cooperation (Bergmüller and Taborsky 2010). Group members of *N. pulcher* differ consistently in their propensity to perform certain tasks such as territory maintenance, defense, and exploration (Bergmüller and Taborsky 2007; Schürch and Heg 2010a; Le Vin et al. 2011). Consistent behavioral variation in helpers implies strategic specialization in different life history stages, and an efficient distribution of tasks

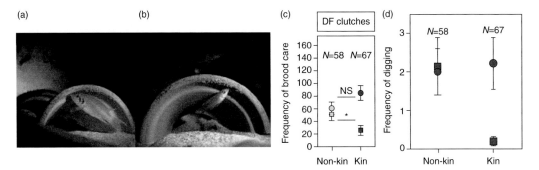

Figure 16.4. Laboratory experiment testing the effect of relatedness on the altruistic egg care of helpers, and their assistance at digging out the breeding shelter (Zöttl et al. 2013a). (a) Female breeder cleaning eggs that she attached to the flower pot serving as breeding shelter. (b) Helper cleaning the female breeder's eggs. (c) Egg cleaning frequencies of female breeders (circles) and helpers (squares) with respect to the relatedness treatment; when helpers were unrelated to the female breeder, they engaged in more egg care than when they were related. (d) Sand removal from the breeding shelter measured in the same experiment; symbols as in (c). Mean ± S.E. and the sample sizes (*N* independent replicates) are depicted. From Zöttl et al. (2013a).

among group members due to the specialized functions fulfilled by different individuals (Bergmüller and Taborsky 2007; Bruintjes and Taborsky 2011). The positive correlation between the propensities to dig and to defend the territory, particularly in immature helpers, suggests the existence of more helpful and more selfish phenotypes (Schürch and Heg 2010a; Le Vin et al. 2011). After sexual maturation, the relationship between helping behavior and different behavioral propensities such as exploration, boldness, and aggression varies between the sexes. In adult female helpers, they are all part of the same behavioral syndrome, whereas in adult male helpers this does not seem to apply; instead, their helping behavior is negatively correlated with the propensity to disperse (Schürch and Heg 2010a).

The behavioral type of individuals can affect dominance relationships and growth (Riebli et al. 2011). The effect of behavioral idiosyncrasies on the likelihood of obtaining dominance and a high quality territory in groups of four similar-sized conspecifics was small, whereas effects on growth and the accumulation of reserves were more pronounced, with low-aggression individuals typically growing faster than more aggressive ones (Riebli et al. 2012). These studies reveal an important modulating effect of the social environment on the link between behavioral

types and life history decisions, in accordance with the social niche hypothesis of animal personality evolution (Bergmüller and Taborsky 2010). This hypothesis proposes that adaptive adjustment to the social environment may generate behavioral consistency, which in turn can have long-lasting effects by diminishing conflict among conspecifics due to reduction of niche overlap between individuals sharing resources. In *N. pulcher*, the behavioral type of individuals during early development were indeed shown to have long-lasting effects, including effects on reproductive decisions and the propensity to accept subordinates in their group after attaining a dominant breeder position (Schürch and Heg 2010b). Furthermore, behavioral types of adults influence which type of subordinates dominants accept in their group, with bold and shy male breeders preferably accepting helpers of similar type (Schürch et al. 2010).

These results reveal that the behavioral type of individuals partly explains interaction patterns within groups and also group composition. Importantly, behavioral types in *N. pulcher* are consistent over a lifetime and heritable (Chervet et al. 2011), suggesting that they are subject to natural selection. Indeed, in *N. pulcher*, personality type explains the propensity to invest in helping behavior even better than does relatedness (Le Vin et al. 2011).

Developmental and maternal effects on helping behavior

Social experience may strongly affect behavioral decisions (Rutte et al. 2006; Champagne 2010). This is of particular importance in group-living species because early social experience can be varied and complex, and potential effects on social behavior may influence social relationships of the individual and the group.

"Social competence" refers to the ability of individuals to respond optimally to available social information, which is a skill largely obtained by prior social experience (Taborsky and Oliveira 2012). In *N. pulcher*, the social experience made during the first 60 days after hatching affects behavioral decisions and social competence throughout life. For example, in experiments using a split brood design, young growing up with adults (dominant breeders with or without helpers) interact more aggressively and submissively among each other than their siblings growing up without adults (Arnold and Taborsky 2010).

Higher social competence apparently results in more efficient conflict resolution (Hick et al. 2014). When two fish of similar size were made owners of the same shelter and competed for it 6 to 12 months after their experimentally controlled rearing conditions, both winners and losers of this contest behaved more adequately (showing more open aggression and submission, respectively), when they had been raised with adults during their first 60 days after hatching than when they had been raised among same-aged peers only (Taborsky et al. 2012). Such competence allowed the socially experienced losers to be tolerated by winners closer to the desired shelter, and later in life to be admitted as subordinates in the territory of unfamiliar and unrelated breeders.

Analysis of gene expression profiles revealed that genes coding for the neuropeptide CRF (corticotrophine-releasing factor) and the steroid hormone receptor GR1 were differently expressed in the fish raised in divergent social environments. Thus, the brains of the fish are affected by their early social experience, which irreversibly alters the expression of these two key gene products regulating the stress response (Taborsky et al. 2013).

The social environment also influences maternal effects that are apparently strategic, with females reducing egg size when assisted by greater numbers of helpers (Taborsky et al. 2007). This corresponds to the productivity increase of females with helpers, which are able to lay larger clutches (Taborsky 1984).

Physiological control of social behavior

One of the key questions regarding the proximate mechanisms of altruistic behavior concerns the hormonal and endocrine mechanisms underlying the motivation and execution of alloparental care (Ziegler 2000). In *N. pulcher*, the cleaning of eggs by nibbling off microorganisms from their surface is a delicate behavior that can easily change into egg eating. The helpers' decision to clean instead of cannibalize eggs depends on their body size or age, dominance status, and previous experience with eggs (Siemens 1990). As brood care behavior in vertebrates, including teleost fishes, is often regulated by prolactin (Whittington and Wilson 2013), this protein is a likely candidate for the proximate causation of direct brood care behavior, which in addition to cleaning involves also fanning of eggs in *N. pulcher*. However, neither the measurement of the expression of prolactin mRNA in the pituitary gland of breeders and helpers, nor the intraperitoneal application of ovine prolactin, have indicated that this hormone is involved in the regulation of direct egg care in this species (Bender et al. 2008a). Brood-caring adult females even showed *lower* gene expression levels of prolactin than adult female nonbreeders. Other candidate neuropeptides for the regulation of altruistic brood care behavior include the nonapeptides isotocin, the teleost homologue to mammalian oxytocin, and the close relative vasotocin, the teleost equivalent to mammalian vasopressin. These trigger a host of social behaviors including cooperation and brood care (Donaldson and Young 2008; Godwin and Thompson 2012; O'Connell et al. 2012). Studies of the potential effects of these neuropeptides on direct brood care and other helping behaviors in *N. pulcher* are currently lacking, but isotocin and arginine vasotocin affect social sensitivity and preference as well as dominance

(Aubin-Horth et al. 2007, Reddon et al. 2012, 2014), which suggests a potential role also in the regulation of socially mediated cooperative behaviors.

Steroid hormones can also trigger brood care, especially in males (Knapp et al. 1999). In *N. pulcher*, however, brood care does not seem to relate to steroid hormone excretion levels (Bender et al. 2008b). Interestingly, cortisol levels are reduced in helpers showing much submissive behavior, suggesting that helpers can reduce social stress by appeasing dominant breeders (Bender et al. 2006). Testosterone and 11-ketotestosterone levels were also reduced in helpers showing high levels of submissive behavior. This connection between signals of submission and the reproductive status of subordinate male helpers indicates that submissive behavior may honestly reveal to male breeders a low reproductive potential of highly submissive male helpers.

Steroidal androgens are important mediators of social behavior, especially aggression and male reproductive behaviors (Ros et al. 2004). In *N. pulcher*, excreted androgen levels were similar between male breeders and male helpers (Oliveira et al. 2003; Bender et al. 2006), whereas plasma 11-ketotestosterone was higher in male breeders than male helpers when groups were sampled in the field (Desjardins et al. 2008b). Females, in contrast, showed the highest testosterone values of all group members, which were positively correlated with their territory maintenance and defense behaviors. In general, dominance interactions in *N. pulcher* seem to be mediated mainly by testosterone in females and 11-ketotestosterone in males (Hirschenhauser et al. 2004, 2008; Aubin-Horth et al. 2007; Taves et al. 2009).

Conclusions

Neolamprologus pulcher is an ideal model for the study of ultimate and proximate mechanisms underlying cooperative breeding due to a combination of complex social traits and unique possibilities for experimentation. These characteristics have allowed us to determine and test experimentally the factors important to cooperative breeding in this species. These include an important role of predation in dispersal decisions, the reciprocal trading of commodities between dominants and subordinates, a relatively minor influence of relatedness on helping decisions compared to reciprocity-based altruism, and a striking efficiency of task sharing based on behavioral specialization of group members. The combination of these traits is evident across populations of *N. pulcher*, an ecologically highly successful species that has colonized Lake Tanganyika all along its shores. Their social dynamics allow the application of experimental approaches both to the fitness-relevant costs and benefits of behavioral and life history decisions and to the proximate mechanisms controlling these decisions at genetic and physiological levels, providing many promising future research avenues.

Acknowledgments

I am very grateful to Janis Dickinson, Joachim Frommen, Arne Jungwirth, Walt Koenig, and Barbara Taborsky for constructive criticism and help with the manuscript, and to the Swiss National Science Foundation for financial support (grants 310030B 138660 and 31003A 156152).

REFERENCES

Aktipis, C. A. (2004). Know when to walk away: contingent movement and the evolution of cooperation. *J. Theor. Biol.*, 231, 249–260.

Arnold, C. and Taborsky, B. (2010). Social experience in early ontogeny has lasting effects on social skills in cooperatively breeding cichlids. *Anim. Behav.*, 79, 621–630.

Aubin-Horth, N., Desjardins, J. K., Martei, Y. M., Balshine, S., and Hofmann, H. A. (2007). Masculinized dominant females in a cooperatively breeding species. *Mol. Ecol.*, 16, 1349–1358.

Awata, S., Munehara, H., and Masanori, K. (2005). Social system and reproduction of helpers in a cooperatively breeding cichlid fish (*Julidochromis ornatus*) in Lake Tanganyika: field observations and parentage analyses. *Behav. Ecol. Sociobiol.*, 58, 506–516.

Balshine, S., Leach, B., Neat, F., Reid, H., Taborsky, M., et al. (2001). Correlates of group size in a cooperatively breeding cichlid fish (*Neolamprologus pulcher*). *Behav. Ecol. Sociobiol.*, 50, 134–140.

Balshine-Earn, S., Neat, F. C., Reid, H., and Taborsky, M. (1998). Paying to stay or paying to breed? Field evidence for direct benefits of helping behavior in a cooperatively breeding fish. *Behav. Ecol.*, 9, 432–438.

Bender, N., Heg, D., Hamilton, I. M., Bachar, Z., Taborsky, M., et al. (2006). The relationship between social status, behaviour, growth and steroids in male helpers and breeders of a cooperatively breeding cichlid. *Horm. Behav.*, 50, 173–182.

Bender, N., Taborsky, M., and Power, D. M. (2008a). The role of prolactin in the regulation of brood care in the cooperatively breeding fish *Neolamprologus pulcher*. *J. Exp. Zool.*, 309A, 515–524.

Bender, N., Heg-Bachar, Z., Oliveira, R. F., Canario, A. V. M., and Taborsky, M. (2008b). Hormonal control of brood care and social status in a cichlid fish with brood care helpers. *Physiol. Behav.*, 94, 349–358.

Bergmüller, R. and Taborsky, M. (2005). Experimental manipulation of helping in a cooperative breeder: helpers "pay to stay" by pre-emptive appeasement. *Anim. Behav.*, 69, 19–28.

Bergmüller, R. and Taborsky, M. (2007). Adaptive behavioural syndromes due to strategic niche specialization. *BMC Ecology*, 7, 12.

Bergmüller, R. and Taborsky, M. (2010). Animal personality due to social niche specialisation. *Trends Ecol. Evol.*, 25, 504–511.

Bergmüller, R., Heg, D., and Taborsky, M. (2005a). Helpers in a cooperatively breeding cichlid stay and pay or disperse and breed, depending on ecological constraints. *Proc. R. Soc. London B*, 272, 325–331.

Bergmüller, R., Heg, D., Peer, K., and Taborsky, M. (2005b). Extended safe havens and between-group dispersal of helpers in a cooperatively breeding cichlid. *Behaviour*, 142, 1643–1667.

Blumer, L. S. (1979). Male parental care in bony fishes. *Q. Rev. Biol.*, 54, 149–161.

Blumer, L. S. (1982). A bibliography and categorization of bony fishes exhibiting parental care. *Zool. J. Linn. Soc.*, 76, 1–22.

Bourke, A. F. G. (2011). *Principles of Social Evolution*. Oxford: Oxford University Press.

Brawand, D., Wagner, C.E., Li, Y. I., Malinsky, M., Keller, I., et al. (2014). The genomic substrate for adaptive radiation in African cichlid fish. *Nature*, 513, 375–381.

Breder, C. M. and Rosen, D. E. (1966). *Modes of Reproduction in Fishes*. Garden City, NY: Natural History Press.

Brichard, P. (1978). *Fishes of Lake Tanganyika*. Neptune City, NJ: T. F. H. Publishers.

Brouwer, L., Heg, D., and Taborsky, M. (2005). Experimental evidence for helper effects in a cooperatively breeding cichlid. *Behav. Ecol.*, 16, 667–673.

Brown, J. L. (1987). *Helping and Communal Breeding in Birds: Ecology and Evolution*. Princeton, NJ: Princeton University Press.

Bruintjes, R. and Taborsky, M. (2008). Helpers in a cooperative breeder pay a high price to stay: effects of demand, helper size and sex. *Anim. Behav.*, 75, 1843–1850.

Bruintjes, R. and Taborsky, M. (2011). Size-dependent task specialization in a cooperative cichlid in response to experimental variation of demand. *Anim. Behav.*, 81, 387–394.

Bruintjes, R., Hekman, R., and Taborsky, M. (2010). Experimental global food reduction raises resource acquisition costs of brood care helpers and reduces their helping effort. *Funct. Ecol.*, 24, 1054–1063.

Bruintjes, R., Bonfils, D., Heg, D., and Taborsky, M. (2011). Paternity of subordinates raises cooperative effort in cichlids. *Plos One*, 6(10), e25673.

Cant, M. A. (2011). The role of threats in animal cooperation. *Proc. R. Soc. London B*, 278, 170–178.

Cant, M. A. and Johnstone, R. A. (2009). How threats influence the evolutionary resolution of within-group conflict. *Am. Nat.*, 173, 759–771.

Champagne, F. A. (2010). Epigenetic influence of social experiences across the lifespan. *Devel. Psychobiol.*, 52, 299–311.

Chervet, N., Zöttl, M., Schürch, R., Taborsky, M., and Heg, D. (2011). Repeatability and heritability of behavioural types in a social cichlid. *Int. J. Evol. Biol.*, 2011, 321729.

Desjardins, J. K., Fitzpatrick, J. L., Stiver, K. A., van der Kraak, G. J., and Balshine, S. (2008a). Costs and benefits of polygyny in the cichlid *Neolamprologus pulcher*. *Anim. Behav.*, 75, 1771–1779.

Desjardins, J. K., Stiver, K. A., Fitzpatrick, J. L., Milligan, N., van der Kraak, G. J., et al. (2008b). Sex and status in a cooperative breeding fish: behavior and androgens. *Behav. Ecol. Sociobiol.*, 62, 785–794.

Desjardins, J. K., Stiver, K. A., Fitzpatrick, J. L., and Balshine, S. (2008c). Differential responses to territory intrusions in cooperatively breeding fish. *Anim. Behav.*, 75, 595–604.

Dey, C. J., Reddon, A. R., O'Connor, C. M., and Balshine, S. (2013). Network structure is related to social conflict in a cooperatively breeding fish. *Anim. Behav.*, 85, 395–402.

Dierkes, P., Taborsky, M., and Kohler, U. (1999). Reproductive parasitism of broodcare helpers in a cooperatively breeding fish. *Behav. Ecol.*, 10, 510–515.

Dierkes, P., Heg, D., Taborsky, M., Skubic, E., and Achmann, R. (2005). Genetic relatedness in groups is sex-specific and declines with age of helpers in a cooperatively breeding cichlid. *Ecol. Lett.*, 8, 968–975.

Donaldson, Z. R. and Young, L. J. (2008). Oxytocin, vasopressin, and neurogenetics of sociality. *Science*, 322, 900–904.

Duftner, N., Sefc, K. M., Koblmüller, S., Salzburger, W., Taborsky, M., et al. (2007). Parallel evolution of facial stripe patterns in the *Neolamprologus brichardi/N. pulcher* species complex endemic to Lake Tanganyika. *Mol. Phyl. Evol.*, 45, 706–715.

Emlen, S. T. (1982). The evolution of helping. 1. An ecological constraints model. *Am. Nat.*, 119, 29–39.

Fischer, S., Zöttl, M., Groenewoud, F., and Taborsky, B. (2014). Group-size-dependent punishment of idle subordinates in a cooperative breeder where helpers pay to stay. *Proc. R. Soc. London B*, 281, 20140184.

Fitzpatrick, J. L., Desjardins, J. K., Stiver, K. A., Montgomerie, R. and Balshine, S. (2006). Male reproductive suppression in the cooperatively breeding fish *Neolamprologus pulcher*. *Behav. Ecol.*, 17, 25–33.

Gashagaza, M. M. (1988). Feeding activity of a Tanganyikan cichlid fish *Lamprologus brichardi*. *African Study Monogr.*, 9, 1–9.

Gaston, A. J. (1978). The evolution of group territorial behavior and cooperative breeding. *Am. Nat.*, 112, 1091–1100.

Godwin, J. and Thompson, R. (2012). Nonapeptides and social behavior in fishes. *Horm. Behav.*, 61, 230–238.

Grantner, A. and Taborsky, M. (1998). The metabolic rates associated with resting, and with the performance of agonistic, submissive and digging behaviours in the cichlid fish *Neolamprologus pulcher* (Pisces: Cichlidae). *J. Comp. Physiol. B*, 168, 427–433.

Griesser, M., Nystrand, M., and Ekman, J. (2006). Reduced mortality selects for family cohesion in a social species. *Proc. R. Soc. London B*, 273, 1881–1886.

Griffin, A. S. and West, S. A. (2003). Kin discrimination and the benefit of helping in cooperatively breeding vertebrates. *Science*, 302, 634–636.

Gross, M. R. and Sargent, R. C. (1985). The evolution of male and female parental care in fishes. *Am. Zool.*, 25, 807–822.

Hager, R. and Jones, C. B., eds. (2009). *Reproductive Skew in Vertebrates: Proximate and Ultimate Causes.* Cambridge: Cambridge University Press.

Hamilton, I. M. and Heg, D. (2008). Sex differences in the effect of social status on the growth of subordinates in a co-operatively breeding cichlid. *J. Fish Biol.*, 72, 1079–1088.

Hamilton, I. M. and Taborsky, M. (2005a). Contingent movement and cooperation evolve under generalized reciprocity. *Proc. R. Soc. London B*, 272, 2259–2267.

Hamilton, I. M. and Taborsky, M. (2005b). Unrelated helpers will not fully compensate for costs imposed on breeders when they pay to stay. *Proc. R. Soc. London B*, 272, 445–454.

Hamilton, I. M., Heg, D., and Bender, N. (2005). Size differences within a dominance hierarchy influence conflict and help in a cooperatively breeding cichlid. *Behaviour*, 142, 1591–1613.

Hamilton, W. D. (1964). The genetical evolution of social behaviour I and II. *J. Theor. Biol.*, 7, 1–52.

Heg, D. (2008). Reproductive suppression in female cooperatively breeding cichlids. *Biol. Lett.*, 4, 606–609.

Heg, D. and Bachar, Z. (2006). Cooperative breeding in the Lake Tanganyika cichlid *Julidochromis ornatus*. *Envir. Biol. Fishes*, 76, 265–281.

Heg, D. and Hamilton, I. M. (2008). Tug-of-war over reproduction in a cooperatively breeding cichlid. *Behav. Ecol. Sociobiol.*, 62, 1249–1257.

Heg, D. and Taborsky, M. (2010). Helper response to experimentally manipulated predation risk in the cooperatively breeding cichlid *Neolamprologus pulcher*. *PLoS One*, 5(5), e10784.

Heg, D., Bachar, Z., Brouwer, L., and Taborsky, M. (2004a). Predation risk is an ecological constraint for helper dispersal in a cooperatively breeding cichlid. *Proc. R. Soc. London B*, 271, 2367–2374.

Heg, D., Bender, N., and Hamilton, I. (2004b). Strategic growth decisions in helper cichlids. *Proc. R. Soc. London B*, 271, S505–S508.

Heg, D., Bachar, Z., and Taborsky, M. (2005a). Cooperative breeding and group structure in the Lake Tanganyika cichlid *Neolamprologus savoryi*. *Ethology*, 111, 1017–1043.

Heg, D., Brouwer, L., Bachar, Z., and Taborsky, M. (2005b). Large group size yields group stability in the cooperatively breeding cichlid *Neolamprologus pulcher*. *Behaviour*, 142, 1615–1641.

Heg, D., Bergmuller, R., Bonfils, D., Otti, O., Bachar, Z., et al. (2006). Cichlids do not adjust reproductive skew to the availability of independent breeding options. *Behav. Ecol.*, 17, 419–429.

Heg, D., Jutzeler, E., Bonfils, D., and Mitchell, J. S. (2008a). Group composition affects male reproductive partitioning in a cooperatively breeding cichlid. *Mol. Ecol.*, 17, 4359–4370.

Heg, D., Heg-Bachar, Z., Brouwer, L., and Taborsky, M. (2008b). Experimentally induced helper dispersal in colonially breeding cooperative cichlids. *Envir. Biol. Fishes*, 83, 191–206.

Heg, D., Rothenberger, S., and Schürch, R. (2011). Habitat saturation, benefits of philopatry, relatedness, and the extent of co-operative breeding in a cichlid. *Behav. Ecol.*, 22, 82–92.

Hick, K., Reddon, A. R., O'Connor, C. M., and Balshine, S. (2014). Strategic and tactical fighting decisions in cichlid fishes with divergent social systems. *Behaviour*, 151, 47–71.

Hirschenhauser, K., Taborsky, M., Oliveira, T., Canario, A. V. M., and Oliveira, R. F. (2004). A test of the "challenge hypothesis" in cichlid fish: simulated partner and territory intruder experiments. *Anim. Behav.*, 68, 741–750.

Hirschenhauser, K., Canario, A. V., Ros, A. F., Taborsky, M., and Oliveira, R. F. (2008). Social context may affect urinary excretion of 11-ketotestosterone in African cichlids. *Behaviour*, 145, 1367–1388.

Hochberg, M. E., Rankin, D. J., and Taborsky, M. (2008). The coevolution of cooperation and dispersal in social groups and its implications for the emergence of multicellularity. *BMC Evol. Biol.*, 8, 238.

Houston, A. I., Szekely, T., and McNamara, J. M. (2005). Conflict between parents over care. *Trends. Ecol. Evol.*, 20, 33–38.

Johnstone, R. A. (2011). Load lightening and negotiation over offspring care in cooperative breeders. *Behav. Ecol.*, 22, 436–444.

Johnstone, R. A., Manica, A., Fayet, A. L., Stoddard, M. C., Rodriguez-Girones, M. A. et al. (2014). Reciprocity and conditional cooperation between great tit parents. *Behav. Ecol.*, 25, 216–222.

Jordan, L. A., Wong, M. Y., and Balshine, S. S. (2010). The effects of familiarity and social hierarchy on group membership decisions in a social fish. *Biol. Lett.*, 6, 301–303.

Kingma, S. A., Santema, P., Taborsky, M., and Komdeur, J. (2014). Group augmentation and the evolution of cooperation. *Trends Ecol. Evol.*, 29, 476–484.

Knapp, R., Wingfield, J. C., and Bass, A. H. (1999). Steroid hormones and paternal care in the plainfin midshipman fish (*Porichthys notatus*). *Horm. Behav.*, 35, 81–89.

Koenig, W. D., Pitelka, F. A., Carmen, W. J., Mumme, R. L., and Stanback, M. T. (1992). The evolution of delayed dispersal in cooperative breeders. *Q. Rev. Biol.*, 67, 111–150.

Kohler, U. (1997). Zur Struktur und Evolution des Sozialsystems von *Neolamprologus multifasciatus* (Cichlidae, Pisces), dem kleinsten Schneckenbuntbarsch des Tanganjikasees. Ph.D. thesis, Ludwig-Maximilians-Universität, München, Germany.

Kokko, H., Johnstone, R. A., and Clutton-Brock, T.H. (2001). The evolution of cooperative breeding through group augmentation. *Proc. R. Soc. London B*, 268, 187–196.

Kokko, H., Johnstone, R. A., and Wright, J. (2002). The evolution of parental and alloparental effort in cooperatively breeding groups: when should helpers pay to stay? *Behav. Ecol.*, 13, 291–300.

Komdeur, J. (2006). Variation in individual investment strategies among social animals. *Ethology*, 112, 729–747.

Komdeur, J. and Ekman, J. (2010). Adaptations and constraints in the evolution of delayed dispersal: implications for cooperation. In: *Social Behaviour: Genes, Ecology and Evolution*, ed. T. Szekely, A. J. Moore and J. Komdeur. Cambridge: Cambridge University Press, pp. 306–327.

Konings, A. (1998). *Tanganyika Cichlids in Their Natural Habitat*. El Paso, TX: Cichlid Press.

Kuwamura, T. (1997). The evolution of parental care and mating systems among Tanganyikan cichlids. In: *Fish Communities in Lake Tanganyika*, ed. H. Kawanabe, M. Hori, and M. Nagoshi), Kyoto, Japan: Kyoto University Press, pp. 57–86.

Le Vin, A., Mable, B., and Arnold, K. (2010). Kin recognition via phenotype matching in a cooperatively breeding cichlid, *Neolamprologus pulcher*. *Anim. Behav.*, 79, 1109–1114.

Le Vin, A., Mable, B., Taborsky, M., Heg, D., and Arnold, K. (2011). Individual variation in helping in a cooperative breeder: relatedness versus behavioural type. *Anim. Behav.*, 82, 467–477.

Lehmann, L. and Keller, L. (2006). The evolution of cooperation and altruism – a general framework and a classification of models. *J. Evol. Biol.*, 19, 1365–1376.

Ligon, J. D. and Ligon, S. H. (1978). Communal breeding in green woodhoopoes as a case for reciprocity. *Nature*, 276, 496–498.

Limberger, D. (1983). Pairs and harems in a cichlid fish, *Lamprologus brichardi*. *Z. Tierpsychol.*, 62, 115–144.

McNamara, J. M., Houston, A. I., Barta, Z., and Osorno, J. L. (2003). Should young ever be better off with one parent than with two? *Behav. Ecol.*, 14, 301–310.

Mileva, V. R., Gilmour, K. M., and Balshine, S. (2011). Effects of maternal stress on egg characteristics in a cooperatively breeding fish. *Comp. Biochem. Physiol. A*, 158, 22–29.

Mitchell, J. S., Jutzeler, E., Heg, D., and Taborsky, M. (2009a). Gender differences in the costs that subordinate group members impose on dominant males in a cooperative breeder. *Ethology*, 115, 1162–1174.

Mitchell, J. S., Jutzeler, E., Heg, D., and Taborsky, M. (2009b). Dominant members of cooperatively-breeding groups adjust their behaviour in response to the sexes of their subordinates. *Behaviour*, 146, 1665–1686.

O'Connell, L. A., Matthews, B. J., and Hofmann, H. A. (2012). Isotocin regulates paternal care in a monogamous cichlid fish. *Horm. Behav.*, 61, 725–733.

Oliveira, R. F., Hirschenhauser, K., Canario, A. V. M., and Taborsky, M. (2003). Androgen levels of reproductive competitors in a co-operatively breeding cichlid. *J. Fish Biol.*, 63, 1615–1620.

Poll, M. (1974). Contribution à la faune ichthyologique du lac Tanganika, d'après les récoltes de P. Brichard. *Rev. Zool. Afri.*, 88, 99–110.

Raihani, N. J., Thornton, A., and Bshary, R. (2012). Punishment and cooperation in nature. *Trends Ecol. Evol.*, 27, 288–295.

Reale, D., Dingemanse, N. J., Kazem, A. J., and Wright, J. (2010). Evolutionary and ecological approaches to the study of personality. *Phil. Trans. R. Soc. London B*, 365, 3937–3946.

Reddon, A. R., Voisin, M. R., Menon, N., Marsh-Rollo, S. E., et al. (2011a). Rules of engagement for resource contests in a social fish. *Anim. Behav.*, 82, 93–99.

Reddon, A. R., Balk, D., and Balshine, S. (2011b). Sex differences in group-joining decisions in social fish. *Anim. Behav.*, 82, 229–234.

Reddon, A. R., O'Connor, C. M., Marsh-Rollo, S. E., and Balshine, S. (2012). Effects of isotocin on social responses in a cooperatively breeding fish. *Anim. Behav.*, 84, 753–760.

Reddon, A. R., Voisin, M. R., O'Connor, C. M., and Balshine, S. (2014). Isotocin and sociality in the cooperatively breeding cichlid fish, *Neolamprologus pulcher*. *Behaviour*, 151, 1389–1411.

Riebli, T., Avgan, B., Bottini, A. M., Duc, C., Taborsky, M., and Heg, D. (2011). Behavioral type affects dominance and growth in staged encounters of cooperatively breeding cichlids. *Anim. Behav.*, 81, 313–323.

Riebli, T., Taborsky, M., Chervet, N., Apolloni, N., Zuercher, Y., et al. (2012). Behavioural type, status and social context affect behaviour and resource allocation in cooperatively breeding cichlids. *Anim. Behav.*, 84, 925–936.

Ros, A. F. H., Bruintjes, R., Santos, R. S., Canario, A. V. M., and Oliveira, R. F. (2004). The role of androgens in the trade-off between territorial and parental behavior in the Azorean rock-pool blenny, *Parablennius parvicornis*. *Horm. Behav.*, 46, 491–497.

Rutte, C., Taborsky, M., and Brinkhof, M. W. G. (2006). What sets the odds of winning and losing? *Trends Ecol. Evol.*, 21, 16–21.

Sargent, R. C. and Gross, M. R. (1986). William's principle: An explanation of parental care in teleost fishes. In: *The Behaviour of Teleost Fishes*, ed. T. J. Pitcher. London: Croom Helm, pp. 275–293.

Schreier, T. (2013). Punishment motivates subordinate helper to pay to stay and to compensate after a period of reduced helping. Bachelor thesis, University of Bern, Switzerland.

Schürch, R. and Heg, D. (2010a). Life history and behavioral type in the highly social cichlid *Neolamprologus pulcher*. *Behav. Ecol.*, 21, 588–598.

Schürch, R. and Heg, D. (2010b). Variation in helper type affects group stability and reproductive decisions in a cooperative breeder. *Ethology*, 116, 257–269.

Schürch, R., Rothenberger, S., and Heg, D. (2010). The building-up of social relationships: behavioural types, social networks and cooperative breeding in a cichlid. *Phil. Trans. R. Soc. London B*, 365, 4089–4098.

Siemens, M. (1990). Broodcare or egg cannibalism by parents and helpers in *Neolamprologus brichardi* (Poll 1986)

(Pisces: Cichlidae): a study on behavioural mechanisms. *Ethology*, 84, 60–80.

Skubic, E., Taborsky, M., McNamara, J. M., and Houston, A. I. (2004). When to parasitize? A dynamic optimization model of reproductive strategies in a cooperative breeder. *J. Theor. Biol.* 227, 487–501.

Solomon, N. G. and French, J. A., eds. (1997). *Cooperative Breeding in Mammals*. Cambridge: Cambridge University Press.

Stacey, P. B. and Koenig, W. D., eds. (1990). *Cooperative Breeding in Birds: Long Term Studies of Ecology and Behavior*. Cambridge: Cambridge University Press.

Stacey, P. B. and Ligon, J. D. (1991). The benefits of philopatry hypothesis for the evolution of cooperative breeding: variance in territory quality and group size effects. *Am. Nat.*, 137, 831–846.

Stiver, K. A., Dierkes, P., Taborsky, M., and Balshine, S. (2004). Dispersal patterns and status change in a co-operatively breeding cichlid *Neolamprologus pulcher*: evidence from microsatellite analyses and behavioural observations. *J. Fish Biol.*, 65, 91–105.

Stiver, K. A., Dierkes, P., Taborsky, M., Gibbs, H. L., and Balshine, S. (2005). Relatedness and helping in fish: examining the theoretical predictions. *Proc. R. Soc. London B*, 272, 1593–1599.

Stiver, K. A., Fitzpatrick, J., Desjardins, J. K., and Balshine, S. (2006). Sex differences in rates of territory joining and inheritance in a cooperatively breeding cichlid fish. *Anim. Behav.*, 71, 449–456.

Stiver, K., Desjardins, J., Fitzpatrick, J., Neff, B., Quinn, J., et al. (2007). Evidence for size and sex-specific dispersal in a cooperatively breeding cichlid fish. *Mol. Ecol.*, 16, 2974–2984.

Stiver, K., Fitzpatrick, J., Desjardins, J., Neff, B., Quinn, J., et al. (2008). The role of genetic relatedness among social mates in a cooperative breeder. *Behav. Ecol.*, 19, 816–823.

Stiver, K., Fitzpatrick, J., Desjardins, J., and Balshine, S. (2009). Mixed parentage in *Neolamprologus pulcher* groups. *J. Fish Biol.*, 74, 1129–1135.

Taborsky, B. and Oliveira, R. F. (2012). Social competence: an evolutionary approach. *Trends Ecol. Evol.*, 27, 679–688.

Taborsky, B., Skubic, E., and Bruintjes, R. (2007). Mothers adjust egg size to helper number in a cooperatively breeding cichlid. *Behav. Ecol.*, 18, 652–657.

Taborsky, B., Arnold, C., Junker, J., and Tschopp, A. (2012). The early social environment affects social competence in a cooperative breeder. *Anim. Behav.*, 83, 1067–1074.

Taborsky, B., Tschirren, L., Meunier, C., and Aubin-Horth, N. (2013). Stable reprogramming of brain transcription profiles by the early social environment in a cooperatively breeding fish. *Proc. R. Soc. London B*, 280, 20122605.

Taborsky, M. (1982). Brutpflegehelfer Beim Cichliden *Lamprologus Brichardi*, Poll (1974): Eine Kosten/Nutzen-Analyse. Ph. D. thesis, Universität Wien, Austria.

Taborsky, M. (1984). Broodcare helpers in the cichlid fish *Lamprologus brichardi*: their costs and benefits. *Anim. Behav.*, 32, 1236–1252.

Taborsky, M. (1985). Breeder-helper conflict in a cichlid fish with broodcare helpers: an experimental analysis. *Behaviour*, 95, 45–75.

Taborsky, M. (1994). Sneakers, satellites, and helpers: parasitic and cooperative behavior in fish reproduction. *Adv. Study Behav.*, 23, 1–100.

Taborsky, M. (2009). Reproductive skew in cooperative fish groups: virtue and limitations of alternative modeling approaches. In: *Reproductive Skew in Vertebrates: Proximate and Ultimate Causes*, ed. R. Hager and C. B. Jones. Cambridge: Cambridge University Press, pp. 265–304.

Taborsky, M. and Grantner, A. (1998). Behavioural time-energy budgets of cooperatively breeding *Neolamprologus pulcher* (Pisces: Cichlidae). *Anim. Behav.*, 56, 1375–1382.

Taborsky, M. and Limberger, D. (1981). Helpers in fish. *Behav. Ecol. Sociobiol.*, 8, 143–145.

Taborsky, M., Hert, E., Siemens, M., and Stoerig, P. (1986). Social behaviour of Lamprologus species: functions and mechanisms. *Ann. Mus. Roy. Afr. Sci. Zool.*, 251, 7–11.

Taves, M. D., Desjardins, J. K., Mishra, S., and Balshine, S. (2009). Androgens and dominance: Sex-specific patterns in a highly social fish (*Neolamprologus pulcher*). *Gen. Comp. Endocrinol.*, 161, 202–207.

Werner, N. Y., Balshine, S., Leach, B., and Lotem, A. (2003). Helping opportunities and space segregation in cooperatively breeding cichlids. *Behav. Ecol.*, 14, 749–756.

Whittington, C. M. and Wilson, A. B. (2013). The role of prolactin in fish reproduction. *Gen. Comp. Endocrinol.*, 191, 123–136.

Wiley, R. H. and Rabenold, K. N. (1984). The evolution of cooperative breeding by delayed reciprocity and queuing for favorable social positions. *Evolution*, 38, 609–621.

Wong, M. and Balshine, S. (2011). The evolution of cooperative breeding in the African cichlid fish, *Neolamprologus pulcher*. *Biol. Rev.*, 86, 511–530.

Wong, M., Jordan, L., Marsh-Rollo, S., St-Cyr, S., Reynolds, J., et al. (2012). Mating systems in cooperative breeders: the roles of resource dispersion and conflict mitigation. *Behav. Ecol.*, 23, 521–530.

Ziegler, T. E. (2000). Hormones associated with non-maternal infant care: a review of mammalian and avian studies. *Folia Primatol.*, 71, 6–21.

Zöttl, M., Heg, D., Chervet, N., and Taborsky, M. (2013a). Kinship reduces alloparental care in cooperative cichlids where helpers pay-to-stay. *Nature Comm.*, 4, 1341.

Zöttl, M., Frommen, J. G., and Taborsky, M. (2013b). Group size adjustment to ecological demand in a cooperative breeder. *Proc. R. Soc. London B*, 280, 20122772.

Zöttl, M., Fischer, S., and Taborsky, M. (2013c). Partial brood care compensation by female breeders in response to experimental manipulation of alloparental care. *Anim. Behav.*, 85, 1471–1478.

Zöttl, M., Chapuis, L., Freiburghaus, M., and Taborsky, M. (2013d). Strategic reduction of help before dispersal in a cooperative breeder. *Biol. Lett.*, 9, 20120878.

17

Meerkats: Cooperative breeding in the Kalahari

Tim Clutton-Brock and Marta Manser

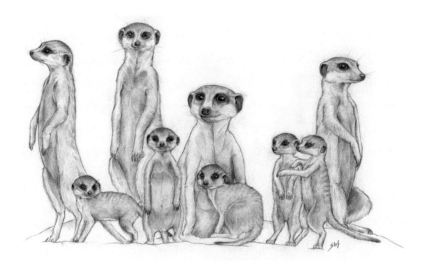

Introduction

The evolution of cooperation has been a focus of interest for evolutionary biologists for over a hundred years (Darwin 1859; Kropotkin 1908; Williams 1966). While all forms of cooperation challenge the centrality of competition in the process of evolution, cooperative and eusocial breeding systems, where offspring produced by a small number of breeding individuals are reared by nonbreeding helpers or workers, raise some of the most fundamental questions about the level at which selection operates the measurement of

fitness and the mechanisms controlling social behavior (Wilson and Sober 1994; Nowak 2006; Abbot et al. 2011; Marshall 2011).

Most detailed studies of cooperative systems have either focused on insects or on birds but cooperative breeding also occurs in mammals with some species showing a level of structural complexity that is intermediate between these two taxa. While the largest groups and the most structurally complex vertebrate cooperative societies occur in mole-rats (Chapter 19), the social mongooses offer unusual advantages for studying cooperation since they are diurnal and terrestrial

Cooperative Breeding in Vertebrates: Studies of Ecology, Evolution, and Behavior, eds W. D. Koenig and J. L. Dickinson.
Published by Cambridge University Press. © Cambridge University Press 2016.

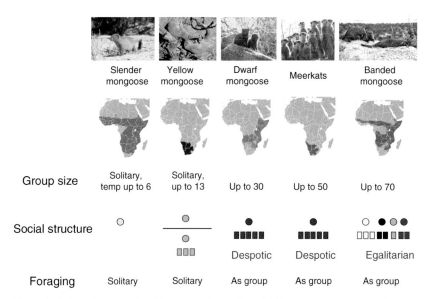

Figure 17.1. Distribution and social structure in five diurnal African mongooses. From Manser et al. (2014). See plate section for color figure.

and habituate to close observation, making it possible to measure individual contributions to different forms of cooperative behavior with considerable precision (Rood 1990; Rasa 1986; Clutton-Brock et al. 2000).

The mongooses (Herpestidae) are an Old World radiation of ~35 species of small carnivores weighing between 320 g and 4 kg. They live on a combination of insects and small vertebrates occasionally eating tubers or bulbs and extend throughout much of Africa including Madagascar, Asia, and parts of southern Europe (Macdonald 2004). The majority of species are nocturnal and solitary but most diurnal species are social and several are cooperative breeders (Rood 1980; Schneider and Kappeler 2013).

This chapter synthesizes the results of our long-term study of Kalahari meerkats (*Suricata suricatta*), one of the most social mongooses along with the banded mongoose (*Mungos mungo*) (Chapter 18, Figure 17.1). Among the social mongooses, Kalahari meerkats are most extensively adapted to living in open country, where vegetation is sparse and foraging groups are easily detectable by predators. Perhaps as a result, they will habituate to close observation (Figure 17.2), although not all do so easily or quickly

and groups can take many months to habituate to close observation.

Our work was initially established to answer three fundamental questions about the evolution of cooperative breeding: Why do helpers delay dispersal? Why do they not breed? And why do they help? Subsequently, it was extended to investigate the organization of cooperation, the communication processes operating between individuals, causes, and consequences of individual differences in cooperative behavior, the hormonal mechanisms underlying reproductive suppression and cooperation, and the effects of cooperative breeding on population demography and dynamics.

Our research on meerkats has now lasted for more than 20 years and has involved detailed studies of more than 60 groups with an average of 15 groups being monitored at any one time. During the first six years of the study we worked in parallel at sites in the Kgalagadi National Park and at one site on unimproved ranch-land 150 km to the east, both in the southern part of the Kalahari Desert of South Africa. At both sites, all individuals in the groups we studied were habituated to observation from within a meter or two, and most individuals have been weighed several times a day, several

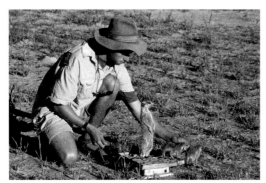

Credit: Tim Clutton-Brock

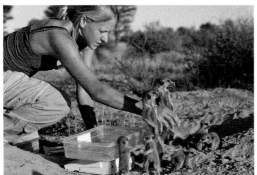

Credit: Tim Clutton-Brock

Figure 17.2. Meerkats habituate to close observation and can be trained with small rewards of water or hard-boiled egg to step onto electronic balances. Photo by T. Clutton-Brock.

days per month throughout their lives. Urine and fecal samples are collected whenever possible and, together with blood samples, are used to measure levels of sex hormones and corticosteroids. Virtually all individuals at the second site (from which our most recent data are drawn) were marked with transponders shortly after emergence and have been sampled for genetic analysis, which has been used to establish their paternity and to construct a multigenerational pedigree.

Social organization

Adult meerkats weigh between 0.5 and 1 kg and are sexually monomorphic (Clutton-Brock et al. 1999a; English et al. 2012). They live in stable groups of 2–50 individuals (Figure 17.3) and show differentiated

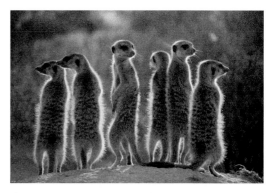

Figure 17.3. Meerkats live in groups of up to 50 in well-defined home ranges which they defend against neighboring groups. Photo by A. Young.

relationships with each other that affect affiliative and aggressive interactions (Thavarajah et al. 2014). Groups typically include one dominant female that is usually either a founding member or has been born in the group and is responsible for most breeding attempts, and one dominant male that is usually an immigrant and that fathers most young born to the dominant female. In addition, groups contain a variable number of subordinate, natal helpers and some contain subordinate immigrant males that are frequently brothers of the dominant male and that either cofounded the group or joined it together with the dominant male (Kutsukake and Clutton-Brock 2008). Female immigration does not occur.

Groups occupy ranges of 2–10 km² that usually include several complex sleeping burrows and more than a thousand bolt-holes that can be used in the event of danger when the group is foraging (Manser and Bell 2004). Ranges are defended against neighboring groups (Mares et al. 2012) (Figure 17.4) and are marked by latrines (Jordan et al. 2007). Groups leave their sleeping burrow shortly after dawn and individuals forage independently for invertebrates and small vertebrates frequently digging substantial holes to access prey living below ground (Barnard 2000; Turbé 2006) (Figure 17.5).

Groups commonly travel several kilometers a day and frequently change sleeping burrows, usually arriving at the burrow where they will sleep around sundown. Individuals do not cooperate to dig for or catch

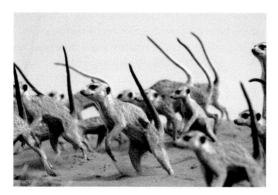

Figure 17.4. Intergroup interactions involve elaborate "war dances" followed, in some cases, by mêlées that can have lethal outcomes. Photo by A. Young.

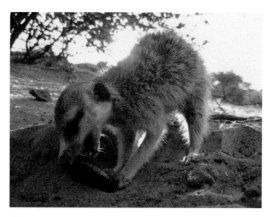

Figure 17.5. Foraging meerkats obtain most of their prey from the top 10 cm of sand. Photo by A. Young.

prey and sometimes compete for prey items or holes. Morning foraging periods usually last for 2–4 hours, after which the animals rest during the heat of the day and forage again in the afternoon before returning to a sleeping burrow at sunset.

Since they forage in an open environment where visibility is high, meerkats are subject to high rates of predation from a wide range of predators and annual rates of mortality are high: in the Kgalagadi Park, a major migration route for raptors, annual rates of mortality was over 50% whereas at the Kuruman River site, annual mortality is around 20%. At both sites, mortality rates were unrelated to sex or status (Clutton-Brock et al. 1999c). Individuals can live for up to 13 years, although the reproductive performance of females begins to decline after they are five years old (Sharp and Clutton-Brock 2011a).

The stable structure of meerkat groups has an important influence on their dynamics, characterized by slow increases in group and population size during the breeding season and relatively sharp declines shortly before the next breeding season as a result of dispersal, especially in dry years. Groups are regulated by a combination of changes in fecundity and emigration in a standard density-dependent fashion and simple models incorporating conventional density dependence and variation in rainfall do a good job of capturing the observed changes in population density (Bateman et al. 2012a, 2012b).

Life histories

Dominant females

Only dominant females breed regularly. While they can breed throughout the year, breeding commonly ceases in midwinter (April-July) and restarts in August or September (Clutton-Brock et al. 1999a). Females can produce 3 or 4 litters of pups per year, with litter sizes ranging from 1 to 7 pups, usually conceiving 5–15 days after giving birth to the previous litter although, in dry years, breeding can cease altogether. Gestation length is approximately 70 days and prenatal growth is slow during the first half of the period and then increases linearly until birth (Sharp and Clutton-Brock 2011a; Huchard et al. 2014).

Pups may be killed soon after birth by other pregnant females that can either be dominant or subordinate (Clutton-Brock et al. 1998b; Young and Clutton-Brock 2006) (Figure 17.6). When infanticide occurs, the entire litter is usually killed: comparisons of ultrasonic scans in late pregnancy and litter size at emergence suggest that partial litter loss is uncommon. There is no indication that resident males ever kill pups, although neighboring groups sometimes raid breeding burrows and will attack and sometimes kill babysitters and pups that may serve to restrict the size and competitiveness of neighboring groups.

Since the breeding success of females depends principally on the number of years for which they hold

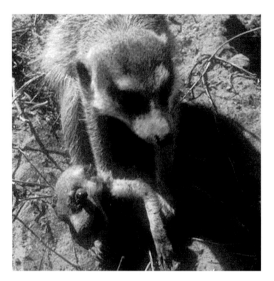

Figure 17.6. Infanticide by pregnant females is common. Here a dominant female has recently killed one of her daughter's pups. Photo by A. Young.

a dominant position, we explored the correlates of dominance. Dominant females have higher levels of estrogen and luteinizing hormone (LH) than subordinates as well as increased levels of cortisol (O'Riain et al. 2000; Moss et al. 2001; Carlson et al. 2004). As in naked mole-rats (*Heterocephalus glaber*), the acquisition of dominant status leads to an almost immediate temporary increase in growth rates in dominant females (Russell et al. 2004). Dominant females are more frequently aggressive than other group members, especially toward older natal females that are forcibly evicted from the group, usually between the ages of 24 and 48 months (Clutton-Brock et al. 1998b, 2010) (Figure 17.7). Females that have been forced out from groups are not accepted into other established groups and can only become breeders by succession in their natal group or by founding a new breeding group, usually together with sisters that have left the same group at the same time.

Age and size affect a female's chances of acquiring a dominant position. When a dominant female dies, the oldest (or heaviest, if from the same litter) resident subordinate female usually succeeds to the dominant position (Clutton-Brock et al. 2006; Thavarajah et al. 2014).

Following the death of a dominant female, subordinate females often compete intensely for the dominant position but once a female establishes and maintains her status for several months, she is rarely displaced unless she is injured (Sharp and Clutton-Brock 2009).

Breeding females can maintain their position for over ten years and produce more than 80 surviving pups. The duration of their tenure as dominant is positively related to their weight relative to that of the heaviest subordinate female in the group and tenure as a breeder has an important effect on their lifetime breeding success (Figure 17.8). Pups born to dominant females are more likely to survive than those born to subordinates and are more likely eventually to acquire dominant status (Russell et al. 2002, 2003a; Clutton-Brock et al. 2006). Nonetheless there is no evidence of differences in the scx ratio of emerging pups in relation to maternal status or other social or environmental parameters, despite the apparent benefit that such sex-ratio biasing would apparently confer (MacLeod and Clutton-Brock 2013b).

Dominant males

Each breeding group includes one clearly dominant male, usually an immigrant that either founded the group or joined it after the death of the previous dominant male. Like females, dispersing males commonly combine with siblings or other close relatives to compete for access to breeding groups and dominant males typically hold their status until their death. Natal dominant males are typically replaced by one or more unrelated immigrant males within a year of their acquisition of the dominant position.

Dominant males are thus seldom closely related to the dominant female, which they guard throughout successive ovulation periods. Extra-pair paternity (EPP) is uncommon and dominant males typically father at least 90% of offspring born to the dominant female in their group (Griffin et al. 2003; Spong et al. 2008) except in rare cases when the breeding individuals are related, in which case EPPs increase in frequency (Leclaire et al. 2013a). Since dominant males father most of the young produced by dominant females, their annual breeding success is similar to that of the dominant female. Their tenure is shorter,

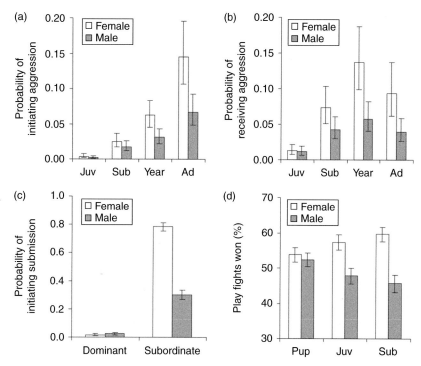

Figure 17.7. Sex differences in aggression and submission. The probability that male and female subordinates of different age categories (a) initiate or (b) receive aggression during a breeding attempt (juvenile, 3–6 months; subadult, 6–12 months; yearling, 12–24 months; adult, >24 months). (c) The probability that dominant and subordinate males and females >1 yr of age will initiate submission. (d) The percentage of play fights involving opposite sexed pups (1–3 months), juveniles (3–6 months) and subadults (6–12 months) won by each sex ($N = 28$ females, 24 males); Graphs show the predicted means ± standard error derived from GLMMs in which group, litter and individual identity were included as random terms.

however, so that variance in their lifetime breeding success is smaller than that in dominant females (Clutton-Brock et al. 2006) (Figure 17.8). Following the death of a dominant male, a natal male sometimes assumes the dominant position in the group. Unlike immigrant males, natal dominant males do not mate guard dominant females (which typically breed outside the group if no immigrant male is available) and rarely father young in the group. Unlike immigrant males, they frequently visit neighboring groups and eventually leave their group to breed elsewhere.

Subordinate Females

In addition to the dominant pair, meerkat groups include a variable number of subordinates of both sexes that assist in rearing offspring. Most helpers are animals that have not yet left their natal group and are typically the offspring of resident breeders or previous dominants, but in newly established groups, some are founding members who have dispersed with the current dominant of the same sex.

Growth rates of pups vary widely and are related to rainfall, the number of helpers present in the group, and their mother's status (English et al. 2013a, 2013b). As individuals increase in age they contribute progressively to different cooperative activities (Figure 17.9). While the growth rate of helpers affects their chance of acquiring dominance status, there is no evidence of discrete differences in growth between individuals that eventually acquire dominance status and those that do not (Carter et al. 2014).

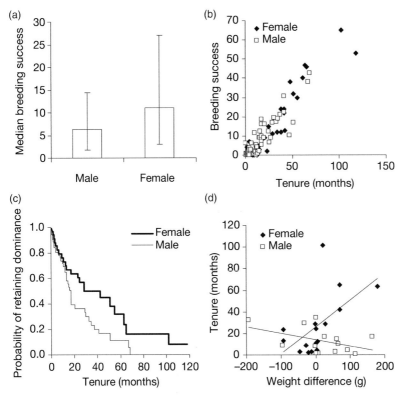

Figure 17.8. Dominance and breeding success in males and females. (a) Breeding success (offspring surviving to 12 months) of 33 dominant females and 53 dominant males. Graph shows medians and interquartile range. (b) The influence of dominance tenure on breeding success in 33 dominant females (linear regression: $F_{1,32} = 226$, $P < 0.001$) and 53 dominant males (linear regression: $F_{1,52} = 186$, $P < 0.001$). (c) Kaplan–Meier estimates of the probability of dominant females ($N = 33$) and males ($N = 53$) retaining their status after different periods of time. (d) The relationship between the difference in body weight between the dominant and the heaviest same-sex competitor and tenure in dominant females ($N = 16$) and dominant males ($N = 14$).

Females typically remain in their natal group for 2–3 years, contributing to cooperative activities (Figure 17.9). As they grow, their social status increases (Thavarajah et al. 2014) and they are progressively more likely to mate with roving males from other groups (see below); thus most subordinate females over two years old attempt to breed at least once a year (Clutton-Brock et al. 2001b, 2010). Older subordinate females suffer increased rates of aggression, have higher abortion rates than dominants, and their pups are commonly killed at birth by other pregnant females (Clutton-Brock et al. 1998b; Young and Clutton-Brock 2006). If pups born to subordinates survive, they are guarded and fed by other group members although dominant females contribute little to rearing them (Clutton-Brock et al. 2001c, 2003, 2004).

During the weeks before the dominant female gives birth, older subordinate females become the targets of increased aggression (Clutton-Brock et al. 2006, 2010; Kutsukake and Clutton-Brock 2006). This overt aggression suggests that there is an underlying conflict between dominant females and older subordinates that is resolved by direct interactions (Stephens et al. 2005). Over 90% of females have left their natal group before they are four years old and all subordinate females are ultimately driven out of their natal groups

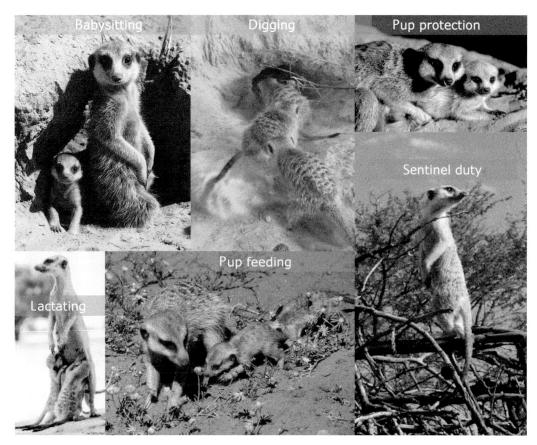

Figure 17.9. All adult helpers contribute to babysitting, pup feeding, burrow renovation, sentinel duty, and the defense of the group's range. Composite photograph by members of the Kalahari Meerkat Project. See plate section for color figure.

unless they acquire dominant status. Subordinate females that have been evicted are sometimes allowed to rejoin the group after the dominant's pups have been born, but the same events are then repeated at subsequent breeding attempts until they leave and eventually fail to return. Dominant females are more likely to evict heavier subordinates, those that are obviously pregnant, and individuals that are more distantly related to them (Clutton-Brock et al. 2010). There is no indication, however, that individuals contributing relatively little to cooperative activities receive a disproportionate share of aggression or are more often evicted than more generous contributors (Santema and Clutton-Brock 2012).

Subordinate females that have been evicted often remain in the vicinity of their natal group for several weeks, but rarely establish new breeding groups unless several females have been evicted together in which case they are more likely to survive and attract roving males to form a new group (Young 2003). When a new group forms, the oldest or heaviest female typically establishes herself as dominant and evicts the other founding females within the first 18 months. Because dispersing females can travel long distances, estimating the proportion of females that leave and successfully breed elsewhere is difficult. Few females, however, have immigrated into the population and less than 10% of females born in our 80 km² study have achieved dominant status after eviction, suggesting that the success rate of dispersers is low (Clutton-Brock et al. 2006).

Subordinate Males

Like females, males usually continue to act as helpers until they leave their natal group. Once they are over two years old, they start to leave their natal group for a day at a time, either alone or in small groups and visit neighboring groups often returning to sleep with their own group. Roving males frequently attempt to mate with unguarded subordinate females and are usually the fathers of pups born to subordinate females or to dominant females in groups that lack immigrant males (Griffin et al. 2003; Spong et al. 2008). Roving has substantial costs, including decreased foraging efficiency, weight loss, and increased cortisol levels (Young et al. 2007; Mares et al. 2012). Groups of resident males commonly attack male intruders and may wound or even kill them. Roving males eventually fail to return to their natal group, either because they have joined an established breeding group, founded a new one, or been killed.

For males, dispersal is a necessary condition for the acquisition of a dominant position and substantial breeding success. Paternity analysis shows that females seldom breed with males reared in the same group and that inbreeding between first-order relatives is rare, even following the death of one of the dominants (Griffin et al. 2003; Nielsen et al. 2012). Instead, dominant females living in groups with a related dominant male generally mate with unrelated, roving males (Spong et al. 2008). As copulations are rarely observed, it is not possible to tell whether subordinate males do not breed in their natal group because natal females reject their attempts to mate, or if males avoid mating with resident (usually related) females. Although incest between first-order relatives is extremely rare, dispersing animals frequently join groups that include either matrilineal or patrilineal relatives and 44% of animals in our population have detectably nonzero inbreeding coefficients. Inbreeding has measurable costs and offspring born as a result of matings between relatives exhibit reduced growth and survival (Nielsen et al. 2012).

Cooperative behavior

Meerkats cannot breed successfully without assistance from helpers, which contribute to eight distinct forms of cooperative behavior (Figure 17.9). Contributions to different activities vary in relation to status, sex, and age but individuals show little evidence of specialization (Clutton-Brock et al. 2003) (Figure 17.10).

Babysitting

During the 3–4 weeks after they are born that pups spend at the natal burrow, one or more "babysitters" remain with the pups at the breeding burrow each day and do not forage with the group (Clutton-Brock et al. 1998a, 2000). Babysitters may be male or female and usually remain at the natal burrow for the entire day, losing 1–2% of body weight in the process. As a result, the same individuals rarely babysit on successive days.

Dominants seldom babysit while, among subordinates, females contribute more than males (Clutton-Brock et al. 2000). Well-fed individuals contribute more than light or hungry ones and experimental feeding of individuals increases their contributions to babysitting (Clutton-Brock et al. 2002). Although there are substantial individual differences in babysitting, these do not appear to be correlated with relatedness to breeding females or their offspring despite evidence that individuals are capable of distinguishing between close kin by smell (LeClaire et al. 2013b).

Allolactation

As in several other social mongooses (Creel et al. 1991), allolactation is common and nearly half of all litters are nursed by one or more subordinate females in addition to their mothers (Doolan and Macdonald 1999; Clutton-Brock et al. 1999b). Allolactators rarely suckle pups for as long as dominant females and their milk production is lower than that of dominants (Scantlebury et al. 2002). Subordinate females are more likely to allolactate if they are or have recently been pregnant and if they are closely related to the dominant female (MacLeod and Clutton-Brock 2013a).

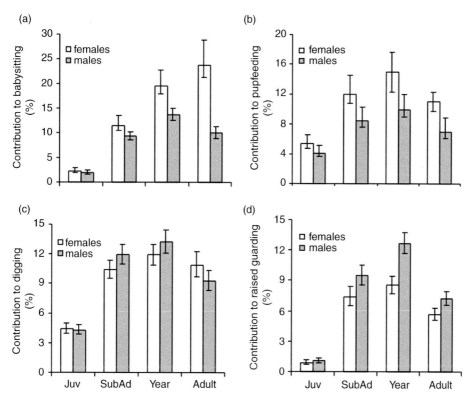

Figure 17.10. Age-related changes in the contributions of male and female helpers to (a) babysitting, (b) pup feeding, (c) social digging, and (d) raised guarding. The level of contributions differed significantly between sexes for all activities except digging. (a) Females contributed more to babysitting than males in all age categories except juveniles (juveniles, $\chi^2 = 0.3$, $df = 1$, $P = 0.61$; subadults, $\chi^2 = 4.4$, $df = 1$, $P = 0.04$; yearlings, $\chi^2 = 12.8$, $df = 1$, $P = 0.001$; adults, $\chi^2 = 32.1$, df = 1, $P < 0.001$). (b) Females contributed more to pup feeding than males in all categories (juveniles, $\chi^2 = 4.6$, $df = 1$, $P = 0.03$; subadults, $\chi^2 = 14.5$, $df = 1$, $P = 0.001$; yearlings, $\chi^2 = 17.1$, $df = 1$, $P = 0.001$; adults, $\chi^2 = 15.5$, $df = 1$, $P = 0.001$). (c) Males and females did not differ in their contributions to social digging in any category (all P values > 0.2). (d) Males contributed more to raised guarding than females in all age categories except juveniles (juveniles, $\chi^2 = 0.1$, df = 1, $P = 0.73$; subadults, $\chi^2 = 6.1$, $df = 1$, $P = 0.01$; yearlings, $\chi^2 = 16.8$, $df = 1$, $P = 0.001$; adults, $\chi^2 = 5.2$, $df = 1$, $P = 0.02$).

Pup feeding

Around 20–25 days after birth, pups leave the natal burrow when the rest of the group leave to forage. Between the ages of ~1–3 months, they are fed solid food and gain weight rapidly. Their rate of weight gain is positively related to the number of helpers in their group as well as to environmental parameters that affect food availability, including rainfall (English et al. 2012, 2013a, 2013b). Breeding females and dominant males contribute relatively less than adult helpers to feeding pups although

their contributions increase when the ratio of helpers to pups is low (Brotherton et al. 2001; Clutton-Brock et al. 2004). Dominant females contribute little to feeding pups produced by subordinate females.

Both male and female subordinates over six months old regularly feed pups, although females do so more frequently than males (Brotherton et al. 2001. Overall, helpers provide pups with around 40% of the food items they find, but this proportion varies with the helper's foraging success and daily weight gain can be increased by experimentally provisioning helpers (Clutton-Brock et al. 2002). In sequential breeding attempts, helpers alternate in "generosity" toward pups, contributing heavily to one breeding attempt and little to the next (Russell et al. 2003b). In contrast to allolactation, there is no evidence that the relative frequency with which helpers feed pups is related to kinship (Clutton-Brock et al. 2001a) and helpers of both sexes readily feed pups born to subordinate females as well as to dominants, although males reduce their relative contributions when subordinates breed (Clutton-Brock et al. 2004).

Helpers typically give food items that they have found to the closest pup and pups compete for access to helpers – especially those individuals that are more generous (Hodge et al. 2007). The frequency of aggression between pups rises when food availability is reduced or pups are experimentally deprived of food and is higher in groups with a lower ratio of helpers to pups (Hodge et al. 2009). Over the period of pup feeding, pups give repeated begging calls, and their rate of calling is associated with their hunger level (Manser et al. 2008), the probability that they will be fed, and whether they are near to a generous adult (Kunc et al. 2007). Individual calling rates are also higher in small groups than in large ones. While one interpretation of this result is that pups cooperate with each other to elevate the level of provisioning by helpers (Bell 2007), a simpler explanation is that pups prefer to call when other pups are silent because this is most likely to elicit a response from adults (Madden et al. 2009b).

Helpers respond to variation in pup begging rates by increasing the frequency with which they feed pups (Manser and Avey 2000). In contrast to banded mongooses, there is no indication that particular helpers are more likely to feed particular pups although some analyses suggest that female, but not male, helpers prefer to feed female pups (Brotherton et al. 2001; Hodge et al. 2007).

As pups get older, their success in finding food for themselves rises and they become increasingly independent. Over the same period, their begging rate falls and adults bring food to them less and less frequently (Manser and Avey 2000; Barnard 2000). The begging calls of dependent pups, 40–60 days old, differ acoustically from those of older pups, and playback experiments demonstrate that changes in call structure affect the rate at which adults provision pups (Madden et al. 2009a).

During pup-feeding, helpers, particularly males, sometimes bring food items to pups but, at the last moment, eat it themselves (Clutton-Brock et al. 2005). One interpretation of these "false-feeding" events is that this gives other group members the impression that individual helpers are contributing more to pup feeding than is actually the case. A simpler alternative, however, is that helpers cannot assess a pup's need for food until they are nearby and, if they discover that pups are satiated, they eat the food themselves. Detailed observations, both in meerkats and other species, suggest that this is the most likely explanation of this phenomenon (Chapter 9).

Teaching

Besides provisioning pups, group members adjust their behavior so as to enhance the foraging skills pups need to survive, initially giving them dead or badly wounded prey and then gradually increasing the prey's ability to escape or strike back (Thornton and McAuliffe 2006). For example, scorpions are initially presented to pups dead or wounded with their stings removed but, as pups' age, they are gradually presented intact while pups learn to kill them and remove the sting. Experiments confirm that presenting pups with active prey improves the rate at which they learn handling skills at some cost to helpers and consequently represents an example of teaching behavior. In addition, helpers preferentially feed rarer food items to pups, which may help to broaden the range of foods they eventually use (Thornton 2008).

Burrow renovation

Both breeders and helpers contribute to removing sand from sleeping burrows and bolt-holes, sometimes forming "chain gangs" to pass the excavated sand back to the burrow entrance (Clutton-Brock et al. 2002; Bousquet 2011). Sex differences in burrow renovation are small but there is a tendency for males to contribute more than females and for dominant individuals to contribute more than subordinates.

Sentinel behavior and alarm calling

Individual meerkats intermittently cease foraging and move to a raised position where they scan the sky and surrounding area. Although there is no regular rotation in sentinel behavior, individuals seldom take successive bouts or go on guard when another individual is already acting as a sentinel (Clutton-Brock et al. 1999b). Individual contributions to sentinel duty vary widely and are positively associated with age, weight, and foraging success, and are higher in males than females. They are higher in males than females and increase when individuals have been artificially provisioned (Clutton-Brock et al. 1999b). Average contributions to sentinel duty increase when the risk of predation is high and rise when pups are foraging with the group (Santema and Clutton-Brock 2013).

When sentinels detect danger, they give graded alarm calls whose structure varies both in relation to the type of predator they have seen and to the urgency of the danger (Manser 2001; Manser et al. 2001, 2002). The likelihood of alarm calling depends on whether other group members are close by (Townsend and Manser 2011; Townsend et al. 2011). Individuals adjust their responses in relation to their own occupation (Amsler 2009) but do not adjust their responses to the identity or reliability of the caller, possibly because the costs of ignoring alarm calls are too high (Schibler and Manser 2007). Sentinels give regular high-pitched calls when they are on "watch" and these are detected by other group members, allowing them to reduce their level of vigilance while foraging (Manser 1999).

Group defense against conspecifics

Both sexes help defend against neighboring groups by scent-marking at latrines (Jordan 2007; Jordan et al. 2007). Scent-marking increases during the peak breeding period and when prospecting males are encountered, indicating that it plays an important role in mate defense. When groups meet, all group members contribute to extended displays that can lead to a mêlée of fighting pairs or trios, in which individuals are sometimes killed (Mares et al. 2012) (Figure 17.4). Strategic scent-marking may help to avoid these costly encounters.

Defense against predators

Both sexes engage in mobbing, which is typically directed at relatively immobile predators, including snakes, monitor lizards, Cape foxes, and other mongoose species that are in burrows (Graw and Manser 2007) as well as at predator cues, such as urine and feces (Zöttl et al. 2013) (Figure 17.11). The intensity and duration of mobbing events rises with the potential risk posed by the predator, group members will also defend each other or pups against predators and groups will bunch and attack predators, including jackals and eagles, that are either posing a threat to the group or have caught a group member.

Organization of cooperative behavior

Individual differences in cooperative behavior

Once juveniles are around six months old, they begin to contribute to feeding subsequent litters of pups, clearing sand from bolt-holes and sleeping burrows and, more gradually, other cooperative activities, including "babysitting" and acting as sentinels (Clutton-Brock et al. 2002; Carter et al. 2014) (Figure 17.9). Contributions to most cooperative activities peak in the second year of life and show a tendency to decline in older individuals as opportunities to disperse increases.

With the exception of allolactation, all group members contribute to all cooperative activities although some individuals contribute substantially more to all cooperative activities than others, and these differences are consistent over time (English et al. 2010). Individual differences are associated with contrasts in early development: heavy juveniles and yearlings contribute more to cooperative activities than light ones (Clutton-Brock et al. 2002) and females that develop in groups with a relatively large number of helpers subsequently contribute less to cooperative activities

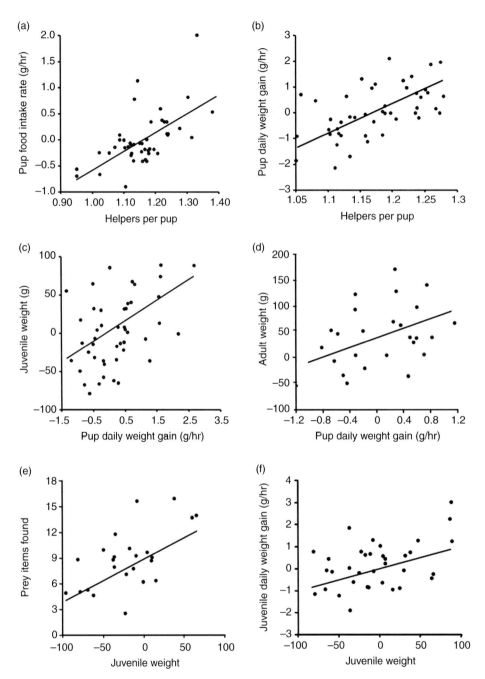

Figure 17.11. Downstream effects of pup feeding by helpers on the daily weight gain of pups, their weight and foraging success at independence, and their weight at adulthood. Analyses were conducted on means for 46 litters [(a) through (c)], 26 litters [(d) through (e)], and 35 litters (f) and controlled for the effects of repeated measures within eight groups. Axes with negative values depict residual values obtained from regressions of the variable in question on age. (a) Correlation between helper:pup ratios

than those that develop in groups with few helpers (English 2010).

Genetic factors may also be involved, for analyses indicate that individual differences in cooperative behavior are partly heritable and, for their age, inbred individuals contribute more to cooperative activities than other group members (Nielsen et al. 2012). One possible explanation of these results is that increases in cooperative behavior in inbred animals are a consequence of increased selection for cooperation among relatives, since inbreeding depresses growth and development. However, an alternative possibility is that the tendency for inbred animals to contribute more is associated with deferred sexual development and an extension of the usual period when individuals contribute heavily to cooperative activities.

Coordination of cooperative behavior

Cooperative behavior needs to be coordinated to enable collective group actions to operate efficiently. Meerkats use several different call types to coordinate spatial organization while foraging, defending against predators, and interacting with peers and offspring. They have evolved one of the most sophisticated vocal repertoires described for mammals and have more than 30 different discrete call types (Manser 1998).

Meerkats forage as a cohesive unit throughout the day and they emit several different call types to maintain group cohesion during their foraging excursions. "Lead calls" are given to coordinate departure from the sleeping burrow and to incite group members to switch foraging patches (Turbé 2006). If more than three individuals are involved in calling, the group moves to the next foraging area, but if just one or no individual replies to the call, the group usually continues to forage on the current foraging patch, suggesting that a quorum has not been reached (Bousquet et al. 2011).

While meerkats are foraging, they regularly emit soft, "close" calls, and are likely to maintain contact among the dispersed group members as well as spacing out themselves to avoid frequent food competition (Engesser 2011). Individuals that get separated from the group emit soft "alert" calls, which turn into loud barks if they cannot see the group. Barking causes other group members to stand bipedally or to move in the direction of the lost animal (Manser 1998).

Vocalizations also play an important role in regulating social relationships within groups. Meerkats express their affiliative or aggressive intentions when approaching each other with appropriate calls. Growls reflect aggression and are given by dominants to subordinate individuals, while subordinates express their submission with higher pitched "groveling" calls (Kutsukake and Clutton-Brock 2006). Close calls are also used to regulate and monitor the movements of other individuals (Townsend et al. 2012). Responses to calls are adjusted to social circumstances. For example, subordinate females that experience aggression from the dominant female and are at risk of being evicted respond very strongly to calls of aggressors (Reber et al. 2013).

Proximate mechanisms

Males that are about to babysit pups have higher levels of prolactin and lower levels of cortisol than males that leave to forage with the group (Carlson et al. 2006a). After pups begin to forage with the group, they beg

Figure 17.11 (*cont.*)

and mean rate of estimated food intake by individual pups between 35 and 75 days old, measured in grams per hour ($F_{1,37} = 21.3$, $P = 0.001$). (b) Correlation between helper:pup ratios and mean daily weight gain of pups between 35 and 75 days old ($F_{1,37} = 12.7$, $P = 0.001$). (c) Correlation between mean daily weight gain of pups between 35 and 75 days old and mean body weight of the same individuals at independence (3 to 4 months) ($F_{1,37} = 10.8$, $P = 0.002$). (d) Correlation between mean daily weight gain of pups between 35 and 75 days old and mean body weight of the same individuals at adulthood (12 to 13 months) ($F_{1,17} = 5.7$, $P = 0.04$). (e) Correlation between the weight of individuals at independence and the number of food items they find per hour at independence ($F_{1,17} = 8.6$, $P = 0.01$). (f) Correlation between the body weight of pups at independence, after pup feeding by helpers had ceased, and their mean residual daily weight gain over the same period ($F_{1,26} = 7.3$, $P = 0.01$).

repeatedly and experimental playback of pup begging calls to male helpers increases their cortisol levels and the rate at which pups are fed (Manser and Avey 2000; Manser et al. 2008; Carlson et al. 2006b). However, intramuscular injection of cortisol in male and female helpers did not increase contributions to cooperative activities, although experimental animals foraged more and tended to spend more time close to pups (Santema et al. 2013).

As in other mammals, cooperative behavior is associated with increased oxytocin levels (Dölen et al. 2013), and intramuscular injection of oxytocin, increased the contributions of individuals to guarding, pup-feeding, and digging, as well as their association with pups (Madden and Clutton-Brock 2011).

The evolution of cooperative breeding

Why don't helpers disperse?

As discussed above, female helpers rarely if ever leave their natal group voluntarily and are generally evicted by force by the dominant breeding females. Their reluctance to leave is apparently associated with the high costs of dispersal and with the fact that groups of dispersing meerkats are seldom able to displace residents or to settle unless they locate a vacant or little-used area between established territories (Clutton-Brock and Lukas 2011). Travelling through unfamiliar areas where they may be attacked either by predators or neighboring groups is dangerous and stressful (Young et al. 2007; Young and Monfort 2009; Mares et al. 2014) and, even after locating a vacant area, small "starter" groups often fail to breed successfully, decline in size, and soon die out. As a result, the best chance that females have of acquiring a breeding position is to remain in their natal group.

The direct fitness benefits that subordinate females derive from remaining in their natal groups and their reluctance to leave home have two important implications. First, it suggests that philopatry increases, rather than reduces, the fitness of individuals and that delayed reproduction caused by remaining in the natal group should not be treated as a cost of cooperation. Second, it indicates that dominant females are unlikely to need to make reproductive concessions to subordinates in

order to retain them in the group (Clutton-Brock et al. 2001b).

Since the presence of subordinates increases the breeding success of dominants and most subordinate females are close relatives of dominants, there are presumably costs to dominants of evicting subordinates, indicating that there must be counteracting benefits. Evicting subordinates probably has multiple benefits to dominant females. If they are pregnant, evicted subordinates commonly abort their litters and eviction may help to reduce the risk of female infanticide and of competition between pups born to the dominant female and those born to subordinates (Young and Clutton-Brock 2006). In addition, subordinate females that have recently aborted frequently nurse pups that are born subsequently to dominants (MacLeod and Clutton-Brock 2013a). Experimental suppression of subordinate fertility shows that controlling subordinate reproduction has energetic costs to dominants that are reduced if subordinates are prevented from breeding (Bell et al. 2014). Finally, evicting older subordinates may also reduce the risk that they will challenge the dominant female in the future (Sharp and Clutton-Brock 2011b).

An associated question is: why do subordinate females seldom challenge and evict dominants? One possible explanation is that subordinates are unlikely to win fights against dominants. Alternatively, it may be to the subordinate's benefit to allow dominants to remain and breed, since dominants are usually close relatives and, because of their greater age and experience, more likely to breed successfully than subordinates. Estimates of the inclusive fitness benefits that helpers would gain by displacing versus tolerating dominants suggest that it is usually in their interests to displace dominants, indicating that their reluctance to challenge dominants is probably associated with a low chance of winning rather than with indirect fitness gains of ceding reproduction to dominants (Sharp and Clutton-Brock 2011b).

Why don't female helpers breed?

The relatively low frequency of breeding by subordinate females appears to be the result of more than one mechanism. The probability that subordinates will breed increases rapidly with their body mass and attempts by heavier animals are much more common than those by lighter ones, indicating that many subordinates may not have reached a stage of development where they have a substantial chance of breeding successfully (Clutton-Brock et al. 2001b). Regular aggression from females depresses levels of LH and estrogen in subordinate females and probably helps to suppress their fertility (O'Riain et al. 2000; Carlson et al. 2004; Young et al. 2006). In addition, subordinate females that lack access to an unrelated male in their group show lower levels of estrogen and are less likely to attempt to breed than those living in groups that include unrelated males (Clutton-Brock et al. 2001a).

Dominant females also interfere directly with breeding attempts by subordinate females. Especially in larger groups, the frequency of aggression directed at subordinates is high and the probability that pregnant subordinates will bring their litters to term is substantially lower than that of dominants (Clutton-Brock et al. 2010). If subordinates give birth successfully, a relatively high proportion of their litters will be killed soon after birth, either by pregnant dominant females or by pregnant subordinates (Clutton-Brock et al. 1998b; Young and Clutton-Brock 2006). As in several other mammals where female infanticide is common, females often kill offspring born not only to more distant relatives or unrelated females, but also offspring born to close relatives, including their sisters' offspring and their own grand-offspring. The relatively low success of subordinates in bringing their litters to term and rearing their offspring and the increased probability that dominant females will evict pregnant subordinates is also likely to reduce the fitness benefits of attempting to breed and to encourage the evolution of delayed reproduction in subordinates.

While the frequency of breeding attempts is lower in subordinate females than in dominants, around 20% of surviving pups are produced by subordinates (Clutton-Brock et al. 2006). So why do dominant females not prevent subordinates from breeding altogether? It seems unlikely that dominant females make reproductive concessions to subordinate females to induce them to remain in the group, since subordinate females do not leave their natal groups unless they are forcibly evicted, as discussed earlier. In addition, subordinates that breed are more, not less, likely to leave their group than those that have not bred (Clutton-Brock et al. 2001b). Subordinate breeding is also most frequent in the months after a new female succeeds to the dominant position and where older, heavier natal subordinates have been allowed to remain in the group, suggesting that subordinates breed when dominants are unable to exert effective control.

The observed distribution of breeding in female meerkats thus does not appear to require any process beyond an incomplete ability in dominance to suppress subordinate reproduction. In this respect, our results resemble those of studies of females in several other cooperative breeding vertebrates that have found little evidence to suggest that transactional processes play an important role in determining the frequency of reproduction in subordinate females (Clutton-Brock et al. 1998a; Haydock and Koenig 2002; Koenig et al. 2009; Holekamp and Engh 2009; Heg et al. 2006).

Since many subordinate females are the offspring of the resident dominant female, an obvious question is: why do dominant females prevent subordinates from breeding? Like eviction, the suppression of subordinate reproduction may help to reduce the risk of female infanticide and of competition between litters (Young and Clutton-Brock 2006). When subordinate reproduction was experimentally prevented by contraceptive injections, pups born to dominants showed increased food intake and growth, factors commonly associated with increased survival (Bell et al. 2014).

Why do helpers help?

To understand why helpers help, it is important to appreciate the diverse consequences of their assistance. The presence of helpers has substantial benefits to pups. The combined contributions of helpers to all cooperative activities (apart from allolactation) substantially exceed those of breeders and the daily weight gain, growth rate, and survival of pups increases with the number of helpers in their group (Russell et al. 2002, 2003a) (Figure 17.12). By experimentally altering helper:pup ratios and artificially provisioning pups, we

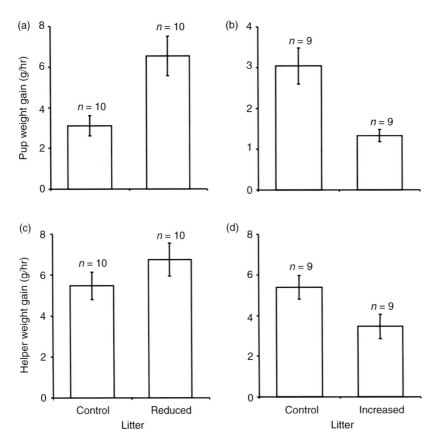

Figure 17.12. Effects of manipulating helper:pup ratios on daily weight gain of pups and helpers. In this experiment, helper:pup ratios were either temporarily increased by removing 75% of pups or were reduced by increasing litter size by 75%. Control values were mean measures of daily weight gain in pups and helpers in the same group within 2 days of the experiment. Analyses used paired t-tests; one-tailed P-values are shown. n = number of temporary removals. (a) Pups in reduced litters (high helper:pup ratios) showed a 100% increase in their daily weight gain ($t_9 = 3.9$, $P = 0.003$) as well as in the number of items they received per hour ($t_9 = 4.7$, $P < 0.001$). (b) Pups in increased litters (low helper:pup ratios) showed a 45% reduction in their daily weight gain ($t_8 = 3.7$, $P = 0.004$) as well as a 34% reduction in items received per hour ($t_8 = 2.8$, $P = 0.02$). Resident pups in increased litters showed a 38% decrease in daily weight gain ($t_8 = 2.2$, $P = 0.02$) as well as a 32% reduction in items received per hour ($t_8 = 1.6$, $P = 0.08$). (c) Helpers feeding reduced litters showed a nonsignificant tendency for daily weight gain to increase as compared with values for the same individuals on the four previous days ($t_9 = -1.2$, $P = 0.12$). (d) Helpers feeding increased litters showed a significant reduction in their daily weight gain of 31% as compared with values for the same individuals on the four previous days ($t_8 = 3.4$, $P = 0.005$).

have shown that the influence of help on fitness of pups is causal (Clutton-Brock et al. 2001c).

The direct fitness of dominant females also increases with helper number. As helper number increases, the contribution of dominant females to feeding pups decreases while their body weight increases (Clutton-Brock et al. 1998a). Breeding females belonging to large groups that include multiple helpers give birth earlier each year and have shorter interbirth intervals, with the result that the total number of litters they produce per year and their annual fecundity is increased (Russell et al. 2003a).

The number of helpers also affects their own fitness. In small groups, the proportion of time that a sentinel is on duty is relatively low and mortality rates are relatively high (Clutton-Brock et al. 1999b, 1999c). As in many other social mammals, the home ranges of small groups are frequently encroached upon and they are often displaced or attacked by larger neighboring groups. As group size rises above 20, growth and breeding success decline (Sharp and Clutton-Brock 2011a), but the costs are probably lower than those experienced by members of small groups, which face heavy per capita expenditure on all cooperative activities, high rates of predation, and regular incursions from neighboring groups (Clutton-Brock et al. 1999c). Increases in group size also raise the size of dispersing parties, which improves the chances of establishing new groups and may have substantial benefits to fitness (Young 2003).

In addition, the costs of helping may not be high. Although helping also has energetic costs to helpers and generous helpers gain less weight than relatively ungenerous individuals, there is little evidence that they suffer increased fitness costs (Russell et al. 2003b; Clutton-Brock 2006). One likely reason for this is that, as in cooperatively breeding birds (Wright et al. 2001), individual investment in helping increases with an individual's foraging success and condition, allowing helpers to minimize the fitness effects of helping (Clutton-Brock et al. 1998a, 2000, 2002; Russell et al. 2003b).

What are the likely evolutionary mechanisms maintaining cooperative behavior in meerkats? The three most commonly suggested explanations of the evolution of helping behavior are that (1) it is maintained by aggression directed by dominants at "lazy" subordinates or by the threat of eviction leading to a "pay-to-stay" situation (Gaston 1977) (Cant and Johnstone 2009; Cant 2011; Kokko et al. 2001; Bergmüller et al. 2005; Bergmüller and Taborsky 2005); (2) it is maintained by kin selection (Hamilton 1964; Brown 1987; Emlen 1991); and (3) it is maintained by mutualistic benefits (Pfeiffer et al. 2005; Hamilton and Taborsky 2005; Nowak 2006; Wilson and Wilson 2007), including generalized reciprocity and selection to increase group size (Kokko et al. 2001; Wilson and Wilson, 2007; Nowak 2006).

There is little evidence that dominant female meerkats direct more frequent aggression at subordinates that contribute relatively little to cooperative activities or that subordinates that receive more aggression subsequently make larger contributions to cooperative activities (Young et al. 2005; Santema and Clutton-Brock 2012). Moreover, such patterns of aggression would not necessarily be favored via inclusive fitness if levels of cooperative behavior reflect individual differences in condition.

Over the past decade there has been continuing debate over the relative importance of indirect fitness benefits (kin selection) versus shared, mutualistic benefits or group selection in maintaining cooperation (Nowak 2006; Wilson and Wilson 2007; Abbot et al. 2011; Marshall 2011). In meerkats, as in several other cooperative vertebrates, there is limited evidence that helpers adjust their contributions to their degree of kinship to the pups they are raising. However, most meerkat groups consist of close relatives: many are offspring of resident breeders and a high proportion are either full or half siblings of the pups they help to raise. Comparative studies show that the extent of discriminatory nepotism declines as average relatedness declines (Cornwallis et al. 2009), so that the limited evidence of nepotism does not argue against a central role for kin selection.

Our work also provides evidence that helping generates mutualistic benefits through its influence on group size and thus on the direct fitness of helpers. Effects of this kind may be common in cooperative societies, and theoretical studies show that a combination of indirect and direct fitness benefits is often likely to generate stronger selection favoring reproductive cooperation than either effect on its own (Kokko et al. 2001). In meerkats, and in many other cooperative breeders, both indirect and direct fitness benefits may be important in maintaining cooperation and their effects are likely to be difficult to separate.

A final question is consequently: does cooperative or eusocial breeding ever evolve in the absence of close kinship between group members and the opportunity for helpers to gain substantial indirect fitness benefits? Phylogenetic reconstructions of the evolution of cooperative and eusocial societies in insects, birds, and mammals now suggest that their evolution has been restricted to species with monogynous or monogamous mating systems where average relatedness between group members is high (Hughes et al. 2008; Boomsma 2009; Cornwallis et al. 2010; Lukas and Clutton-Brock 2012) and, with the exception of humans, there is no firm evidence that systems of this kind have evolved where relatedness among helpers is low. High relatedness between group members and opportunities for helpers to gain inclusive fitness benefits consequently seem likely to be a precondition for the evolution of cooperative or eusocial breeding.

Acknowledgments

We are grateful to the Kotze family for access to their land; to the Trustees of the Kalahari Research Trust for access to the Kuruman River Reserve; and to all past and present members of the Kalahari Meerkat Project especially Grant McIlrath, Lynda Sharpe, Elissa Cameron, Andrew Young, Neil Jordan, Tom Flower, Rob Sutcliffe, Dave Bell, Megan Price, Christle Bourgond, Jamie Samson, Nathan Thavarajah, Lewis Howell; Sky Bischoff-Mattson, Lyndsey Marris, and David and Nanine Gaynor for their role in maintaining the long-term data; to Josephine Pemberton, Ashleigh Griffin, Goran Spong, and Johanna Nielsen for their contributions to the genetic analysis; to Ian Stevenson for database management and to Andy Russell and Stuart Sharp for contributions to the research; to Nigel Bennett, Anne Carlson, Steve Monfort, and Christine Drea for their role in hormonal analyses; and to Walt Koenig and Janis Dickinson for comments on earlier drafts and for introducing us to a minimalist approach to punctuation. The research has been funded by grants from the NERC, the BBSRC, the Earthwatch Foundation, the European Research Council, the Swiss National Science Foundation, and the University of Zurich.

REFERENCES

Abbot, P., Abe, J., Alcock, J., Alizon, S., Alpedrinha, J. A., et al. (2011). Inclusive fitness theory and eusociality. *Nature*, 471, E1–E4.

Amsler, V. (2009). How urgency levels in alarm calls influence the forager's response in meerkats *(Suricata suricatta)*. M.Sc. thesis, University of Zürich, Zürich, Switzerland.

Barnard, J. A. (2000). Costs and benefits of group foraging in cooperatively breeding meerkats. Ph.D. thesis, University of Cambridge, Cambridge, U.K.

Bateman, A. W., Ozgul, A., Coulson, T., and Clutton-Brock, T. H. (2012a). Density dependence in group dynamics of a highly social mongoose, *Suricata suricatta*. *J. Anim. Ecol.*, 81, 628–639.

Bateman, A. W., Ozgul, A., Nielsen, J., Coulson, T., and Clutton-Brock, T. H. (2012b). Social structure mediates environmental effects on group size in an obligate cooperative breeder, *Suricata suricatta*. *Ecology*, 94, 587–597.

Bell, M. B. V. (2007). Cooperative begging in banded mongoose pups. *Curr. Biol.*, 17, 717–721.

Bell, M. B., Cant, M. A., Borgeaud, C., Thavarajah, N., Samson, J., et al. (2014). Experimentally suppressing subordinate reproduction in cooperative mammals provides benefits to dominants. *Nature Comm.*, 5, 4499.

Bergmüller, R. and Taborsky, M. (2005). Experimental manipulation of helping in a cooperative breeder: helpers "pay to stay" by pre-emptive appeasement. *Anim. Behav.*, 69, 19 28.

Bergmüller, R., Heg, D., and Taborsky, M. (2005). Helpers in a cooperatively breeding cichlid stay and pay or disperse and breed, depending on ecological constraints. *Proc. R. Soc. London B*, 272, 325–331.

Boomsma, J. J. (2009). Lifetime monogamy and the evolution of eusociality. *Phil. Trans. R. Soc. B*, 364, 3191–3208.

Bousquet, C. A. H. (2011). Group decision-making in meerkats *(Suricata suricatta)*. Ph.D. thesis, University of Zürich, Zürich, Switzerland.

Bousquet, C. A. H., Sumpter, D. J. T., and Manser, M. (2011). Moving calls: a vocal mechanism underlying quorum decisions in cohesive groups. *Proc. R. Soc. London B*, 278, 1482–1488.

Brotherton, P. N. M., Clutton-Brock, T. H., O'riain, M. J., Gaynor, D., Sharpe, L., et al. (2001). Offspring food allocation by parents and helpers in a cooperative mammal. *Behav. Ecol.*, 12, 590–599.

Brown, J. L. (1987). *Helping and Communal Breeding in Birds: Ecology and Evolution*. Princeton, NJ: Princeton University Press.

Cant, M. A. (2003). Patterns of helping effort in cooperatively breeding banded mongooses (*Mungos mungo*). *J. Zool.*, 259, 115–121.

Cant, M. A. (2011). The role of threats in animal cooperation. *Proc. R. Soc. London B*, 278, 170–178.

Cant, M. A. and Johnstone, R. A. (2009). How threats influence the evolutionary resolution of conflicts. *Am. Nat.*, 173, 759–771.

Carlson, A. A., Young, A. J., Russell, A. F., Bennett, N. C., Mcneilly, A. S., et al. (2004). Hormonal correlates of dominance in meerkats (*Suricata suricatta*). *Horm. Behav.*, 46, 141–150.

Carlson, A. A., Russell, A. F., Young, A. J., Jordan, N. R., Mcneilly, A. S., et al. (2006a). Elevated prolactin levels immediately precede decisions to babysit by male meerkat helpers. *Horm. Behav.*, 50, 94–100.

Carlson, A. A., Manser, M. B., Young, A. J., Russell, A. F., Jordan, N. R., et al. (2006b). Cortisol levels are positively associated with pup-feeding rates in male meerkats. *Proc. R. Soc. London B*, 273, 571–577.

Carter, A. J., English, S., and Clutton-Brock, T. H. 2014. Cooperative personalities and social niche specialization in female meerkats. *J. Evol. Biol.*, 27, 815–825.

Clutton-Brock, T. H. (2006). Cooperative breeding in mammals. In *Cooperation in Primates and Humans*, ed. P. M. Kappeler and C. P. Van Schaik. Berlin: Springer Verlag, pp. 173–190.

Clutton-Brock, T. H. and Lukas, D. (2011). The evolution of social philopatry and dispersal in female mammals. *Mol. Ecol.*, 21, 472–492.

Clutton-Brock, T. H., Gaynor, D., Kansky, R., Maccoll, A. D. C., Mcilrath, G., et al. (1998a). Costs of cooperative behaviour in suricates, *Suricata suricatta*. *Proc. R. Soc. London B*, 265, 185–190.

Clutton-Brock, T. H., Brotherton, P. N. M., Smith, R., Mcilrath, G., Kansky, R., et al. (1998b). Infanticide and expulsion of females in a cooperative mammal. *Proc. R. Soc. London B*, 265, 2291–2295.

Clutton-Brock, T. H., Maccoll, A. D. C., Chadwick, P., Gaynor, D., Kansky, R., et al. (1999a). Reproduction and survival of suricates (*Suricata suricatta)* in the southern Kalahari. *African J. Ecol.*, 37, 69–80.

Clutton-Brock, T. H., O'riain, M. J., Brotherton, P. N. M., Gaynor, D., Kansky, R., et al. (1999b). Selfish sentinels in cooperative mammals. *Science*, 284, 1640–1644.

Clutton-Brock, T. H., Gaynor, D., McIlrath, G. M., Maccoll, A. D. C., Kansky, R., et al. (1999c). Predation, group size and mortality in a cooperative mongoose, *Suricata suricatta*. *J. Anim. Ecol.*, 68, 672–683.

Clutton-Brock, T. H., Brotherton, P. N. M., O'riain, M. J., Griffin, A. S., Gaynor, D., et al. (2000). Individual contributions to babysitting in a cooperative mongoose, *Suricata suricatta*. *Proc. R. Soc. London B*, 267, 301–305.

Clutton-Brock, T. H., Brotherton, P. N. M., O'riain, M. J., Griffin, A. S., Gaynor, D., et al. (2001a). Contributions to cooperative rearing in meerkats. *Anim. Behav.*, 61, 705–710.

Clutton-Brock, T. H., Brotherton, P. N. M., Russell, A. F., O'riain, M. J., Gaynor, D., et al. (2001b). Cooperation, conflict and concession in meerkat groups. *Science*, 291, 478–481.

Clutton-Brock, T. H., Russell, A. F., Sharpe, L., Brotherton, P. N. M., McIlrath, G. M., et al. (2001c). Effects of helpers on juvenile development and survival in meerkats. *Science*, 293, 2446–2449.

Clutton-Brock, T. H., Russell, A. F., Sharpe, L. L., Young, A. J., Balmforth, Z., et al. (2002). Evolution and development of sex differences in cooperative behavior in meerkats. *Science*, 297, 253–256.

Clutton-Brock, T. H., Russell, A. F., and Sharpe, L. L. (2003). Meerkat helpers do not specialize in particular activities. *Anim. Behav.*, 66, 531–540.

Clutton-Brock, T. H., Russell, A. F., and Sharpe, L. L. (2004). Behavioural tactics of breeders in cooperative meerkats. *Anim. Behav.*, 68, 1029–140.

Clutton-Brock, T. H., Russell, A. F., Sharpe, L. L., and Jordan, N. R. (2005). "False-feeding" and aggression in meerkat societies. *Anim. Behav.*, 69, 1273–1284.

Clutton-Brock, T. H., Hodge, S. J., Spong, G., Russell, A. F., Jordan, N. R., et al. (2006). Intrasexual competition and sexual selection in cooperative mammals. *Nature*, 444, 1065–1068.

Clutton-Brock, T. H., Hodge, S. J., Flower, T. P., Spong, G. F., and Young, A. J. (2010). Adaptive suppression of subordinate reproduction in cooperative mammals. *Am. Nat.*, 176, 664–673.

Cornwallis, C. K., West, S. A., and Griffin, A. S. (2009). Routes to indirect fitness in cooperatively breeding vertebrates: kin discrimination and limited dispersal. *J. Evol. Biol.*, 22, 2445–2457.

Cornwallis, C. K., West, S. A., Davis, K. E., and Griffin, A. S. (2010). Promiscuity and the evolutionary transition to complex societies. *Nature*, 466, 969–972.

Creel, S. R., Monfort, S. L., Wildt, D. E., and Waser, P. M. (1991). Spontaneous lactation is an adaptive result of pseudopregnancy. *Nature*, 351, 660–662.

Darwin, C. (1859). *On the Origin of Species by Means of Natural Selection*. London: John Murray.

Dölen, G. Darvishzadeh, A., Huang, K. W., and Malenka, R. C. (2013). Social reward requires coordinated activity of nucleus accumbens oxytocin and serotonin. *Nature*, 501, 179–184.

Doolan, S. P. and MacDonald, D. W. (1999). Cooperative rearing by slender-tailed meerkats (*Suricata suricatta*) in the southern Kalahari. *J. Ethol.*, 105, 851–866.

Emlen, S. T. (1991). Evolution of cooperative breeding in birds and mammals. In: *Behavioural Ecology: an Evolutionary Approach*. 3rd edn, ed. J. R. Krebs and N. B. Davies. Oxford: Blackwell Scientific Publications.

Engesser, S. (2011). Function of "close" calls in a group foraging carnivore, *Suricata suricatta*. M.Sc. thesis, University of Zürich, Zürich, Switzerland.

English, S. E. (2010). Individual variation in helping behaviour in meerkats. Ph.D. thesis, University of Cambridge, Cambridge, U.K.

English, S., Nakagawa, S., and Clutton-Brock, T. H. (2010). Consistent individual differences in cooperative behaviour in meerkats (*Suricata suricatta*). *J. Evol. Biol.*, 23, 1597–1604.

English, S., Bateman, A. W., and Clutton-Brock, T. H. (2012). Lifetime growth in wild meerkats: incorporating life history and environmental factors into a standard growth model. *Oecologia*, 169, 143–153.

English, S., Bateman, A. W., Mares, R., Ozgul, A., and Clutton-Brock, T. H. (2013a). Maternal, social and abiotic environment effects on growth vary across life stages in a cooperative mammal. *J. Anim. Ecol.* 83, 332–342.

English, S., Huchard, E., Nielsen, J., and Clutton-Brock, T. H. (2013b). Early growth, dominance acquisition and lifetime reproductive success in male and female cooperative meerkats. *Ecol. Evol.* 3, 4401–4407.

Gaston, A. J. (1977). Social behaviour within groups of jungle babblers (*Turdoides striatus*). *Anim. Behav.*, 25, 828–848.

Graw, B. and Manser, M. B. (2007). The function of mobbing in cooperative meerkats. *Anim. Behav.*, 74, 507–517.

Griffin, A. S., Pemberton, J. M., Brotherton, P. N. M., Gaynor, D., and Clutton-Brock, T. H. (2003). A genetic analysis of breeding success in the cooperative meerkat (*Suricata suricatta*). *Behav. Ecol.*, 14, 472–480.

Hamilton, I. M. and Taborsky, M. (2005). Contingent movement and cooperation evolve under generalized reciprocity. *Proc. R. Soc. London B*, 272, 2259–2267.

Hamilton, W. D. (1964). The genetical evolution of social behaviour. I. II. *J. Theor. Biol.*, 7, 1–52.

Haydock, J. and Koenig, W. D. (2002). Reproductive skew in the polygynandrous acorn woodpecker. *Proc. Natl. Acad. Sci. (USA)*, 99, 7178–7183.

Heg, D., Bergmüller, R., Bonfils, D., Otti, O., Bachar, Z., et al. (2006). Cichlids do not adjust reproductive skew to the availability of independent breeding options. *Behav. Ecol.*, 17, 419–429.

Hodge, S. J., Flower, T. P., and Clutton-Brock, T. H. (2007). Offspring competition and helper associations in cooperative meerkats. *Anim. Behav.*, 74, 957–964.

Hodge, S. J., Thornton, A., Flower, T. P., and Clutton-Brock, T. H. (2009). Food limitation increases aggression in juvenile meerkats. *Behav. Ecol.*, 20, 930–935.

Holekamp, K. E. and Engh, A. L. (2009). Reproductive skew in female-dominated mammalian societies. In *Reproductive Skew in Vertebrates: Proximate and Ultimate Causes*, ed. R. Hager and C. B. Jones. Cambridge: Cambridge University Press, pp. 53–83.

Huchard, E., Charmantier, A., English, S., Bateman, A., Nielsen, J. F., et al. (2014). Additive genetic variance and developmental plasticity in growth trajectories in a wild cooperative mammal. *J. Evol. Biol.*, 27, 1893–1904.

Hughes, W. O. H., Oldroyd, B. P., Beekman, M., and Ratnieks, F. L. W. (2008). Ancestral monogamy shows kin selection is key to the evolution of eusociality. *Science*, 320, 1213–1216.

Jordan, N. (2007). Scent-marking investment is determined by sex and breeding status in meerkats. *Anim. Behav.*, 74, 531–540.

Jordan, N. R., Cherry, M. I., and Manser, M. B. (2007). The spatial and temporal distribution of meerkat latrines reflects intruder diversity and suggests a role of mate defence. *Anim. Behav.*, 73, 613–622.

Koenig, W. D., Shen, S.-F., Krakauer, A. H., and Haydock, J. (2009). Reproductive skew in avian societies. In: *Reproductive Skew in Vertebrates: Proximate and Ultimate Causes*, ed R. Hager and C. B. Jones. Cambridge: Cambridge University Press, pp. 227–264.

Kokko, H., Johnstone, R. A., and Clutton-Brock, T. H. (2001). The evolution of cooperative breeding through group augmentation. *Proc. R. Soc. London B*, 268, 187–196.

Kropotkin, P. (1908). *Mutual Aid*. London: William Heinneman.

Kunc, H. P., Madden, J. R., and Manser, M. B. (2007). Begging signals in a mobile feeding system: the evolution of different call types. *Am. Nat.*, 170, 617–624.

Kutsukake, N. and Clutton-Brock, T. H. (2006). Aggression and submission reflect reproductive conflict between females in cooperatively breeding meerkats *Suricata suricatta*. *Behav. Ecol. Sociobiol.*, 59, 541–548.

Kutsukake, N. and Clutton-Brock, T. H. (2008). The number of subordinates moderates intrasexual competition among males in cooperatively breeding meerkats. *Proc. R. Soc. London B*, 275 (209–216).

Leclaire, S., Nielsen, J. F., Sharp, S. P., and Clutton-Brock, T. H. (2013a). Mating strategies in dominant meerkats: evidence for extra-pair paternity in relation to genetic relatedness between pair mates? *J. Evol. Biol.*, 26, 1499–1507.

Leclaire, S., Nielsen, J. F., Thavarajah, N. K., Manser, M., and Clutton-Brock, T. H. (2013b). Odour-based kin discrimination in the cooperatively breeding meerkat. *Biol. Lett.*, 9, 20121054.

Lukas, D. and Clutton-Brock, T. H. (2012). Cooperative breeding and monogamy in mammalian societies. *Proc. R. Soc. London B*, 279, 2151–2156.

Macdonald, D. W. (2004). *The New Encyclopedia of Mammals*. Oxford: Oxford University Press.

MacLeod, K. J. and Clutton-Brock, T. H. (2013a). Factors predicting the frequency, likelihood and duration of allonursing in the cooperatively breeding meerkat. *Anim. Behav.* 86, 1059–1067.

MacLeod, K. J. and Clutton-Brock, T. H. (2013b). No evidence for adaptive sex ratio variation in the cooperatively breeding meerkat, *Suricata suricatta. Anim. Behav.* 85, 645–653.

Madden, J. R. and Clutton-Brock, T. H. (2011). Experimental peripheral administration of oxytocin elevates a suite of cooperative behaviours in a wild social mammal. *Proc. R. Soc. London B*, 278, 1189–1194.

Madden, J. R., Kunc, H.-J. P., English, S., and Clutton-Brock, T. H. (2009a). Why do meerkat pups stop begging? *Anim. Behav.*, 78, 85–89.

Madden, J. R., Kunc, H. P., English, S., Manser, M. B., and Clutton-Brock, T. H. (2009b). Calling in the gap: competition or cooperation in littermates' begging behaviour. *Proc. R. Soc. London B*, 276, 1255–1262.

Manser, M. B. (1998). The evolution of auditory communication in suricates *Suricata suricatta*. Ph.D. thesis, University of Cambridge, Cambridge, U.K.

Manser, M. B. (1999). Response of foraging group members to sentinel calls in suricates, *Suricata suricatta. Proc. R. Soc. London B*, 266, 1013–1019.

Manser, M. B. (2001). The acoustic structure of suricates' alarm calls varies with predator type and the level of response urgency. *Proc. R. Soc. London B*, 268, 2315–2324.

Manser, M. B. and Avey, G. (2000). The effect of pup vocalisations on food allocation in a cooperative mammal, the meerkat (*Suricata suricatta*). *Behav. Ecol. Sociobiol.*, 48, 429–437.

Manser, M. B. and Bell, M. B. (2004). Spatial representation of shelter locations in meerkats, *Suricata suricatta. Anim. Behav.*, 68, 151–157.

Manser, M. B., Bell, M. B., and Fletcher, L. B. (2001). The information that receivers extract from alarm calls in suricates. *Proc. R. Soc. London B*, 268, 2485–2491.

Manser, M. B., Seyfarth, R. M., and Cheney, D. L. (2002). Suricate alarm calls signal predator class and urgency. *Trends Cogn. Sci.*, 6, 55–57.

Manser, M. B., Madden, J. R., Kunc, H.-P., English, S., and Clutton-Brock, T. H. (2008). Signals of need in a cooperatively breeding mammal with mobile offspring. *Anim. Behav.*, 76, 1805–1813.

Manser, M. B., Jansen, D. A. W. A. M., Graw, B., Hollén, L. I., Bousquet, C. A. H., et al. (2014). Vocal complexity in meerkats and other mongoose species. *Adv. Stud. Behav.*, 46, 281–310.

Mares, R., Young, A. J., and Clutton-Brock, T. H. (2012). Individual contributions to territory defence in a cooperative breeder: weighing up the benefits and costs. *Proc. R. Soc. London B*, 279, 3989–3995.

Mares, R., Bateman, A. W., English, S., Clutton-Brock, T. H., and Young, A. J. (2014). Timing of pre-dispersal prospecting forays in meerkat societies: the importance of environmental, social and state-dependent factors. *Anim. Behav.*, 88, 185–193.

Marshall, J. A. R. (2011). Group selection and kin selection: formally equivalent approaches. *Trends Ecol. Evol.*, 26, 325–332.

Moss, A. M., Clutton-Brock, T. H., and Monfort, S. L. (2001). Longitudinal gonadal steroid excretion in free-living male and female meerkats (*Suricata suricatta*). *Gen. Comp. Endocrin.*, 122, 158–171.

Nielsen, J. F., English, S. E., Goodall-Copestake, W. P., Wang, J., Walling, C. A., et al. (2012). Inbreeding and inbreeding depression of early life traits in a cooperative mammal. *Mol. Ecol.*, 21, 2788–2804.

Nowak, M. A. (2006). Five rules for the evolution of cooperation. *Science*, 314, 1560–1565.

O'Riain, M. J., Bennett, N. C., Brotherton, P. N. M., McIlrath, G., and Clutton-Brock, T. H. (2000). Reproductive suppression and inbreeding avoidance in wild populations of cooperatively breeding meerkats (*Suricata suricatta*). *Behav. Ecol. Sociobiol.*, 48, 471–477.

Pfeiffer, T., Rutte, C., Killingack, T., Taborsky, M., and Benhoeffer, S. (2005). Evolution of cooperation by generalized reciprocity. *Proc. R. Soc. London B*, 272, 1115–1120.

Rasa, O. A. E. (1986). Ecological factors and their relationship to group size, mortality and behaviour in the dwarf mongoose *Helogale undulata*. *Cimbebasia*, 8, 15–21.

Reber, S. A., Townsend, S. W., and Manser, M. B. (2013). Odour-based kin discrimination in the cooperatively breeding meerkat. *Proc. R. Soc. London B*, 280.

Rood, J. P. (1980). Mating relationships and breeding suppression in the dwarf mongoose. *Anim. Behav.*, 28, 143–150.

Rood, J. P. (1990). Group size, survival, reproduction, and routes to breeding in dwarf mongooses. *Anim. Behav.*, 39, 566–572.

Russell, A. F., Clutton-Brock, T. H., Brotherton, P. N. M., Sharpe, L. L., McIlrath, G. M., et al. (2002). Factors affecting pup growth and survival in co-operatively breeding meerkats *Suricata suricatta. J. Anim. Ecol.*, 71, 700–709.

Russell, A. F., Brotherton, P. N. M., McIlrath, G. M., Sharpe, L. L., and Clutton-Brock, T. H. (2003a). Breeding success in cooperative meerkats: effects of helper number and maternal state. *Behav. Ecol.*, 14, 486–492.

Russell, A. F., Sharpe, L. L., Brotherton, P. N. M., and Clutton-Brock, T. H. (2003b). Cost minimization by helpers in cooperative vertebrates. *Proc. Natl. Acad. Sci. (USA)*, 100, 3333–3338.

Russell, A. F., Carlson, A. A., McIlrath, G. M., Jordan, N. R., and Clutton-Brock, T. (2004). Adaptive size modification by dominant female meerkats. *Evolution*, 58, 1600–1607.

Santema, P. and Clutton-Brock, T. (2012). Dominant female meerkats do not use aggression to elevate work rates of helpers in response to increased brood demand. *Anim. Behav.* 83, 827–832.

Santema, P. and Clutton-Brock, T. (2013). Meerkat helpers increase sentinel behaviour and bipedal vigilance in the presence of pups. *Anim. Behav.* 85, 655–661.

Santema, P., Teitel, Z., Manser, M., Bennett, N., and Clutton-Brock, T. (2013). Effects of cortisol administration on cooperative behavior in meerkat helpers. *Behav. Ecol.*, 24, 1122–1127.

Scantlebury, M., Russell, A. F., McIlrath, G. M., Speakman, J. R. and Clutton-Brock, T. H. (2002). The energetics of lactation in cooperatively breeding meerkats *Suricata suricatta. Proc. R. Soc. London B*, 269, 2147–2153.

Schibler, F. and Manser, M. B. (2007). The irrelevance of individual discrimination in meerkat alarm calls. *Anim. Behav.*, 74, 1259–1268.

Schneider, T. C. and Kappeler, P. M. (2013). Social systems and life history characteristics of mongooses. *Biol. Rev.* 89, 173–198.

Sharp, S. P. and Clutton-Brock, T. H. (2009). Reproductive senescence in a cooperatively breeding mammal. *J. Anim. Ecol.*, 79, 176–183.

Sharp, S. P. and Clutton-Brock, T. H. (2011a). Competition, breeding success and ageing rates in female meerkats. *J. Evol. Biol.*, 24, 17561762.

Sharp, S. P. and Clutton-Brock, T. H. (2011b). Reluctant challengers: why do subordinate female meerkats rarely displace their dominant mothers? *Behav. Ecol.*, 22, 1337–1343.

Spong, G. F., Hodge, S. J., Young, A. J., and Clutton-Brock, T. H. (2008). Factors affecting reproductive success of dominant male meerkats. *Mol. Ecol.*, 17, 2287–2299.

Stephens, P. A., Russell, A. F., Young, A. J., Sutherland, W. J., and Clutton-Brock, T. H. (2005). Dispersal, eviction, and conflict in meerkats (*Suricata suricatta*): an evolutionarily stable strategy model. *Am. Nat.*, 165, 120–135.

Thavarajah, N. K., Fenkes, M., and Clutton-Brock, T. H. (2014). The determinants of dominance relationships among subordinate females in the cooperatively breeding meerkat. *Behaviour*, 151, 89–102.

Thornton, A. (2008). Early body condition, time budgets and the acquisition of foraging skills in meerkats. *Anim. Behav.*, 75, 951–962.

Thornton, A. and McAuliffe, K. (2006). Teaching in wild meerkats. *Science*, 313, 227–229.

Townsend, S. W. and Manser, M. B. (2011). The function of non-linear phenomena in meerkat alarm calls. *Biol. Lett.*, 7, 47–49.

Townsend, S. W., Zöttl, M., and Manser, M. B. (2011). All clear? Meerkats attend to contextual information in close calls to coordinate vigilance. *Behav. Ecol. Sociobiol.*, 65, 1927–1934.

Townsend, S. W., Allen, C., and Manser, M. B. (2012). A simple test of vocal individual recognition in wild meerkats. *Biol. Lett.*, 8, 179–182.

Turbé, A. (2006). Habitat use, ranging behaviour and social control in meerkats. Ph.D. thesis, University of Cambridge, Cambridge, U.K.

Williams, G. C. (1966). Natural selection, the costs of reproduction, and a refinement of Lack's principle. *Am. Nat.*, 100, 687–690.

Wilson, D. S. and Sober, E. (1994). Re-introducing group selection to the human behavioral sciences. *Behav. Brain Sci.*, 17, 585–654.

Wilson, D. S. and Wilson, E. O. (2007). Rethinking the theoretical foundation of sociobiology. *Q. Rev. Biol.*, 82, 327–348.

Wright, J., Berg, E., De Kort, S. R., Khazin, V., and Maklakov, A. A. (2001). Cooperative sentinel behaviour in the Arabian Babbler. *Anim. Behav.*, 62, 973–979.

Young, A. J. (2003). Subordinate tactics in cooperative meerkats: breeding, helping and dispersal. Ph.D. thesis, University of Cambridge, Cambridge, U.K.

Young, A. J. and Clutton-Brock, T. H. (2006). Infanticide by subordinates influences reproductive sharing in cooperatively breeding meerkats. *Biol. Lett.*, 2, 385–387.

Young, A. J. and Monfort, S. L. (2009). Stress and the costs of extra-territorial movement in a social carnivore. *Biol. Lett.*, 5, 439–441.

Young, A. J., Carlson, A. A., and Clutton-Brock, T. (2005). Trade-offs between extraterritorial prospecting and helping in a cooperative mammal. *Anim. Behav.*, 70, 829–837.

Young, A. J., Carlson, A. A., Monfort, S. L., Russell, A. F., Bennett, N. C., et al. (2006). Stress and the suppression of subordinate reproduction in cooperatively breeding meerkats. *Proc. Natl. Acad. Sci. (USA)*, 103, 12005–12010.

Young, A. J., Spong, G., and Clutton-Brock, T. H. (2007). Subordinate male meerkats prospect for extra-group paternity: alternative reproductive tactics in a cooperative mammal. *Proc. R. Soc. London B*, 274, 1603–1609.

Zöttl, M., Lienert, R., Clutton-Brock, T., Millesi, E., and Manser, M. B. (2013). The effects of recruitment to direct predator cues on predator responses in meerkats. *Behav. Ecol.*, 24, 198–204.

18

Banded mongooses: Demography, life history, and social behavior

Michael A. Cant, Hazel J. Nichols, Faye J. Thompson, and Emma Vitikainen

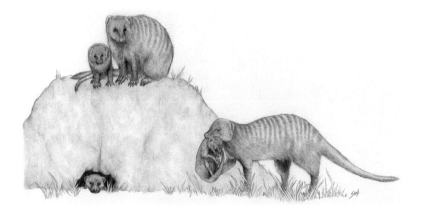

Introduction

The banded mongoose (*Mungos mungo)* is a small (~1.5 kg) cooperative mammal (Carnivora: Herpestidae) which is distributed widely throughout sub-Saharan Africa (Figure 18.1). The species has been studied at sites in the Serengeti (Waser et al. 1995), South Africa (Hiscocks and Perrin 1991), and Botswana (Alexander et al. 2002, 2010; Laver et al. 2012), but most of what is known about the life history and social behavior of this species comes from a long-term study of a population living on and around Mweya peninsula in western Uganda.

Jon Rood of the Smithsonian Institute initiated study of banded mongooses at Mweya in the early 1970s and provided tantalizing insights into its social and reproductive behavior. For example, Rood confirmed earlier reports that multiple females in each group became pregnant in each breeding attempt (Rood 1975); discovered that males guard young offspring at the den while lactating females go off to forage (Rood 1974); and described striking examples of altruism, such as one case where an adult mongoose scaled a tree to rescue a groupmate from the clutches (literally) of a martial eagle (Rood 1983). Unfortunately, political instability in the region prevented further work until the early 1990s, when Daniela de Luca from the Institute of Zoology in London returned to continue Rood's research (De Luca and Ginsberg 2001). The current project was started in 1995 by Mike Cant and Tim Clutton-Brock, and the population has been studied continuously since then.

Cooperative Breeding in Vertebrates: Studies of Ecology, Evolution, and Behavior, eds W. D. Koenig and J. L. Dickinson.
Published by Cambridge University Press. © Cambridge University Press 2016.

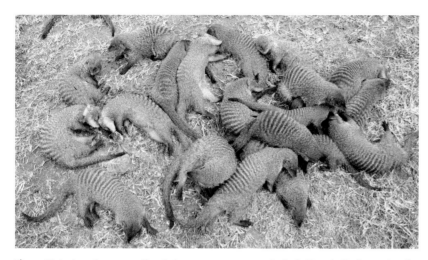

Figure 18.1. A resting group of banded mongooses at our study site in Uganda. Each morning the group leaves the den to forage for 3 or 4 hours before retiring to rest in shade during the hottest part of the day. One individual in each pack wears a radiocollar (note the individual on the far left). Other group members are identified by small fur shavings on the rump. Photo by M. Cant. See plate section for color figure.

Our initial motivation to study banded mongooses was to understand why groups feature multiple breeding females, whereas in closely related dwarf mongooses (*Helogale parvula*) and meerkats (*Suricata suricatta*) there is typically only a single breeding female per group (Creel and Waser 1991; Keane et al. 1996; Clutton-Brock et al. 2001). This difference in the pattern of female reproduction among mongooses with similar cooperative breeding systems offered a good opportunity to test reproductive skew models, developed to understand why the distribution of reproduction varies within cooperative groups. It soon became apparent, however, that banded mongooses were unusual in several other respects. As we now know, they exhibit extreme within-group birth synchrony, male-biased helping, female-biased eviction, and a unique "escort" system of alloparental care (Cant 1998; Gilchrist 2004). Escorts are helpers that form one-to-one caring relationships with pups and act as cultural role models, leading to the coexistence of multiple foraging "traditions" within groups (Müller and Cant 2010).

In addition to having escorts, banded mongooses have three additional attributes that distinguish them: (1) dispersal is relatively rare, and new groups form by fusion of dispersing same-sex cohorts; (2) groups commonly attack natal dens of rival groups and can kill their entire litter (Cant et al. 2002), yet groups also sometimes kidnap and rear pups from neighboring groups (Müller and Bell 2009); (3) males start breeding later, and live substantially longer than females. Together, these unusual features of the banded mongoose system make this a particularly useful species to test the generality of theoretical models of social behavior and life history evolution, to highlight restrictive assumptions of existing models, and to suggest alternatives.

The aim of this chapter is to collate information from the last 20 years of research on four main topics: the demography and structure of the population, intergroup competition, helping behavior, and reproductive conflict within groups. In the discussion we evaluate our findings against new developments in social evolution theory. In particular, we relate our results to recent "demographic" models of inclusive fitness in structured populations, discuss intergroup competition as a mechanism promoting cooperation within groups (Choi and Bowles 2007; Reeve and Hölldobler 2007; Eaton et al. 2011), and examine the implications of our results for models of reproductive conflict.

Study site and population

Mweya Peninsula is a 5 km² heart-shaped promontory extending into Lake Edward on the border of Uganda with the Democratic Republic of Congo. It is connected to the mainland by a narrow isthmus. The habitat is medium-height grassland interspersed with candelabra trees (*Euphorbia candelabrum)* and dense thickets of the woolly caper bush (*Capparis tomentosa*) and needle bush *(Azima tetracantha)*. The peninsula is divided into lower and upper halves by a 40 m-high grassy fault. The lower peninsula is uninhabited by humans but the upper peninsula is the site of a village of approximately 300 people and 100 buildings, including a large tourist lodge. Major herbivores include hippopotamus (*Hippopotamus amphibious*), warthog (*Phacochoerus africanus*), waterbuck (*Kobus ellipsiprymnus*), Cape buffalo (*Syncerus caffer*), and African elephant (*Loxodonta africana*). The climate is equatorial, with little seasonal fluctuation in temperature or day length. Annual precipitation is typically 800–900 mm, with two dry periods in January–February and June–July.

At any one time the population of banded mongooses consists of around 250 individuals living in 10 to 12 groups. Typically seven of these groups occupy the peninsula proper, with the remaining groups inhabiting the adjoining mainland (Figure 18.2). The mean home range area is 0.84 km⁻² (range 0.30–1.32), with a mean perimeter of 5.2 km (range 3.7–7.5) (Jordan et al. 2010). Each group sleeps together in an underground or sheltered den, typically an erosion gully or abandoned termite mound. Just after dawn the group leaves the den on a foraging trip, digging up millipedes, beetles, and other insects, and occasionally taking small vertebrate prey (Rood 1975). The group rests in shade during the hottest part of the day before a second foraging trip that lasts 2–3 hours and takes them back to the same or to a different den. Groups change dens every 2–3 days, except when they have just given birth, and each group utilizes 20–40 different den sites within the home range.

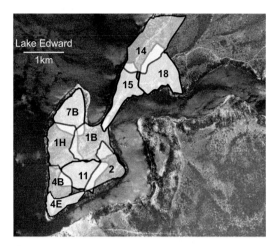

Figure 18.2. (a) Satellite image of Mweya peninsula overlayed with the approximate home ranges of ten groups (as of November 2012). Note the extensive areas of overlap between home ranges. Neighboring groups encounter each other frequently and engage in violent fights in which adults and offspring may be injured or killed. From Cant et al. (2013)

Demography and population structure

Group composition

Group sizes are highly variable, ranging from 5 to 75 individuals, although groups of around 20 adults plus offspring are more typical (median group size = 18; Cant 2000). Groups consist of a core of 1–5 breeding females and 3–7 breeding males that reproduce on average four times per year along with a subset of younger adult females (older than one year) that breed less frequently (Cant et al. 2010; Nichols et al. 2010, 2012b). Older females are classified as socially "dominant" because they contribute to the forcible eviction of younger females; younger females by contrast do not evict older females. Males and females of all age classes, including breeders, nonbreeding males, and juveniles (6 months to 1 year), help to rear the communal litter. While most females start to breed regularly once they are one year old, males form a strict dominance hierarchy in which the oldest two to four males monopolize reproduction and lower ranked individuals are excluded from breeding. While males are capable of reproduction from one year of age, they typically do not achieve paternity until they are at least 3 or 4 years old. Consequently, the fertility schedules of males and females are very different (Figure 18.3a). The median age of reproducing males is 50 months, compared to 37 months for females (Figure 18.3a).

Unusually for a mammal, males outlive females in our population (Cox regression: Wald = 5.23, $P = 0.02$). Of the individuals surviving to one year, males lived on average 42 months ($N = 544$) and females 38 months ($N = 397$; Figure 18.3b). The sex difference in longevity contributes to the significant male bias in the adult sex ratio of the population (mean proportion of males = 0.62, $N = 222$; $\chi^2 = 11.3$, df = 1, $P < 0.001$). Within groups there are more males than females in almost all age classes. This disparity is particularly high for the youngest adults (aged 1 to 2 years), where over a period of nine years there were 1.46 times as many males than females (proportion male = 0.69). The imbalance in sex ratio becomes steadily more pronounced over time during the period of growth and development up to one year of age, starting at 0.51 males among emergent pups, increasing to 0.56 among nutritionally independent pups, and 0.58 among 6-month old juveniles. The cause of these mortality differences in the first year of life, and in later adulthood, is unclear. We can unequivocally rule out dispersal as a cause of female disappearance in the first year of life because female (and male) banded mongooses always disperse in same-sex groups, as described in the next section.

Patterns of eviction

Almost all individuals of both sexes remain in their natal group past the age of sexual maturity (i.e., one year old). Both males and females commonly breed in their natal group prior to dispersal, and most remain as breeders in their natal group for their entire lives. As a consequence, inbreeding is a regular part of the breeding system (see "Genetic structure"). Despite the risk of inbreeding, banded mongoose females have never been observed to leave their natal group voluntarily. Dominant females typically forcibly evict younger females before the age of four years (Cant et al. 2001). Eviction involves the sudden onset of aggression directed at multiple younger females, which continues over a period of 1–4 days. During this time females that are singled out for eviction are repeatedly chased, harassed, and bitten. While each eviction "event" appears to be initiated by older females, other members of the group, including adult males, juveniles, and even infants commonly join in the attacks until the victims are expelled.

Females are more likely to be evicted from natal groups than are males. Forty-seven eviction events were observed in the population between December 1996 and January 2013. In the 46 events where we knew the sex and identities of evictees, evictions led to the expulsion of 274 females and 170 males. In 25 (53%) of these eviction events only females were evicted, with a mean of 5.7 females evicted per event. In the remaining 22 events both males and females were evicted, with a mean of 6.0 females and 7.7 males evicted in each event. Groups of males were never evicted without females. All evictions occurred during periods of intense reproductive conflict; 70% occurred in the latter stages of group pregnancy (after 35 days postestrus); and the remaining 30% of eviction events occurred during estrus (Cant et al. 2010). For both females and males, the probability of being evicted rises sharply with age, peaking at age 2–3 years in females, and 3–4 years in males, before declining (Figure 18.3c). Eviction probability rises again for very old males (age 8+ years).

Eviction of females is not always permanent. In 11 (44%) of the 25 female-only eviction events, the eviction was temporary in that all evicted females eventually rejoined the group. In these cases a group of females was attacked and driven away from the group but continued to follow the group at a distance for up to a week, sleeping nearby each night in a separate den. During this time the evictees were attacked if they came too close to the main group, but the intensity of aggression declined over time and all the females were eventually reassimilated into the group. Females that were pregnant when evicted typically aborted before they rejoined the group, suggesting that dominant females may use eviction as a means of reducing reproductive competition (Cant et al. 2010). In the remaining eviction events, some or all of the evicted females dispersed permanently and attempted to form a new group.

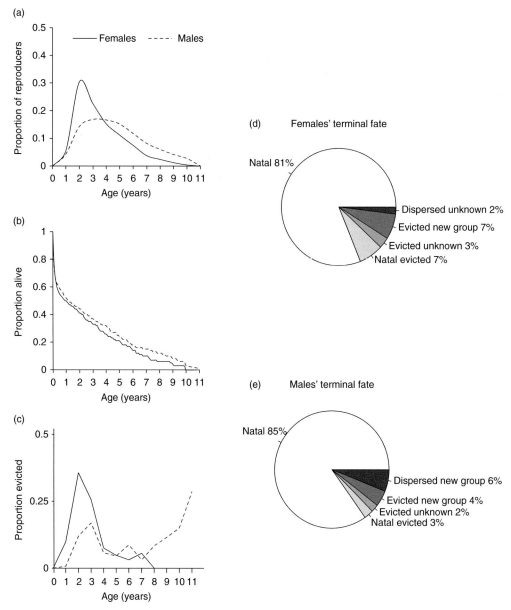

Figure 18.3. Fertility, survival and eviction in the Uganda population. (a) Fertility (females: [number of litters produced by females of age x] / [total number of litters produced in the population]; males: [number of males attaining dominant "mate guarding" status at age x] / [total mate guards in the population]). (b) Survival of 397 females and 544 males for which exact birth and death dates were known. (c) Annual probability of eviction (number of evictees of age i years) / (number of individuals of age i years in the population). (d) and (e) Terminal fate of females ($N = 895$) and males ($N = 1,091$). Category definitions: "natal": individuals that were born and died in their natal group, and were never evicted; "natal evicted": individuals that were born and died in their natal group, and were evicted at least once in their lifetime; "evicted unknown": final fate unknown; "evicted new group": founded a new group in the study area; "dispersed unknown": died in a nonnatal group, but method of dispersal unknown; "dispersed new group": dispersed voluntarily, founded a new group in the study area.

Overall, 115 of the 274 evicted females (42%) dispersed permanently and the remaining 159 (58%) rejoined their group. In the 22 events where males were also evicted alongside females, 78 (46%) of the 170 evicted males left their natal group permanently, either forming a new group with unrelated females, or dispersing in a male coalition away from the study site.

Finally, the eviction of females from one group may have a destabilizing influence on the other groups because groups of low ranking males have been observed to leave their natal group voluntarily to join groups of evicted females, thereby forming a new group (see the following section).

Terminal fate

The great majority of males (85% of 925) and females (81% of 720) lived and died in their natal group without ever being subjected to an eviction attempt (Figures 18.3d and 18.3e). Males were sometimes observed to voluntarily disperse from their natal group, usually after encountering a group of young adult females that had been evicted permanently. In a sample of 53 males and 29 females that were evicted permanently, 6 males (13%) and 9 females (27%) joined or formed a new group within the study area. This suggests either that females are more successful at attracting mates and founding new groups, or that males disperse farther than females.

Group formation

The mode by which groups form is a key determinant of the genetic structure of populations. In banded mongooses, new groups form either when a cohort of evicted females is joined by voluntarily dispersing males from a different group, or when a cohort of same-sex evictees or invades a different group and supplants the same-sex breeders. For the 10 new groups that formed in the study population between 1997 and 2009, three were formed by the fusion of single-sex cohorts and established a new territory. In the remaining seven cases, a new group was formed when a cohort of evicted females (5 cases) or evicted males (2 cases) displaced same-sex adults from an existing group

(Nichols et al. 2012c). In one further case, a cohort of evicted females established a territory and reproduced despite never being joined permanently by a coalition of males. Females in this group, which lasted less than two years, mated with males from neighboring groups. Once formed, groups are stable and migration between established groups is virtually absent, with only three individuals having been detected immigrating into existing groups since 1997.

Genetic structure

Genetic analysis has revealed a high degree of population structuring, with relatively strong differentiation between groups despite their close proximity (F_{ST} = 0.129) (Nichols et al. 2012c). Neighboring groups with spatially overlapping territories are not more genetically similar than are nonneighboring groups, consistent with the observation that the rate of migration between neighboring groups is very low for both sexes. In contrast, genetic distance between groups (pairwise F_{ST}) is highly correlated with time since group fission – that is, since a cohort of dispersers left their "parent" group and formed a new group – allowing historical relationships between groups to be traced through genetic similarity. These patterns are consistent with our behavioral observations of high rates of natal philopatry in both sexes, coupled with the coalition-based dispersal of cohorts of males and females.

Inbreeding is common in banded mongooses, and includes cases of father-daughter and brother-sister incest (Nichols et al. 2014). The majority (64%) of pups are born to females reproducing in their natal group. Of these within-group matings, 26.7% of females conceived to a male related by ≥ 0.25, and 7.5% conceived to a male related by ≥0.5 (Nichols et al. 2014).

All of the groups in the study area contain close relatives, but the pattern of relatedness within and between sexes changes over time (Nichols et al. 2012c). In newly founded groups, same-sex group members are related to one another, but males are not related to females, so the potential for inbreeding is initially low (Figure 18.4a). As groups age, however, the degree of relatedness between male and female adults in each group increases as original group founders of

(a)

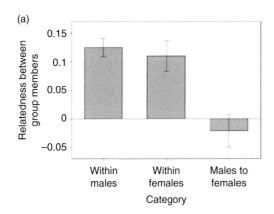

(b)

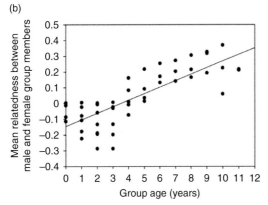

Figure 18.4. Patterns of genetic relatedness within groups. (a) Relatedness between males and females in newly formed groups. (b) Relatedness between male and female group members (> 2 years old) as a function of time since group founding. The graph shows mean values per group year and a linear regression fitted to the data. Data are from 1,250 mongooses living in 12 groups between 2000 and 2009. From Nichols et al. (2012c).

both sexes die and are replaced as breeders by philopatric offspring. However, this pattern of increasing relatedness between breeders does not translate into increased levels of homozygosity among offspring, perhaps because females in established groups mate nonrandomly with respect to relatedness (Sanderson et al. 2015), or because the offspring from incestuous mating die earlier, and are less likely to be sampled (at 1 month old) than outbred offspring.

There is some evidence that females take steps to counter the negative impacts of rising within-group relatedness. In particular, females are known to engage in extra-group matings with males from neighboring groups. Usually these matings take place in the middle of an aggressive intergroup encounter (Cant et al. 2002; Nichols et al. 2015). However, in a few cases estrus females have been observed to lead their group on a foray deep into the core territory of a neighboring group and mate with the males there. While these extra-group matings are not sufficiently frequent to undermine the strong genetic structuring between neighboring groups, recent analyses suggest that the frequency of intergroup fertilizations may increase with the time since group founding. Thus, females may offset problems of inbreeding in long-established groups by seeking extra-group matings.

Intergroup competition

Fighting between groups

On average, around 40% of the home range of each group overlaps with the home range of a neighbor, although for some groups this overlap is as high as 81% (Jordan et al. 2010). Neighboring groups encounter each other frequently, about 2–10 times per month, particularly in areas of overlap, and fights between neighboring groups are common (Cant et al. 2002). Mongooses respond to the sight or smell of other mongooses by standing upright and giving a "screeching call" that alerts the rest of the group and causes them to bunch up and prepare to attack. Playback experiments of these screeching calls show that group size and the location of the playback affect the fighting response to these calls: specifically, individuals are more likely to attack or advance toward the loudspeaker if they are members of a large group and the playback is located in the core of the home range, rather than in an area of overlap (Furrer et al. 2011). Furthermore, scent translocation experiments suggest that mongooses recognize the scents of neighbors and respond more aggressively to known, neighboring groups than to scents from unknown individuals (Müller and Manser 2007). Mongooses may be primed to respond more aggressively to the scents of neighbors because these represent a constant territorial threat, whereas scents from unknown individuals, on the rare occasions that they are encountered, are most likely to derive from transient dispersing cohorts.

Fighting is particularly likely if the groups are evenly matched in size (Cant et al. 2002). Where one group is much smaller than the other, the smaller group usually runs away before there is any physical confrontation. Fights between evenly matched groups are violent and can last for an hour or more, with animals repeatedly chasing, scratching, and biting each other. Injuries and bleeding wounds are common, and in some cases animals have later died from the injuries sustained in fighting. Intergroup fighting is responsible for 8% of adult mortality in cases where the cause of death is known (Jordan et al. 2010). The gains of intergroup fighting appear to be increased territory and resources to sustain a large group, which in turn is more resistant to attacks from neighboring groups. Thus intergroup conflict may involve an element of positive feedback and selection for altruistic fighting and helping behaviors that improve the future security and productivity of the group through a form of group augmentation (Kokko et al. 2001).

Intergroup infanticide

Pups that are foraging with the group are sometimes killed in the midst of fighting between rival groups. More commonly, rival groups discover the natal den and kill the pups prior to their emergence at one month of age. Like other social mongooses, banded mongooses protect very young offspring in the den by leaving adult guards or "babysitters" behind while the rest of the group goes off to forage. If a rival group encounters one of these dens, they attack the babysitters, enter the den and kill the offspring, sometimes dragging the young pups out screaming prior to dispatching and eating them. Over a 29-month period studying 10 groups, Müller and Bell (2009) observed 12 incidences of infanticide involving the death of 17 pups. These authors also observed two kidnapping events over the same period, where pups under two weeks old were removed from the natal den and carried off by female members of the attacking group

without any signs of aggression. On one of these occasions the female kidnappers were later confirmed to allosuckle the pups, despite not being pregnant or having dependent pups of their own at the time. Pied babblers (*Turdoides bicolor*) also acquire group members by kidnapping and nurture them as a means of augmenting group size (Chapter 7).

Evaluating the true rate of pup loss to intergroup infanticide is inherently difficult because many encounters occur in thick bush and infanticide is difficult to observe. We suspect, however, that intergroup competition and infanticide of young pups is a major selective force in the life of banded mongooses (Nichols et al. 2015). Groups smaller than 10 adults are repeatedly attacked by larger neighboring groups, and rarely succeed in raising litters to emergence from the den. The failure to recruit litters leads to the steady attrition of small groups through predation of adults or injury and death during intergroup encounters. Thus there appear to be strong Allee effects (Courchamp et al. 1999) in banded mongooses, whereby small groups become increasingly susceptible to mortality, driven primarily by intergroup fighting and infanticide. Intergroup competition is also the main barrier to successful group formation. Groups that attempt to set up a new territory are vulnerable to attack and injury from larger established groups (Cant et al. 2002). Overall, these patterns suggest that between-group competition exerts an important selective force on within-group cooperation in banded mongooses, and with the exception of pied babblers, distinguishes them from the majority of cooperative breeders in this book.

Helping behavior

Babysitting and escorting

Banded mongooses exhibit two main forms of helping behavior: "babysitting" of offspring at the den in the first month of life; and "escorting" of offspring after they emerge from the den and accompany the group on foraging trips. Most group members over 6 months old take part in one or both of these activities. Each day after birth, 1–5 adults and juveniles remain behind at the den as babysitters to guard neonatal offspring while the rest of the group goes off to forage. Typically the main group returns to the natal den in the middle part of the day and some or all of the babysitters may be exchanged prior to a second foraging trip in the late afternoon.

The number of babysitters left to guard young has a strong impact on the survival of litters in the first month of life. In particular, groups that chronically fail to leave a babysitter never successfully raise pups to emergence (Figure 18.5). By contrast, the mean survivorship of pups in dens for groups that leave a mean of two or more babysitters per foraging trip is 36%. Small groups are constrained to leave fewer babysitters, which explains why Allee effects in this population may be particularly strong.

"Escorting" behavior begins at around 3–4 weeks of age, when pups begin to accompany adults, starting with short excursions around the den and progressing quickly to full morning or afternoon foraging trips. During this time pups receive food from adults and some pups start to follow particular adults consistently, aggressively defending access to these escorts by chasing or attacking other pups that attempt to follow the same individual. While pups initiate the pup–escort bond by monopolizing access to a particular adult (Gilchrist 2008), later on in the provisioning period escorts actively maintain this relationship. Escorts recognize and respond to the experimental presentation of "their" pup (Gilchrist et al. 2008), and respond particularly strongly to playbacks of their pup's distress calls (Müller and Manser 2008). Being escorted has a large fitness benefit to pups: pups that are frequently escorted are more likely to survive to nutritional independence, grow faster, and reproduce earlier than pups that are not escorted (Hodge 2005).

Individual contributions to helping

Across all age classes 6 months or older, males spend more time babysitting than females. Subordinate males (males that do not engage in mate-guarding during estrus) are particularly likely to babysit in the morning session, which is longer and more energetically demanding than the afternoon session (Cant 2003).

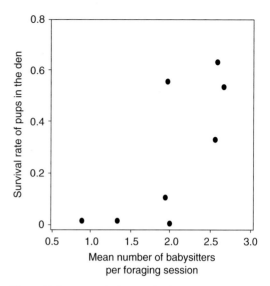

Figure 18.5. Pup survival rate in the den as a function of the mean number of babysitters left behind to guard them. Survival rate was calculated as (number of pups emerging from the den at 1 month) / (estimated communal litter size at birth). Communal litter size at birth was estimated from the number of females that were known to have given birth and the age-specific fetal litter sizes of these females measured using palpation. Means are shown for 8 groups observed between 1995 and 1997. Each point represents a group. From Cant (2003).

Males of all age classes are also more likely to escort pups than are females (Gilchrist and Russell 2007). Almost half of males escort a pup in any given litter compared to 37% of females (Nichols et al. 2012a). Males also feed pups more frequently than females, and this sex difference is particularly pronounced for juveniles and young adults (Hodge 2007).

Relatedness does not explain much of the variation in helping behavior in our population (Nichols et al. 2012a). The hardest working babysitters are usually nonbreeding, subordinate males that are no more closely related to the communal litter than randomly selected group members. Escorts are usually not the parents of the pups that they guard and provision, and preliminary analysis suggests that pup-escort pairs are not more closely related than the average background relatedness within groups.

Instead, variation within and between sexes in helping effort is best explained by variation in the fitness costs of helping (Heinsohn and Legge 1999; Clutton-Brock et al. 2000; Hodge 2007). Since the period of babysitting typically overlaps the postpartum estrus, subordinate males with little chance of gaining paternity have less to lose from remaining at the den than do dominant, mate-guarding males. In other words, the opportunity cost of babysitting is much lower for nonbreeding males.

Individuals of both sexes suffer weight loss as a consequence of investing in babysitting and escorting behavior, but the fitness consequences of this weight loss are particularly severe for females. This is because there is a strong maternal effect of body weight on offspring success, with the weight of females when they conceive being positively correlated with the weight of their offspring at emergence from the den 3 months later (Figure 18.6); furthermore, heavier pups are more likely to survive to adulthood. In contrast, paternity success among males is strongly related to age but not weight, and males are usually able to regain their weight during the nonbreeding period (Hodge 2007).

A final difference between males and females is the degree to which helpers discriminate between potential recipients of care. While male escorts tend to provision larger offspring irrespective of their sex, female escorts preferentially feed light-weight, poor quality female pups that have most to gain from extra food (Hodge 2003). For females, the decision of whether and how much to help appears to depend on how much a given unit of help will boost the future success of the offspring that receive it. The greater cost of helping for females compared to males may have selected for females to discriminate among potential recipients of their help and target their investment where it will generate the most benefit for a given level of cost (Hamilton 1963).

Social learning by helpers as a possible route to cultural transmission

Having an escort not only boosts survival and growth of pups in their care, it even affects their future

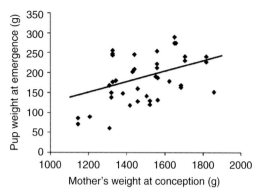

Figure 18.6. Pup weight at first emergence from the den (1 month old) versus their mother's weight at conception (i.e., 3 months previously). Data are shown for 39 pups for which maternity was assigned using microsatellite markers. Babysitting usually overlaps with estrus and the onset of gestation of the next litter, so energetic costs incurred during babysitting may have a negative impact on the weight of pups in the next litter. From Hodge et al. (2009).

behavior: we have shown experimentally that pups observe and later imitate the particular foraging techniques of their escort. Specifically, escorts were given an artificial food item (a plastic "Kinder egg" containing fish/rice paste) that the escort could open in front of its dependent pup in one of several different ways. Some escorts consistently smashed the Kinder egg against a hard surface (a technique used naturally to open eggs, snails, and some hardbodied insects); other escorts consistently used their jaws to bite the egg open. Later, as 5–7 month-old independent juveniles and as yearling adults, the grown-up pups were presented with the Kinder egg problem. When pups had observed their escort consistently use the smash technique or the bite technique, they were more likely to use the same technique themselves (Müller and Cant 2010; Figure 18.7).

Studies of foraging traditions in animal societies are usually based on the premise that social learning leads to behavioral uniformity within groups and differences in behavior between groups because members of the same group copy one another (Whiten et al. 1999; van Schaik et al. 2003; Laland and Janik 2006). Our experiment shows that this premise may

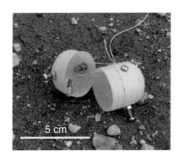

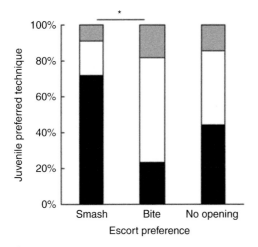

Figure 18.7. Cultural transmission via imitation in escort-pup pairs. Escorts were presented with a foraging problem which required them to open a modified Kinder egg to obtain a food reward inside (top photo). Escorts used two distinct techniques to open the egg: *smash*, which involved hurling the egg repeatedly at a hard surface until it broke open; and *bite*, which involved prying the egg open using the jaws. The graph shows the preference for particular foraging techniques used by grown pups (5–7 months old) as a function of the technique they observed their escort to use when they were 1–3 months old. Percentage of trials in which juveniles used the *smash* and *bite* technique are shown as black bars and white bars respectively; grey bars are the percentage of trials in which there was no clear preference. Escorts were assigned to *smash* and *bite* categories depending on the technique they employed consistently when presented with the Kinder egg 10 times. The "No opening" category is a control that combines treatments where the egg was already opened and where no food was encountered. Juveniles (and yearlings) copied the technique they had observed their escort to use when they were young. From Müller and Cant (2010).

be incorrect. Specifically, the one-on-one nature of the pup–escort relationship means that escorts can act as role models for individual pups, with the consequence that individual variation in foraging techniques among escorts may be passed on to the next generation. In contrast, where individuals learn from multiple teachers or where everyone learns from the same teacher, social learning is expected to erode behavioral heterogeneity within groups and promote heterogeneity between groups (Boyd and Richerson 1987; Müller and Cant 2010).

Reproductive competition

Patterns of reproduction

Banded mongooses are a particularly interesting cooperative breeder because of their unusual plural breeding system. On average, 83% of females conceive in each breeding attempt, and 93% of these females carry their litter to term (Cant 2000; Gilchrist et al. 2004). In 64% of litters, all pregnant females in the group synchronize birth to the same day (Hodge et al. 2011); on one occasion 12 females in a group all gave birth on the same day. When females give birth on different days ("asynchronous" litters), females still give birth within 1–30 days of each other.

After birth, females leave the den to forage in the mornings, but return to suckle pups underground in the afternoons. Females usually come into estrus again 7–10 days after giving birth while they are still suckling their current litter. We suspect that pseudopregnancy and allolactation is common: the minority of adult females that do not become pregnant in a given breeding attempt show very similar progesterone and estrogen profiles to their pregnant group mates.

Birth synchrony and escape from suppression

The extreme birth synchrony we observe in banded mongooses is consistent with selection to evade the threat of infanticide by dominant females (Cant 2000; Gilchrist 2006). Birth synchrony requires explanation because females could in principle gain an advantage in pup-pup competition by giving birth a few days before their group mates (Hodge et al. 2011). When females give birth asynchronously, however, the first-born litters are killed within days of birth, most likely by other pregnant females. Early life pup survivorship in asynchronous litters is around half that in synchronous litters, and females that conceive particularly early appear to extend gestation by up to two weeks in order to achieve birth synchrony with the rest of their group. Our working hypothesis is that synchronous birth allows females to escape the threat of infanticide because it removes or scrambles the usual temporal or spatial cues that are used to identify the maternity of offspring, thereby increasing the risk that females, if they were to commit infanticide, would mistakenly kill their own young.

Recently we carried out an experimental test of this hypothesis by manipulating which females contributed to communal litters using contraceptive injections (Cant et al. 2014). Our design consisted of three treatments: in Treatment A we switched off all subordinate females for a single breeding attempt, so that only dominant females gave birth. In Treatment B we switched off all except a single dominant breeding female, thereby mimicking the high skew pattern seen in meerkats and dwarf mongooses. Finally, in Treatment C we switched off all dominant female breeders and allowed subordinates to breed. In each case we compared the reproductive success and patterns of early life pup mortality in experimental breeding attempts (EXP) with the breeding attempts in the same group before (PRE) and after (POST) treatment.

Results showed that experimental suppression of subordinate females in Treatment A had little influence on the reproductive success of dominant females (Figure 18.8d). When some or all of the dominant females were prevented from breeding in Treatments B and C, however, there was a sharp spike in the probability that litters failed in the first week after birth (Figure 18.8h and 18.8i), consistent with whole litter infanticide. Thus it appears that dominant females that reproduced on their own and communal litters of subordinate females were victims of infanticide, most likely by dominant females that had not given birth themselves.

These results support our hypothesis that dominant females kill litters that are certain not to contain their own young, and hence that other females can escape from the threat of infanticide by synchronizing parturition to the same day as dominant females. While dominant females suffer little immediate cost when other females breed alongside them (Figure 18.8d), they do have an incentive to kill whole litters that are certain not to contain their own young because this removes competitors of their next litter: pups are more likely to survive to independence and are heavier at independence when there are no older pups present in the group when they are born (Cant et al. 2014). Selection to avoid the threat of infanticide can explain the evolution of both (a) extreme birth synchrony and (b) the absence of reproductive suppression in banded mongooses.

Reproductive control via eviction

Although dominant females suffer little immediate fitness cost when only a few other females breed at the same time, reproductive competition becomes intense when many females reproduce within a group because this results in large numbers of emergent pups all competing for food and a limited number of escorts (Cant et al. 2010). Competition is particularly intense during periods with little rainfall when there is less invertebrate prey on which to feed pups (Nichols et al. 2012b). Dominant females respond to this reproductive competition by evicting younger, subordinate females from the group. However, females that remain on the territory when the risk of eviction is high are no less likely to mate or become pregnant, and females that are evicted and allowed to return are no less likely to reproduce in the subsequent breeding attempt.

Thus, there is no evidence that the threat of eviction is effective in deterring subordinates from breeding as assumed by the "restraint" model of reproductive skew (Johnstone and Cant 1999). Eviction threats are unlikely to be effective in this system because dominants target both pregnant and nonpregnant subordinates for eviction and thus there is little to be gained by exercising preemptive reproductive restraint, and because pregnant subordinates that are evicted often

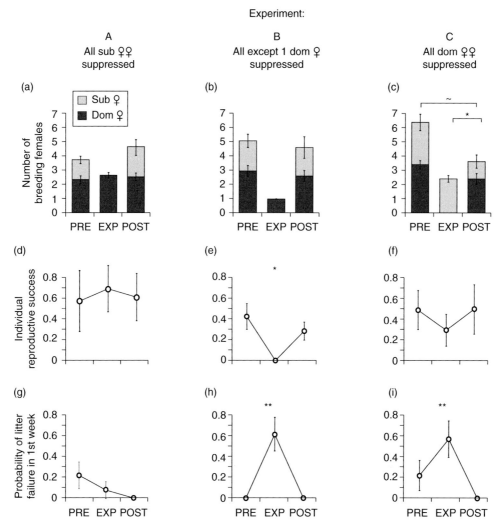

Figure 18.8. The effects of manipulating which females contribute to communal litters. Top row, panels (a)-(c): number of dominant and subordinate breeders in breeding attempts before treatment with contraceptive ('PRE'), the treatment breeding attempt ('EXP'), and the breeding attempt subsequent to the treatment ('POST'). Middle row, panels (d)-(f): (d) individual reproductive success (measured as the number of pups reared to independence) of dominant females that reproduced in Experiment A; (e) reproductive success of the single dominant female left untreated in Experiment B; (f) individual reproductive success of subordinate females in Experiment C. Bottom row, panels (g)-(i): probability of whole litter failure in the first week after birth. Symbols: * $P < 0.05$; ** $P < 0.01$; ~ $P=0.06$. Experiment A: $N = 12$ breeding attempts in each of PRE, EXP, POST; Experiment B: $N = 8$; Experiment C: $N = 9$. Bars show one standard error. From Cant et al. (2014)

spontaneously abort their litter within days of being thrown out of the group, at which point they are readily accepted back into the group. Since the threat of eviction is ineffective at deterring subordinate reproduction, acts of eviction are carried out and observed frequently (Cant et al. 2010).

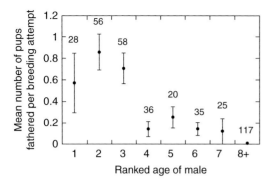

Figure 18.9. Male reproductive success (*N* surviving pups fathered per successful breeding attempt) as a function of male age rank within groups (oldest male = rank 1). Data are from 90 males from 5 groups in 44 breeding attempts. Numbers above points indicate *N* males. Older males monopolize paternity because they mate guard older females, which produce more surviving pups. From Nichols et al. (2010).

Reproductive competition among males

In contrast to females, reproductive skew among males is high. Males form an age-based dominance hierarchy in which the oldest males aggressively monopolize access to females during estrus. These "mate-guarding" males follow receptive females around all day, sometimes for two or three days at a time, obtaining 83% of observed matings (Cant 2000). This behavioral dominance translates directly into fertilization success: paternity analyses indicate that the three oldest individuals in each group sire 85% of pups in the communal litter (Figure 18.9).

Two other observations explain how the same two or three males are able to dominate paternity despite the fact that almost all adult females in the group reproduce synchronously in each breeding attempt. First, while females usually give birth on the same day, they do not all mate on the same day (Cant 2000). The staggered pattern of female mating allows the same few males to monopolize access to females during the 1–2 days during which they are maximally fertile. Second, while younger males frequently manage to gain matings, such matings are often with younger subordinate females whose pups are at a competitive disadvantage compared to the offspring of older females.

The eviction of young males also appears to be linked to reproductive competition. Unlike dominant females, however, dominant males can exclude younger males from paternity, so these younger males do not represent a major threat to their reproductive monopoly. When males are evicted, it is always as part of an eviction event in which females are also evicted. These males could be merely collateral damage, but we think it more likely that the eviction of females changes the landscape of reproductive competition for males, so that staying suddenly becomes a much less attractive option than accepting eviction. Males are clearly not evicted to support the success of dispersing groups of females, because in every case that we have observed males and females to be permanently evicted together, the animals immediately split into same-sex groups and dispersed separately. Older males are particularly likely to be evicted, possibly by middle-aged, nondominant males who stand to gain most from their expulsion.

Discussion

Demography, population structure, and the evolution of cooperative breeding

The past twenty years have seen rapid progress in theoretical understanding of how natural selection acts on social traits in structured or viscous populations, that is, populations in which dispersal is limited and hence most social interactions occur between kin (Lehmann and Rousset 2010). Most of these models are based on the island population genetic framework of Wright (1931), developed for social traits by (Taylor 1992), which assumes an asexual population divided into an infinite number of "islands" (or groups) each containing a fixed number of breeders. Each generation a fraction of offspring disperse away from their natal group, after which both natal offspring and dispersers compete to obtain one of the limited number of breeding positions in the group.

These models may be particularly useful to understanding the evolution of social behavior and life history traits in cooperative vertebrates, including both birds and mammals, because these species live in highly viscous groups in which there are often strong constraints on dispersal for one or both sexes, and often intense local competition for resources and breeding positions (Cant et al. 2009; Johnstone and Cant 2010). To date, however, these models have received relatively little attention from empiricists working on cooperatively breeding species.

How do our findings compare to the assumptions and predictions of these models? Johnstone and Cant (2008) predicted that where there are sex differences in successful dispersal, members of the philopatric sex should be selected to engage in helping behavior, while members of the dispersing sex should be selected to harm other group members. Our results are consistent with this prediction: successful dispersal appears to be biased toward females, and males clearly contribute more to helping behavior. This pattern is reversed in dwarf mongooses and meerkats: females are more likely to remain in their natal group and also provide most of the care (Creel and Waser 1994; Waser et al. 1994; Clutton-Brock et al. 2000; Stephens et al. 2005).

At a broader comparative level, cooperative mammals typically exhibit male-biased dispersal and female-biased helping, whereas birds typically exhibit female-biased dispersal and male-biased helping (Cockburn 1998; Russell 2004). It is important to examine the logic that underscores the model predictions, however. In Johnstone and Cant's (2008) model, female-biased dispersal selects for male-biased helping because, while male and female parents produce offspring that experience the same average level of kin competition, female members of the population have less to gain from altruism because they tend to interact with groups of nonrelatives. This prediction may not hold, however, if females disperse with other female relatives, as occurs in banded mongooses, since in this case dispersing females may be equally or possibly even more closely related to group offspring than nondispersing males.

Dispersing in sibling coalitions should erode the effect of sex-differences in dispersal on selection for helping. Dispersal of same-sex coalitions is common in social vertebrates (Koenig et al. 1998; Stephens et al. 2005; Sharp et al. 2008; Port et al. 2010), but current models of coalitional dispersal have considered only asexual populations (Gardner and West 2006; Gardner et al. 2009). The effect of sex-biases in budding (or coalition-based) dispersal on selection for helping and harming has yet to be explored.

Intergroup competition and cooperation

Recent theoretical models aimed at explaining the evolution of cooperation in humans have suggested that intergroup competition, and in particular the potential for lethal intergroup killing, can maintain selection for altruistic behavior within groups. For example, Choi and Bowles (2007) used a simulation model to show that the potential for intergroup fighting can select for the coevolution of two allelic traits: "parochialism" P (a tendency to attack other groups) and "altruism" A (a tendency to help members of one's own group). According to this model the estimated mortality risk attributable to intergroup fighting in ancestral human groups – around 10% of individuals each generation – is more than enough to favor parochial altruists (P-A individuals) over nonparochial, nonaltruistic types in the population. In banded mongooses, adult deaths due to fighting between groups make up around 10% of all known causes of death, suggesting that intergroup competition may be sufficiently intense to influence selection for both helping and intergroup hostility in the manner assumed by the model (Nichols et al. 2015).

The main conclusion from these models is that levels of conflict among groups seen in banded mongooses, meerkats (Chapter 17), and other social vertebrates, such as pied babblers (Chapter 7) are probably intense enough to influence selection for helping behavior and intergroup hostility. Intergroup hostility may also affect constraints on dispersal and the mode of group founding, thereby amplifying (or dampening) the effects other demographic factors influencing behavior in structured population models, such as sex-biased dispersal, "budding" dispersal, and the expandability (or "elasticity") of territories (Lehmann and Rousset 2010). The primary need now is to incorporate some of the life history features of cooperative vertebrates into models of intergroup fighting (Lehmann 2011) and to test the assumptions and predictions of these models using data from long-term studies.

The evolution and maintenance of helping

Recent comparative analyses of mammals (Lukas and Clutton-Brock 2012) and birds (Cornwallis et al. 2010) indicate that most cooperatively breeding species evolved from monogamous ancestors, suggesting that high levels of genetic relatedness between helpers and offspring are critical for the transition to sociality. While this may be true, our data suggest that it is not required for the maintenance of cooperative breeding in banded mongooses (Nichols et al. 2012c). Rather, selection for helping appears to be maintained by a combination of indirect and direct fitness benefits.

First, helpers gain indirect fitness benefits because they boost the survival of genetically related offspring, and may increase the likelihood that these offspring disperse successfully or inherit breeding status in the future. In addition, there are likely to be strong direct fitness benefits of helping because this ensures that groups remain large and able to defend themselves against attack and infanticide by neighboring groups, reducing the probability of group extinction and hence increasing the success with which reproductives export copies of their alleles through the wider population.

The question remains, however, as to why there is so much individual variation in helping effort, even among individuals that were born in the same litter and are the same weight, sex, and dominance status. Our working hypothesis (based on preliminary data) is that these differences in helping effort are driven by variation in early life care and access to escorts, which affects the hormonal state of offspring and their subsequent life history trajectory. We are currently conducting experiments to test this idea. Banded mongooses are an ideal species to tease out genetic versus developmental influences on adult behavior and life history because there is extreme variation within communal litters: some pups gain access to hardworking escorts while their siblings and other littermates receive little help.

The evolution of reproductive skew

Our observations and experimental results provide no support for "restraint" or "concessions" models of reproductive skew that assume the distribution of reproduction within groups is determined by threats of departure or eviction (Vehrencamp 1983; Johnstone and Cant 1999; Reeve 2000). In particular, none of the suppression experiments described above had any detectable effects on the stability of social groups (Cant et al. 2014). Suppression of dominant females did not lead to the eviction of subordinate females, and suppression of subordinates did not cause them to disperse. Indeed, no female has ever been observed to leave its group voluntarily.

While transactional skew models have played an important role in focusing attention on the use of threats to influence behavior, our results suggest that it is the threat of infanticide, not the threat of group breakup, which is most important in the resolution of conflict over reproduction. This conclusion fits with theoretical arguments that threats of departure or eviction are unlikely to be credible in cooperatively breeding vertebrates. In turn, this is because in these systems groups consist of close relatives and helpers can have a large positive impact on group productivity, so neither dominant nor subordinate group members stand to gain from breaking up the group (Cant and Johnstone 2009; Johnstone and Cant 2009).

The idea that threats and punishment can mediate conflict resolution has implications on sexual selection in cooperative species. Threats of infanticide are expected to be particularly effective at enforcing reproductive skew among female cooperative birds and mammals because the cost of producing offspring is high, so even a small risk of infanticide may be enough to deter a subordinate from breeding (Cant et al. 2014). Compared to males, dominant females may frequently enforce control over reproduction using threats rather than actions, at relatively little cost and with little overt sign of aggression (Cant and Young 2013). This may explain why females in cooperative vertebrate societies often show higher reproductive skew, longer dominance tenures, and higher variance in reproductive success than males (Hauber and Lacey 2005; Clutton-Brock et al. 2006; Rubenstein and Shen 2009), but this higher variance in reproductive success rarely translates into female-biased size dimorphism.

Conclusion and future prospects

Our detailed, longitudinal study of life history and behavior of banded mongooses highlights some of the strengths, and the weaknesses, of current theoretical approaches to the study of social evolution. Our data fit some basic predictions of structured population genetic models, for example, that selection for helping should be stronger in members of the philopatric sex. But our observations of eviction also highlight how unrealistic it is to assume that dispersal probability is a fixed, genetically encoded trait, identical for all group members (or, in more recent models, all the members of one or the other sex; Johnstone and Cant 2008). Our data provide strong support for models of reproductive skew based on threats of infanticide, and more limited support for kin selection models of helping that take into account current and future costs of helping. There remains considerable variation in helping effort that we cannot yet explain.

One limitation of current models is that they typically look for the drivers of social behavior within the group, and ignore causes that might originate outside the group such as intergroup competition or variation in the mechanism of dispersal and the traits of dispersers. All models are limited, but in the study of social evolution there is a disconnect between models of behavior that focus on social interaction at the level of the individual (e.g., reproductive skew theory, models of optimum helping effort), and population genetic models that focus on the selective consequences of a given demography (Lehmann and Rousset 2010). We lack a coherent understanding of how within-group behavior and population processes link up. As a first step, it should be possible to add simple behavioral detail (such as the behavioral processes of eviction, or behaviorally responsive dispersal) to structured population models, and to study the population consequences of individual-focused models of conflict resolution and helping effort. Long-term studies of cooperative breeders can be at their most valuable in guiding such future theoretical endeavors.

More broadly, the study of cooperative breeders can help to advance fundamental understanding of the evolution of biological complexity. The "major transitions" perspective on evolution (Buss 1988; Maynard Smith and Szathmary 1995), which seeks to explain the evolution of biological complexity from RNA replicators to complex animal societies, suggests that there are two ways that cooperation can result in the emergence of new levels of biological organization (Queller 2000): "fraternal" transitions in which within-group conflict is reduced or eradicated via high relatedness; and "egalitarian" major transitions, in which group members are unrelated, and hence other mechanisms to suppress conflict must be invoked, such as reproductive leveling (Alexander 1987). But recent reproductive conflict models show that high levels of conflict are expected in certain circumstances even among close kin, and conversely that peaceful conflict resolution may be evolutionarily stable even among nonrelatives with completely divergent interests (Cant 2012). Many cooperative breeding species form groups containing a mixture of related and unrelated individuals, which employ a range of strategies to reduce or escape within-group conflict. Empirical studies on these species may be particularly useful to elucidate the different ways that divergent interests can be aligned and conflicts suppressed in the evolution of cooperation.

Acknowledgments

We are grateful to Uganda Wildlife Authority (UWA) and Uganda National Council for Science and Technology (UNCST) for permission to conduct our research since 1995, and the wardens of Queen Elizabeth National Park for logistical support throughout this period. The research is made possible by the exceptional skill and effort of the Uganda field team: Francis Mwanguhya, Solomon Kyabulima, Kenneth Mwesige, Robert Businge, and Solomon Ahabyoona. We thank the staff of UWA, Uganda Institute of Ecology, Mweya Safari Lodge, and Makerere University Veterinary School for help over the lifetime of the project, in particular Dr Margaret Driciru, Nelson Guma, Prof Derek Pomeroy, Dr Ludwig Siefert, Aggrey Rwetsiba, Dr Gladys Kalema-Zikusoka, Henry Busulwa, Tom Okello, Amooti Latif, and Onen Marcello. We thank Tim Clutton-Brock for his continuous logistical and intellectual input throughout the project and for ensuring the continuity of the long-term dataset; and to Marta Manser for her numerous contributions. For help in the field we thank Jennifer Sanderson, David Jansen, Roman Furrer, Bonnie Metherell, Corsin Müller, and Harry Marshall. The long-term database was created thanks to the generosity of four independent researchers who shared their data: Jason Gilchrist, Sarah Hodge, Matthew Bell, and Neil Jordan. The project is funded by grants to MAC from the Natural Environment Research Council of the U.K., the Royal Society, and the European Research Council.

REFERENCES

Alexander, K. A., Pleydell, E., Williams, M. C., Lane, E. P., Nyange, J. F., et al. (2002). *Mycobacterium* tuberculosis: an emerging disease of free-ranging wildlife. *Emerg. Infec. Dis.*, 8, 598–601.

Alexander, K. A., Laver, P. N., Michel, A. L., Williams, M., van Helden, P. D., et al. (2010). Novel *Mycobacterium* tuberculosis complex pathogen, *M. mungi. Emerg. Infec. Dis.*, 16, 1296.

Alexander, R. D. (1987). *The Biology of Moral Systems*. New York: Aldine de Gruyter.

Boyd, R. and Richerson, P. (1987). *Culture and the Evolutionary Process*. Chicago, IL: University of Chicago Press.

Buss, L. W. (1988). *The Evolution of Individuality*. Princeton, NJ: Princeton University Press.

Cant, M. A. (1998). Communal breeding in banded mongooses and the theory of reproductive skew. Ph.D. thesis, University of Cambridge, Cambridge, U.K.

Cant, M. A. (2000). Social control of reproduction in banded mongooses. *Anim. Behav.*, 59, 147–158.

Cant, M. A. (2003). Patterns of helping effort in co-operatively breeding banded mongooses (*Mungos mungo*). *J. Zool.*, 259, 115–121.

Cant, M. A. (2012). Suppression of social conflict and evolutionary transitions to cooperation. *Am. Nat.*, 179, 293–301.

Cant, M. A. and Johnstone, R. A. (2009). How threats influence the evolutionary resolution of within-group conflict. *Am. Nat.*, 173, 759–771.

Cant, M. A. and Young, A. J. (2013). Resolving social conflict among females without overt aggression. *Phil. Trans. R. Soc. London B*, 368, 20130076.

Cant, M. A., Otali, E., and Mwanguhya, F. (2001). Eviction and dispersal in co-operatively breeding banded mongooses (*Mungos mungo*). *J. Zool.*, 254, 155–162.

Cant, M. A., Otali, E., and Mwanguhya, F. (2002). Fighting and mating between groups in a cooperatively breeding mammal: the banded mongoose. *Ethology*, 108, 541–555.

Cant, M. A., Johnstone, R. A., and Russell, A. F. (2009). Reproductive conflict and the evolution of menopause. In: *Reproductive Skew in Vertebrates, Proximate and Ultimate Causes*, ed. R. Hager and C. B. Jones. Cambridge: Cambridge University Press, pp. 24–50.

Cant, M. A., Hodge, S. J., Gilchrist, J. S., Bell, M. B. V., and Nichols, H. J. (2010). Reproductive control via eviction (but not the threat of eviction) in banded mongooses. *Proc. R. Soc. London B*, 277, 2219–2226.

Cant, M. A., Vitikainen, E., and Nichols, H. J. (2013). Demography and social evolution of banded mongooses. *Adv. Study Behav.*, 45, 407–445.

Cant, M. A., Nichols, H. J., Johnstone, R. A., and Hodge, S. J. (2014). Policing of reproduction by hidden threats in a cooperative mammal. *Proc. Natl. Acad. Sci. (USA)*, 111, 326–330.

Choi, J.-K. and Bowles, S. (2007). The coevolution of parochial altruism and war. *Science*, 318, 636–640.

Clutton-Brock, T. H., Brotherton, P. N. M., O'Riain, M. J., Griffin, A. S., Gaynor, D., et al. (2000). Individual contributions to babysitting in a cooperative mongoose, *Suricata suricatta*. *Proc. R. Soc. London B*, 267, 301–305.

Clutton-Brock, T. H., Brotherton, P. N. M., Russell, A. F., O'Riain, M. J., Gaynor, D., et al. (2001). Cooperation, conflict and concession in meerkat groups. *Science*, 291, 478–481.

Clutton-Brock, T. H., Hodge, S. J., Spong, G., Russell, A. F., Jordan, N. R., et al. (2006). Intrasexual competition and sexual selection in cooperative mammals. *Nature*, 444, 1065–1068.

Cockburn, A. (1998). Evolution of helping behavior in cooperatively breeding birds. *Annu. Rev. Ecol. Syst.*, 29, 141–177.

Cornwallis, C. K., West, S. A., Davis, K. E., and Griffin, A. S. (2010). Promiscuity and the evolutionary transition to complex societies. *Nature*, 466, 969–972.

Courchamp, F., Clutton-Brock, T., and Grenfell, B. (1999). Inverse density dependence and the Allee effect. *Trends Ecol. Evol.*, 14, 405–410.

Creel, S. R. and Waser, P. M. (1991). Failures of reproductive suppression in dwarf mongooses (*Helogale parvula*): accident or adaption? *Behav. Ecol.*, 2, 7–15.

Creel, S. R. and Waser, P. M. (1994). Inclusive fitness and reproductive strategies in dwarf mongooses. *Behav. Ecol.*, 5, 339–348.

De Luca, D. W. and Ginsberg, J. R. (2001). Dominance, reproduction and survival in banded mongooses: towards an egalitarian social system? *Anim. Behav.*, 61, 17–30.

Eaton, B. C., Eswaran, M., and Oxoby, R. J. (2011). "Us" and "Them": the origin of identity, and its economic implications. *Can. J. Econ.*, 44, 719–748.

Furrer, R. D., Kyabulima, S., Willems, E. P., Cant, M. A., and Manser, M. B. (2011). Location and group size influence decisions in simulated intergroup encounters in banded mongooses. *Behav. Ecol.*, 22, 493–500.

Gardner, A. and West, S. A. (2006). Demography, altruism, and the benefits of budding. *J. Evol. Biol.*, 19, 1707–1716.

Gardner, A., Arce, A., and Alpedrinha, J. (2009). Budding dispersal and the sex ratio. *J. Evol. Biol.*, 22, 1036–1045.

Gilchrist, J. S. (2004). Pup escorting in the communal breeding banded mongoose: behavior, benefits, and maintenance. *Behav. Ecol.*, 15, 952–960.

Gilchrist, J. S. (2006). Female eviction, abortion, and infanticide in banded mongooses (*Mungos mungo*): implications for social control of reproduction and synchronized parturition. *Behav. Ecol.*, 17, 664–669.

Gilchrist, J. S. (2008). Aggressive monopolization of mobile carers by young of a cooperative breeder. *Proc. R. Soc. London B*, 275, 2491–2498.

Gilchrist, J. S. and Russell, A. F. (2007). Who cares? Individual contributions to pup care by breeders vs. non-breeders in the cooperatively breeding banded mongoose (*Mungos mungo*). *Behav. Ecol. Sociobiol.*, 61, 1053–1060.

Gilchrist, J. S., Otali, E., and Mwanguhya, F. (2004). Why breed communally? Factors affecting fecundity in a communal breeding mammal: the banded mongoose (*Mungos mungo*). *Behav. Ecol. Sociobiol.*, 57, 119–131.

Gilchrist, J. S., Otali, E., and Mwanghuya, F. (2008). Caregivers recognize and bias response towards individual young in a cooperative breeding mammal, the banded mongoose. *J. Zool.*, 275, 41–46.

Hamilton, W. D. (1963). The evolution of altruistic behavior. *Am. Nat.*, 97, 354–365.

Hauber, M. E. and Lacey, E. A. (2005). Bateman's principle in cooperatively breeding vertebrates: the effects of non-breeding alloparents on variability in female and male reproductive success. *Integr. Comp. Biol.*, 45, 903–914.

Heinsohn, R. and Legge, S. (1999). The cost of helping. *Trends Ecol. Evol.*, 14, 53–57.

Hiscocks, K. and Perrin, M. R. (1991). Den selection and use by dwarf mongooses and banded mongooses in South Africa. *S. Afr. J. Wildl. Res.*, 21, 119–122.

Hodge, S. J. (2003). The evolution of cooperation on the communal breeding banded mongoose Ph.D. thesis. University of Cambridge, Cambridge, U.K.

Hodge, S. J. (2005). Helpers benefit offspring in both the short and long-term in the cooperatively breeding banded mongoose. *Proc. R. Soc. London B*, 272, 2479–2484.

Hodge, S. J. (2007). Counting the costs: the evolution of male-biased care in the cooperative breeding banded mongoose. *Anim. Behav.*, 74, 911–919.

Hodge, S. J., Bell, M. B. V., Mwanghuya, F., Kyabulima, F., Waldick, R. C., et al. (2009). Maternal weight, offspring competition and the evolution of communal breeding. *Behav. Ecol.*, 20, 729–735.

Hodge, S. J., Bell, M. B., and Cant, M. A. (2011). Reproductive competition and the evolution of extreme birth synchrony in a cooperative mammal. *Biol. Lett.*, 7, 54–56.

Johnstone, R. A. and Cant, M. A. (1999). Reproductive skew and the threat of eviction: a new perspective. *Proc. R. Soc. London B*, 266, 275–279.

Johnstone, R. A. and Cant, M. A. (2008). Sex differences in dispersal and the evolution of helping and harming. *Am. Nat.*, 172, 318–330.

Johnstone, R. and Cant, M. A. (2009). Models of reproductive skew: outside options and the resolution of reproductive conflict. *Reproductive Skew in Vertebrates*. ed. R. Hager and C. B. Jones. Cambridge: Cambridge University Press, pp. 3–23.

Johnstone, R. A. and Cant, M. A. (2010). The evolution of menopause in cetaceans and humans: the role of demography. *Proc. R. Soc. London B*, 277, 3765–3771.

Jordan, N. R., Mwanguhya, F., Kyabulima, S., Ruedi, P., and Cant, M. A. (2010). Scent marking within and between groups of wild banded mongooses. *J. Zool.*, 280, 72–83.

Keane, B., Creel, S. R., and Waser, P. M. (1996). No evidence of inbreeding avoidance or inbreeding depression in a social carnivore. *Behav. Ecol.*, 7, 480–489.

Koenig, W. D., Haydock, J., and Stanback, M. T. (1998). Reproductive roles in the cooperatively breeding acorn woodpecker: incest avoidance versus reproductive competition. *Am. Nat.*, 151, 243–255.

Kokko, H., Johnstone, R. A., and Clutton-Brock, T. H. (2001). The evolution of cooperative breeding through group augmentation. *Proc. R. Soc. London B*, 268, 187–196.

Laland, K. N. and Janik, V. M. (2006). The animal cultures debate. *Trends Ecol., Evol.*, 21, 542–547.

Laver, P. N., Ganswindt, A., Ganswindt, S. B., and Alexander, K. A. (2012). Non-invasive monitoring of glucocorticoid metabolites in banded mongooses (*Mungos mungo*) in response to physiological and biological challenges. *Gen. Comp. Endocrinol.*, 179, 178–183.

Lehmann, L. (2011). The demographic benefits of belligerence and bravery: defeated group repopulation or victorious group size expansion? *PLoS One* 6, e21437.

Lehmann, L. and Rousset, F. (2010). How life history and demography promote or inhibit the evolution of helping behaviours. *Phil. Trans. R. Soc. London B*, 365, 2599–2617.

Lukas, D. and Clutton-Brock, T. H. (2012). The evolution of mammalian societies: cooperative breeding monogamy and polytocy. *Proc. R. Soc. London B*, 279, 4065–4070.

Maynard Smith, J. and Szathmary, E. (1995). *The Major Transitions in Evolution*. Oxford: Oxford University Press.

Müller, C. A. and Bell, M. B. V. (2009). Kidnapping and infanticide between groups of banded mongooses. *Mammal. Biol.* 74, 315–318.

Müller, C. A. and Cant, M. A. (2010). Imitation and traditions in wild banded mongooses. *Curr. Biol.*, 20, 1–5.

Müller, C. A. and Manser, M. B. (2007). "Nasty neighbours" rather than "dear enemies" in a social carnivore. *Proc. R. Soc. London B*, 274, 959–965.

Müller, C. A. and Manser, M. B. (2008). Mutual recognition of pups and providers in the cooperatively breeding banded mongoose. *Anim. Behav.*, 75, 1683–1692.

Nichols, H. J., Amos, W., Cant, M. A., Bell, M. B. V., and Hodge, S. J. (2010). Top males gain high reproductive success by guarding more successful females in a cooperatively breeding mongoose. *Anim. Behav.*, 80, 649–657.

Nichols, H. J., Amos, W., Bell, M. B. V., Mwanguhya, F., Kyabulima, S., et al. (2012a). Food availability shapes patterns of helping effort in a cooperative mongoose. *Anim. Behav.*, 83, 1377–1385.

Nichols, H. J., Bell, M. B. V., Hodge, S. J., and Cant, M. A. (2012b). Resource limitation moderates the adaptive suppression of subordinate breeding in a cooperatively breeding mongoose. *Behav. Ecol.*, 23, 635–642.

Nichols, H. J., Jordan, N. R., Jamie, G. A., Amos, W., Cant, M. A., et al. (2012c). Fine-scale spatiotemporal patterns of genetic variation in a cooperatively breeding mammal. *Mol. Ecol.*, 21, 5348–5362.

Nichols, H. J., Cant, M. A., Hoffman, J. I., and Sanderson, J. L. (2014). Evidence for frequent incest in a cooperatively breeding mammal. *Biol. Lett.*, 10, 20140898.

Nichols, H. J., Cant, M. A., and Sanderson, J. L. (2015). Adjustment of costly extra-group paternity according to inbreeding risk in a cooperative mammal. *Behav. Ecol.*, doi:10.1093/beheco/arv095.

Port, M., Johnstone, R. A., and Kappeler, P. M. (2010). Costs and benefits of multi-male associations in redfronted lemurs (*Eulemur fulvus rufus*). *Biol. Lett.*, 6, 620–622.

Queller, D. C. (2000). Relatedness and the fraternal major transitions. *Phil. Trans. R. Soc. London B*, 355, 1647–1655.

Reeve, H. K. (2000). A transactional theory of within-group conflict. *Am. Nat.*, 155, 365–382.

Reeve, H. K. and Hölldobler, B. (2007). The emergence of a superorganism through intergroup competition. *Proc. Natl. Acad. Sci. (USA)*, 104, 9736–9740.

Rood, J. P. (1974). Banded mongoose males guard young. *Nature*, 248, 176.

Rood, J. P. (1975). Population dynamics and food habits of the banded mongoose. *E. Afr. Wildl. J.* 13, 89–111.

Rood, J. P. (1983). Banded mongoose rescues pack member from eagle. *Anim. Behav.*, 31, 1261–1262.

Rubenstein, D. R. and Shen, S.-F. (2009). Reproductive conflict and the costs of social status in cooperatively breeding vertebrates. *Am. Nat.*, 173, 650–661.

Russell, A. F. (2004). Mammals: comparisons and contrasts. In: *Ecology and Evolution of Cooperative Breeding in Birds*, ed W. D. Koenig and J. L. Dickinson. Cambridge: Cambridge University Press, pp. 210–227.

Sanderson, J. L., Wang, J., Vitikainen, E. I., Cant, M. A., and Nichols, H. J. (2015). Banded mongooses avoid inbreeding when mating with members of the same natal group. *Mol. Ecol.*, 24, 3738–3751.

Sharp, S. P., Simeoni, M., and Hatchwell, B. J. (2008). Dispersal of sibling coalitions promotes helping among immigrants in a cooperatively breeding bird. *Proc. R. Soc. London B*, 275, 2125–2130.

Stephens, P. A., Russell, A. F., Young, A. J., Sutherland, W. J., and Clutton-Brock, T. H. (2005). Dispersal, eviction, and conflict in meerkats (*Suricata suricatta*): an evolutionarily stable strategy model. *Am. Nat.*, 165, 120–135.

Taylor, P. D. (1992). Altruism in viscous populations: an inclusive fitness approach. *Evol. Ecol.*, 6, 352–356.

van Schaik, C. P., Ancrenaz, M., Borgen, G., Galdikas, B., Knott, C. D., et al. (2003). Orangutan cultures and the evolution of material culture. *Science*, 299, 102–105.

Vehrencamp, S. L. (1983). A model for the evolution of despotic versus egalitarian societies. *Anim. Behav.*, 31, 667–682.

Waser, P. M., Creel, S. R., and Lucas, J. R. (1994). Death and disappearance: estimating mortality risks associated with philopatry and dispersal. *Behav. Ecol.*, 5, 135–141.

Waser, P. M., Elliott, L. F., Creel, N. M., and Creel, S. R. (1995). Habitat variation and mongoose demography. In: *Serengeti II: Dynamic, Management and Conservation of an Ecosystem*, ed. A. R. E. Sinclair and P. Arcese. Chicago, IL: University of Chicago Press, pp. 421–448.

Whiten, A., Goodall, J., McGrew, W. C., Nishida, T., Reynolds, V., et al. (1999). Cultures in chimpanzees. *Nature*, 399, 682–685.

Damaraland and naked mole-rats: Convergence of social evolution

Chris G. Faulkes and Nigel C. Bennett

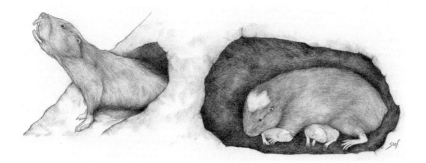

Introduction

African mole-rats (Family: Bathyergidae) have become well established as a model taxon with which to investigate the evolutionary origins and maintenance of cooperative breeding. They occupy an unusual position among vertebrates in having members whose breeding systems range from solitary to eusocial, defined by Michener (1969) and later generalized by Wilson (1971) as having overlapping generations, cooperative brood care, and reproductive division of labor. Following the first report of "eusociality" in naked mole-rats, *Heterocephalus glaber*, more than 30 years ago (Jarvis 1981), similar eusocial behavior was observed in Damaraland mole-rats, *Fukomys damarensis*, paving the way for phylogenetically controlled comparative studies (Bennett and Jarvis 1988; Jarvis and Bennett 1993).

The use of genetic techniques to reconstruct molecular phylogenies and reassess evolutionary relationships and biodiversity within the family has indicated that the Bathyergidae are an extensive adaptive radiation of subterranean rodents. Current estimates suggest that there are more than 30 species comprising six genera that range from strictly solitary to eusocial species, including the eusocial genus, *Heterocephalus* (with the monotypic naked mole-rat), solitary dwelling *Heliophobius*, *Bathyergus*, and *Georychus*, social *Cryptomys*, and social/eusocial *Fukomys* (Figure 19.1). Of particular significance to comparative studies is the fact that there have been convergent gains and losses of sociality within the family, which makes the Bathyergidae an excellent group with which to investigate the evolution of sociality and cooperative behavior. Given the phylogenetic reconstruction in Figure 19.1a, it is apparent that irrespective

Cooperative Breeding in Vertebrates: Studies of Ecology, Evolution, and Behavior, eds W. D. Koenig and J. L. Dickinson.
Published by Cambridge University Press. © Cambridge University Press 2016.

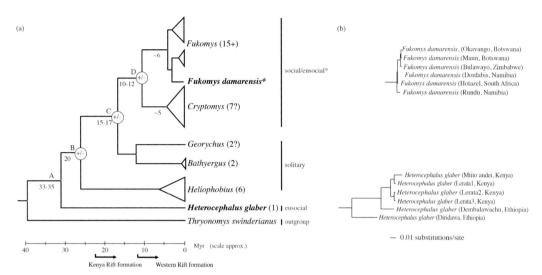

Figure 19.1. (a) Simplified phylogeny for the Bathyergidae indicating the six main clades/genera, together with the closest extant outgroup (the cane rat *Thryonomys swinderianus*), based on mitochondrial 12S rRNA and cyt-*b* sequence data. Numbers on internal nodes and scale bar represent divergence times in millions of years ago (Myr) estimated using a molecular clock approach, and using the Bathyergid fossil *Proheliophobius* for calibration of genetic distances. Numbers in parentheses indicate current estimates of species numbers in each genus. Circles with +/– at nodes represent common ancestors where sociality/a solitary lifestyle may potentially have been gained or lost, depending on the social status of the common ancestor of the family at node A. Further elaboration of social behavior is apparent along the *H. glaber* and *F. damarensis* lineages, and as a result they are often termed eusocial mammals. (b) *H. glaber* and *F. damarensis* clades sampled across their respective ranges, expanded to show the relatively deep branches of the former, compared with the shallow branches of *F. damarensis*, indicative of a recent radiation. Data and figure adapted from Faulkes et al. (1997a, 2004, 2010, 2011); Faulkes and Bennett (2013); Ingram et al. (2004).

of the status of the common ancestor of the family at Node A of the phylogeny, there have been phylogenetically independent gains and/or losses of social/solitary behavior and cooperative breeding at some or all of Nodes B, C, and D. In particular, naked and Damaraland mole-rats are highly divergent within the family, and it is likely that further social elaboration has occurred along their respective lineages, although on different timescales.

Heterocephalus is the basal lineage within the family and constitutes an ancient divergence, with the molecular phylogeny forming relatively deep branches among populations across its range. Molecular clock estimates of divergence times suggest that *Heterocephalus* separated from the common ancestor of the Bathyergidae more than 30 million

years ago (MYA), and fossils resembling naked mole-rats have been dated to approximately 18 MYA or earlier (Bishop 1962). Conversely, molecular phylogenies reveal that *F. damarensis* has small genetic differences and thus very shallow branches separating populations across the distributional range, indicating that the origin of the Damaraland mole-rat clade is much more recent, possibly within the last one million years (Van Daele et al. 2007). These differences in divergence between naked and Damaraland mole-rats are interesting in the context of the convergence of their social behavior (Table 19.1), and this chapter will compare and contrast both ultimate and proximate factors implicated in the evolutionary origin and proximate mechanisms of cooperative breeding and eusociality in these two species.

Table 19.1. Comparison of the characteristic features of the Damaraland mole-rat and the naked mole-rat

	Damaraland mole-rat	Naked mole-rat
Habitat/rainfall/soil type	Arid; high temperatures (>28°C) and low irregular rainfall (ca. 200–400 mm annually); red Kalahari arenosols and a range of coarse sandy soils	Arid; high temperatures and low and irregular rainfall (ca. 200–400 mm annually); hard, consolidated, lateritic loams, sometimes fine sand, pure gypsum, and laterite
Burrow size (tunnel length)	300m to 1km	595m to 3.0km
Colony size range (mean)	2 to ≥ 41 (12)	≤ 10 to ≥ 290 (80)
Body size (mean) g	100–281 (165)	9–69 (34)
Reproduction	Obligate outbreeding; spontaneous ovulation; no seasonality; gestation 78 days, litters 1–5 (mean = 3)	Facultative inbreeding, but outbreeding preferred; spontaneous ovulation; no seasonality; gestation 72 days, litters 1–28 (mean = 11)
Reproductive skew/lifetime reproductive success	1 female and 1–2 males; multiple paternity of litters possible; In a 5-year study, 92% of nonbreeding females never bred	1 female and 1–3 males; multiple paternity of litters possible; 99.9% of >4,000 nonbreeders caught were re-caught as nonbreeders
Extra-colony paternity	Yes	Unknown
Reproductive suppression	Clear physiological suppression in nonreproductive females only	Clear physiological suppression in nonreproductive females and males
Divisions of labor	Primary: reproductive Secondary: work related based on body size (foraging, defense, pup care)	Primary: reproductive Secondary: work related based on body size (foraging, defense, pup care)

Distribution and geographical ecology

African mole-rats are widely distributed across sub-Saharan Africa, occurring from the extreme tip of the Cape region of South Africa through to disjunct and isolated populations in Southern Sudan in the north, Somalia in the east, and Ghana in West Africa. Over much of their range, speciation and diversity within the family appears to have been influenced by the physical, ecological, and climatic changes associated with the formation of the African Rift Valley, with cladogenesis associated with major episodes of volcanism (Faulkes et al. 2004, 2010, 2011).

In the Zambezian region of south-central Africa, shifting patterns of river drainage are of particular significance for populations of *Fukomys*, resulting in extensive vicariance and possible incipient speciation events (Van Daele et al. 2004, 2007). Within the family, the distributions of naked and Damaraland mole-rats are allopatric and geographically distant, but both are characterized by an arid habitat where rainfall can be unpredictable and typically averages no more than 200–400 mm per

year (Figure 19.2). Naked mole-rats are endemic to hot, dry regions of eastern Africa, encompassing much of Somalia, central Ethiopia, and parts of northern and eastern Kenya, extending south as far as the eastern edge of Tsavo West National Park. The soil types they inhabit are most frequently hard packed lateritic loams, although they may be found in fine sand, pure gypsum, and pure laterite (Hill et al. 1957; Jarvis 1985; Brett 1991a). Damaraland mole-rats are endemic to southern Africa, specifically the drier regions of northern South Africa, central and northern Namibia, Botswana, western Zimbabwe, and western Zambia; this is the widest distribution in southern Africa of any species of *Fukomys* or *Cryptomys*. Much of their distribution is characterized by red Kalahari arenosols, but they can also occur in a wide range of coarse sandy soils (Bennett and Jarvis 2004).

Burrow architecture

The disjunct occurrence of African mole-rats across their distributional range is predominantly determined

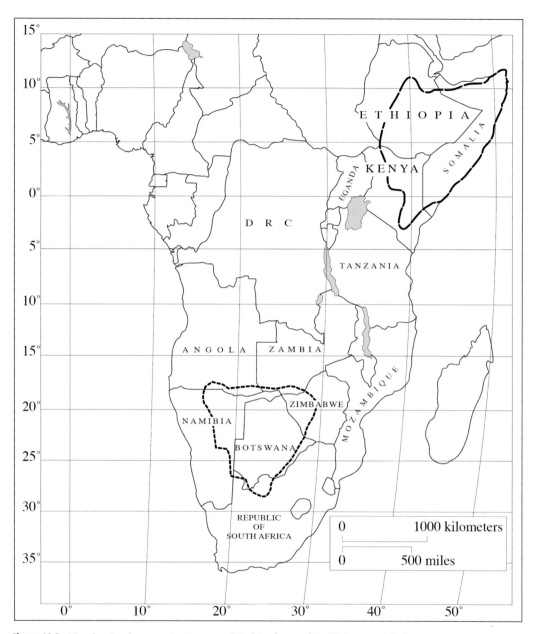

Figure 19.2. Map showing the approximate ranges of *H. glaber* (– – – – –) and *F. damarensis* (---).

Adapted from Bennett and Faulkes (2000).

by the presence of their principle food resource which comprises geophytes – plants with underground storage organs such as bulbs, corms, and tubers. Furthermore, the spatial pattern of these resources is thought to play a major role in shaping cooperative breeding and sociality. The distribution and size of geophytes dictates the overall burrow architecture, but there are a number of common features. Most of the burrow consists of superficial foraging tunnels that are excavated in search of food, and therefore occur at a depth of 5–25 cm (depth and chambers). Interspersed among these tunnels is a communal nest and toilet chambers that are up to 2.5 m in depth. Normally only one nest chamber is occupied at a time and these form important focal points where animals interact socially on a regular basis within the labyrinth of the burrow.

While the Damaraland mole-rat also has chambers that are used for food storage (where the food resources are small enough to gather), these are not found in naked mole-rat burrows, possibly because in the habitat of the latter the geophytes often form very large tubers that cannot be retrieved whole and stored. The food caches of the Damaraland mole-rat may represent resources that can be utilized by the queen when she is gravid and her mobility in the tunnel system is constrained. It is possible that they also represent a short-term emergency source of food to mitigate against periods of unsuccessful foraging. It has been calculated that the geophytes in the store may support a colony for a period of about 10 days (N. C. Bennett, unpubl. data).

Because of the difficulties involved in studying a subterranean animal, relatively few burrows have been fully mapped for either naked or Damaraland mole-rats. From those that have, it is apparent that they represent a considerable and largely permanent resource that is aggressively defended. Brett (1991a) radio-tracked individuals in a colony of 87 naked mole-rats and found that the total length of tunnels was 3–4 km, with 3,660–4,570 kg of soil being excavated in a single year, the equivalent of 2.3–2.9 km of new tunnels. These are impressive statistics for a rodent whose average body mass is 34 g.

Damaraland mole-rats are equally industrious, and while they occur in smaller groups, they are larger,

averaging 140 g in mass. During a two-week period that followed significant rainfall, a colony of 16 animals extruded 3,048 kg of soil, equivalent to approximately 1 km of tunnels (Jarvis et al. 1998). Clearly, rapid and dynamic changes to burrows in response to rainfall and food availability are possible in both species during the cooperative pursuit and exploration of the habitat for food resources, yet the central core of the burrow may remain static for many years if food remains available, and colonies of both Damaraland and naked mole-rats may occupy the same home range for many years (>6 and >7 years respectively; (Jarvis et al. 1998; Brett 1991b).

Thus, burrows represent a valuable, defendable, and long-term resource in terms of the food reserves contained within its range and as a safe nest site. This in itself may promote philopatry and the elaboration of sociality (Alexander et al. 1991). Aggression is apparent between adjacent colonies of naked mole-rats, and there is no evidence of adjacent colonies mixing, apart from occasional dispersers joining established colonies, although these may be rare occurrences (Brett 1991b; Braude 2000).

The importance of the burrow is further evidenced by an increased likelihood of survival in large established colonies. Of 21 nascent colonies of naked mole-rats containing 1–4 emigrants from nearby colonies, only one colony survived for longer than one year (O'Riain and Braude 2001). Similar observations have been made in Damaraland mole-rats: there are significant positive effects of group size on offspring recruitment and survival (A. J. Young et al. unpubl. data) and survival increases with group size (Jarvis et al. 1998).

Group size, composition, and divisions of labor

The establishment and maintenance of a large burrow system necessitates, or is at least facilitated by, large group size. Among cooperative breeders, African mole-rats are exceptional in this respect. In the naked mole-rat, colonies may range from as few as 10 to as many as 295 individuals, with an average of 75–80 animals per colony (Braude 1991, 2000; Brett 1991a).

Average biomass per colony is approximately 2.4 kg (for three complete colonies with over 50 individuals), while biomass ranged from 0.31–3.39 kg (with group sizes of 13 and 97, respectively) over 26 colonies from northern and southern Kenya (Brett 1991b). Group size in Damaraland mole-rats average 11 (range 2–41), with a modal size from 110 complete colonies of 12. Although the absolute numbers within a colony may be less than for naked mole-rats, the total biomass of animals is comparable at approximately 2 kg (Bennett and Jarvis 2004).

In both species large colony sizes are attained through natal philopatry arising from what appear to be the high risks and associated costs of dispersal. As a consequence, overlapping litters of nonbreeding individuals remain with their parents and adopt various helper roles, including cooperative care of the offspring of the breeding queen and 1–3 males (a reproductive division of labor), thereby fulfilling the definition of eusociality derived from social insects (Jarvis 1981; Brett 1991b; Jarvis and Bennett 1993). This characteristic reproductive division of labor within colonies, or reproductive skew, also translates into high skew in lifetime reproductive success (see "Nature and extent of reproductive skew").

Arguably other mole-rat species may also meet the aforementioned basic conditions of eusociality, and there has been much debate about the usefulness of categorical definitions in this context (Bennett and Faulkes 2000; Burda et al. 2000). Unlike other species studied to date, however, both naked and Damaraland mole-rats exhibit a body size (and to some extent age) dependent behavioral division of labor among the nonbreeding helper cohort within the colony, with both sexes contributing equally to care of newborns and to maintenance and defense of the burrow system.

In Damaraland mole-rats, smaller individuals form a "frequent worker" group (Bennett and Jarvis 1988; Bennett 1990; Scantlebury et al. 2006). In newly established colonies, however, it is the larger animals in the colony that constitute the work force (Gaylard et al. 1998). In naked mole-rats, the frequency of work described as colony maintenance, including foraging for food, digging, and maintaining the burrow system, shows a negative trend with increasing body mass.

Nonbreeders also huddle with pups, handle and groom them, retrieve them if they wander out of the nest, and evacuate them during disturbances, and again small (usually younger) animals are the most active in pup care.

Conversely, defense-related activities such as guarding and patrolling increase in frequency with body mass (Faulkes et al. 1991a; Lacey and Sherman 1991), and larger individuals are the most active "volcanoers," producing the molehills (Braude 1991). This is a risky activity as animals are potentially exposed to predators when near the surface. Individuals gradually switch from maintenance to defense activities as they age and grow larger. However, a strict age polyethism may frequently be obscured by behavioral and body size changes associated with variation in colony composition and within-colony competition to fill reproductive vacancies (Lacey and Sherman 1991, 1997). For example, individuals born to mature colonies may remain small and therefore maintain their role as frequent workers for many years, whereas individuals born in nascent colonies attain a higher body mass more rapidly and move out of the worker role to become defenders, dispersers, or, more rarely, breeders (O'Riain and Jarvis 1998). Thus, although the largest individuals in a naked mole-rat colony are usually the oldest, early social influences can affect growth rates and hence the precise role an individual occupies in the colony's work force.

Although morphological caste determination is rare in mammals, there is evidence for a male disperser morph in naked mole-rats (O'Riain et al. 1996; Braude 2000), and naked mole-rat queens exhibit morphological differences in their vertebrae compared to workers (O'Riain et al. 2000). In the Damaraland mole-rat, breeding females are also morphologically different from the nonbreeding females within a colony (Young and Bennett 2010), and physiological castes are also discernable (Scantlebury et al. 2006). Regarding the latter, during the dry season larger "infrequent workers" have lower metabolic rates than "frequent worker" colony members. During the wet season, however, there are no differences. This implies that larger mole-rats become physiologically distinct and more active prior to dispersal. Physiological differences have also been recorded in naked mole-rats, in which disperser males have reproductive hormones that resemble those of breeder males. Table 19.1 summarizes and compares some of the social and reproductive characteristics for both species.

Ultimate factors shaping social evolution

As an explanation for sociality in the Bathyergidae, the "aridity food distribution hypothesis" (AFDH) has received much attention. The AFDH is specific version of the ecological constraints hypothesis, and posits that increased natal philopatry, cooperative breeding, and ultimately eusocial behavior in African mole-rats have evolved in response to patterns of rainfall and their interaction with the geology and vegetation of habitats occupied by this group of organisms. Rainfall affects soil hardness and therefore the energetics of burrowing, and importantly also influences the patterns of mole-rat food distribution and the subsequent costs and risks of foraging and dispersal (Bennett 1988; Lovegrove and Wissell 1988; Lovegrove 1991; Jarvis et al. 1994, 1998). In arid habitats it is easy to see how sociality and cooperation could be adaptive, as cooperative foraging divides the energetic costs of burrowing and increases the chances of finding food in the form of underground roots and tubers. The clumped nature of these geophytes and, in some cases, their large size once found, are sufficient to provide the energy needed to sustain large groups of animals.

Empirical evidence from the field in support of the AFDH comes from both inter- and intraspecific studies across the family. Interspecifically, phylogenetically controlled comparative analysis of the Bathyergidae reveal a significant positive correlation between social group size and the coefficient of variation in rainfall, while mean distances between food sources and numbers of months in which rainfall exceeds 25 cm, the amount required to penetrate to the depth of foraging tunnels, are inversely correlated with colony size, as predicted by the AFDH (Faulkes et al. 1997a).

Analyses of the architecture of burrow systems demonstrates that in the arid habitats inhabited by naked and Damaraland mole-rats, colonies containing larger numbers of individuals are able to explore their habitat and search for food more efficiently with a greater degree of complexity (calculated as fractal dimension) of the foraging tunnels than smaller groups (Le Comber et al. 2002). Furthermore, a long-term field study of Damaraland mole-rats has shown that larger colonies are less likely to fail when environmental conditions are at their most extreme and challenging, such as during droughts, again emphasizing the adaptive advantage of sociality (Jarvis et al. 1998).

The prediction of AFDH that increased aridity should reduce dispersal and increase within-group relatedness (R) has also found support. Hess (2004) used microsatellite genotyping to estimate relatedness in colonies across an aridity gradient in Kenya, finding a weak but statistically significant positive correlation in support of the hypothesis that aridity constrains dispersal. Similarly, comparison of intracolony relatedness in Damaraland mole-rats revealed, as predicted, a lower R-value at a field site in Hotazel, South Africa, compared to a more arid site at Dordabis, Namibia (mean $\pm$ 95% confidence interval: 0.40 $\pm$ 0.02 versus 0.54 $\pm$ 0.04 respectively; Burland et al. 2002).

Intraspecific comparisons of philopatry and dispersal in arid and mesic-dwelling common mole-rats (*Cryptomys hottentotus*), a sister clade to *Fukomys* found in South Africa, have also shown that immigration and emigration were lower at an arid site than at a mesic one, indicating that constraints on dispersal are higher in areas of low and unpredictable rainfall (Spinks et al. 2000). Despite these differences, however, estimates of intracolony relatedness were not found to differ between sites (mean $\pm$ standard error [S.E.] = 0.23 $\pm$ 0.02 at Somerset West, South Africa (mesic site) vs. 0.28 $\pm$ 0.03 at Steinkopf, South Africa, an arid site).

While the aforementioned studies offer support for the AFDH as a means of understanding the ecological drivers of mammalian eusociality, these environmental factors are operating within the context of life history traits that facilitate cooperative breeding. Clearly an ancestral tendency for monogamy and the ability to form social bonds, a subterranean lifestyle that constrains dispersal, and longevity are all vital prerequisites for social elaboration and cooperation in kin groups (Burda et al. 2000; Lukas and Clutton-Brock 2012).

Proximate factors maintaining high reproductive skew and cooperative breeding

The nature and extent of reproductive skew

In colonies of all cooperatively breeding mole-rats studied to date, a single female – the queen – normally breeds with one, and rarely two or three resident breeding males. This indicates that at any one point in time within a colony, all social mole-rat groups have extreme reproductive division of labor and high reproductive skew among females, with somewhat lower skew among males. "Snapshot" data such as this can be misleading, however, and it is important to consider a temporal component, since skew in terms of lifetime reproductive success (LRS) can differ considerably among species depending on the chances of dispersal and independent breeding.

The AFDH predicts that skew in LRS will be greater in species such as naked and Damaraland mole-rats, which inhabit harsher habitats where ecological constraints are higher. In such habitats, while individual reproduction may be prevented over relatively long time periods, longer lifespans may allow mole-rats to breed during periods when environmental pressures on individual reproduction are relaxed.

In Damaraland mole-rats, 89% of 18 colonies had just one breeding male resident at any particular time (Burland et al. 2004). These individuals can be readily distinguished by morphological characteristics as well as paternity analysis. In more than half (53% of 17 colonies), however, no father could be assigned to at least one of the resident offspring. This indicates that the breeding female has contact with other nonresident males either by temporarily leaving the colony, or more likely by transient males passing through the colony. Given that plural breeding among female Damaraland mole-rats has not been observed, either in captivity or in the wild, skew in lifetime reproductive success among males appears to be potentially much less than in females. In the longer term, estimates from a mark-release-recapture study in Namibia have revealed that over a five-year period, 370 of 403 (92%) of nonbreeding females did not breed at all (Jarvis and Bennett 1993; Jarvis et al. 1994).

Very high skew in both the short-term and long-term is also found in naked mole-rats. In captive colonies of naked mole-rats up to three males can mate with the queen (Lacey and Sherman 1991), and molecular analyses confirm that up to three males may sire offspring in a single litter (Faulkes et al. 1997b). Unlike in Damaraland mole-rats, plural breeding has been found in both captive and wild colonies, although it is apparently rare. For example, Braude (1991) recorded only two instances of plural breeding from an extensive field study of 2,051 naked mole-rats from 23 colonies in Meru National Park, Kenya, and only a single breeding queen was detected in wild colonies in Kenya studied by Brett (1991b) and Jarvis (1985).

In captivity, Jarvis (1991) reported groups containing two queens but offspring produced were rarely reared successfully and often there was intense conflict between the breeding females. She also reported that in some of these captive colonies, plural breeding followed periods of high offspring recruitment and suggested that in the wild, such favorable environmental conditions may trigger dispersal of rival females and new colony formation. Overall, skew in LRS in naked mole-rats is even more extreme than in Damaraland mole-rats, with fewer than 0.1% of over 4,000 recaptured nonbreeders eventually becoming queens (Jarvis et al. 1994).

Kin structure of colonies, reproductive suppression and reproductive skew

Of the social mole-rats in the genera *Cryptomys* and *Fukomys* studied to date, both in the wild and in captivity, all appear to have a mating system that involves obligate outbreeding. Hence a colony of social mole-rats comprised of parents and offspring will by default exhibit a reproductive division of labor and high reproductive skew simply as a result of there being no unrelated mates accessible for adult offspring of breeding age. This effect is so strong that in both wild and captive colonies of Damaraland mole-rats in which the breeding female has died, all individuals will remain reproductively quiescent, sometimes for years, until a new, unrelated, individual becomes available, or until fragmentation of the colony occurs (Jarvis and Bennett

1993; Rickard and Bennett 1997; Bennett et al. 1996; Bennett and Faulkes 2000).

In contrast, naked mole-rats have been shown to adopt a mating strategy of facultative inbreeding: the incest avoidance mechanisms observed in *Cryptomys* and *Fukomys* are not present, and if no suitable unrelated mates are available, mating with close relatives within the colony may readily occur. These incestuous tendencies may be an adaptive trait enabling reproduction to continue when environmental conditions prevent dispersal and outbreeding, and were originally proposed as an important factor in explaining eusociality by Reeve et al. (1990), who argued that inbreeding produces a within-kin-group genetic structure analogous to haplodiploidy in the Hymenoptera. Specifically, Reeve et al. (1990) estimated intracolony relatedness in some groups at 0.8, a value greater than the average 0.75 relatedness in haplodiploid organisms where the queen is singly mated (Faulkes and Bennett 2009). The observation of normal familial levels of relatedness in Damaraland mole-rats, however, argues against high relatedness per se as a prerequisite for the emergence of eusociality (Burland et al. 2002).

The contrasting mating patterns of inbreeding and outbreeding among the social mole-rat genera provide insight into species differences in the proximate control of reproductive skew. Molecular genetic studies combined with mark-release-recapture data from *Cryptomys* and *Fukomys* show that intergroup movements may be common, giving rise to the potential for reproductive conflict between the breeding and nonbreeding members of the colony (Burland et al. 2004; Bishop et al. 2004). In Damaraland mole-rats, immigrants of both sexes were identified and opposite-sex nonbreeding animals were present at the same time in some colonies (Burland et al. 2004). Nonetheless, only a single queen was found to be breeding, begging the question of what proximate factors prevent these unrelated nonbreeding animals from reproducing.

In such cases, inbreeding avoidance alone is not sufficient to explain skew. In the case of females, the proximate mechanism driving skew is a physiological block to reproduction in the form of disruption of gonadotrophin releasing hormone (GnRH), leading ultimately to a failure to ovulate (Bennett et al. 1996,

1999; Molteno and Bennett 2000). Curiously, in female Damaraland mole-rats there are no differences in the number, morphology, or size of the cell bodies of the GnRH neurosecretory cells between reproductive and nonreproductive female Damaraland mole-rats (Molteno et al. 2004). There is, however, a significant difference in the amount of GnRH that is retained in the hypothalamic neurosecretory cells of these two groups, with GnRH concentrations in the median eminence and proximal pituitary stalk significantly higher in nonreproductive compared to reproductive females. These findings imply that the GnRH release is physiologically inhibited in nonreproductive females and accumulates in the cells, leading to the observed increase in GnRH concentrations. Such an inhibition mechanisms could be favored by the fitness costs of attempting to breed in the presence of a more dominant, reproductive individual.

The social cues that lead to the suppression of GnRH and subsequent state of anovulation in Damaraland mole-rats remain unknown, since in captivity this species is typically kept in family groups where incest avoidance maintains skew; behavioral interactions between unrelated nonbreeding adults have not been studied. Nonbreeding males are not physiologically suppressed to the same extent as females, but they do possess increased proportions of sperm with morphological defects (Maswanganye et al. 1999), although the significance of these abnormalities for fertility is unclear. Furthermore, in contrast to females, the mean concentration of GnRH in the hypothalami of reproductive and nonreproductive male Damaraland mole-rats is similar (Molteno et al. 2004).

Among cooperative breeders, naked mole-rats exhibit the most extreme of socially induced infertility, with nonbreeders of both sexes being physiologically suppressed in the presence of the dominant queen. In females, gonadal development is much less than that observed in nonbreeding Damaraland mole-rats, leaving them in an apparent prepubertal state with gonads almost embryonic in appearance. As in Damaraland mole-rats, ovarian cyclicity and ovulation are ultimately blocked.

In male naked mole-rats, most nonbreeders have spermatozoa within the reproductive tract, but they are both reduced in number and lack normal levels of motility. In both sexes, these gonadal deficiencies appear to arise from reduced secretion of luteinizing hormone (Faulkes et al. 1990a, 1990b, 1991a, 1991b; Faulkes and Abbott 1991).

While incest avoidance, together with other factors, may explain how reproductive division of labor is maintained in Damaraland mole-rats, the proximate control of reproductive skew in naked mole-rats is mediated through dominance: the extreme (but potentially rapidly reversible) reproductive blocks are brought about specifically by behavioral contact with the dominant breeding queen (Faulkes and Abbott 1993; Clarke and Faulkes 1997, 1998; Smith et al. 1997). Why have subordinate naked mole-rats evolved to "accept" such extreme physiological suppression of reproduction? High reproductive skew and a large nonbreeding workforce are clearly adaptive in this species. Facultative inbreeding occurs both in captivity and in the wild (Faulkes and Bennett 2009), largely due to ecological constraints that preclude dispersal and result in a near zero chance of encountering an unrelated mating partner. In the face of within-colony competition to mate, a control mechanism has evolved whereby social cues bring about suppression of reproductive physiology in both sexes. Without such suppression, reproductive conflict among related individuals attempting to breed would likely be rampant by opting out subordinates likely avoid costly competition. Debate continues with respect to the extent to which suppression is "imposed" (dominant control) or "accepted" (so called self-restraint), and how these concepts fit into theoretical models of optimal reproductive skew. Within this discussion it is important to consider mechanistically how suppression is mediated, irrespective of the relative costs and benefits of suppression to the subordinate nonbreeder. For example, it is possible to understand a dominant control model in the context of stress physiology, but more difficult to explain how a restraint model may operate from a neuroendocrine or physiological point of view (Faulkes and Bennett 2009).

Among other species of African mole-rats, including the common, Mashona, and giant mole-rats, no physiological suppression of reproduction is observed (Bennett et al. 1997; Bennett et al. 2000; Spinks et al. 2000). In these taxa, opportunities for individual reproduction following dispersal are apparently greater and incest avoidance alone is apparently sufficient to maintain reproductive skew within colonies. The Damaraland mole-rat is intermediate between these species and the naked mole-rat, with suppression of reproductive physiology restricted to nonbreeding females (Bennett et al. 1996; Molteno et al. 2004). A possible explanation is that this trait may have evolved as a result of reproductive conflict as a potential control mechanism by the queen preventing unrelated immigrant males from mating with other females in the colony, thus maintaining the high skew observed among females.

The neurobiology of living together

A critical but until recently largely overlooked proximate factor driving sociality in African mole-rats is the ability to modulate tolerance and social affiliation among both breeding and nonbreeding animals within a colony. Not all mole-rat species have this trait, as the solitary species are highly aggressive toward one another, pairing only briefly to mate, with young being expelled from the natal burrow immediately after weaning (Bennett and Jarvis 1988; Bennett et al. 1991). Among mammals generally, the evolution of cooperative breeding is restricted to socially monogamous species (Lukas and Clutton-Brock 2012) in which pair-bonding behavior is dependent on particular neurobiological phenotypes (Young and Wang 2004).

In rodents, two neuropeptides, oxytocin (OXT) and vasopressin (AVP), act centrally in the brain to modulate sociality, pair bonding, and aggression (Lim and Young 2006). More specifically, the location, pattern, and density of receptors for OXT and AVP differ significantly between promiscuous and monogamous species of voles (*Microtus montanus* and *M. ochrogastor* respectively) and mice (*Peromyscus* spp.; Curtis et al. 2007). Recent studies have determined that the naked mole-rat exhibits higher levels of OXT receptor binding than the solitary and promiscuous Cape mole-rat (*Georychus capensis*) in several significant regions of

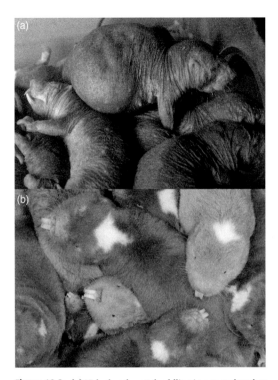

Figure 19.3. (a) Naked mole-rats huddling in a nest chamber. The pregnant queen is on top of the pile of animals, and below her two large animals guard one entrance to the nest. (b) Damaraland mole-rats in a nest chamber. Photographs by C. Faulkes and T. Jackson. See plate section for color figure.

the forebrain. As with social voles, OXT receptor levels in naked mole-rats are intense and extensive in an area known as the nucleus accumbens. Conversely, OXT receptors are not detectable in the Cape mole-rat in this area, consistent with a paucity of prosocial behaviors exhibited by this species (Kalamatianos et al. 2010).

The interpretation of these findings is that abundance of OXT receptor densities in the nucleus accumbens of naked mole-rats reflects their high levels of sociality, alloparenting behavior, and potential for reproductive pair bonding. As the queen may have up to three male consorts with which she mates during a particular estrus period, the mating system is polyandrous rather than monogamous, but bonding is nonetheless simultaneous and long-term, rather than sequential. In that sense it resembles the bonds

that form in a monogamous relationship. Preliminary studies confirm that the Damaraland mole-rat, which is convergently social (Figure 19.3), resembles both naked mole-rat (and social voles), with OXT receptor binding being present in the nucleus accumbens (Coen et al. 2011).

Conclusions

Within the extensive adaptive radiation of African mole-rats endemic to sub-Saharan Africa, naked and Damaraland mole-rats are two key species divergent within the family, but convergent in their highly social cooperative breeding behavior. As well as revealing possible gains and losses of sociality across the family, molecular phylogenies have enabled comparative analyses and the investigation of the ultimate drivers and proximate maintenance of social behavior. Such studies indicate that sociality and cooperative breeding require the correlated evolution of a mosaic of characteristics, set against a backdrop of phylogenetically constrained life-history traits such as a subterranean lifestyle and relatively long lifespan. These include the appropriate neurobiological phenotype facilitating the ability to form social bonds followed by a number of behavioral and reproductive adaptations including inbreeding avoidance, behavioral division of labor, and socially induced suppression of reproduction.

Ultimately the social lifestyle of mole-rats is driven by natal philopatry, most likely imposed by the high costs of dispersal and the risks involved in foraging singly or in small groups where food resources are dispersed. These problems become exaggerated in arid habitats such as those exploited by naked and Damaraland mole-rats, where the soil is also compact and energetically costly to excavate. Under these conditions the best strategy is to stay and help, delaying breeding rather than attempting to increase individual fitness.

This reproductive cost is offset by gains in inclusive fitness, as the majority of colony members are closely related (Reeve et al. 1990; Faulkes et al. 1997b; Burland et al. 2002). Given the prevalence of natal philopatry and sociality across the family, and the advantages of such behavior, a major question is: why have some species gained a solitary and aggressive phenotype along with its underlying neurobiology or, alternatively, lost the social phenotype? Perhaps relatively common mutations occurring in a few key genes underlie the pair-bonding observed in the social phenotype. These may be under strong selection in certain habitats, but neutral in others, and thus lost relatively easily.

Although convergence within the family has produced similar social phenotypes in naked and Damaraland mole-rats, identifying the similarities and differences in the underlying proximate mechanisms are of interest in understanding common mechanisms and neurobiological substrates that underpin behavior. Whether the differential expression of such mechanisms in asocial and social African mole-rats is structured genetically, in a similar way to that seen in voles, remains a fascinating question that still requires answering.

Adaptations to the subterranean niche have not only given rise to sociality, but also to a host of unexpected traits that have become of great interest to researchers into human health. In naked mole-rats, these include extreme longevity and lack of senescence (Sherman and Jarvis 2002; Buffenstein 2008), insensitivity to certain kinds of pain (Park et al. 2008; Smith et al. 2011), and resistance to cancer (Kim et al. 2011; Yu et al. 2011; Tian et al. 2013). Future research in African mole-rats will likely focus on understanding these adaptations, which are unique and of general interest. Their discovery through basic, exploratory research is significant, and future explorations stand to gain much by integrating evolutionary theory with exploration of these interesting, applied, research contexts.

Acknowledgments

We acknowledge research grants from the National Research Foundation, the University of Pretoria as well as a DST-NRF South African Research Chair of Mammal Behavioural Ecology and Physiology award to NCB. Neurobiological work was supported by BBSRC project grant no. BBD5231861 (CGF).

REFERENCES

Alexander, R. D., Noonan, K. M., and Crespi, B. J. (1991). The evolution of eusociality In: *The Biology of the Naked Mole-rat*, ed. P. W. Sherman, J. U. M. Jarvis and R. D. Alexander. Princeton, NJ: Princeton University Press, pp. 3–44.

Bennett, N. C. (1988). The trend towards sociality in three species of southern African mole-rats (Bathyergidae): causes and consequences. Ph.D. thesis. University of Cape Town, Cape Town, South Africa.

Bennett, N. C. (1990). Behaviour and social organization in a colony of the Damaraland mole-rat *Cryptomys damarensis*. *J. Zool.*, 220, 225–248.

Bennett, N. C. and Faulkes, C. G. (2000). *African Mole-rats: Ecology and Eusociality*. Cambridge: Cambridge University Press.

Bennett, N. C. and Jarvis, J. U. M. (1988). The social structure and reproductive biology of colonies of the mole-rat, *Cryptomys damarensis* (Rodentia, Bathyergidae). *J. Mammal.*, 69, 293–302.

Bennett, N. C. and Jarvis, J. U. M. (2004). *Cryptomys damarensis*. *Mammal. Species*, 756, 1–5.

Bennett, N. C., Jarvis, J. U. M., Aguilar, G. H., and McDaid, E. (1991). Growth rates and development in six species of African mole-rats (Family; Bathyergidae). *J. Zool.*, 225, 13–26.

Bennett, N. C., Faulkes, C. G., and Molteno, A. J. (1996). Reproductive suppression in subordinate, non-breeding female Damaraland mole-rats: two components to a lifetime of socially-induced infertility. *Proc. R. Soc. London B*, 263, 1599–1603.

Bennett, N. C., Faulkes, C. G., and Spinks, A. C. (1997). LH responses to single doses of exogenous GnRH by social Mashona mole-rats: a continuum of socially-induced infertility in the family Bathyergidae. *Proc. R. Soc. London B*, 264, 1001–1006.

Bennett, N. C., Faulkes, C. G., and Jarvis, J. U. M. (1999). Socially-induced infertility, incest avoidance and the monopoly of reproduction in cooperatively breeding African mole-rats (Family Bathyergidae). *Adv. Study Behav.*, 28, 75–114.

Bennett, N. C., Molteno, A. J., and Spinks, A. C. (2000). Pituitary sensitivity to exogenous GnRH in giant Zambian mole-rats, *Cryptomys mechowi* (Rodentia: Bathyergidae): support for the "socially-induced infertility continuum." *J. Zool.*, 252, 447–452.

Bishop, W. W. (1962). The mammalian fauna and geomorphological relations of the Napak volcanics, Karamoja. *Uganda Geological Survey, Records 1957–58*, 1–18.

Bishop J. M., Jarvis, J. U. M., Spinks, A. C., Bennett, N. C., and O'Ryan, C. (2004). Molecular insight into patterns of colony composition and paternity in the common mole–rat *Cryptomys hottentotus hottentotus*. *Mol. Ecol.*, 13, 1217–1229.

Braude, S. (1991). The behavior and demographics of the naked mole-rat, *Heterocephalus glaber*. Ph.D. Thesis, University of Michigan, Ann Arbor, Michigan.

Braude, S. (2000). Dispersal and new colony formation in wild naked mole-rats: evidence against inbreeding as the system of mating. *Behav. Ecol.*, 11, 7–12.

Brett, R. A. (1991a). The ecology of naked mole-rat colonies: burrowing, food and limiting factors. In: *The Biology of the Naked Mole-rat*, ed. P. W. Sherman, J. U. M. Jarvis and R. D. Alexander. Princeton, NJ: Princeton University Press, pp. 137–184.

Brett, R. A. (1991b). The population structure of naked mole-rat colonies In: *The Biology of the Naked Mole-rat*, ed. P. W. Sherman, J. U. M. Jarvis and R. D. Alexander, Princeton, NJ: Princeton University Press, pp. 97–136.

Buffenstein, R. (2008). Negligible senescence in the longest living rodent, the naked mole-rat: insights from a successfully aging species. *J. Comp. Physiol. B*, 178, 439–445.

Burda, H., Honeycutt, R. L., Begall, S., Locker-Grütjen, O., and Scharff, A. (2000). Are naked and common mole-rats eusocial and if so, why? *Behav. Ecol. Sociobiol.*, 47, 293–303.

Burland, T. M., Bennett, N. C., Jarvis, J. U. M., and Faulkes, C. G. (2002). Eusociality in African mole–rats: new insights from patterns of genetic relatedness in the Damaraland mole-rat (*Cryptomys damarensis*). *Proc. R. Soc. London B*, 269, 1025–1030.

Burland, T. M., Bennett, N. C., Jarvis, J. U. M., and Faulkes, C. G. (2004). Colony structure and parentage in wild colonies of co-operatively breeding Damaraland mole-rats suggest incest avoidance alone may not maintain reproductive skew. *Mol. Ecol.*, 13, 2371–2379.

Clarke, F. M. and Faulkes, C. G. (1997). Hormonal and behavioural correlates of dominance and queen succession in captive colonies of the eusocial naked mole-rat, *Heterocephalus glaber*. *Proc. R. Soc. London B*, 264, 993–1000.

Clarke, F. M. and Faulkes, C.G. (1998). Hormonal and behavioural correlates of male dominance and reproductive status in captive colonies of the naked mole-rat, *Heterocephalus glaber*. *Proc. R. Soc. London B*, 265, 1391–1399.

Coen, C. W., Zhou, S, Kalamatianos, T., Faulkes, C. G., and Bennett, N. C. (2011). Telencephalic distribution of oxytocin and vasopressin and their binding sites in Damaraland mole-rats: implications for eusocial behavior. In: *Society for Neuroscience Annual Meeting, Washington, DC, 12–16 November 2011*. 186.11/SS10. Society for Neuroscience.

Curtis, J. T., Liu, Y., Aragona, B. J., and Wang, Z. (2007). Neural regulation of social behavior in rodents. In: *Rodent Societies: An Ecological and Evolutionary Perspective*, ed. J. O. Wolff and P. W. Sherman, Chicago, IL: University of Chicago Press, pp. 185–194.

Faulkes, C. G. and Abbott, D. H. (1991). Social control of reproduction in both breeding and non-breeding male naked mole-rats, *Heterocephalus glaber*. *J. Repro. Fert.*, 93, 427–435.

Faulkes, C. G. and Abbott, D. H. (1993). Evidence that primer pheromones do not cause social suppression of reproduction in male and female naked mole-rats, *Heterocephalus glaber*. *J. Repro. Fert.*, 99, 225–230.

Faulkes, C. G. and Bennett, N. C. (2009). Reproductive skew in African mole-rats: Behavioural and physiological mechanisms to maintain high skew. In: *Reproductive Skew in Vertebrates: Proximate and Ultimate Causes*, ed. R. Hager and C. B. Jones. Cambridge: Cambridge University Press, pp. 369–396.

Faulkes, C. G. and Bennett, N. C. (2013). Plasticity and constraints on social evolution in African mole-rats: ultimate and proximate factors. *Phil. Trans. R. Soc. London B*, 368 (1618).

Faulkes, C. G., Abbott, D. H., and Jarvis, J.U. M. (1990a). Social suppression of ovarian cyclicity in captive and wild colonies of naked mole-rats, *Heterocephalus glaber*. *J. Repro. Fert.*, 88, 559–568.

Faulkes, C. G., Abbott, D. H., Jarvis, J. U. M., and Sherrif, F. E. (1990b). LH responses of female naked mole-rats, *Heterocephalus glaber* to single and multiple doses of exogenous GnRH. *J. Repro. Fert.*, 89, 317–323.

Faulkes, C. G., Abbott, D. H. Liddell, C., George, L. M., and Jarvis, J. U. M. (1991a). Hormonal and behavioral aspects of reproductive suppression in female naked mole-rats. In: *The Biology of the Naked Mole-rat*, ed. P. W. Sherman, J. U. M. Jarvis, and R. D. Alexander. Princeton, NJ: Princeton University Press, pp. 426–444.

Faulkes, C. G., Abbott, D. H., and Jarvis, J. U. M. (1991b). Social suppression of reproduction in male naked mole-rats, *Heterocephalus glaber*. *J. Repro. Fert.*, 91, 593–604.

Faulkes, C. G., Bennett, N. C., Bruford, M. W., O'Brien, H. P., Aguilar, G. H., et al. (1997a). Ecological constraints drive social evolution in the African mole-rats. *Proc. R. Soc. London B*, 264, 1619–1627.

Faulkes, C. G., Abbott, D. H., O'Brien, H. P., Lau, L., Roy, M. R., et al. (1997b). Micro- and macro-geographic genetic structure of colonies of naked mole-rats, *Heterocephalus glaber*. *Mol. Ecol.*, 6, 615–628.

Faulkes, C. G., Verheyen, E., Verheyen, W., Jarvis, J. U. M., and Bennett, N. C. (2004). Phylogeographical patterns of genetic divergence and speciation in African mole-rats (Family: Bathyergidae). *Mol. Ecol.*, 13, 613–629.

Faulkes, C. G., Mgode, G. F., Le Comber, S. C., and Bennett, N. C. (2010). Cladogenesis and endemism in Tanzanian mole-rats, genus *Fukomys*:(Rodentia Bathyergidae): a role for tectonics? *Biol. J. Linn. Soc.*, 100, 337–352.

Faulkes, C. G., Bennett, N. C., Cotterill, F. P. D., Mgode, G. F., and Verheyen, E. (2011). Phylogeography and cryptic diversity of the solitary-dwelling silvery mole-rat, genus *Heliophobius* (family: Bathyergidae). *J. Zool.*, 285, 324–338.

Gaylard, A., Harrison, Y., and Bennett, N. C. (1998). Temporal changes in the social structure of a captive colony of the Damaraland mole-rat, *Cryptomys damarensis*: the relationship of sex and age to dominance and burrow maintenance activity. *J. Zool.*, 244, 313–321.

Hess, J. (2004). A population genetic study of the eusocial naked mole-rat (*Heterocephalus glaber*). Ph.D. thesis, University of Washington, Seattle, Washington.

Hill, W. C. O., Porter, A., Bloom, R. T., Seago, J., and Southwick, M. D. (1957). Field and laboratory studies on the naked mole-rat (*Heterocephalus glaber*). *Proc. Zool. Soc. London*, 128, 455–513.

Ingram, C., Burda, H., and Honeycutt, R. L. (2004). Molecular phylogenetics and taxonomy of the African mole-rats, genus *Cryptomys* and the new genus *Coetomys* Gray, 1864. *Mol. Phyl. Evol.*, 31, 997–1014.

Jarvis, J. U. M. (1981). Eusociality in a mammal: cooperative breeding in naked mole-rat colonies. *Science*, 212, 571–573.

Jarvis, J. U. M. (1985). Ecological studies on *Heterocephalus glaber*, the naked mole-rat, in Kenya. *Nat. Geo. Soc. Res. Rep.*, 20, 429–437.

Jarvis J. U. M. (1991). Reproduction of naked mole-rats. In: *The Biology of the Naked Mole-rat*, ed. P. W. Sherman, J. U. M. Jarvis, and R. D. Alexander. Princeton, NJ: Princeton University Press, pp. 384–425.

Jarvis, J. U. M. and Bennett, N. C. (1993). Eusociality has evolved independently in two genera of bathyergid mole-rats – but occurs in no other subterranean mammal. *Behav. Ecol. Sociobiol.*, 33, 253–260.

Jarvis, J. U. M., O'Riain, M. J., Bennett, N. C., and Sherman, P. W. (1994). Mammalian eusociality: a family affair. *Trends Ecol. Evol.*, 9, 47–51.

Jarvis, J. U. M., Bennett, N. C., and Spinks, A. C. (1998). Food availability and foraging by wild colonies of Damaraland mole-rats (*Cryptomys damarensis*): implications for sociality. *Oecologia*, 113, 290–298

Kalamatianos T., Faulkes, C. G, Oosthuizen, M. K., Bennett, N. C., and Coen, C. W. (2010). Telencephalic binding sites for oxytocin reflect social organisation: evidence from eusocial naked mole-rats and solitary Cape mole-rats. *J. Comp. Neurol.*, 518, 1792–1813.

Kim, E. B., Fang, X., Fushan, A. A., Huang, Z., Lobanov, A. V., et al. (2011). Genome sequencing reveals insights into physiology and longevity of the naked mole rat. *Nature*, 479, 223–227.

Lacey, E. A. and Sherman, P. W. (1991). Social organization of naked mole-rat colonies: evidence for divisions of labor. In: *The Biology of the Naked Mole-rat*, ed. P. W. Sherman, J. U. M. Jarvis, and R. D. Alexander. Princeton, NJ: Princeton University Press, pp. 275–336.

Lacey, E. A. and Sherman, P. W. (1997). Cooperative breeding in naked mole-rats: implications for vertebrate and invertebrate sociality. In: *Cooperative Breeding in Mammals*, ed. N. G. Solomon and J. A. French. Cambridge: Cambridge University Press, pp. 267–301.

Le Comber, S. C., Spinks, A. C., Bennett, N. C., Jarvis, J. U. M., and Faulkes, C. G. (2002). Fractal dimension of African mole-rat burrows. *Can. J. Zool.*, 80, 436–441.

Lim, M. M. and Young, L. J. (2006). Neuropeptidergic regulation of affiliative behavior and social bonding in animals. *Horm. Behav.*, 50, 506–517.

Lovegrove, B. G. (1991). The evolution of eusociality in mole–rats (Bathyergidae): a question of risks, numbers and costs. *Behav. Ecol. Sociobiol.*, 28, 37–45.

Lovegrove, B. G. and Wissel, C. (1988). Sociality in mole–rats: metabolic scaling and the role of risk sensitivity. *Oecologia*, 74, 600–606.

Lukas, D. and Clutton-Brock, T. (2012). Cooperative breeding and monogamy in mammalian societies. *Proc. R. Soc. London B*, 279, 2151–2156.

Maswanganye, K. A., Bennett, N. C., Brinders, J., and Cooney, R. (1999). Oligospermia and azoospermia in non-reproductive male Damaraland mole-rats (*Cryptomys damarensis*) (Rodentia: Bathyergidae). *J. Zool.*, 248, 411–418.

Michener, C. D. (1969). Comparative social behavior of bees. *Annu. Rev. Entomol.*, 14, 299–342.

Molteno, A. J. and Bennett, N. C. (2000). Anovulation in non-reproductive female Damaraland mole-rats (*Cryptomys damarensis*). *J. Repro. Fert.*, 119, 35–41.

Molteno A.J., Kallo, I., Bennett, N.C., King, J.A., and Coen, C.W. (2004). A neuroanatomical and neuroendocrinological study into the relationship between social status and the GnRH system in cooperatively breeding female Damaraland mole- rats, *Cryptomys damarensis*. *Reproduction*, 127, 13–21.

O'Riain, M. J. and Braude, S. (2001). Inbreeding versus outbreeding in captive and wild populations of naked mole-rats. In: *Dispersal*, ed. J. Clobert, E. Danchin, A. A. Dhondt, and J. D. Nichols, Oxford: Oxford University Press, pp. 143–154.

O'Riain, M. J. and Jarvis, J. U. M. (1998). The dynamics of growth in naked mole-rats: the effects of litter order and changes in social structure. *J. Zool.*, 246, 49–60.

O'Riain, M. J., Jarvis, J. U. M., and Faulkes, C. G. (1996). A dispersive morph in the naked mole-rat. *Nature* 380, 619–621.

O'Riain, M. J., Jarvis, J. U. M., Buffenstein, R., Alexander, R. D., and Peeters. C. (2000). Morphological castes in a vertebrate. *Proc. Natl. Acad. Sci. (USA)*, 97, 13194–13197.

Park, T. J., Lu, Y., Jüttner, R., Smith, E. S., Hu, J., et al. (2008). Selective inflammatory pain insensitivity in the African naked mole-rat (*Heterocephalus glaber*). *PLoS Biology*, 6(1), e13.

Reeve, H. K., Westneat, D. F., Noon, W. A., Sherman, P. W., and Aquadro, C. F. (1990). DNA "fingerprinting" reveals high levels of inbreeding in colonies of the eusocial naked mole-rat. *Proc. Natl. Acad. Sci. (USA)*, 87, 2496–2500.

Rickard, C. A. and Bennett, N. C. (1997). Recrudescense of sexual activity in a reproductively quiescent colony of the Damaraland mole-rat, by the introduction of a genetically unrelated male – a case of incest avoidance in "queenless" colonies. *J. Zool.*, 241, 185–202.

Scantlebury, M., Speakman, J. R., Oosthuizen, M. K., Roper, T. J., and Bennett, N. C. (2006). Energetics reveals physiologically distinct castes in a eusocial mammal. *Nature* 440, 795–797.

Sherman, P. W. and Jarvis, J. U. M. (2002). Extraordinary life spans of naked mole-rats (*Heterocephalus glaber*). *J. Zool.*, 258, 307–311.

Smith, E. S. J., Omerbasic, D., Lechner, S. G., Anirudhan, G., Lapatsina, L., et al. (2011). The molecular basis of acid insensitivity in the African naked mole-rat. *Science*, 334, 1557–1560.

Smith, T. E., Faulkes, C. G., and Abbott, D. H. (1997). Combined olfactory contact with the parent colony and direct contact with non-breeding animals does not maintain suppression of ovulation in female naked mole-rats. *Horm. Behav.*, 31, 277–288.

Spinks, A. C., Jarvis, J. U. M., and Bennett, N.C. (2000). Comparative patterns of philopatry and dispersal in two common mole-rat populations: implications for the evolution of mole-rat sociality. *J. Anim. Ecol.*, 69, 224–234.

Tian, X., Azpurua, J., Hine, C., Vaidya, A., Myakishev-Rempel, M., et al. (2013). High-molecular-mass hyaluronan mediates the cancer resistance of the naked mole rat. *Nature*, 499, 346–349.

Van Daele, P. A. A. G., Dammann, P., Meier, J. L., Kawalika, M., Van De Woestijne, C., et al. (2004). Chromosomal diversity in mole-rats of the genus Cryptomys (Rodentia: Bathyergidae) from the Zambezian region: with descriptions of new karyotypes. *J. Zool.*, 264, 317–326.

Van Daele, P. A. A. G., Verheyen, E., Brunain, M., and Adriaens, D. (2007). Cytochrome b sequence analysis reveals differential molecular evolution in African mole-rats of the chromosomally hyperdiverse genus Fukomys (Bathyergidae, Rodentia) from the Zambezian region. *Mol. Phyl. Evol.*, 45, 142–157.

Wilson, E.O. (1971). *The Insect Societies*. Cambridge, MA: Harvard University Press.

Young, A. J. and Bennett, N. C. (2010). Morphological specialization among queens in Damaraland mole-rat societies. *Evolution*, 64, 3190–3197.

Young, L. J. and Wang, Z. (2004). The neurobiology of pair bonding. *Nature Neuroscience*, 7, 1048–1054.

Yu, C., Li, Y., Holmes, A. Szafranski, K., Faulkes, C. G., Coen, C. W., et al. (2011). RNA sequencing reveals differential expression of mitochondrial and oxidation reduction genes in the long-lived naked mole-rat when compared to mice. *PLoS One*, 6(11), e26729.

Synthesis: Cooperative breeding in the twenty-first century

Walter D. Koenig, Janis L. Dickinson, and Stephen T. Emlen

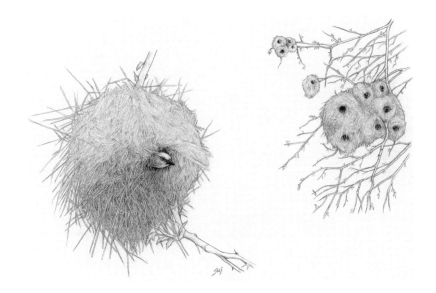

Introduction

One result of putting together this book was the realization that the field is less unified than it was 25 years ago when the prior book summarizing studies of cooperative breeding was published (Stacey and Koenig 1990). The focus at that time was largely on territoriality and ecological constraints as drivers of cooperative breeding in birds. Since then, the field has diversified both empirically and theoretically, encompassing an ever-widening range of social organizations from a broader suite of habitats and geographic locations. We were surprised to discover how enlightening, yet difficult, it was to try to integrate this amalgam of long-term studies into a coherent framework. We admit that this was somewhat disappointing for us, who, as senior workers in the field, had hoped to generate a "grand synthesis." It bodes well, however, for students interested in pursuing studies of cooperative breeding, because it indicates significant potential for further discovery and innovation.

As the grand synthesis remains elusive, we have instead elected to summarize a subset of issues

Cooperative Breeding in Vertebrates: Studies of Ecology, Evolution, and Behavior, eds W. D. Koenig and J. L. Dickinson.
Published by Cambridge University Press. © Cambridge University Press 2016.

drawing from the chapters in this book, moving beyond a summary in two ways. First, we emphasize the importance of distinguishing different kinds of group members based on their reproductive options; this is critical for generating the correct comparisons needed to understand which factors drive the evolution of cooperative breeding. Second, we analyze hypotheses that have been proposed for the ecological factors important to the evolution of delayed (or local) dispersal and helping behavior, two of the key features of cooperative breeding. Our goal is to provide a framework in these key areas that will facilitate future advances.

Forms of cooperative breeding and key factors in its evolution

Group structure and ecology

As already pointed out, cooperative breeding is not a unified phenomenon. At one end of complexity are nonbreeding helpers that are offspring of the breeders and have delayed, or at least localized, dispersal, while at the other are species exhibiting cooperative polygamy and various forms of plural breeding. Not infrequently, nonbreeding helpers co-occur with cooperative polygamy and plural breeding with variation in whether there is delayed dispersal, localized dispersal, or even coloniality.

Cooperative polygamy and plural breeding are particularly variable phenomena (Brown 1987), and we still do not have a good handle on all their various forms, because only a fraction of species known to exhibit such behavior have been studied in detail and because no doubt many have yet to be discovered. This book thus represents the range of cooperative breeding systems that are currently being studied intensively, not the diversity of all such systems. Preliminary studies of species such as the greater vasa parrot (*Caracopsis vasa*) of Madagascar, in which females copulate with and are fed by multiple unrelated and nonterritorial males (Ekstrom et al. 2007), the moustached warbler (*Acrocephalus melanopogon*), in which unrelated floater males assist in incubation, feeding of nestlings,

and defense of chicks (Fessl et al. 1996), and several of the other species mentioned by Cockburn (2004) suggest that many variants of cooperatively breeding remain to be investigated.

In the earlier volume of long-term studies, Smith (1990) pointed out that most cooperative breeders live on relatively stable, all-purpose territories, and this remains true for the majority of species discussed here, at least during the breeding season. Notable exceptions, however, include the long-tailed tit (*Aegithalos caudatus*; Chapter 3), which is non-territorial even when breeding; chestnut-crowned babblers (*Pomatostomus ruficeps*; Chapter 9), which have large, overlapping home ranges; and the grey-capped social weaver (*Pseudonigrita arnudi*), which is also nonterritorial and lives in relatively stable colonies (S. T. Emlen, unpubl. data; see illustration at beginning of chapter). Group sizes of many cooperative breeders are relatively small (<10; Smith 1990), but the spatiotemporal distribution of resources favors larger aggregations in others. Such species include the superb starling (*Lamprotornis superbus*; Chapter 11), in which groups can contain up to at least 40 birds, and some of the species discussed in the later chapters of this book, in which group sizes range from several dozen (in the fish *Neolamprologus pulcher*; Chapter 16) to upward of 75–80 individuals in banded mongoose (*Mungos mungo*; Chapter 18) and several hundred individuals in naked mole-rats (*Heterocephalus glaber*; Chapter 19). Cooperative breeding in vertebrates is clearly not just restricted to small groups of territorial species.

Extra-group parentage and its relationship to kinship

In the past 25 years significant advances to our understanding of cooperative breeding have come from molecular parentage analysis. In some cases it has turned out that the genetic mating system parallels the social mating system, and thus the molecular era has made little difference in terms of understanding social behavior. In red-cockaded woodpeckers (*Picoides borealis*; Chapter 4) and Florida scrub-jays (*Aphelocoma coerulescens*; Chapter 5), breeding pairs are socially *and* genetically monogamous, whereas extra-pair paternity occurs, but is relatively uncommon, in long-tailed tits (Chapter 3). In other species, however, data on extra-pair paternity have led to significant reinterpretation of the breeding system.

Two of the more notable species where parentage analysis has altered our understanding of the social system are the Seychelles warbler (*Acrocephalus sechellensis*; Chapter 12) and the superb fairy-wren (*Malurus cyaneus*; Chapter 8). In Seychelles warblers, 44% of subordinate females lay eggs, although they were originally thought to be nonbreeding helpers, and a similar proportion of offspring are fathered by males from outside the group, thus altering earlier conclusions about the fitness benefits of helping in this species. In the superb fairy-wren, the incidence of extra-pair parentage is such that the genetic and social mating systems bear almost no relationship to each other. With extra-pair parentage on the order of 61% of offspring, among the highest found in any wild population, monogamy is clearly not required for the maintenance of cooperative breeding, despite evidence, supported by comparative phylogenetic analyses, that monogamy is associated with the evolutionary transition to complex societies in both birds and mammals (Cornwallis et al. 2010; Lukas and Clutton-Brock 2012).

The rationale for the hypothesis that monogamy is fundamental for the evolutionary transition to cooperative breeding is based on the assumption that genetic monogamy enhances relatedness between helpers and the offspring they help raise (Boomsma 2009). While this is true in some social insects, in which breeder turnover can be low enough that relatedness is unlikely to change significantly during the lifetime of a helper, it does not apply to vertebrates, whose relatedness to potential recipients of help frequently changes, most commonly when a parent dies and is replaced, thereby cutting relatedness of a helper to subsequent nestlings in half (Emlen 1995, 1997).

A second problem with this assumption is that it fails to consider the effect of extra-pair paternity on outside options. In such situations, what matters, in addition to the costs and benefits of helping, is relatedness of helpers to the young they would help raise, compared to their relatedness to the young they would parent were they to breed independently. In particular, a son's

relatedness to half-sibs resulting from extra-pair paternity is $r = 0.25$, whereas his relatedness to extra-pair young in his own nest is $r = 0$ (Dickinson et al. 1996). Thus, counterintuitively, extra-pair paternity can lead to the situation in which sons in cooperatively breeding vertebrates are *more* closely related to young in their parents' nest than they would be to young in their own nest (Dickinson et al. 1996; Kramer and Russell 2014). Indeed, if success at extra-pair paternity increases with age, as postulated by the delayed extra-pair benefits hypothesis described in Chapter 2, female promiscuity can actually *increase*, rather than decrease, the future direct and the future indirect benefits of helping for young males. This can be true even if helpers are unable to discriminate extra-pair from within-pair young and instead base their decision to help on their presumed relationship to the breeders, as is typically the case for cooperatively breeding vertebrates (Kramer and Russell 2014).

Inbreeding avoidance and reproductive skew

When cooperative breeding groups are extended families, a primary factor that restricts breeding on the part of helpers is incest avoidance (Koenig and Haydock 2004). The value of using incest avoidance to make a priori assumptions about the breeding status of different kinds of "helpers" is discussed in greater detail in the next section.

In most cases, incest is reduced through immigration, which provides unrelated individuals that can be chosen over kin as mates. Three species discussed here provide intriguing counterexamples, however. First are, once again, superb fairy-wrens (Chapter 8), in which social pairs are often first-order relatives; nonetheless, the high incidence of extra-pair fertilizations avoids any significant cost to such incestuous social pairings. Second is the banded mongoose (Chapter 18), in which groups are founded by unrelated individuals, but the permanent retention of philopatric offspring of both sexes leads to increased relatedness between breeders within groups over time, resulting in an extraordinarily high incidence of brother-sister and father-daughter incest. Last but not least is the naked mole-rat

(Chapter 19), where the mating system appears to be one of facultative incest.

The evolutionary implications of incest in these two latter species are, however, unclear. In the mongoose, the strikingly high levels of incest do not appear to lead to increasing levels of homozygosity among offspring, perhaps because of lower survivorship (inbreeding depression) among inbred offspring. Meanwhile, eusociality in Damaraland mole-rats (*Fukomys damarensis*), for which there is no indication of high levels of incest (Chapter 19), counters the hypothesis that inbreeding has played a key role in the evolution of eusociality in this taxon (Reeve et al. 1990). Indeed, whether inbreeding leads to increased relatedness and thus plays an important role in driving social behavior in any vertebrate remains an open question, whereas incest avoidance is clearly important in nearly all systems in which adult relatives find themselves in a position to potentially mate with each other.

Eliminating individuals constrained by incest avoidance leads to more insightful examination of reproductive competition (skew) within groups (Emlen 1996), which remains an important issue relying heavily on genetic analyses. Reproductive skew is examined in several of the species in this book that exhibit some form of cooperative polygamy. As with other aspects of cooperative breeding, skew is highly variable, with reproduction being largely or entirely monopolized by a dominant pair in western bluebirds (*Sialia mexicana*; Chapter 2) southern pied babblers (*Turdoides bicolor*; Chapter 7) and meerkats (*Suricata suricatta*; Chapter 17), less strongly monopolized by a dominant pair in chestnut-crowned babblers (Chapter 9) and banded mongooses (Chapter 18), and shared equally among joint-nesting females and cobreeding males in acorn woodpeckers (*Melanerpes formicivorus*; Chapter 13), at least when taking into consideration "switching" of paternity across nesting attempts. Currently we still have relatively little understanding of the factors driving these differences, although it is by means of such studies that our empirical knowledge of reproductive skew may eventually catch up with the plethora of theoretical models addressing this issue (Magrath et al. 2004; Shen and Reeve 2010; Nonacs and Hager 2011).

What is a helper?

Distinguishing different kinds of helpers

The above example highlights a key issue concerning not only family dynamics, but the very definition of helpers (often referred to as "subordinates" or "auxiliaries"). In particular, there are several categories of "helpers" in cooperative breeding systems that are frequently not clearly distinguished, despite the fact that the potential and means of gaining fitness within groups have long been known to be very different.

As a relatively simple example, consider white-browed scrubwrens (*Sericornis frontalis*). Whittingham et al. (1997) and Magrath and Whittingham (1997) described the behavior and differing degrees of paternity achieved by subordinate "helper" males in three contrasting circumstances. The first (Figure 20.1a) is a subordinate male that is the offspring of the dominant female. Such individuals, which may or may not also be the offspring of the dominant male, feed young at the nest but never achieve any paternity. The second (Figure 20.1b) is a subordinate male that is unrelated to the dominant female because its mother has died and been replaced by a stepmother. Subordinates in this situation achieve paternity *in some nests*; that is, they share reproduction with the dominant male, but unequally, and contribute to nestling care even when they have no paternity in the nest. The third (Figure 20.1c) is a subordinate male that is unrelated to both dominants, most commonly (but not necessarily) because he is an immigrant. Subordinates in this position share paternity more or less equally with the dominant male and, once again, provision offspring (i.e., help). Note that in all three cases we assume no extra-group paternity and thus the social parents are also the genetic parents; we will return to the case of extra-group parentage later.

Although there are multiple ways that the subordinates in Figure 20.1 can be categorized, a criterion that is key to interpreting helping behavior is whether the subordinate male helper is or is not the offspring of the dominant female, since this determines whether he potentially shares paternity, as in Figures 20.1b and 20.1c, or not, as in Figure 20.1a. In other words,

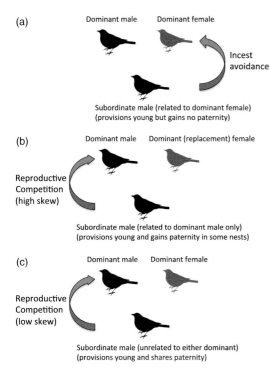

(a)

Dominant male   Dominant female

Incest
avoidance

Subordinate male (related to dominant female)
(provisions young but gains no paternity)

(b)

Dominant male   Dominant (replacement) female

Reproductive
Competition
(high skew)

Subordinate male (related to dominant male only)
(provisions young and gains paternity in some nests)

(c)

Dominant male   Dominant female

Reproductive
Competition
(low skew)

Subordinate male (unrelated to either dominant)
(provisions young and shares paternity)

Figure 20.1. Different kinds of "helpers" illustrated by the three social situations in which subordinate male white-browed scrub-wrens find themselves. (a) A subordinate male living with a breeding pair, the female of which is the subordinate's mother. The subordinate is constrained from breeding by incest avoidance with the dominant female; he provisions young but never gains paternity within the group. (b) A subordinate male living with a breeding pair, the male of which is the subordinate's father and the female of which is a replacement (stepmother). The subordinate's successful reproduction is limited by reproductive competition with the dominant male; the subordinate provisions young and gains paternity in some nests. (c) A subordinate male living with a pair, neither of which is related to the subordinate. As in (b), the subordinate provisions young and competes for paternity with the dominant male. However, he is more successful (skew is lower), and the subordinate shares paternity relatively equally with the dominant male.

the classification scheme most relevant to biological insight determines status based on whether the subordinate is a nonbreeding helper due to incest avoidance with the opposite-sex dominant (Figure 20.1a) or

reproductive competition with the same-sex dominant (Figures 20.1b and 20.1c).

This distinction defines two kinds of subordinates in a way that has been around at least since Reyer's (1980, 1990) work on pied kingfishers (*Ceryle rudis*) describing "primary" helpers that are offspring helping to raise younger siblings (subordinates that do not breed because of incest avoidance) and "secondary" helpers that are unrelated immigrants whose helping behavior is part of a strategy by which they may eventually replace the dominant male and mate with the breeder female (subordinates that do not breed due to reproductive competition). Failure to recognize the difference between the two types means failing to acknowledge two very different and critically important evolutionary factors driving their helping behavior: primary helpers gain indirect fitness benefits while secondary helpers help in order to gain the future direct fitness benefits of breeding if and when they succeed in replacing the dominant male.

Although we use white-browed scrubwrens and pied kingfishers as our examples, the distinction between different types of subordinates is quite general and applicable to almost any cooperative breeding system, regardless of its complexity. It is therefore important to emphasize what does and does not distinguish the two kinds of subordinates.

First, the evolutionarily interesting distinction between the two types of subordinate helpers is *not* whether they are or are not successful at reproduction. Note that the subordinate in Figure 20.1b only sires offspring in *some* broods, and thus his status could easily be misconstrued if determination was based on genetic information alone. Conclusions based solely on parentage analyses are potentially misleading, even in the absence of extra-group paternity (see also Chapter 7).

A problem arises, however, when reproductive skew is strong and subordinates, despite being unrelated to the opposite-sex breeder at a nest, never (or at least very rarely) parent offspring, as is the case for secondary helpers in pied kingfishers and subordinates in species such as western bluebirds (Chapter 2), long-tailed tits (Chapter 3), pied babblers (Chapter 7), and meerkats (Chapter 17). Such nonbreeding individuals can reasonably be (and often are) referred to as nonbreeding helpers, but are nonetheless distinct from helpers whose reproduction is limited by incest avoidance rather than reproductive competition.

Second, the distinction between the different kinds of subordinate helpers is only partly determined by whether they are helping to raise related offspring or not. In general, subordinate male helpers that are offspring of the breeding female (Figure 20.1a) are helping to raise what are at least half-siblings. Subordinate male helpers that are unrelated to the breeding female may or may not be helping related nestlings, depending on whether they are (Figure 20.1b) or are not (Figure 20.1c) related to the dominant male. Making these distinctions leads to interesting predictions about how much effort these different kinds of helpers should devote to cooperative behaviors and whether they should stay in the group at all.

Third, the distinction between subordinate helpers is possibly behavioral and physiological, but there is no guarantee of either. Physiologically, there may be hormonal differences between the two types of helpers, but such differences are generally transient consequences of status, rather than predictive (Schoech et al. 2004).

Fourth, although many studies, including that of white-browned scrubwrens, refer to helpers based on their status as subordinate to a dominant breeder, behavioral subordinance is not, in general, a reliable means of distinguishing different kinds of helpers. Indeed, behavioral dominance may or may not be evident in a particular system, and even if it is, there is no guarantee that it will correspond to breeding status. For example, in superb fairy-wrens, males that have acquired dominant status do not mate with the dominant female when she is their mother (Chapter 8).

Fifth and last, subordinate helpers are not necessarily distinguishable on the basis of sex. Thus far we have used subordinate males to illustrate our points, and male helpers are generally more common than female helpers, at least in birds. But either or both can be subordinate helpers in some systems, and when the latter is the case, the criteria we propose to distinguish different kinds of helpers are likely to be the same (Koenig et al. 1998).

The distinction among helpers is critical for recognizing what factors are important to test in a particular system. When helpers are constrained from breeding by incest avoidance, current and future indirect fitness benefits are a priori likely to be important to why they help. The importance of future direct fitness benefits to such individuals are also of interest to test, just as they would be for helpers that are not constrained from breeding within the group.

In contrast, subordinates that are *unrelated* to the opposite-sex breeder and therefore constrained by reproductive competition fall into at least three categories. Those that rarely or never reproduce while an auxiliary and are thus "nonbreeding helpers" may gain indirect fitness benefits if they are related to the dominant breeder of the same sex. Those that do reproduce – that is, share breeding status with the dominant, even if unequally, asynchronously, or infrequently – are breeders (or cobreeders) and should not be considered "helpers" at all. Finally, those that do not reproduce but are unrelated to the dominant breeders, as is the case for secondary helpers in pied kingfishers, clearly cannot gain indirect fitness benefits by helping. Such individuals are nonbreeding helpers, but are just as reasonably thought of as "hopeful breeders" whose behavior is driven by current or future direct fitness benefits.

What is problematic is when researchers confound the different types of helpers, several of which may be present in the same system. In particular, it is not novel or surprising to show that direct fitness benefits are important to "helpers" that are unrelated to the breeder of the opposite sex and that they share breeding status to some extent with the dominant of the same sex. Rather than reporting that such "helpers" have direct fitness benefits, authors of such studies should recognize that what they thought were helpers aren't helpers afterall. Reviews emphasizing the importance of direct fitness benefits to the evolution of helping behavior are potentially misleading unless the type of helper is clearly defined (Clutton-Brock 2002; Riehl 2013; Kingma et al. 2014).

Extra-group mating, high mortality, and incest

There are three nuances with regard to the above generalizations that we will consider in more detail.

Extra-group mating

In general, extra-group mating does not alter our conclusions, even when it is frequent. Animals do not necessarily know what we as researchers are now able to determine from molecular analyses, and although there may be exceptions, most appear to base their behavior on social criteria – that is, on the social mating system – rather than on the far more cryptic genetic mating system (see, for example, Chapters 2 and 3). Thus, the distinction made here between different kinds of subordinates is unlikely to be affected by the extent of extra-group parentage or other means by which parentage is obscured.

However, extra-group mating potentially confounds conclusions when the status of a particular individual is based *solely* on genetic data. For example, a subordinate female helper may be unrelated to the dominant breeder male and still function as if constrained by incest avoidance if she was the product of an extra-pair mating on the part of the dominant female. Analogously, a subordinate male helper that was "kidnapped" from a neighboring group (as described for pied babblers in Chapter 7, banded mongooses in Chapter 18, and white-winged choughs [*Corcorax melanorhamphos*] by Heinsohn [1991]) may nonetheless behave as if constrained from mating within the group by incest avoidance, despite being unrelated to either of the dominants. In such situations, kidnapping works because it takes advantage of the rules normally used to recognize and discriminate kin.

An additional consequence of extra-group mating is that it opens up a new path for direct fitness benefits by helpers that are otherwise constrained to be nonbreeders because of incest avoidance, reproductive competition, or both. Such a path to direct fitness can increase the potential for sexual selection (Webster et al. 1995), and provides an additional route to direct fitness benefits for helpers, especially if remaining in the natal group facilitates a male helper's access to extra-pair matings.

Incest

The biggest difficulty with distinguishing the different types of subordinates arises when incest takes place, since under such circumstances relatedness to the opposite-sex breeders by definition no longer constrains breeding. This is not true if incest is the incidental result of limited dispersal, which can bring unfamiliar kin into close proximity, in which case individuals, again basing their actions on social rather than genetic cues, are likely to behave as unrelated mates.

Given that one of the key criteria for distinguishing among subordinates is based on incest avoidance, it is unsurprising that our categorization of helpers breaks down when incest occurs. Fortunately, the frequency of incest in vertebrates, in both cooperative and noncooperative breeders, is generally quite low (Rowley et al. 1993; Koenig and Haydock 2004), with banded mongooses and naked mole-rats being the only two species currently known that exhibit a mating system of facultative incest.

Adult mortality

High adult mortality and turnover are demographic factors that reduce relatedness and the indirect fitness benefits of helping behavior (Riehl 2013). However, as illustrated in Figure 20.1b and discussed in the context of family dynamics more generally by Emlen (1995, 1997), adult turnover and replacement is a key route by which one type of "helper" can transition to another (e.g., related to unrelated) or, more importantly, transition to breeding (or cobreeding) status. For example, a nonbreeding helper male in the acorn woodpeckers, whose parent of the opposite sex has died and been replaced by new, unrelated immigrants, can be viewed as "inheriting" cobreeding status and will subsequently breed (at least potentially) alongside his brother or father (Chapter 13), leading to questions about his relative benefits as a cobreeder, and render discussion of his benefits as a helper superfluous.

Recommendations

Any individual that provisions or otherwise assists in the raising of an offspring that is not his or her own has been defined as a helper (Brown 1987), but failing to distinguish among such individuals based on the factors limiting their reproduction is likely to result in

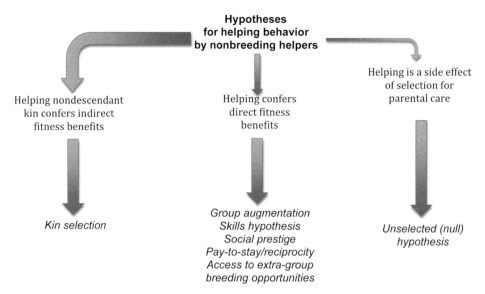

Figure 20.2. Hypotheses potentially selecting for helping behavior by nonbreeding helpers (offspring in the situation illustrated by Figure 20.1a that are constrained from breeding by incest avoidance). Indirect (kin selected) benefits are generally very important; direct fitness benefits may be significant but have rarely been confirmed. No recent authors support the null hypothesis that helping behavior is an unselected side effect of selection for parental care.

misinterpretation as to the significance of their role in the group. This is particularly important with respect to claims that "helpers" gain current direct fitness benefits (i.e., reproduce within their natal group), since such cases nearly always refer to individuals that have inherited breeding status due to turnovers and are thus no longer helpers at all, but rather cobreeders. Considering them to be helpers can lead to the erroneous conclusion that kinship is not important to helping, rather than viewing helping as a route to independent breeding within the group (i.e., future direct fitness benefits). As already discussed, such turnovers can be relatively common.

For the remainder of this chapter, "nonbreeding helpers" (or just "helpers") will refer *only* to the first type of helper discussed: individuals that provide assistance in raising young, none of which is their own offspring, and are constrained from breeding due to incest avoidance. Individuals that are constrained from breeding by reproductive competition may or may not actually breed, and thus it will generally be prudent to avoid referring to such individuals as "helpers" unless

it is known that they rarely if ever successfully parent offspring. (Such absolute skew occurs, for example, in western bluebirds [Chapter 2], where no brothers or sons that help have yet been found by genetics to cobreed.) Even if they do not cobreed, new questions may arise from distinguishing them from nonbreeding helpers constrained by incest avoidance.

Evolution of helping behavior

Now that we have defined what we mean by a helper, let's consider what they do – specifically their helping behavior – and why (Figure 20.2). The presence of nonbreeding helpers has almost always been found to benefit the individuals they assist in some way, either by facilitating the production of more young or by allowing breeders to lessen their breeding effort, generally by reducing their provisioning ("load-lightening"; Heinsohn 2004). In several cases, including superb fairy-wrens (Russell et al. 2007), carrion crows (*Corvus corone*; Chapter 6), and

Neolamprologus pulcher (Chapter 16), helping allows breeder females to lay smaller, and in the case of fairy-wrens, lower-quality, eggs.

Thus, given that helpers (as we have just restricted them) are assisting putative relatives, indirect fitness benefits – those gained by assisting in the production of nondescendant kin – are likely to be important to helping behavior in all species where helping is found, a conclusion further bolstered by evidence of kin recognition and kin discrimination, which have been found to be important in several of the species covered in this book. What is not always clear is whether observed benefits are a result of helping per se rather than a by-product of helpers being in the group (e.g., a group size effect) – a critical assumption that is easily overlooked. Nonetheless, the benefits associated with helpers, along with the variability in helping behavior frequently associated with relatedness and evidence that helping is costly (Heinsohn and Cockburn 1994; see also Chapter 17), counters the hypothesis that helping behavior is an "unselected" phenomenon (Craig and Jamieson 1990).

Paradoxically, however, attempts to quantify kin-selected benefits of helping by nonbreeding helpers have often revealed that they are small relative to what the same individual would be expected to gain by breeding independently; this is, for example, the case in western bluebirds and long-tailed tits (Chapters 2 and 3). Along the same lines, the high incidence of extra-pair fertilizations in superb fairy-wrens means that initial estimates of the inclusive fitness benefits gained by helpers in this species were considerably optimistic (Chapter 8).

In contrast to strong evidence for at least some indirect fitness benefits, evidence that the provisioning behavior of helpers confers direct fitness benefits through mechanisms such as reciprocity ("pay-to-stay"), social prestige, the "skills hypothesis," or group augmentation remains scarce (Dickinson and Hatchwell 2004; Chapter 10), despite attempts to explicitly test for such phenomena in western bluebirds (Chapter 2), red-cockaded woodpeckers (Chapter 4), chestnut-crowned babblers (Chapter 9), bell miners (*Manorina melanophyrs*; Chapter 10), and acorn woodpeckers (Chapter 13). Again, distinguishing between the different kinds of subordinates is important, as

illustrated by Seychelles warblers, where earlier work indicating that helping behavior conferred experience, allowing birds to be more successful in their first breeding attempt, turns out to be confounded by the finding that many of the "helpers" were most likely subordinate cobreeders (Chapter 12).

Two cases in which researchers have found an important role for direct fitness benefits are worth mentioning. First is the superb fairy-wren, where experiments suggest that dominants coerce helpers into helping by punishing them when they are temporarily removed from the territory to simulate defection (Mulder and Langmore 1993). Such experiments sorely need repeating in order to demonstrate not only that helpers are punished when they fail to help, but that aggression causes "lazy" individuals to increase their helping behavior (Raihani et al. 2012). The second is *Neolamprologus pulcher*, where detailed experimental work by Taborsky and his colleagues has demonstrated that pay-to-stay is an important mechanism by which helpers are allowed to remain in groups (Chapter 16). Note, however, that although delayed dispersal occurs and some subordinates are related in this species, breeding turnovers are common and thus a majority of subordinates are no longer helpers as we have defined them above, but likely to be aspiring, at least at some level, to breeding status within the group.

The evolutionary origins of cooperative breeding

The most general hypothesis in the category of evolutionary origins is the "life-history" hypothesis, which proposes that low annual mortality predisposes lineages to exhibit delayed dispersal and cooperative breeding by driving low territory turnover and thus strengthening ecological constraints (Arnold and Owens 1998, 1999; Figure 20.3). This hypothesis is supported by evidence that the incidence of cooperative breeding within families of birds is associated with decreases in annual adult mortality and modal clutch size, and that the proportion of cooperatively breeding species per family is correlated with a low family-typical value of annual mortality. Arnold and

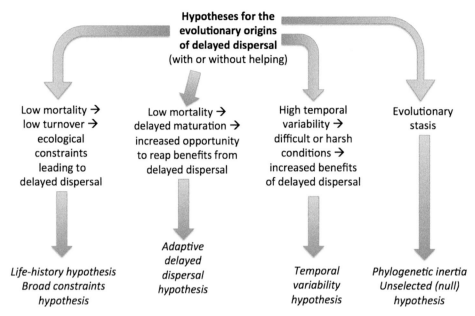

Figure 20.3. Hypotheses for the evolutionary origins of delayed dispersal with or without helping behavior.

Owens (1998) interpreted these results as indicating that low mortality predisposes cooperative breeding rather than vice versa.

Two aspects of this hypothesis are worth noting. First, being phylogenetically based, it is at a different level of analysis and thus does not refute the functional-level explanations we discuss later. Second, although its primary focus is on the life-history factors that predispose a population to evolve delayed dispersal and cooperative breeding, it involves an ecological component, specifically that the life-history trait of high longevity drives strong demographic constraints in the form of high competition for relatively few breeding opportunities in the population (Rowley and Russell 1990).

Related to the life-history hypothesis are the "broad constraints" hypothesis of Hatchwell and Komdeur (2000) and the "adaptive delayed dispersal" hypothesis of Covas and Griesser (2007). Both accept the importance of low mortality rates and go on to postulate that this trait works in conjunction with ecological factors to predispose certain lineages in the direction of cooperative breeding. Hatchwell and Komdeur (2000) stress the importance of a suite of life-history factors working

in conjunction with each other to facilitate constraints and delayed dispersal, while Covas and Griesser (2007) focus on how life-history factors associated with cooperative breeding might interact with various benefits of philopatry to enhance offspring survival and lead to the situation where parents gain by having young stay – that is, to mutual benefits of delayed dispersal outweighing the costs.

One other hypothesis that we place in the category of evolutionary origins is the "temporal variability" hypothesis (Rubenstein and Lovette 2007; Jetz and Rubenstein 2011; Chapter 11), which proposes that high temporal variability predisposes lineages to exhibit cooperative breeding by setting the stage for strategies that maximize the social benefits of delayed dispersal and group living when conditions are poor. In contrast to the other life-history hypotheses, however, the temporal variability hypothesis puts the ecological component first, identifying it as the driver of the key life-history traits that are associated with cooperative breeding rather than vice versa.

Finally, the null hypothesis for the evolutionary origins of delayed dispersal and cooperative breeding is the "phylogenetic inertia" hypothesis put forth by Edwards and Naeem (1993). This hypothesis proposes that cooperative breeding is not driven by any specific life history or ecological driver, but is the consequence of evolutionary stasis resulting in the retention of these traits in certain lineages. As with any evolutionary null hypothesis, it can only be tested by the elimination of alternatives.

Ecological factors and the evolution of delayed dispersal

We now turn to the particularly vexing and contentious question of what ecological factors are important to the evolution of delayed dispersal by nonbreeding helpers. Everyone, we believe, can agree that delayed dispersal, which does not inevitably go along with helping (Chapter 1), occurs when two criteria are met. First, the average lifetime benefit gained by an individual remaining in its natal group is greater than or equivalent to the benefit of dispersing and trying to achieve an independent breeding position; and second, the average lifetime benefit to the dominant breeders of allowing those offspring to remain and, at least potentially, help is greater than or equivalent to the benefit of forcing them to disperse. (All alternatives are assumed to take into consideration the inclusive fitness costs of the behavior as well as the benefits.) Measuring these costs and benefits, especially in terms of lifetime fitness, is difficult and one reason why long-term studies are so vital.

Beyond these somewhat obvious (as well as onerous) conditions, there are several assumptions that we believe are important to embrace in order to understand delayed dispersal. First, given any particular ecological circumstance, it is always better to breed than to be a nonbreeding helper. Consequently, if nonbreeding helpers exist, it is at least in part because of some constraint on their ability to breed.

Second, constraints are universal, and thus simply acknowledging the existence of constraints on dispersal and independent breeding does little to illuminate the ecological drivers of these phenomena. There are, however, different kinds of constraints that vary in their relative strength depending on ecological, environmental,

and social circumstances. Thus, despite their ubiquity, identifying the constraints important in a particular system is an important part of understanding the ecological drivers of delayed dispersal.

Third, the benefits of delayed dispersal, like the benefits associated with any kind of group living, are not automatic (Alexander 1974). There are, however, a wide variety of social benefits that potentially become available to individuals that delay dispersal or disperse locally and maintain proximity to kin, one of which is the potential to provision or otherwise help and be helped by close relatives.

Fourth, there are exceptions to almost any generalization that is made concerning delayed dispersal and cooperative breeding. Our goal here is to organize and frame our knowledge about these phenomena in a way that is conceptually useful and applicable to a large proportion of cases. We have tried to cast our thoughts as generally as possible, but they are nonetheless unlikely to apply to every species or every situation.

Based on these postulates, we propose that the ecological factors important to delayed dispersal are profitably visualized as a continuum. The inability to breed independently is important for all species that exhibit delayed dispersal; what varies more widely is the degree to which they are able to accrue the potential benefits associated with continued access to the natal group or the natal territory. When such benefits are small, ecological factors constitute the main limits on opportunities to breed independently from the natal group; we call these "resource constraints" since most authors envision them as involving access to a resource such as a cavity, territory, or mate. When benefits of being in a group are large, reproductive competition and other social factors are likely to limit opportunities to reproduce, both within or outside the natal group; we refer to these as "social benefits," but they can just as plausibly be thought of as "social constraints," as we discuss below in the section "Constraints and benefits act in concert to favor cooperative breeding."

At one end of the cooperative-breeding continuum where the net benefit of delayed dispersal and helping is low, delayed breeding is primarily driven by shortage of resources, mates, or breeding space. Helpers are "making the best of a bad job" and the natal territory is the best place to wait for breeding opportunities. At the other end are species for which the relative benefit associated with delayed dispersal is considerable and delayed reproduction is driven by social constraints or social competition. Delayed dispersal in such species can reasonably be thought of as being driven by the benefits of philopatry and the critical importance of socially produced benefits such as helping behavior. Although authors often stress factors falling into one end or the other of this continuum, constraints and benefits can be detected in nearly all cooperative breeding systems (Table 20.1).

Constraints-based systems

Constraints on access to resources

Resource-access constraints postulate that the key factor driving delayed dispersal and cooperative breeding is access to some resource that limits the ability of individuals to breed successfully, and, in addition, their potential to leave and become "floaters" in the population (Koenig et al. 1992). In some cases the limiting resource is a breeding territory, but it can also be an engineered resource such as the roosting cavities of red-cockaded woodpeckers (Chapter 4), the granaries and nesting cavities of acorn woodpeckers (Chapter 13), or, to the extent that it is farmed by the birds that live on a site over many generations, the mistletoe that serves as winter food for western bluebirds (Chapter 2). The key is that restricted access to the resource is the primary constraint increasing the costs of dispersal to such an extent that individuals are better off remaining on their natal territory, and, at least potentially, helping to raise younger siblings, rather than assuming the costs of floating or dispersing into a situation where obtaining the resources necessary for breeding is unlikely and their survivorship low. Benefits of helping, while potentially small, still provide indirect fitness advantages compensating for being, at least temporarily, unable to breed.

The fundamental characteristic of cooperative breeders in this category is that the inclusive fitness of a helper is less than what the same or a comparable individual would achieve by breeding in the absence of the limitation. In the absence of such a test or comparison, an alternative prediction is that the per capita reproductive success of groups is less than that of unaided pairs (Koenig 1981; see also Chapter 14). Such comparisons are not conclusive, even when confounding factors such as experience, territory quality, and group composition are carefully controlled. But in many cases, comparing the per capita reproductive success of groups versus pairs can provide a useful and often underappreciated starting point for further investigation of the ecological drivers of delayed dispersal and cooperative breeding.

The idea of constraints driving delayed dispersal has frequently been called the "ecological constraints" hypothesis; however, given the ubiquity of constraints, this term should be used with caution. Cooperative breeders that face resource constraints are typically territorial and live in relatively small groups, and when the limiting resource appears to be space or suitable territories (see, for example, Chapter 5), constraints arguments imply that all suitable territories are occupied and thus that cooperative breeding is driven by "habitat saturation." This latter term is also fraught with problems (Koenig et al. 1992), but is nonetheless useful for conveying the idea that individuals that stay home are making the best of a bad job because of their inability to compete successfully for a suitable breeding territory or space encompassing sufficient resources to breed.

A corollary of the prediction that the inclusive fitness of a helper is less than what could be achieved by breeding in the absence of the limitation is that helpers should attempt to disperse when given access to a suitable territory or limiting resource. Empirical evidence for this prediction comes from Florida scrub-jays (Chapter 5) and acorn woodpeckers (Chapter 13), where birds regularly fight to fill reproductive vacancies. Experimental evidence exists for red-cockaded woodpeckers (Chapter 4), where helpers quickly disperse and colonize artificial cavities when they are provided, and Seychelles warblers (Chapter 12), in which birds transplanted to uninhabited islands forgo group

Table 20.1. The primary factors driving sociality and cooperative breeding in the species discussed in this volume

Species	Key benefits of delayed dispersal or group living	Key constraints to natal dispersal and/or independent breeding	Comments
Siberian jay	Nepotism (access to food and protection against predators); natal territory a safe haven	High-quality territories (unthinned spruce forest) limited	Delayed dispersal but no helping
Western bluebird	Access to mistletoe and reduced aggression by mothers	Female mates	Redirected helpers common; adult helpers all males; simultaneous breeder-helpers occur
Long-tailed tit	Communal roosting	Short breeding season with very high nest predation; seasonal decline in reproductive success	All helpers failed breeders; 85% are males
Florida scrub-jay	Access to year-round food, enhanced juvenile survival and dispersal opportunities	Habitat saturation; limited post-fire successional habitat	Intense competition for unusually large territories in habitat-limited, fire-prone ecosystem
Red-cockaded woodpecker	Living on or acquiring a high-quality territory	Roosting and nesting cavities	Experimental support for importance of cavities
Carrion crow	Nepotism (access to food); natal territory a safe haven	Shortage of territories constrains independent breeding	Differences between populations not due to differences in constraints
Southern pied babbler	Buffering against harsh conditions	Highly variable conditions	"Kidnapping" of helpers; groups merge during droughts
Superb fairy-wren	Access to within- and extra-group reproduction	Female mates	Experimental support for shortage of females
Chestnut-crowned babbler	Reduced predation; thermoregulatory benefits of huddling	Inability to breed as a pair in most years	Obligate group living
Bell miner	Significant benefits of group sociality; breeding positions for males only within natal coterie	Collective food resource defence (against allospecifics); possibly collective anti-predator defence	Live in large colonies divided into coteries; complex helping patterns; kin-selected helping crucial
Superb starlings	Reduced fecundity variance; increased offspring provisioning and enhanced nest defense	Highly variable conditions and heterogeneous landscape	Obligate group living; bet-hedging important
Seychelles warbler	Access to high-quality territories; higher survival; higher future reproductive success; both direct and indirect benefits	Saturation of high-quality habitat	Experimental evidence for importance of high-quality territories
Acorn woodpecker	Some indirect fitness benefits for helpers	Nesting cavities and acorn-storage facilities	Intense competition for reproductive vacancies expressed through "power struggles"
Taiwan yuhina	Lower parental cost of nesting in a harsh environment	High nest failure risk due to predation and severe weather	Non-kin based groups

(cont.)

Table 20.1 (*cont.*)

Species	Key benefits of delayed dispersal or group living	Key constraints to natal dispersal and/or independent breeding	Comments
Guira cuckoo	Indirect fitness and reduced competition in kin-based groups; enhanced foraging and protection against predators	Reproductive competition intense	No apparent habitat saturation; egg ejection and infanticide common
Neolamprologus pulcher	Protection against predation; participation in reproduction	High predation pressure	Obligate group living; cooperation payment for being allowed to stay in the group
Meerkat	Enhanced survival and increased chance of breeding	Absence of unrelated mates for males; reproductive suppression by dominant for females	Obligate group living
Banded mongoose	Enhanced competitiveness; protection against predation	Intergroup competition	Obligate group living; "kidnapping" of offspring
Naked mole-rat	Protection against predation and reduced risk of unsuccessful foraging	Harsh environmental conditions	Obligate group living; aridity food distribution hypothesis

living until the population increases to the point that high-quality territories are occupied and the habitat is again saturated.

One of the long-recognized difficulties with the concepts of ecological constraints and habitat saturation is that they do a poor job of distinguishing cooperative breeders from noncooperative species. One attempt to make such a distinction was the "marginal habitat" hypothesis, which suggests that delayed dispersal results from a shortage of suboptimal habitat or territories, thus producing relatively many offspring fledging from high-quality territories that have few options to disperse to territories of lesser quality (Koenig and Pitelka 1981). This idea was subsequently turned around by Stacey and Ligon (1991) in a paper hypothesizing that even when territory quality varies continuously, rather than declining precipitously, high variance in territory quality can drive delayed dispersal and cooperative breeding. Following Doerr and Doerr (2006), we call this the "variance" hypothesis.

Regardless of the validity of these hypotheses as ways to envision the specific ecological conditions potentially facilitating delayed dispersal in different populations, neither has thus far been particularly useful empirically, in part because quantifying the complete distribution of territory quality within or between populations is challenging (but see Chapter 2 for a within-population example). Meanwhile, despite some advances (Cockburn and Russell 2011; Jetz and Rubenstein 2011), our ability to predict interspecific differences in cooperative breeding beyond a clear relationship with sedentariness (Arnold and Owens 1999) remains poor (Cockburn 2014), and is clearly an area in which significant progress stands to be made in the future.

Shortage of mates

Whether or not resource constraints are important in a population, independent breeding can be limited by a shortage of available mates (Chapter 2). A landmark experiment on superb fairy-wrens demonstrated that both territories and mates are important constraints on independent breeding in this species (Pruett-Jones and Lewis 1990). When breeder males were removed, helpers moved in to replace them within hours; when both members of a pair were removed, replacement did not take place until the female was returned to the territory two to three days later. Further discussion of this example is provided by Cockburn et al. (Chapter 8), who point out some of the difficulties of generalizing it to other fairy-wren species.

Benefits-based systems

Socially produced benefits and the hard-life hypothesis

Where the benefits associated with delayed dispersal and helping augment fitness, remaining in the group is potentially superior to breeding independently. Such social benefits may be produced through nepotism (Ekman et al. 2004), parental facilitation (Brown and Brown 1984), the "safe-haven" effect of living on a high-quality and familiar territory (Kokko and Ekman 2002), or an enhanced potential for inheriting the territory in the future and becoming a breeder. In more extreme (and presumably derived) cases, benefits may consist largely of the indirect fitness coming from provisioning kin or group augmentation, which involves helpers later being assisted by group members (often kin) that were added as a function of their help (Kokko et al. 2001; Kingma et al. 2014). As suggested by Russell in Chapter 9, such cases may be distinct in that helping behavior has become so important that it is driving delayed dispersal rather than (as is more commonly envisioned) the reverse.

Benefits-based hypotheses propose that the key constraint leading to delayed dispersal is not gaining access to suitable space or a mate, but rather the ability to survive and breed successfully independent of a group despite access to other critical resources. Species for which delayed dispersal is benefits-based often live in relatively large aggregations or colonies comprised of a mix of kin and nonkin. Often, the benefit driving delayed dispersal in such cases is socially produced, specifically the presence of additional individuals and/or the availability of potential helpers from within the group or colony. In such cases, the group itself is in effect the resource limiting the ability of individuals to breed on their own.

The fundamental characteristic of benefits-based cooperative breeding is that the mean inclusive fitness benefits of delayers increase with group size up to some empirical maximum greater than the mean for a pair of individuals. Examples where such social benefits are likely to be important include species in which high predation risk has resulted in the evolution of sophisticated babysitting and sentinel systems such as in pied babblers (Chapter 7), meerkats (Chapter 17), and banded mongooses (Chapter 18). Striking evidence of such social benefits is provided by the phenomenon of "kidnapping" young from neighboring groups, as found in the babblers and mongooses.

Intuitively, the most straightforward benefits-based hypothesis is that successful breeding is so difficult that it cannot be accomplished by a pair of individuals alone, but rather can be done only by cooperative groups of individuals (Emlen 1982), an idea that has been referred to as the "hard-life" hypothesis (Koenig and Mumme 1987; Koenig et al. 2011). The importance of large group sizes for successful breeding need not be this extreme, however, and the hard-life hypothesis is potentially applicable to any case in which the difficulties of breeding successfully are mitigated by additional help to an extent that helping compensates for the loss in fitness helpers forgo by not breeding independently. Such conditions may only occur intermittently as in populations subject to conditions that vary dramatically from year to year, leading to helpers having very different effects from year to year and breeding group sizes that vary depending on the ecological circumstances.

Benefits of philopatry

Starting with Stacey and Ligon (1987, 1991), "benefits of philopatry" has been used in two very different ways. First, it is often used in the sense of *any* benefit gained by individuals living in a cooperative, breeding group, whether or not those benefits outweigh the advantages of independent reproduction. Second, the term is also used to refer to the variance hypothesis, as described earlier.

These two concepts are, however, distinct. Stacey and Ligon's focus on variance in territory quality leads to the important general point that the costs and benefits of dispersal compared to independent reproduction can differ among individuals based on their relative options. Variance in territory quality as a particular kind of condition potentially facilitating delayed dispersal should not, however, be conflated with the more general use of "benefits of philopatry" to describe the many ways individuals of a particular species benefit from delayed dispersal. Just as all cooperative breeders are subject to constraints, most accrue at least some benefits from delayed dispersal and helping behavior. In other words, virtually all cooperative-breeding species gain some "benefits of philopatry," regardless of whether delayed dispersal is primarily constraints-driven or benefits-driven.

Bet-hedging and environmental variability

Another potentially important benefits-based hypothesis is that cooperative breeding is a bet-hedging strategy (Rubenstein 2011) selected for because the reduced (arithmetic) mean fitness suffered by helpers is more than compensated by a decrease in fecundity variance through time (Starrfelt and Kokko 2012). Thus, both bet-hedging and the hard-life hypotheses propose that delayed dispersers gain significant inclusive fitness benefits potentially outweighing those of independent breeding, the difference being whether the benefit results from lifetime increases in inclusive fitness (hard-life hypothesis) or reduced fecundity variance (bet-hedging). Bet-hedging has been proposed to be important to cooperative breeding in superb starlings (Chapter 11); its potential importance to other cooperative breeders remains to be determined, however (Koenig and Walters 2015).

Benefits-based hypotheses in general, and the hard-life and bet-hedging hypotheses in particular, propose that delayed dispersal and cooperative breeding are favored by harsh, variable, and unpredictable conditions (Emlen 1982; Rubenstein 2011). To the extent that this is the case, a prediction of benefits-based hypotheses is that helpers should have a greater effect on reproductive success when conditions are poor than when they are good, a result found in several cooperatively breeding species (Magrath 2001) including pied babblers (Chapter 7), superb starlings (Chapter 11) and grey-capped social weavers (S. T. Emlen, unpubl. data),

as well as sociable weavers, *Philetairus socius* (Covas et al. 2008) and white-fronted bee-eaters, *Merops bullockoides* (Emlen 1990; Emlen and Wrege 1991). Surprisingly, the opposite result is observed in acorn woodpeckers: helper males have a greater effect on reproductive success following good, rather than poor, acorn crops (Koenig et al. 2011; Chapter 13).

When conditions vary greatly among individuals or from one year to the next, a potential response is plasticity and the ability to switch between delayed dispersal and independent breeding as conditions permit. Such fluid moving back and forth between helping and breeding independently also occurs in species that live in kin neighborhoods, suggesting that understanding the ecological drivers of more dispersed aggregations of kin could provide new insights into where such species fit on the constraints/benefits-based continuum.

Obligate cooperative breeding

Benefits-based delayed dispersal is most evident in obligate cooperative breeders – species in which individuals are always or nearly always found in groups, including chestnut-crowned babblers (Chapter 9), bell miners (Chapter 10), meerkats (Chapter 17), banded mongooses (Chapter 18), and mole-rats (Chapter 19). Although constraints are, as usual, important to delayed dispersal in such species, the social benefits of delayed dispersal and living in a group clearly outweigh the costs of independent breeding. In the chestnut-crowned babblers, it is further hypothesized that the benefits associated with helping per se are sufficient to explain delayed dispersal (Chapter 9), a possibility that had previously been thought to be rare (Ekman et al. 2004).

Constraints and benefits act in concert to favor cooperative breeding

One lesson from the studies summarized in this book is that it is challenging to categorize and distinguish cooperative breeders based on ecological constraints and benefits of philopatry, since both are frequently, and perhaps typically, important (Table 20.1). While the field has emphasized these as distinct causal factors, ecological constraints are not unique to cooperative breeders; indeed, it is not even obvious that constraints are greater for cooperative breeders than for noncooperative species (Hatchwell and Komdeur 2000). More useful is to focus on how the net benefit of helping for parents and their offspring compares with outside options and why in cooperative breeders this differential leads to delayed dispersal and helping.

An illustrative example is that of the importance of the natal territory as a safe haven for Siberian jays (Chapter 1). In this species, offspring commonly delay breeding and those that also delay dispersal reap nepotistic benefits, surviving longer and having higher lifetime reproductive success compared to immigrants that have joined their group as nonbreeders. Nonetheless, these benefits of philopatry are not necessarily the primary reason why young Siberian jays delay dispersal and fail to breed independently. Instead, a key factor is the limited availability of high-quality breeding sites, which constrains the ability of young to breed for up to three years. Delayed dispersal in this species is driven importantly by ecological constraints, but the natal territory is the best place for offspring to wait for the opportunity to breed, largely due to nepotism. Similar issues involving both constraints and benefits can be identified for many, if not all, the species considered in this book (Table 20.1).

This point is particularly evident in obligate cooperative breeders; indeed, constraints and benefits are arguably indistinguishable in such cases. Consider naked mole-rats (Chapter 19). The currently accepted hypothesis for natal philopatry, cooperative breeding, and ultimately the evolution of eusociality in this species is the "aridity food distribution hypothesis," which proposes that the suite of characters that comprise the cooperative breeding syndrome have evolved in response to the hardness of the soil, the costs of making new burrows, and the risks associated with foraging and dispersal. These factors can clearly be considered resource constraints that render it difficult for individuals to disperse and obtain a breeding position. Just as reasonably, however, the existence of a burrow system for safe foraging and safe living are benefits associated with group-living that make it impossible for

individuals to breed successfully on their own even if they disperse to a suitable site.

As these examples show, the dichotomy that has frequently been made in the literature between benefits of philopatry and ecological constraints is a red herring; constraints and benefits act in concert to shape cooperative breeding systems and to produce the variety of social systems described in this book. This does not mean that we cannot draw any generalizations, but it argues for a pluralistic approach to investigation of the drivers of cooperative breeding that is less linear and more complex than previously acknowledged.

What are the outside options?

Few studies have provided insights on the benefits of remaining in the natal group relative to floating or dispersing to another group in which to live. One example where such options have been examined is that of the Siberian jay, where young birds exhibit higher survival when they remain on their natal territory than when they join new groups (Chapter 1). In contrast, overwinter survival of first-winter male western bluebirds is strikingly high (95%) whether they remain on their natal territory or disperse locally, leading to the hypothesis that males dispersing locally distribute themselves in a way that approximates an ideal-free distribution across habitat that is generally of high quality (with respect to overwinter survival), but that habitat quality varies importantly at the landscape scale (Chapter 2).

At least as important as the relative costs and benefits of delayed dispersal to offspring are the costs and benefits to parents, which are generally assumed to have the ability to either tolerate offspring or evict them. This is an area where additional field studies could contribute significantly and where insights may arise with new models that vary the level of parental control and treat delayed dispersal as an interaction between parents and offspring in which fitness effects on both can vary. Particularly exciting are new tracking technologies that promise to transform what we know about dispersal and the poorly understood period between fledging and first breeding (Koenig et al. 1996). Such methods will allow researchers to measure the fitness of dispersers, and equally importantly, floaters, whose fitness is likely to play a vital role in understanding why animals remain near home and/or near kin.

Delayed dispersal is not a prerequisite for kin-based cooperative breeding

Although delayed dispersal and helping are commonly associated, studies of western bluebirds (Chapter 2) and long-tailed tits (Chapter 3), and acorn woodpeckers (Chapter 13) illustrate that delayed dispersal is not a necessary precursor to kin-based helping behavior. In western bluebirds, males settle near kin in both migratory and resident populations, all but a few offspring disperse to breed, and helping appears to be making the best of a bad job due to a shortage of females or loss of a mate midseason (Chapter 2). In long-tailed tits, all offspring disperse, but many remain in the vicinity of their natal site and subsequently have the opportunity to help at the nests of relatives when their own nests fail, which they often do (Chapter 3). Helping in this species is compensated by future indirect fitness benefits that arise when helpers lighten the workload of male relatives they assist (Meade et al. 2010). Last but not least, a significant fraction of acorn woodpeckers inheriting their natal territory do so *after* dispersing and attempting to breed elsewhere (Chapter 13). In all three of these cases, opportunities to help are provided by remaining in close proximity to kin, and thus further exploration of the selective factors, both social and otherwise, of maintaining close proximity to kin is clearly needed.

Where to go from here

The four factors important to the decision of an individual to delay dispersal are: (1) the constraints limiting outside options; (2) the benefits of group living; (3) relatedness to other individuals in the group in which the individual stays or potentially interacts; and (4) whether they are tolerated by the dominant group members. Of these factors, relatedness can now be determined with some precision using a combination of social genealogies and molecular techniques or, more coarsely, with molecular techniques alone. The benefits of group living have been investigated in many

species, but numerous questions remain concerning the kinds of fitness benefits helpers may be gaining in different systems. As for the constraints limiting outside options such as floating or settling in groups of nonkin, we know strikingly little in most cases. We have a similarly poor understanding of what ecological factors prompt parents in some species to tolerate the continued presence of their offspring.

Drilling into the details of such factors is one of the great benefits of a system such as *Neolamprologus pulcher*, on which experiments can be conducted under relatively realistic conditions in the laboratory (Chapter 16). For the other species in this book, we can only hope that continued long-term studies combined with emerging technologies will begin to fill this gap by allowing workers to follow individuals and quantify the fitness consequences of their behavior as they engage in pursuing options that up until now have been challenging to observe. We expect that a hypothetical third volume in this series, published in another 25 years, will have much to say about the costs and benefits of alternative strategies in ways that we can only dream about today.

It is also worth noting that the four factors we have identified as key to delayed dispersal above are essentially the same factors determining reproductive partitioning in optimal skew models (Keller and Reeve 1994). Such models have already been adapted to address the issues of delayed dispersal and living in kin neighborhoods (Stern 2012). Of course, many of the same issues that have made it difficult to test skew models using empirical data on reproductive sharing (Magrath et al. 2004) are likely to apply to testing similar types of models for delayed dispersal. Nonetheless, such modeling efforts have the potential to add significantly to, and help guide, future empirical work in the field of cooperative breeding.

Unanswered questions

This synthesis discusses only a small set of the unanswered questions raised by the studies of cooperative breeding included in this book. Consider the variability in the levels of extra-group paternity observed in cooperative breeders, which range from near zero in the Florida scrub-jay (Chapter 5) to 61% in the superb fairy-wren, possibly the most genetically promiscuous, socially monogamous species in existence. Some hints as to what might be driving such variability can be gleaned from chapters here: for example, Cockburn et al. (Chapter 8) make a strong case for how sexual selection drives the frequency of extra-pair fertilizations in fairy-wrens, and Dickinson et al. (Chapter 2) point to how extra-pair fertilizations favoring older males can potentially augment delayed fitness benefits and thus favor helping. Nonetheless, our understanding of such variation remains poor.

Another notable problem has to do with the considerable variability in cooperative behavior exhibited by helpers, which in at least some species range from individuals providing more help than do the breeders themselves to helpers that apparently devote little or no effort to cooperative activities (Chapter 9). Although some of the variation is attributable to genetic relatedness, or in some cases need (Chapter 6), much remains unexplained, and the evolution of such "flexible parenting" (or, in this case, "flexible alloparenting"), within a class of individuals that otherwise seem to be similar, is a problem that has only recently begun to be explored (Brouwer et al. 2014; Royle et al. 2014). Our suggestions for differentiating helpers from potential cobreeders will hopefully help workers address this problem using increasingly informative comparison groups in the future.

At the very least, one issue all workers in this field can probably agree on is that much work remains to be done, and that the primary innovations in this field are likely to come from the kinds of long-term studies highlighted in this book. We hope that the chapters in this book will help pave the way for future workers to reveal answers to the many unresolved issues in this field, which we expect to continue to excite behavioral ecologists through the end of the twenty-first century and beyond.

Acknowledgments

We thank all the authors of chapters in this book for providing the food for thought that went into this chapter and our many colleagues over the years for their contributions both to our thinking and to the field of cooperative breeding in general. We particularly acknowledge Andy Russell and Andrew Cockburn for commenting on the chapter. WDK would also like to thank Michael Griesser, Michael Taborsky, Andy Russell, Carel van Schaik, and the participants in the Trogan ProDoc Workshop of January 2014 for their help in discussing some of the ideas presented here, and STE would like to thank Natalia Demong for her help during the writing of this chapter. The work of all the authors has been supported by the National Science Foundation.

REFERENCES

Alexander, R. D. (1974). The evolution of social behavior. *Annu. Rev. Ecol. Syst.*, 5, 325–383.

Arnold, K. E. and Owens, I. P. F. (1998). Cooperative breeding in birds: a comparative test of the life history hypothesis. *Proc. R. Soc. London B*, 265, 739–745.

Arnold, K. E. and Owens, I. P. F. (1999). Cooperative breeding in birds: the role of ecology. *Behav. Ecol.*, 10, 465–471.

Boomsma, J. J. (2009). Lifetime monogamy and the evolution of eusociality. *Phil. Trans. R. Soc. London B*, 364, 3191–3207.

Brouwer, L., van de Pol, M., and Cockburn, A. (2014). The role of social environment on parental care: offspring benefit more from the presence of female than male helpers. *J. Anim. Ecol.*, 83, 491–503.

Brown, J. L. (1987). *Helping and Communal Breeding in Birds: Ecology and Evolution*. Princeton, NJ: Princeton University Press.

Brown, J. L. and Brown, E. R. (1984). Parental facilitation: parent-offspring relations in communally breeding birds. *Behav. Ecol. Sociobiol.*, 14, 203–209.

Clutton-Brock, T. H. (2002). Breeding together: kin selection and mutualism in cooperative vertebrates. *Science*, 296, 69–72.

Cockburn, A. (2004). Mating systems and sexual conflict. In: *Ecology and Evolution of Cooperative Breeding in Birds*, ed. W. D. Koenig and J. L. Dickinson. Cambridge: Cambridge University Press, pp. 81–101.

Cockburn, A. (2014). Behavioral ecology as big science: 25 years of asking the same questions. *Behav. Ecol.*, 25, 1283–1286.

Cockburn, A. and Russell, A. F. (2011) Cooperative breeding: a question of climate? *Curr. Biol.*, 21, R195–R197.

Cornwallis, C. K., West, S. A., Davis, K. E., and Griffin, A. S. (2010). Promiscuity and the evolutionary transition to complex societies. *Nature*, 466, 969–972.

Covas, R. and Griesser, M. (2007). Life history and the evolution of family living in birds. *Proc. R. Soc. London B*, 274, 1349–1357.

Covas, R., Du Plessis, M. A., and Doutrelant, C. (2008) Helpers in colonial cooperatively breeding sociable weavers *Philetairus socius* contribute to buffer the effects of adverse breeding conditions. *Behav. Ecol. Sociobiol.*, 63, 103–112.

Craig, J. L. and Jamieson, I. G. (1990). Pukeko: different approaches and some different answers. In: *Cooperative Breeding in Birds: Long-term Studies of Ecology and Behavior*, ed. P. B. Stacey and W. D. Koenig. Cambridge: Cambridge University Press, pp. 385–412.

Dickinson, J. L. and Hatchwell, B. J. (2004). Fitness consequences of helping. In: *Ecology and Evolution of Cooperative Breeding in Birds*, ed. W. D. Koenig and J. L. Dickinson. Cambridge: Cambridge University Press, pp. 48–66.

Dickinson, J. L., Koenig, W. D., and Pitelka, F. A. (1996). Fitness consequences of helping behavior in the western bluebird. *Behav. Ecol.*, 7, 168–177.

Doerr, E. D. and Doerr, V. A. J. (2006). Comparative demography of treecreepers: evaluating hypotheses for the evolution and maintenance of cooperative breeding. *Anim. Behav.*, 72, 147–159.

Edwards, S. V. and Naeem, S. (1993). The phylogenetic component of cooperative breeding in perching birds. *Am. Nat.*, 141, 754–789.

Ekman, J., Dickinson, J. L., Hatchwell, B. J., and Griesser, M. (2004). Delayed dispersal. In: *Ecology and Evolution of Cooperative Breeding in Birds*, ed. W. D. Koenig and J. L. Dickinson. Cambridge: Cambridge University Press, pp. 35–47.

Ekstrom, J. M. M., Burke, T., Randrianaina, L., and Birkhead, T. R. (2007). Unusual sex roles in a highly promiscuous parrot: the greater vasa parrot *Caracopsis vasa*. *Ibis*, 149, 313–320.

Emlen, S. T. (1982). The evolution of helping I. An ecological constraints model. *Am. Nat.*, 119, 29–39.

Emlen, S. T. (1990). White-fronted bee-eaters: helping in a colonially nesting species. In: *Ecology and Evolution of Cooperative Breeding in Birds*, ed. W. D. Koenig and J. L. Dickinson. Cambridge: Cambridge University Press, pp. 487–526.

Emlen, S. T. (1995). An evolutionary theory of the family. *Proc. Natl. Acad. Sci. (USA)*, 92, 8092–8099.

Emlen, S. T. (1996). Reproductive sharing in different types of kin associations. *Am. Nat.*, 148, 756–763.

Emlen, S. T. (1997). Predicting family dynamics in social vertebrates. In: *Behavioural Ecology: An Evolutionary Approach, 4th ed.*, ed. J. R. Krebs and N. B. Davies. Oxford: Blackwell, pp. 228–253.

Emlen, S. T. and Wrege, P. H. (1991). Breeding biology of white-fronted bee-eaters at Nakuru: the influence of helpers on breeder fitness. *J. Anim. Ecol.*, 60, 309–326.

Fessl, B., Kleindorfer, S., Hoi, H., and Lorenz, K. (1996). Extra male parental behaviour: evidence for an alternative mating strategy in the moustached warbler *Acrocephalus melanopogon*. *J. Avian Biol.*, 27, 88–91.

Hatchwell, B. J. and Komdeur, J. (2000). Ecological constraints, life history traits and the evolution of cooperative breeding. *Anim. Behav.*, 59, 1079–1086.

Heinsohn, R. G. (1991). Kidnapping and reciprocity in cooperatively breeding white-winged choughs. *Anim. Behav.*, 41, 1097–1100.

Heinsohn, R. G. (2004). Parental care, load-lightening, and costs. In: *Ecology and Evolution of Cooperative Breeding in Birds*, ed. W. D. Koenig and J. L. Dickinson. Cambridge: Cambridge University Press, pp. 67–80.

Heinsohn, R. G. and Cockburn, A. (1994). Helping is costly to young birds in cooperatively breeding white-winged choughs. *Proc. R. Soc. London B*, 256, 293–298.

Jetz, W. and Rubenstein, D. R. (2011). Environmental uncertainty and the global biogeography of cooperative breeding in birds. *Curr. Biol.*, 21, 72–78.

Keller, L. and Reeve, H. K. (1994). Partitioning of reproduction in animal societies. *Trends Ecol. Evol.*, 9, 98–102.

Kingma, S. A., Santema, P., Taborsky, M., and Komdeur, J. (2014). Group augmentation and the evolution of cooperation. *Trends Ecol. Evol.*, 29, 476–484.

Koenig, W. D. (1981). Reproductive success, group size, and the evolution of cooperative breeding in the acorn woodpecker. *Am. Nat.*, 117, 421–443.

Koenig, W. D. and Haydock, J. (2004). Incest and incest avoidance. In: *Ecology and Evolution of Cooperative Breeding in Birds*, ed. W. D. Koenig and J. L. Dickinson. Cambridge: Cambridge University Press, pp. 142–156.

Koenig, W. D. and Mumme, R. L. (1987). *Population Ecology of the Cooperatively Breeding Acorn Woodpecker*. Princeton, NJ: Princeton University Press.

Koenig, W. D. and Pitelka, F. A. (1981). Ecological factors and kin selection in the evolution of cooperative breeding in birds. In: *Natural Selection and Social Behavior: Recent Research and New Theory*, ed. R. D. Alexander and D. W. Tinkle. Concord, MA: Chiron press, pp. 261–280.

Koenig, W. D. and Walters, E. L. (2015). Temporal variability and cooperative breeding: testing the bet-hedging hypothesis in the acorn woodpecker. *Proc. R. Soc. London B*, 282, 20151742.

Koenig, W. D., Pitelka, F. A., Carmen, W. J., Mumme, R. L., and Stanback, M. T. (1992). The evolution of delayed dispersal in cooperative breeders. *Q. Rev. Biol.*, 67, 111–150.

Koenig, W. D., Van Vuren, D., and Hooge, P. N. (1996). Detectability, philopatry, and the distribution of dispersal distances in vertebrates. *Trends Ecol. Evol.*, 12, 514–517.

Koenig, W. D., Haydock, J., and Stanback, M. T. (1998). Reproductive roles in the cooperatively breeding acorn woodpecker: incest avoidance versus reproductive competition. *Am. Nat.*, 151, 243–255.

Koenig, W. D., Walters, E. L., and Haydock, J. (2011). Variable helpers effects, ecological conditions, and the evolution of cooperative breeding in the acorn woodpecker. *Am. Nat.*, 178, 145–158.

Kokko, H. and Ekman, J. (2002). Delayed dispersal as a route to breeding: territorial inheritance, safe havens, and ecological constraints. *Am. Nat.*, 160, 468–484.

Kokko, H., Johnstone, R. A., and Clutton-Brock, T. H. (2001). The evolution of cooperative breeding through group augmentation. *Proc. R. Soc. London B*, 268, 187–196.

Kramer, K. L. and Russell, A. F. (2014). Kin-selected cooperation without lifetime monogamy: human insights and animal implications. *Trends Ecol. Evol.*, 29, 600–606.

Lukas, D. and Clutton-Brock, T. H. (2012). Cooperative breeding and monogamy in mammalian societies. *Proc. R. Soc. London B*, 279, 2151–2156.

Magrath, R. D. (2001). Group breeding dramatically increases reproductive success of yearling but not older female scrubwrens: a model for cooperatively breeding birds? *J. Anim. Ecol.*, 70, 370–385.

Magrath, R. D. and Whittingham, L. A. (1997). Subordinate males are more likely to help if unrelated to the breeding female in cooperatively breeding white-browed scrubwrens. *Behav. Ecol. Sociobiol.*, 41, 185–192.

Magrath, R. D., Johnstone, R. A., and Heinsohn, R. G. (2004). Reproductive skew. In: *Ecology and Evolution of Cooperative Breeding in Birds*, ed. W. D. Koenig and J. L. Dickinson. Cambridge: Cambridge University Press, pp. 157–176.

Meade, J., Nam, K.-B., Beckerman, A. P., and Hatchwell, B. J. (2010). Consequences of "load-lightening" for future indirect fitness gains by helpers in a cooperatively breeding bird. *J. Anim. Ecol.*, 79, 529–537.

Mulder, R. A. and Langmore, N. E. (1993). Dominant males punish helpers for temporary defection in superb fairy-wrens. *Anim. Behav.*, 45, 830–833.

Nonacs, P. and Hager, R. (2011). The past, present and future of reproductive skew theory and experiments. *Biol. Rev.*, 86, 271–298.

Pruett-Jones, S. G. and Lewis, M. J. (1990). Sex ratio and habitat limitation promote delayed dispersal in superb fairy-wrens. *Nature*, 348, 541–542.

Raihani, N. J., Thornton, A., and Bshary, R. (2012). Punishment and cooperation in nature. *Trends Ecol. Evol.*, 27, 288–295.

Reeve, H. K., Westneat, D. F., Noon, W. A., Sherman, P. W., and Aquadro, C. F. (1990). DNA "fingerprinting" reveals high levels of inbreeding in colonies of the eusocial naked mole-rat. *Proc. Natl. Acad. Sci. (USA)*, 87, 2496–2500.

Reyer, H.-U. (1980). Investment and relatedness: a cost/benefit analysis of breeding and helping in the pied kingfisher (*Ceryle rudis*). *Anim. Behav.*, 32,1163–1178.

Reyer, H.-U. (1990). Pied kingfishers: ecological causes and reproductive consequences of cooperative breeding. In: *Cooperative Breeding in Birds: Long-term Studies of Ecology and Behavior*, ed. P. B. Stacey and W. D. Koenig. Cambridge: Cambridge University Press, pp. 527–557.

Riehl, C. (2013). Evolutionary routes to non-kin cooperative breeding in birds. *Proc. R. Soc. London B*, 280, 20132245.

Rowley, I. and Russell, E. (1990). Splendid fairy-wrens: demonstrating the importance of longevity. In: *Cooperative Breeding in Birds: Long-term Studies of Ecology and Behavior*, ed. P. B. Stacey and W. D. Koenig. Cambridge: Cambridge University Press, pp. 2–30.

Rowley, I., Russell, E., and Brooker, M. (1993). Inbreeding in birds. In: *The Natural History of Inbreeding and Outbreeding*, ed. N. W. Thornhill. Chicago, IL: University of Chicago Press, pp. 304–328.

Royle, N. J., Russell, A. F., and Wilson, A. J. (2014). The evolution of flexible parenting. *Science*, 345, 776–781.

Rubenstein, D. R. (2011). Spatiotemporal environmental variation, risk aversion and the evolution of cooperative breeding in birds. *Proc. Natl. Acad. Sci. (USA)*, 108, 10816–10822.

Rubenstein, D. R. and Lovette, I. J. (2007). Temporal environmental variability drives the evolution of cooperative breeding in birds. *Curr. Biol.*, 17, 1414–1419.

Russell, A. F., Langmore, N. E., Cockburn, A., Astheimer, L. B., and Kilner, R. M. (2007). Reduced egg investment can conceal helper effects in cooperatively breeding birds. *Science*, 317, 941–944.

Schoech, S. J., Reynolds, S. J., and Boughton, R. K. (2004). Endocrinology. In: *Ecology and Evolution of Cooperative Breeding in Birds*, ed. W. D. Koenig and J. L. Dickinson. Cambridge: Cambridge University Press, pp. 128–141.

Shen, S.-F. and Reeve, H. K. (2010). Reproductive skew theory unified: the general bordered tug-of-war model. *J. Theor. Biol.*, 263, 1–12.

Smith, J. N. M. (1990). Summary. In: *Cooperative Breeding in Birds: Long-term Studies of Ecology and Behavior*, ed. P. B.

Stacey and W. D. Koenig. Cambridge: Cambridge University Press, pp. 593–611.

Stacey, P. B. and Koenig, W. D. (eds.) (1990). *Cooperative Breeding in Birds: Long-term Studies of Ecology and Behavior.* Cambridge: Cambridge University Press.

Stacey, P. B. and Ligon, J. D. (1987). Territory quality and dispersal options in the acorn woodpecker, and a challenge to the habitat-saturation model of cooperative breeding. *Am. Nat.*, 130, 654–676.

Stacey, P. B. and Ligon, J. D. (1991). The benefits-of-philopatry hypothesis for the evolution of cooperative breeding: variation in territory quality and group size effects. *Am. Nat.*, 137, 831–846.

Starrfelt, J. and Kokko, H. (2012). Bet-hedging – a triple trade-off between means, variances and correlations. *Biol. Rev.*, 87, 742–755.

Stern, C. A. (2012). Cooperation and competition in kin associations. Ph.D. thesis, Cornell University, Ithaca, New York.

Webster, M. S., Pruett-Jones, S., Westneat, D. F., and Arnold, S. J. (1995). Measuring the effects of pairing success, extra-pair copulations and mate quality on the opportunity for sexual selection. *Evolution*, 49, 1147–1157.

Whittingham, L. A., Dunn, P. O., and Magrath, R. D. (1997). Relatedness, polyandry and extra-group paternity in the cooperatively-breeding white-browed scrubwren (*Sericornis frontalis*). *Behav. Ecol. Sociobiol.*, 40, 261–270.

Index

acorn crop, 79, 87, 90, 92, 219, 226–228, 230–232, 232t13.4

acorn woodpecker, 20, 73, 190, 217–234, 263, 268, 356, 359, 361, 365t20.1, 368

Acridotheres tristis. See common myna

Acrocephalus melanopogon. See moustached warbler

Acrocephalus sechellensis. See Seychelles warbler

adaptive delayed dispersal hypothesis, 362

additive care, 158

Aegithalos caudatus. See long-tailed tit

African lion, 224

alarm calling, 28, 42, 44, 126, 127, 161, 187, 268, 305

Allee effect, 325, 326

allolactation, 302, 304, 305, 328

Aphelocoma californica. See western scrub-jay

Aphelocoma coerulescens. See Florida scrub-jay

Aphelocoma insularis. See island scrub-jay

Aphelocoma wollweberi. See Mexican jay

Arabian babbler, 7, 115, 116, 117, 168

aridity food distribution hypothesis, 344, 366t20.1, 369

Australian magpie, 128

auxiliary. *See* helper

babysitting, 301f17.9, 302, 303f17.10, 305, 307, 325, 326, 326f18.5, 327, 327f18.6, 367

banded mongoose, 295, 304, 318–334, 354, 355, 356, 359, 366t20.1, 367, 368

Bateman gradient, 23

begging, 106, 118, 124, 126, 142, 168, 169, 171, 252f14.10, 304, 308

behavioral syndrome, 83

bell miner, 165–178, 361, 365t20.1, 368

benefits of philopatry,17, 20, 72, 100, 161, 162, 201, 203, 254, 280, 362, 367–369

bet-hedging, 191–192, 232, 365t20.1, 368

birth synchrony, 319, 328–329

blue jay, 79

Printed in the United States
By Bookmasters